Mastering Competencies in Family Therapy

A PRACTICAL APPROACH TO THEORIES AND CLINICAL CASE DOCUMENTATION

Mastering Competencies in Family Therapy

A PRACTICAL APPROACH TO THEORIES AND CLINICAL CASE DOCUMENTATION

First Edition

Diane Gehart
California State University, Northridge

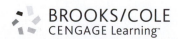
BROOKS/COLE
CENGAGE Learning™

Australia • Brazil • Japan • Korea • Mexico • Singapore • Spain • United Kingdom • United States

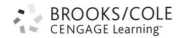

Mastering Competencies in Family Therapy: A Practical Approach to Theories and Clinical Case Documentation, First Edition

Diane Gehart

Acquisitions Editor: Seth Dobrin

Assistant Editor: Allison Bowie

Editorial Assistant: Rachel McDonald

Media Editor: Andrew Keay

Marketing Manager: Trent Whatcott

Marketing Coordinator: Darlene Macanan

Marketing Communications Manager: Tami Strang

Content Project Manager: Rita Jaramillo

Creative Director: Rob Hugel

Art Director: Caryl Gorska

Print Buyer: Rebecca Cross

Rights Acquisitions Account Manager, Text: Bob Kauser

Production Service: Matrix Productions

Text Designer: Anne Draus

Copy Editor: Susan Zorn

Cover Designer: Gia Giasullo

Compositor: Integra

For product information and technology assistance, contact us at **Cengage Learning Customer & Sales Support, 1-800-354-9706.**

For permission to use material from this text or product, submit all requests online at **www.cengage.com/permissions.**

Further permissions questions can be e-mailed to **permissionrequest@cengage.com.**

Library of Congress Control Number: 2008939485

ISBN-13: 978-0-495-59724-7

ISBN-10: 0-495-59724-4

Brooks/Cole
10 Davis Drive
Belmont, CA 94002-3098
USA

Cengage Learning is a leading provider of customized learning solutions with office locations around the globe, including Singapore, the United Kingdom, Australia, Mexico, Brazil, and Japan. Locate your local office at **www.cengage.com/international.**

Cengage Learning products are represented in Canada by Nelson Education, Ltd.

To learn more about Brooks/Cole, visit **www.cengage.com/brookscole**

Purchase any of our products at your local college store or at our preferred online store **www.ichapters.com.**

Printed in Canada
1 2 3 4 5 6 7 13 12 11 10 09

Brief Table of Contents

Detailed Table of Contents

Dedication

In the past few years, the field of family therapy has lost many whose contributions are our mainstay. This book is dedicated to those who have paved the way for the next generation. We are forever in their debt.

Gianfranco Cecchin
Whose laughter, humility, and acceptance transformed me

Tom Andersen
Whose presence was angelic: the most "gentle" man I have ever met

Paul Watzlawick
Whose courage and kind words I shall never forget

Steve de Shazer
Whose brilliance dazzled me

Insoo Kim Berg
Whose energy and enthusiasm inspired the best in me

Michael White
Whose ideas opened new worlds for me

Jay Haley
Who taught me the logic of paradox

Ivan Boszormenyi-Nagy
Who reminded me to focus on what really matters

Acknowledgments

*I would like to thank the following **content experts** who gave their time and energy to ensure that the information in this textbook was accurate and current:*

Scott Miller: Outcome and Session Rating Scales (Chapter 5)
Michael Lambert: Outcome Questionnaire (Chapter 5)
Wendel Ray and his doctoral students, **Todd Gunter** and **Allison Lux:** Philosophical Foundations and Systemic Therapies (Chapters 8 and 9)
Marion Lindblad-Goldberg: Structural Therapy/Ecosystemic Structural Family Therapy (Chapter 10)
Michael Chafin: Symbolic-Experiential Therapy (Chapter 11)
Lynne M. Azpeitia: Satir Growth Model (Chapter 11)
Scott Woolley: Emotionally Focused Therapy (Chapter 11)
Michael Kerr and Cynthia Larkby: Bowen Intergenerational Therapy (Chapter 12)
Naomi Knoble: Gottman's Marriage Clinic Approach (Chapter 13)
Bill O'Hanlon: Solution-Based Therapies (Chapter 14)
Harlene Anderson: Collaborative Therapy (Chapter 15)
Gerald Monk: Narrative Therapy (Chapter 15)
Eric McCollum: Group Therapy (Chapter 16)
Ron Chenail: Competencies Assessment System and Thoughtful Introduction
Thorana Nelson: Competencies Assessment System
William Northey: Competencies Assessment System
Julie Diaz: Clinical Forms

The following reviewers provided invaluable feedback on making this book work for faculty:

William F. Northey, Jr. (Bill Northey): Former AAMFT Staff
John K. Miller: University of Oregon
Joshua M. Gold: University of South Carolina
Brent Taylor: San Diego State
Randall Lyle: St. Mary's University
Cynthia T. Walley: Old Dominion University

The following students and former students assisted in the development of the Instructors' Manual:

Brandy Lucus: Syllabi, test bank, and video lists
Tricia Lethcoe: PowerPoints and test bank
Karen Graber: Reference checks and CACREP rubrics
Julie Woodworth: Test bank
Alina Whitmore: Test bank

I would also like to thank the following people for their generous assistance:

Bill O'Hanlon: Whose Writing Bootcamp made this book happen much more easily and quickly and whose encouragement kept me going

Michael Bowers: Who provided permission to reprint the AAMFT Core Competencies

Marquita Flemming: The book's initial editor at Cengage who helped develop its vision and focus

Marcus Boggs: Who supported and helped shepherd the book at Cengage

Seth Dobrin: The book's second editor at Cengage who helped bring it to its final form

Trent Whatcott: Whose creative promotional efforts got the book into your hands

Seth Miller: Who oversaw production of this complex text at Matrix Productions

Susan Zorn: Copyeditor who kept me consistent and grammatically in line

Guenther and Anna Gehart: My parents, whose proofreading and editing kept the drafts clean

Joseph McNicholas: My husband, whose editing and writing assistance made Chapter 1 sing and whose encouragement, support, and understanding made the process fun

Foreword By Ronald J. Chenail, Ph.D.

Becoming Competent with Competencies, or What I Have Learned About Learning

Even though I have been teaching in one form or another since 1978, I was never formally schooled in educational concepts like student learning outcomes, rubrics, and competencies. I, like many of my colleagues, followed a tried-and-true method of teaching—how I remembered being taught by those teachers I admired the most and not teaching how I recalled being instructed by those teachers I dreaded the most. (With this steadfast educational philosophy intact, I, along with my fellow teachers in the elementary, middle, and high schools and community colleges and universities, would approach the latest, greatest new educational theory, model, or fad rolled out by well-meaning, earnest administrators and instructional specialists with the same disinterest as some of our students would embrace our own zealous pronouncements of the importance of mastering algebra, knowing who Charlemagne was, and differentiating between first- and second-order change.) Funny as it seems, we as teachers and students both appeared to share the same lament—what does all this learning stuff have to do with being successful in the real world? Now looking back 30 years later, I have come to the realizations that learning has everything to do with being successful and that learning is not the same thing as teaching.

Learning About Learning

I have always loved learning, although I was not always crazy about school. I was one of those students who lived by the proverb to never let my schooling get in the way of my education. Today I live by another proverb when it comes to working—to never let my job get in the way of my career, but that is a preface for another book.

It was this apparent paradox of loving learning but not loving school that led me to think about what made the two processes so different in my mind and life. For me, the main difference to making a difference between learning and schooling seemed to be predicated on who decided what needed to be learned and who directed the learning process. When I was able to explore what interested me, acquire information I felt I needed to master, and access mentors who could help facilitate my learning, I was always more successful in achieving my goals and objectives.

With this new revelation filling my head, I started to think how I could share this way of learning with my students. The first step in this epiphany was to see that my students were not that different from me. They too liked to learn what they liked to learn, so I made this insight the centerpiece of my learning-centric approach. The second step was to see learning, not as an epic dyadic struggle between me as the omniscient and omnipotent teacher who possessed all knowledge and wisdom and the students as reluctant, empty opponents needing to be directed and taught, but rather as a triadic arrangement involving three interrelated parts: the student, a body of knowledge or group of skills, and me. In this configuration I find I am no longer in conflict with students, forcing them to learn what I deem as privileged knowledge; instead I now try to learn what students aspire to become; help them define this aspiration into goals, objectives, and competencies; and work with them to support and facilitate their learning journeys.

Taking this approach was liberating for me and startling for many of the students. In their formal schooling, many of them had never been asked to be proactive with their learning, but like me, they all found they could learn well when they could be in charge of their own learning. Having confidence that students were really like me and could learn very well on their own was an insight I wanted to put into practice in my work with marriage and family therapy (MFT) graduate students.

Being Competent with Competencies

Most students who choose to matriculate in therapy programs like counseling, clinical psychology, social work, or family therapy really want to be therapists or counselors. The challenge is that students usually do not know all the things they will want to know before they know them. We always wish we knew *then* what we know now. Students wanting to become competent marriage and family therapists are no different.

We now seem to be in the world of competencies for marriage and family therapists. The American Association for Marriage and Family Therapy (AAMFT) initiated a dialogue in which marriage and family therapists reflected on what they knew about being effective therapists and shared these insights with one another. Through this ongoing, collaborative process the AAMFT Core Competencies were born (Nelson, Chenail, Alexander, Crane, Johnson, & Schwallie, 2007), with the result that therapists can now clearly define what competent marriage and family therapists should be able to accomplish in their work with clients.

The effort to create this set of competencies originated within a number of critical contexts. Health care policymakers in Washington wanted providers to be clearer about what they did and did not do as practitioners with their patients and clients. Consumers also wanted clarity in what they could expect licensed professionals to deliver. Higher education accreditation professionals and policymakers wanted educators to take an outcomes-based approach to learning and to become more accountable to students and employers so that all interested parties could know what could be expected from graduates of specific degree and training programs.

The good news was that the competencies were here. We as MFT educators could work from a system that was specific enough to communicate learning objectives and outcomes so that we, along with our students, could have reasonable expectations of what becoming competent family therapists would entail, while being generic enough for us to be creative in facilitating and supporting our students as they began the journey to become therapists.

Of course, the bad news was also that the competencies were here. Most of us had not been educated in this style of learning when we were training to become therapists. We also had not been trained as faculty members and supervisors to educate our students in this manner. The challenge before us was how to become competent with the competencies.

And that is where Diane Gehart's delightful new book comes in.

To meet this challenge, Diane, like many of us, has had to learn about learning to become competent with the competencies! She has taken the best of the learning-centered approaches and has woven in the latest clinical innovations and scholarship from the world of marriage and family therapy to create a clear and concise set of learning outcomes that can become that third partner with students and faculty to form a triadic learning model.

In the first part of the book Diane introduces her readers to this wonderful world of learning in which teachers and students work together to learn new knowledge and skills in the pursuit of transparent and mutually beneficial goals. She then deconstructs the Core Competencies into the basics of case conceptualization, clinical assessment, treatment planning, evaluation, and documentation, making them more readily apparent to the beginning marital and family therapist. Finally, she reconstructs MFT learning by bringing modern and postmodern approaches into this world of learning outcomes and competencies so that we can skillfully conceptualize, assess, treat, evaluate, and document our work, regardless of the clinical approach we embrace.

I encourage you to learn how Diane has learned how to learn marriage and family therapy so that you too can become proficient with the MFT competencies. If you do, I think you will come away from this book with a new appreciation and affection for learning.

Ronald J. Chenail, Ph.D.
Ft. Lauderdale, Florida

Reference

Nelson, T. S., Chenail, R. J., Alexander, J. F., Crane, D. R., Johnson, S. M., & Schwallie, L. (2007). The development of core competencies for the practice of marriage and family therapy. *Journal of Marital and Family Therapy, 33*(4), 417–438. doi:10.1111/ j.1752-0606.2007.00042.x

About the Author

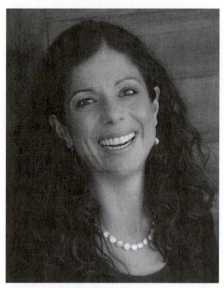

Photo by Jones Photo Art

Dr. Diane R. Gehart is Professor in the Marriage and Family Therapy Program at California State University, Northridge. Having taught and supervised students in family therapy for fifteen years, she is known as an energetic, fun, yet challenging instructor. In addition to the current text, she authored *The Complete MFT Core Competency Assessment System*, co-edited *Collaborative Therapy: Relationships and Conversations that Make a Difference*, and co-authored *Theory-Based Treatment Planning for Marriage and Family Therapists*. She has also written extensively on postmodern therapies, mindfulness, sexual abuse treatment, gender issues, children and adolescents, client advocacy, qualitative research, and education in family therapy. She speaks internationally, having given workshops to professional and general audiences in the United States, Canada, Europe, and Mexico. Her work has been featured in newspapers, radio shows, and television worldwide. She is an associate faculty member at two international post-graduate training institutes: the Taos Institute and the Marburg Institute for Collaborative Studies in Germany. Additionally, she is an active leader in state and national professional organizations. She maintains a private practice in Thousand Oaks, California, specializing in couples, families, trauma, life transitions, and difficult to treat cases. For fun, she enjoys hiking or going to the beach with her family, trail running, Bikram yoga, meditation, whole food cooking, traveling, and dark chocolate in any form.

Author's Introduction: On Saying "Yes" and Falling in Love

I never envisioned myself writing a book such as this. Up to this point, I have focused my career less on the science and more on the heart and soul of therapy, choosing to train as a collaborative therapist who works side-by-side with clients to create new understandings (Chapter 15; Anderson & Gehart, 2007), to conduct postmodern qualitative research that introduces the voices of clients into professional literature (Gehart & Lyle, 1999), and to incorporate Buddhist psychology, mindfulness, and spiritual principles and practices into my work (Gehart & McCollum, 2007). Except for my earlier book on treatment planning (Gehart & Tuttle, 2003), nothing in my background points in the direction of writing a book on the competencies or the science-based aspects of family therapy. So, how did I get here? Ironically, what led me here were the very things that one would assume would have prevented it: namely, my postmodern and Buddhist training. More specifically, their practices of saying "yes."

One of the hallmark principles of collaborative therapy, and most family therapies for that matter, is to honor the perspectives of all participants, saying "yes, I hear you and take your concerns to heart." The Buddhist practice of "saying yes" is the practice of softening and moving toward "what is," even if it is uncomfortable, undesirable, or painful. As a professional, saying "yes" involves taking seriously the perspectives of our colleagues, our clients, third-party payers, state and federal legislatures, licensing boards, professional organizations, and the general public. How do they see us? What questions and concerns do they have about what we do?

Over the years, voices from outside our profession have increasingly demanded clarity on and evidence for what we do. Answering to these demands while maintaining integrity with my training is often challenging because the working assumptions of what "counts" as evidence in human relations are not as simple or straightforward as one might think. What an insurance company considers as evidence of successful therapy (i.e., a particular score on an assessment form) is quite different from what a therapist might emphasize (i.e., observing the client move with the ceaseless stream-of-life stressors more gracefully).

As part of our profession's response to the demand for greater accountability, family therapists generated a list of Core Competencies that detail the knowledge and skills that define the practice of family therapy (see Chapter 1). For faculty members such as myself, this is essentially a "to do" list of what we need to teach our students. As a member of this community, I recognized that I needed to find a positive, respectful way to work with these external priorities and balance them with my own. This book is my answer, my "yes," to these concerns.

My Other Purpose: Falling in Love

I must confess that I had another intention for writing this book: to help you to fall in love. And, preferably to do so again and again—making even Casanova envious. I want you to fall in love with not one but all of the family therapy theories in this book, enthusiastically embracing each while seeing both its beauty and its limitations, much in the same way we help our clients to love each other. I hope you cultivate a profound respect for the brilliant minds that have paved the way for us to help clients with their most complex and intimate problems—their couple and family relationships—or, more essentially, to teach them how to love. I hope you find yourself passionate about the insight each approach offers in understanding human relationships as well as about helping people create the relationships they desire. As family therapists, we inherit a stunning and profound body of knowledge that is difficult to fully appreciate in the beginning. I personally believe that some of the greatest wisdom in the Western world is captured in the philosophical foundations of family therapy. Although these ideas sometimes seem surprising or even objectionable at first, if you sincerely try to put them into practice, I believe you will find that each touches upon a useful truth and reality. Should you choose to seriously study it, the field of family therapy offers an ever-widening exploration of the human experience that cannot but transform you both personally and professionally. I hope this book inspires you on a passionate journey of discovery that lasts a lifetime.

What You Will Find

This book is divided into two sections: the first on the *competencies* and the second on *theories*. In the competencies section, you will learn how to conceptualize a case, conduct a clinical and diagnostic assessment, write a detailed treatment plan, evaluate client progress, and write progress notes. These are the most common written documents in the field.

In the second half of the book, you will learn about the major family therapy theories, both the traditional theories and the newer evidence-based therapies. The theories are divided into seven major schools or related approaches: systemic, structural, experiential, intergenerational and psychoanalytic, behavioral and cognitive-behavioral, solution-based, and postmodern. Each chapter includes a complete set of the clinical documentation introduced in the first half of the book. Before introducing specific theories, I introduce you to the philosophical foundations, the common factors debate, and the evidence-based trend to provide a frame of reference for understanding the role of theory in the field. I also include a chapter on couple and family groups to provide an overview of this increasingly popular treatment format.

The Invitation

I invite you to passionately and enthusiastically embrace each perspective, concept, and theory that follows. Savor the big-picture view of case conceptualization while also taking time to examine the intricate matters of clinical assessment. Appreciate the unique wisdom of each theory while also recognizing the *common factors* (Chapter 7) that they share. Get excited about research and the evidence base of our work (Chapter 7), while honoring the philosophical foundations (Chapter 8). Be open to theories that rely on technique and content to promote change as well as to those that rely on process and relationship, knowing that each has its place when working with diverse clients. Say "yes" to all that comes your way, and take pleasure in the incredible journey of becoming a family therapist.

Enjoy the adventure.

Diane R. Gehart, Ph.D., LMFT
Thousand Oaks, California
June 2008

References

Anderson, H., & Gehart, D. (2007). *Collaborative therapy: Relationships and conversations that make a difference.* New York: Brunner/Routledge.

Gehart, D. R., & Lyle, R. R. (1999). Client and therapist perspectives of change in collaborative language systems: An interpretive ethnography. *Journal of Systemic Therapy, 18*(4), 78–97.

Gehart, D., & McCollum, E. (2007). Engaging suffering: Towards a mindful re-visioning of marriage and family therapy practice. *Journal of Marital and Family Therapy, 33,* 214–226.

Gehart, D. R., & Tuttle, A. R. (2003). *Theory-based treatment planning for marriage and family therapists: Integrating theory and practice.* Pacific Grove, CA: Brooks/Cole.

Mastering Competencies in Family Therapy

A PRACTICAL APPROACH TO THEORIES AND CLINICAL CASE DOCUMENTATION

CHAPTER

1

Competency in Family Therapy

The Secret to Competent Therapy

There is a secret to providing competent family therapy. Fortunately, it is an open secret, and the goal of this chapter is to sketch a map showing where and, more importantly, how to look for it. You are probably familiar with the basic landscape. You may recognize therapy's more promising pathways and some of the dead-end routes. But like everyone setting out on a journey, your choice between the high road and the low road would be easier if you knew what was in store for you beforehand.

Since I know you will race ahead if I make you wait too much longer, let's lay our map on the table right now and get a better sense of this secret on the first page. Mapping a successful therapeutic journey involves five steps:

THE FIVE STEPS TO COMPETENT THERAPY

Step 1. Map the Territory: Conceptualize the situation with the help of theory (Chapter 2).

Step 2. Identify Oases and Obstacles: Assess the client's mental status and provide case management (Chapter 3).

Step 3. Select a Path: Develop a treatment plan with therapeutic tasks—including how to build a working therapeutic relationship—and measurable client goals (Chapter 4).

Step 4. Track Progress: Evaluate the client's response to treatment (Chapter 5).

Step 5. Leave a Trail: Document the work (Chapter 6).

Mapping a Successful Therapeutic Journey

These five steps follow a classic method used by all explorers in uncharted territory. And that's what each new therapeutic relationship is: uncharted territory, an unknown region, a *terra incognita*. Although it may seem that clients can be easily lumped into groups—depressed clients, distressed couples, children with ADHD, for example—any experienced therapist can tell you that each client's journey is unique. The excitement—and secret—to competent therapy is mapping the distinctive terrain of each client's life and charting a one-of-a-kind journey through it.

The first step is to delineate as much of the terrain as possible: to get the big picture. What are the contours of the relationships? Where are the comfort zones? Where is the page marked "Here Be Dragons?" As with all maps, the bigger and more detailed the record, the easier it is to move through the territory. In family therapy, our maps are our *case conceptualizations*, assessments of the client using family therapy theories. Once you have a map, you identify the landmarks, the oases and obstacles. You notice where the rest stops are and identify what dangers lie ahead. In therapy, you can recognize the oases as client resources: anything that can be used to strengthen and support the client. The obstacles appear as those potential or existing hindrances to creating change in the client's life: Are there really dragons there, or is the region just unfamiliar?

Like a cartographer surveying the landscape, therapists assess potential hindrances carefully, ruling out possible medical issues in consultation with physicians, identifying psychiatric issues by conducting a *mental status exam*, and considering basic life needs, such as financial or social resources, through *case management*. When actual or probable impediments are addressed early in the therapeutic process through *clinical assessment*, the therapeutic journey is likely to proceed more easily and smoothly.

Once you have your map with oases and obstacles clearly identified, you can confidently select a realistic path toward the client's chosen destination or *goal*. If you have done a good job mapping, you will be able to choose from among several different paths, depending on what works best for those on the journey: namely, you and the client. This translates to being able to choose a therapeutic theory and style that suit all involved. Seasoned clinicians distinguish themselves from newer therapists in their ability to identify and successfully navigate through numerous terrains: forests, seas, deserts, plains, paradises, and wastelands. The greater a therapist's repertoire of skills, the more able the therapist is to move through each terrain. Once a preferred path is chosen, the therapist generates a *treatment plan*, a general set of directions for how to address client concerns. Like any set of travel plans, treatment plans are subject to change due to weather, natural disaster, human error, and other unforeseeable events, otherwise known as "real life." Therapists can rest assured that unexpected detours, delays, and short cuts (yes, unexpected good stuff happens also) will be part of any therapeutic journey.

Once you select a course of action, you need to check frequently to make sure that (a) the plan is working and (b) you are sticking with it. In therapy, this translates to *assessing client progress* along the way. If the client is not making progress, the therapist needs to go back and reassess (a) the accuracy of the map and (b) the wisdom of the plan. Almost always, it is easy to make improvements in both areas that will get things back on course. The key is assessing client progress often enough to notice when you are off course as soon as possible.

Finally, you need to leave a trail to track where you have been. Leaving a trail always helps you find your way back if you get lost: others (as well as yourself) can see why and how you proceeded. Therapists leave a trace of their path by generating thorough *clinical documentation*, which helps in two highly prized aspects of therapy: getting paid by third-party payers (i.e., insurance) and avoiding lawsuits (i.e., the state lets you practice). By making it clear where you are going, you can help everyone concerned better understand your specific route of treatment.

From Trainee to Seasoned Therapist

The difference between trainees and seasoned therapists can be found in the quality of the map, the effectiveness of the path of treatment, and the speed with which it takes to move through the steps. A seasoned therapist may move through the five steps of competent therapy in the first few minutes of a session, whereas a trainee may take more time, collecting information and trying various options. How long it takes is less important than the quality of the journey. This book is designed to help you move through these five steps more effectively, whether you are just starting out or have been doing therapy for years.

On Becoming Competent

Therapists love to talk. They talk with clients about their private lives, wildest thoughts, deepest fears, darkest secrets, and outrageous dreams. They talk with colleagues about what works, what does not, and how reality is too unbelievable for a Hollywood movie. For years, therapists have been trained primarily through talk: they have discussed theories and ideas about how to assess, diagnose, and treat clients with various disorders.

But what happens when the garrulous graduates enter the therapy room? Are they able to translate classroom chatter into meaningful, helpful treatments? Sometimes it seems that the gap between class and practice feels more like the Grand Canyon than the next logical step. New therapists soon learn that talk is not enough. It takes real-world skills to be a competent therapist. Thankfully, marriage and family therapists have recently completed a list of the 128 skills needed to be a competent therapist. This list of skills provides a clear and specific map for becoming an effective clinician. So that is where we will turn our attention for the remainder of this chapter.

The Marriage and Family Therapy Core Competencies

In December 2002, the American Association for Marriage and Family Therapy (AAMFT) created the Core Competency Task Force

> to define the domains of knowledge and requisite skills in each domain that comprise the practice of marriage and family therapy… outlining core competencies [that] would define knowledge and skill levels… as well as any characteristics that might be defined that would pre-dispose one for success as a marriage and family therapist. (AAMFT, 2002, p. 1)

Two years later, AAMFT (2004) published a list of 128 distinct competencies that enable a therapist to work independently as a licensed professional. These competencies create a comprehensive template for becoming a successful therapist in today's marketplace and are increasingly used by government and insurance companies to define what it means to be a licensed marriage and family therapist. The competencies are divided into six domains, each with five subdomains.

Core Competency Domains

The Core Competencies include six general domains. The first four address the process of treatment, and the last two address (a) legal and ethical issues and (b) research and evaluation.

THE SIX DOMAINS OF THE MFT CORE COMPETENCIES

1. **Admission to Treatment:** Getting therapy started
2. **Clinical Assessment and Diagnosis:** Assessing individual and family functioning
3. **Treatment Planning and Case Management:** Developing a plan of care and coordinating care with other professionals
4. **Therapeutic Interventions:** Effecting change in the therapy session

(continued)

(continued)

> 5. **Legal Issues, Ethics, and Standards:** Understanding the legal and ethical aspects of practice
> 6. **Research and Program Evaluation:** Knowing the relevant research and how to evaluate one's effectiveness

Core Competency Subdomains

Each of these domains is divided into five subdomains that describe the type of knowledge or skill to be developed:

> ## THE FIVE SUBDOMAINS OF THE MFT CORE COMPETENCIES
>
> 1. **Conceptual:** Factual knowledge—what we expect to learn from a book
> 2. **Perceptual:** Ability to perceive or see what is going on with clients and in the therapy process
> 3. **Executive:** Skills and actions: ability to "execute" knowledge
> 4. **Evaluative:** Ability to assess one's *own* abilities and performance accurately
> 5. **Professional:** Ability to adhere to professional and ethical standards

CACREP Competency-Based Standards

In addition to the Family Therapy Core Competencies developed by the American Association for Marriage and Family Therapy, the Council on Accreditation of Counseling and Related Educational Programs (CACREP; related to the American Counseling Association) has also developed a list of competency-based standards that students in their marriage, couple, and family counseling programs must master before graduating. Because these define the knowledge and skills needed to complete a master's degree rather than to gain a license, they are less demanding and more academically focused than the Family Therapy Core Competencies. However, they overlap closely, creating a clear consensus on the basic competencies and making life easier for students, faculty, lawmakers, and third-party payers. The complete list of marriage, couple, and family counseling standards is included in the appendix.

The New Educational Paradigm: Learning-Centered Pedagogy

The competency movement is shaping how future generations of family therapists will teach and learn professional skills. Too often, traditional classroom experiences have been *textbook-centered*, organized around chapter-by-chapter textbook content (Gehart, 2007), or *teaching-centered*, focused on the process of teaching rather than learning (Chenail, 2008). Students read, talked, and wrote about the ideas in the book, and faculty focused on their own teaching more than on student learning, assuming that excellent teaching automatically results in learning.

In contrast, learning-centered pedagogy is based on the premise that instructors must continually focus on *learning outcomes:* Are students learning what instructors hope to teach? (Blumberg & Gonzalez-Major, 2006; Chenail, 2008; Koester, Hellenbrand, & Piper, 2005; Nelson, 2005; Weimer, 2002). Instruction is organized around a single question: What do students need to be able to do or know at the end of this course? Instructors then design practical assignments, select relevant readings, and develop learning-focused activities to enable students to demonstrate real-world knowledge or skills. Rather than summarize or analyze readings, learning-centered assignments require students to practice specific professional skills. For example, rather than writing a well-cited academic paper on a favorite theory, the student uses the same academic resources to create a well-developed clinical assessment, treatment plan, or case conceptualization for a case the student is working on (hint: you will be doing this soon). Similarly, Chenail (2008) had his students in a research course develop an evidence-based practice project (see Chapter 7) in which they systematically and thoughtfully examined the research literature to support their clinical practice and address specific client concerns. In this new learning paradigm, academic coursework becomes the foundation for real-world skills.

To further explore the possibilities of this new approach, in 2005 the AAMFT assembled a Beta-Test Group of eight universities from around the country to adopt the Core Competencies: Alliant International University, Christian Theological Seminar, St. Mary's University, Saybrook Graduate School, Southern Connecticut State University, University of Akron, University of Oregon, and Utah State University. Faculty at these universities are developing various tools for evaluating student learning, using activities such as live interviews and role play (Allgood, Brown, Bruff, Linville, Northey, & Parr, 2007; see Gehart, 2007, for a more complete discussion of the pedagogical issues related to teaching the Core Competencies). In the years to come, the education and training of family therapists will increasingly employ learning-centered activities to enable students to more quickly learn the competencies required in today's practice environments.

Implications for Students

In a learning-centered classroom, students are not passive containers of academic knowledge, needing only to memorize or analyze information. Instead, learning is *active:* it involves applying ideas to real situations, completing formal clinical forms, and developing treatment strategies for actual cases, all of which is grounded in academic literature. Classrooms are transformed into living laboratories, foreshadowing clinical practice. Learning-centered education may not be as safe and comfortable as traditional pedagogy, but it certainly is more exciting, more thorough, and more likely to get you out of your seat and moving.

Implications for Instructors

Instructors also have something new to learn. In the past, providing comprehensive content was the hallmark of successful university teaching. The Core Competencies invite faculty to take another step by helping students understand how the content relates to and informs clinical practice. At first, this appears to be a daunting task and may be somewhat awkward for those who have perfected their lectures over the years. It is my hope that this text provides a roadmap for bringing the excitement of the clinic alive and into the classroom, for faculty and students alike. I believe faculty will find that learning-centered education is more fun than traditional pedagogical styles and, surprisingly, often requires less faculty time and energy while accelerating the learning process.

Core Competencies in This Book

To help faculty and trainers integrate the Core Competencies into their teaching, this book focuses on four different learning tasks, which represent the most common written documents in clinical practice:

- Theoretical case conceptualizations (Chapter 2)
- Clinical assessments (Chapter 3)
- Treatment plans (Chapter 4)
- Case notes (Chapter 6)

These four clinical documents measure 43 of the Family Therapy Core Competencies *in full* and 57 *in part*. At the end of this chapter is an inventory of all 128 competencies, with the 100 entries either fully or partially addressed in this text listed in **bold-faced** font. The remaining 28 competencies are fully assessed in four other instruments available separately as part of *The Complete Marriage and Family Therapy Core Competencies Assessment System* (Gehart, 2007).

For those of you reading the Core Competencies for the first time, they are long and overwhelming. The more you work with them, the more their logic and organization start to become second nature. I recommend you find a time when your mind is particularly clear to sit down and read through these to get a sense of the roadmap your faculty and supervisors are using to teach you to be a competent therapist. I will leave you here with a highlighter and cup of tea to get acquainted with the road ahead.

ONLINE RESOURCES

American Association for Marriage and Family Therapy
More information on the Core Competencies; downloadable version of the competencies

www.aamft.org

Marriage and Family Therapy Core Competencies Assessment System
More information on assessing the Core Competencies

www.mftcompetencies.org

REFERENCES

Allgood, S., Brown, S., Bruff, B., Linville, D., Northey, B., & Parr, P. (2007, October). *Tools for evaluating core competencies.* Workshop (2 hour) presented at the Annual Conference of the American Association for Marriage Family Therapy, Long Beach, CA.

American Association for Marriage and Family Therapy. (2002). *Competencies task force: Scope and charge.* Alexandria, VA: Author.

American Association for Marriage and Family Therapy. (2004). *Marriage and therapy core competencies.* Alexandria, VA: Author.

Blumberg, P., & Gonzalez-Major, J. (2006, October). *Using rubrics to foster learning-centered practices.* Presented at EDUCAUSE Annual Conference. www.connect.educause.edu.

Chenail, R. (2008). *Learning marriage and family therapy in the time of competencies.* Manuscript submitted for publication.

Gehart, D. (2007). *The complete marriage and family therapy core competencies assessment system: Eight outcome-based instruments for assessing student learning.* Available at www.mftcompetencies.org

Koester, J., Hellenbrand, H., & Piper, T. (2005). Exploring the actions behind the words "learning-centered institution." *About Campus, 10*(4), 10–16.

Nelson, T. S. (2005). Core competencies and MFT education. *Family Therapy Magazine,* 4(4), 20–23.

Weimer, M. (2002). *Learner-centered teaching: Five key changes to practice.* New York: Jossey-Bass.

THE FAMILY THERAPY CORE COMPETENCIES

HOW TO READ THE CORE COMPETENCIES

- **Number:** Each competency is identified with a three-part number.
  First number: Domains 1–6
  Second number: Subdomains 1–5
  Third number: The specific competency in the subdomain
- **Subdomain:** The second column refers to the subdomain: conceptual, perceptual, executive, evaluative, or professional.
- **Competence:** The third column is the specific competence or skill.
- **Form:** The last column identifies the form or assignment where the competency is measured in *The Complete Marriage and Family Core Competencies Assessment System* (Gehart, 2007). A competency may be measured on one or more forms and may be measured more than once; *the number of measurements is indicated in parentheses, such as (2).* Only four of the eight forms are included in this book. These are abbreviated as follows:
  CC = Case Conceptualization (Chapter 2)
  CA = Clinical Assessment (Chapter 3)
  TP = Treatment Plan (Chapter 4)
  PN = Progress Notes (Chapter 6)
- The remaining competencies (not included in this book) are measured in the following forms:
  PD = Professional Development Plan
  LI = Live Interview
  LE = Live Interview Evaluation
  RP = Research Proposal
- **Bold-Text Competencies:** Boldface indicates that this competency is taught and measured in a form included in this book.

DOMAIN 1: ADMISSION TO TREATMENT

NUMBER	SUBDOMAIN	COMPETENCE	FORM
1.1.1	Conceptual	**Understand systems concepts, theories, and techniques that are foundational to the practice of marriage and family therapy.**	CC (10)
1.1.2	Conceptual	**Understand theories and techniques of individual, marital, couple, family, and group psychotherapy.**	TP
1.1.3	Conceptual	**Understand the behavioral health care delivery system, its impact on the services provided, and the barriers and disparities in the system.**	TP

(continued)

DOMAIN 1:   **ADMISSION TO TREATMENT** *(continued)*

NUMBER	SUBDOMAIN	COMPETENCE	FORM
1.1.4	Conceptual	**Understand the risks and benefits of individual, marital, couple, family, and group psychotherapy.**	TP
1.2.1	Perceptual	**Recognize contextual and systemic dynamics (e.g., gender, age, socioeconomic status, culture/ race/ethnicity, sexual orientation, spirituality, religion, larger systems, social context).**	CC
1.2.2	Perceptual	**Consider health status, mental status, other therapy, and other systems involved in the clients' lives (e.g., courts, social services).**	CA
1.2.3	Perceptual	**Recognize issues that might suggest referral for specialized evaluation, assessment, or care.**	CA
1.3.1	Executive	**Gather and review intake information, giving balanced attention to individual, family, community, cultural, and contextual factors.**	CA
1.3.2	Executive	**Determine who should attend therapy and in what configuration (e.g., individual, couple, family, extrafamilial resources).**	CA (2) TP
1.3.3	Executive	**Facilitate therapeutic involvement of all necessary participants in treatment.**	TP LI
1.3.4	Executive	Explain practice setting rules, fees, rights, and responsibilities of each party, including privacy, confidentiality policies, and duty to care to client or legal guardian.	LI
1.3.5	Executive	Obtain consent to treatment from all responsible persons.	LI
1.3.6	Executive	**Establish and maintain appropriate and productive therapeutic alliances with the clients.**	TP LI
1.3.7	Executive	**Solicit and use client feedback throughout the therapeutic process.**	PN LI
1.3.8	Executive	**Develop and maintain collaborative working relationships with referral resources, other practitioners involved in the clients' care, and payers.**	PN
1.3.9	Executive	Manage session interactions with individuals, couples, families, and groups.	LI
1.4.1	Evaluative	**Evaluate case for appropriateness for treatment within professional scope of practice and competence.**	TP
1.5.1	Professional	Understand the legal requirements and limitations for working with vulnerable populations (e.g., minors).	LI
1.5.2	Professional	**Complete case documentation in a timely manner and in accordance with relevant laws and policies.**	PN
1.5.3	Professional	**Develop, establish, and maintain policies for fees, payment, record keeping, and confidentiality.**	CA PN (2) LI

DOMAIN 2: **CLINICAL ASSESSMENT AND DIAGNOSIS**

NUMBER	SUBDOMAIN	COMPETENCE	FORM
2.1.1	Conceptual	Understand principles of human development; human sexuality; gender development; psychopathology; psychopharmacology; couple processes; and family development and processes (e.g., family, relational, and system dynamics).	CC CA
2.1.2	Conceptual	Understand the major behavioral health disorders, including the epidemiology, etiology, phenomenology, effective treatments, course, and prognosis.	CA (2)
2.1.3	Conceptual	Understand the clinical needs and implications of persons with comorbid disorders (e.g., substance abuse and mental health; heart disease and depression).	TP
2.1.4	Conceptual	Comprehend individual, marital, couple, and family assessment instruments appropriate to presenting problem, practice setting, and cultural context.	TP RP
2.1.5	Conceptual	Understand the current models for assessment and diagnosis of mental health disorders, substance use disorders, and relational functioning.	CA
2.1.6	Conceptual	Understand the strengths and limitations of the models of assessment and diagnosis, especially as they relate to different cultural, economic, and ethnic groups.	CA RP
2.1.7	Conceptual	Understand the concepts of reliability and validity, their relationship to assessment instruments, and how they influence therapeutic decision making.	RP
2.2.1	Perceptual	Assess each client's engagement in the change process.	LI
2.2.2	Perceptual	Systematically integrate client reports, observations of client behaviors, client relationship patterns, reports from other professionals, results from testing procedures, and interactions with client to guide the assessment process.	CC
2.2.3	Perceptual	Develop hypotheses regarding relationship patterns, their bearing on the presenting problem, and the influence of extra-therapeutic factors on client systems.	CC (11)
2.2.4	Perceptual	Consider the influence of treatment on extra-therapeutic relationships.	CA
2.2.5	Perceptual	Consider physical/organic problems that can cause or exacerbate emotional/interpersonal symptoms.	CA
2.3.1	Executive	Diagnose and assess client behavioral and relational health problems systemically and contextually.	CA
2.3.2	Executive	Provide assessments and deliver developmentally appropriate services to clients, such as children, adolescents, elders, and persons with special needs.	TP (2) LI
2.3.3	Executive	Apply effective and systemic interviewing techniques and strategies.	TP LI

(continued)

DOMAIN 2: CLINICAL ASSESSMENT AND DIAGNOSIS *(continued)*

NUMBER	SUBDOMAIN	COMPETENCE	FORM
2.3.4	Executive	Administer and interpret results of assessment instruments.	CA RP
2.3.5	Executive	Screen and develop adequate safety plans for substance abuse, child and elder maltreatment, domestic violence, physical violence, suicide potential, and dangerousness to self and others.	CA PN LI
2.3.6	Executive	Assess family history and dynamics using a genogram or other assessment instruments.	CC (2)
2.3.7	Executive	Elicit a relevant and accurate biopsychosocial history to understand the context of the clients' problems.	CC (3) LI
2.3.8	Executive	Identify clients' strengths, resilience, and resources.	CC (2)
2.3.9	Executive	Elucidate presenting problem from the perspective of each member of the therapeutic system.	CC (2) LI
2.4.1	Evaluative	Evaluate assessment methods for relevance to clients' needs.	CA LE
2.4.2	Evaluative	Assess ability to view issues and therapeutic processes systemically.	CA LE
2.4.3	Evaluative	Evaluate the accuracy and cultural relevance of behavioral health and relational diagnoses.	CA LE
2.4.4	Evaluative	Assess the therapist-client agreement of therapeutic goals and diagnosis.	CA LE
2.5.1	Professional	Utilize consultation and supervision effectively.	PN LI

DOMAIN 3: TREATMENT PLANNING AND CASE MANAGEMENT

NUMBER	SUBDOMAIN	COMPETENCE	FORM
3.1.1	Conceptual	Know which models, modalities, and/or techniques are most effective for presenting problems.	TP
3.1.2	Conceptual	Understand the liabilities incurred when billing third parties, the codes necessary for reimbursement, and how to use them correctly.	PN
3.1.3	Conceptual	Understand the effects that psychotropic and other medications have on clients and the treatment process.	CA
3.1.4	Conceptual	Understand recovery-oriented behavioral health services (e.g., self-help groups, 12-step programs, peer-to-peer services, supported employment).	TP LI
3.2.1	Perceptual	Integrate client feedback, assessment, contextual information, and diagnosis with treatment goals and plan.	TP PN LI

3.3.1	Executive	Develop, with client input, measurable outcomes, treatment goals, treatment plans, and aftercare plans with clients utilizing a systemic perspective.	TP
3.3.2	Executive	Prioritize treatment goals.	TP
3.3.3	Executive	Develop a clear plan of how sessions will be conducted.	TP (2)
3.3.4	Executive	Structure treatment to meet clients' needs and to facilitate systemic change.	TP
3.3.5	Executive	Manage progression of therapy toward treatment goals.	TP
3.3.6	Executive	Manage risks, crises, and emergencies.	TP CA LI
3.3.7	Executive	Work collaboratively with other stakeholders, including family members, other significant persons, and professionals not present.	PN
3.3.8	Executive	Assist clients in obtaining needed care while navigating complex systems of care.	TP LI
3.3.9	Executive	Develop termination and aftercare plans.	TP
3.4.1	Evaluative	Evaluate progress of sessions toward treatment goals.	PN
3.4.2	Evaluative	Recognize when treatment goals and plan require modification.	PN
3.4.3	Evaluative	Evaluate level of risks, management of risks, crises, and emergencies.	CA TP LI
3.4.4	Evaluative	Assess session process for compliance with policies and procedures of practice setting.	LE
3.4.5	Professional	Monitor personal reactions to clients and treatment process, especially in terms of therapeutic behavior, relationship with clients, process for explaining procedures, and outcomes.	LE
3.5.1	Professional	Advocate with clients in obtaining quality care, appropriate resources, and services in their community.	TP LI
3.5.2	Professional	Participate in case-related forensic and legal processes.	CA
3.5.3	Professional	Write plans and complete other case documentation in accordance with practice setting policies, professional standards, and state/provincial laws.	TP PD (2) LE (2) RP (2)
3.5.4	Professional	Utilize time management skills in therapy sessions and other professional meetings.	LI

(continued)

DOMAIN 4: **THERAPEUTIC INTERVENTIONS** *(continued)*

NUMBER	SUBDOMAIN	COMPETENCE	FORM
4.1.1	Conceptual	Comprehend a variety of individual and systemic therapeutic models and their application, including evidence-based therapies and culturally sensitive approaches.	TP LE
4.1.2	Conceptual	Recognize strengths, limitations, and contraindications of specific therapy models, including the risk of harm associated with models that incorporate assumptions of family dysfunction, pathogenesis, or cultural deficit.	TP LE
4.2.1	Perceptual	Recognize how different techniques may impact the treatment process.	TP (2)
4.2.2	Perceptual	Distinguish differences between content and process issues, their role in therapy, and their potential impact on therapeutic outcomes.	TP LI
4.3.1	Executive	Match treatment modalities and techniques to clients' needs, goals, and values.	TP LI
4.3.2	Executive	Deliver interventions in a way that is sensitive to special needs of clients (e.g., gender, age, socioeconomic status, culture/race/ethnicity, sexual orientation, disability, personal history, larger systems issues of the client).	PN LI
4.3.3	Executive	Reframe problems and recursive interaction patterns.	TP (2) LI
4.3.4	Executive	Generate relational questions and reflexive comments in the therapy room.	TP (2) LI
4.3.5	Executive	Engage each family member in the treatment process as appropriate.	TP (2) LI
4.3.6	Executive	Facilitate clients developing and integrating solutions to problems.	TP (2) PN LI
4.3.7	Executive	Defuse intense and chaotic situations to enhance the safety of all participants.	LI
4.3.8	Executive	Empower clients and their relational systems to establish effective relationships with each other and larger systems.	TP (2) LI
4.3.9	Executive	Provide psychoeducation to families whose members have serious mental illness or other disorders.	TP (2) LI
4.3.10	Executive	Modify interventions that are not working to better fit treatment goals.	PN LI
4.3.11	Executive	Move to constructive termination when treatment goals have been accomplished.	TP
4.3.12	Executive	Integrate supervisor/team communications into treatment.	PN LI
4.4.1	Evaluative	Evaluate interventions for consistency, congruency with model of therapy and theory of change, cultural and contextual relevance, and goals of the treatment plan.	TP LE (2)

4.4.2	**Evaluative**	**Evaluate ability to deliver interventions effectively.**	**PN** LE
4.4.3	**Evaluative**	**Evaluate treatment outcomes as treatment progresses.**	**PN** LE
4.4.4	**Evaluative**	**Evaluate clients' reactions or responses to interventions.**	**PN** LI LE
4.4.5	**Evaluative**	**Evaluate clients' outcomes for the need to continue, refer, or terminate therapy.**	**TP PN** LE
4.4.6	Evaluative	Evaluate reactions to the treatment process (e.g., transference, family of origin, current stress level, current life situation, cultural context) and their impact on effective intervention and clinical outcomes.	LE
4.5.1	**Professional**	**Respect multiple perspectives (e.g., clients, team, supervisor, practitioners from other disciplines who are involved in the case).**	**PN** LI
4.5.2	Professional	Set appropriate boundaries, manage issues of triangulation, and develop collaborative working relationships.	LI
4.5.3	**Professional**	**Articulate rationales for interventions related to treatment goals and plan, assessment information, and systemic understanding of clients' context and dynamics.**	**TP** LE

DOMAIN 5: LEGAL ISSUES, ETHICS, AND STANDARDS

NUMBER	SUBDOMAIN	COMPETENCE	FORM
5.1.1	Conceptual	**Know state, federal, and provincial laws and regulations that apply to the practice of marriage and family therapy.**	**CA** LI
5.1.2	Conceptual	**Know professional ethics and standards of practice that apply to the practice of marriage and family therapy.**	**CA** LI
5.1.3	Conceptual	Know policies and procedures of the practice setting.	LI
5.1.4	Conceptual	**Understand the process of making an ethical decision.**	**CA PN** LE
5.2.1	Perceptual	**Recognize situations in which ethics, laws, professional liability, and standards of practice apply.**	**CA PN** LI
5.2.2	Perceptual	**Recognize ethical dilemmas in practice setting.**	**PN** LE
5.2.3	Perceptual	**Recognize when a legal consultation is necessary.**	**PN** LE

(continued)

DOMAIN 5:   **LEGAL ISSUES, ETHICS, AND STANDARDS** *(continued)*

NUMBER	SUBDOMAIN	COMPETENCE	FORM
5.2.4	**Perceptual**	**Recognize when clinical supervision or consultation is necessary.**	**PN** **LI**
5.3.1	**Executive**	**Monitor issues related to ethics, laws, regulations, and professional standards.**	**PN** **LI**
5.3.2	**Executive**	**Develop and assess policies, procedures, and forms for consistency with standards of practice to protect client confidentiality and to comply with relevant laws and regulations.**	**CA**
5.3.3	Executive	Inform clients and legal guardian of limitations to confidentiality and parameters of mandatory reporting.	LI
5.3.4	**Executive**	**Develop safety plans for clients who present with potential self-harm, suicide, abuse, or violence.**	**CA** **PN** **LI**
5.3.5	**Executive**	**Take appropriate action when ethical and legal dilemmas emerge.**	**CA** **PN** **LI**
5.3.6	**Executive**	**Report information to appropriate authorities as required by law.**	**CA** **PN** **LI**
5.3.7	**Executive**	**Practice within defined scope of practice and competence.**	**TP**
5.3.8	Executive	Obtain knowledge of advances and theory regarding effective clinical practice.	PD
5.3.9	Executive	Obtain license(s) and specialty credentials.	PD (2)
5.3.10	Executive	Implement a personal program to maintain professional competence.	PD (3)
5.4.1	Evaluative	Evaluate activities related to ethics, legal issues, and practice standards.	LE
5.4.2	Evaluative	Monitor attitudes, personal well-being, personal issues, and personal problems to ensure they do not impact the therapy process adversely or create vulnerability for misconduct.	PD
5.5.1	**Professional**	**Maintain client records with timely and accurate notes.**	**PN**
5.5.2	**Professional**	**Consult with peers and/or supervisors if personal issues, attitudes, or beliefs threaten to adversely impact clinical work.**	**PN** PD
5.5.3	Professional	Pursue professional development through self-supervision, collegial consultation, professional reading, and continuing educational activities.	PD
5.5.4	**Professional**	**Bill clients and third-party payers in accordance with professional ethics, relevant laws, and policies, and seek reimbursement only for covered services.**	**PN**

DOMAIN 6: RESEARCH AND PROGRAM EVALUATION

NUMBER	SUBDOMAIN	COMPETENCE	FORM
6.1.1	**Conceptual**	**Know the extant MFT literature, research, and evidence-based practice.**	**TP** **RP**
6.1.2	Conceptual	Understand research and program evaluation methodologies, both quantitative and qualitative, relevant to MFT and mental health services.	RP
6.1.3	Conceptual	Understand the legal, ethical, and contextual issues involved in the conduct of clinical research and program evaluation.	RP
6.2.1	Perceptual	Recognize opportunities for therapists and clients to participate in clinical research.	RP
6.3.1	Executive	Read current MFT and other professional literature.	PD (2)
6.3.2	**Executive**	**Use current MFT and other research to inform clinical practice.**	**CC** **TP**
6.3.3	Executive	Critique professional research and assess the quality of research studies and program evaluation in the literature.	RP
6.3.4	Executive	Determine the effectiveness of clinical practice and techniques.	LE RP
6.4.1	Evaluative	Evaluate knowledge of current clinical literature and its application.	PD RP
6.5.1	Professional	Contribute to the development of new knowledge.	PD

Note: The Core Competencies have been reproduced with permission from AAMFT.

Case Conceptualization

Step 1: Mapping the Territory

There are few moments as exciting or neuroses-inducing in a therapist's training as "the first session": seeing your first client and losing your therapeutic "virginity," so to speak. We know the questions that follow: "Was it good for you?" "Did I get it right?" "Was I okay?" Before the session, there are other predictable questions: "What do I say?" "What do I do?" "What if I can't remember X?" Although logical, these questions can quickly get a new therapist lost and off course. That is why the first step in therapy is to map the territory. To develop a good map, therapists need to master the art of *viewing*, which in a talking profession like therapy refers to knowing where to focus your attention while listening.

The heart of therapy—the seeming brilliance of a great therapist—has always been in the viewing. The most useful question for new therapists to ask their supervisors is: *What should I be noticing and listening for when I talk with this client?* Thankfully, this is much easier than trying to memorize what to say. The apparent magic that distinguishes master therapists from average therapists and average therapists from the average person lies in what the person attends to when another is speaking. Essentially, the better you get at knowing how to focus your viewing, the better therapist you will be. I believe it is a skill that great therapists continually develop and refine over the course of their careers—so don't plan on mastering it anytime soon.

Case conceptualization is the technical term for the therapeutic art of viewing. Although it is also sometimes called *assessment, assessment* is a tricky term because it can refer to two different therapeutic tasks: a case conceptualization approach to assessing individual and family dynamics (covered in this chapter) or a diagnostic approach to assessing symptomology (covered in Chapter 3, Clinical Assessment). To reduce confusion, I refer to a theory-informed assessment as *case conceptualization* and to a diagnostic assessment as *clinical assessment*.

Theories provide therapists with unique lenses through which to view clients' problems. Like a detailed map, they place problems in a broader and more comprehensive context that allows therapists to see how pieces fit together and that provides clues to the best path out of a tangled situation.

Case Conceptualization and the Art of Viewing

Case conceptualization enables therapists to generate new perspectives that enable them to be helpful to clients. For example, Ron and Suzie have been arguing for months. They seek out a therapist hoping that somehow, some way, the therapist can help them resolve their differences. When they enter therapy, each is thinking: "I hope the therapist can help my spouse see what he/she is doing wrong and encourage him/her to fix it. I know I have problems too, but I am sure that as soon as my spouse changes, it will be easy for me to change." They have told this and less benevolent versions of their stories to their family and friends, yet no one has been able to help either Ron or Suzie to make meaningful changes. So what makes the therapist different from the family, friends, and hairdressers who listen to this story? Does the therapist have special knowledge that will allow him/her to provide the "answer" to the couple's problem? Or does the therapist simply serve as a socially sanctioned referee to this dispute? Or does the therapist do something more?

Although some therapists define themselves as "educators" or "mediators," most define their roles as promoting change through a transformational interpersonal process that is far more nuanced than education or mediation. Therapists differ from friends, educators, and mediators in their ability to view the situation in new and useful ways. From these new perspectives, possibilities for intervention emerge that did not arise in any of the previous conversations between the partners or with their family and friends.

Overview of Case Conceptualization

As therapists become more experienced, case conceptualization takes place primarily in their heads—while clients are talking. It happens so fast that often they have difficulty tracing their steps. However, new therapists must take things more slowly. Similar to learning a new dance step, the new move needs to be broken down into small pieces with specific instructions for where the hands and feet go; with practice, the dancer is able to put the pieces together more quickly and smoothly until it becomes "natural." That is what we are going to do here with case conceptualization. So, let's start with identifying the components of a systemic case conceptualization:

1. **Introduction to Client**
2. **Presenting Concern**
3. **Background Information**
4. **Systemic Assessment**
5. **Genogram**
6. **Client Perspectives**

The complete form for case conceptualization is included at the end of this chapter, and in the following paragraphs you will find instructions for completing each section. Examples of how to complete a case conceptualization are found at the end of each of the theoretical chapters in Part II of this text.

Introduction to Client

Case conceptualization starts by identifying (a) who the client is (individual, couple, or family) and (b) the most salient demographic features that relate to treatment. Common demographic information includes the following.

- Age
- Ethnicity

- Gender
- Sexual orientation
- Current occupation/work status or grade in school

I. Introduction to Client *(Define client as individual, couple, or family; include age, ethnicity, occupation, grade, etc.)*

This initial introduction to the client defines the type of therapy—individual, couple, or family—as well as provides the reader with a basic sketch of the client that will be elaborated upon as the case conceptualization unfolds.

Presenting Concern

The presenting concern is a description of how all parties involved are defining the problem: client, family, friends, school, workplace, legal system, and society.

II. Presenting Concern
- *Clients'/Family's Descriptions of Problem(s)*
- *Broader System Problem Descriptions*

Often new and even experienced therapists assume that this description is a straightforward and clear-cut matter. Though sometimes it is, usually it is surprisingly complex. Anderson and Goolishian (Anderson, 1997; Anderson & Gehart, 2006) developed a unique means of conceptualizing the presenting problem in their Collaborative Language Systems Approach, also referred to as collaborative therapy (Chapter 15). This postmodern approach maintains that each person who is talking about the problem is part of the problem-generating system, the set of relationships that produced the perspective or idea that there is a problem. Each person involved has a different definition of the problem; sometimes the difference is slight and sometimes it is stark. For example, when parents bring a child to therapy, the mother, father, siblings, grandparents, teachers, school counselors, doctors, and friends have different ideas of what the problem actually is. The mother may think it is a medical problem, such as ADHD; the father may believe it is related to his wife's permissiveness; the teacher may say it is poor parenting; and the child may think there really is not a problem at all.

Historically, therapists have moved rapidly to define the problem according to their theoretical worldview—either a formal diagnosis (ADHD, depression, etc.) or another mental health category (such as parenting style, defense mechanism, family dynamics, etc.)—with little reflection on the contradictory opinions and descriptions of the various people involved. Although this may be practical at one level, the more therapists can remain open to the family's alternative descriptions of the problem, the more they can remain adaptable and creative. They can maintain stronger rapport with each person involved, honoring each person's perspective and referring to it throughout treatment. Furthermore, being mindful of the multiple problem definitions gives the therapist greater maneuverability when treatment stagnates or conditions do not improve.

A description of the presenting problem should include the following:

1. The reason(s) each client states he/she is seeking counseling or has been referred
2. Any information from the referring agent (teacher, doctor, psychiatrist, etc.) and his/her description of the problem

3. A brief history of the problem and family (if applicable)
4. Descriptions of the attempted solutions and the outcome of these attempts
5. Any other problem-related information that may be relevant to the situation

Background Information

Obtaining background information about the problem is the next step. Traditionally, therapists have included information such as the following:

- Education/grade in school
- Relevant family history
- Recent life changes
- Health situation and medications
- History of mental disorders and/or substance abuse
- History of previous counseling
- History of childhood abuse
- History of trauma

III. Background Information

- *Recent Background*: Life changes, precipitating events, first symptoms, other stressors, etc.
- *Related Historical Background*: Family history, related issues, past abuse, trauma, previous counseling, medical/mental health history, etc.

Often, this background information is considered the "facts" of the case. However, as family therapists have historically cautioned, how we describe the facts makes all the difference (Anderson, 1997; O'Hanlon & Weiner-Davis, 1989; Watzlawick, Weakland, & Fisch, 1974). For example, whether you begin by saying that the client "recently won a state-level academic decathlon" or whether you begin with "her mother recently divorced her alcoholic father" paints two very different pictures of the same client for both you, the therapist, and anyone else who reads the assessment. Therefore, although this may seem like the "factual" part of the report in which you as a professional are not imposing any bias, in fact, therapists impose bias by their subtle choice of words, their ordering of information, and their emphasis on particular details.

Based on research about the importance of the therapeutic relationship and of hope (Lambert & Ogles, 2004; Miller, Duncan, & Hubble, 1997), I recommend that therapists write the background section so that they and anyone reading the report, including potentially the client, will have a positive impression of the client and hope for the client's recovery; these two factors affect the outcome of treatment.

Systemic Assessment

The systemic assessment—identifying the interactional and relational patterns in the client's family and social network—is the heart of case conceptualization and the longest part. It includes the following subparts, each of which are discussed in more detail in the rest of this chapter:

1. Client and Relational Strengths
2. Family Structure and Interaction Patterns
3. Intergenerational Patterns
4. Previous Solutions
5. Narratives and Social Discourses

IV. Systemic Assessment

Client/Relational Strengths

- Personal/Individual
- Relational/Social
- Spiritual

Family Structure and Interaction Patterns

Couple Subsystem Functioning

- Couple Boundaries: Internal and External
- Problem Interaction Patterns
- Complementary Patterns
- Satir's Communication Stances
- Gottman's Divorce Indicators

Parental Subsystem

- Parental and Sibling Subsystem Boundaries
- Family Life Cycle Stages
- Hierarchy Between Child and Parents
- Emotional Boundaries with Children
- Problem Interaction Patterns
- Triangles/Coalitions
- Communication Stances

Systemic Hypothesis

A hypothesis regarding the role of the symptom in maintaining family-relational-individual homeostasis (norms)

Intergenerational Patterns

- Substance/Alcohol Abuse
- Sexual/Physical/Emotional Abuse
- Parent/Child Relations
- Physical/Mental Disorders
- Historical Incidents of Presenting Problem

Previous Solutions

- That DID NOT Work
- That DID Work

Narratives and Social Discourses

- Dominant Discourses (cultural, gender, and social influences, etc.)
- Identity Narratives
- Local and Preferred Discourses

This assessment can be used with individuals, couples, or families. The approach presented here draws from the major theories in family therapy. Consistent with both systemic (earlier family therapies) and postmodern (later forms of family therapy) practices, it uses multiple descriptors to generate a complete, "both/and" perspective (Keeney, 1983) and a rich, multivoiced depiction of the problem (Anderson, 1997).

Client and Relational Strengths

Client strengths and resources should be the first thing assessed. This is a lesson I learned the hard way. When I began teaching systemic assessment, I put the client strength section at the end because it is more clearly associated with solution-based and postmodern approaches (Chapters 14 and 15; Anderson, 1997; de Shazer, 1988; White & Epston, 1990), which were developed later historically. What I discovered is that after reading about the presenting problem, history, and problematic family dynamics, I was often feeling quite hopeless about the case. However, often upon reading the strengths section at the end, I would immediately perk up and find myself having hope, deep respect, and even excitement about the clients and their future. I have since decided to start by assessing strengths and believe it puts the therapist in a more resourceful mindset, whether working from either a systemic or postmodern perspective.

Emerging research supports the importance of identifying client strengths and resources. Researchers who developed the *common factors model* (discussed in Chapter 7; Lambert & Ogles, 2004; Miller, Duncan, & Hubble, 1997) estimate that 40% of outcomes can be attributed to client factors, such as severity of symptoms, access to resources, and support system; the remaining factors include the therapeutic relationship (30%), therapist interventions (15%), and the client's sense of hope (15%). Assessing for resources leverages client factors (40%), strengthens the therapeutic relationship (30%), and instills hope (15%), thus drawing on three of the four common factors. Thus, the benefit of assessing strengths is hard to overestimate.

To conceptualize a full spectrum of client strengths and resources, therapists can include strengths at several levels:

1. Personal/individual strengths
2. Relational/social strengths and resources
3. Spiritual resources

Personal or Individual Strengths

When assessing for personal or individual strengths and resources, the therapist can begin by reviewing two general categories of strengths: abilities and personal qualities.

- **Abilities:** Where and how are clients functioning in daily life? How do they get to sessions? Are they able to maintain a job, a hobby, or a relationship? Do they have any special talents, either now or in the past? If you look, you will always find a wide range of abilities with even the most "dysfunctional" of clients, especially if you consider the past as well as the present and future.

  Naming their abilities can increase clients' sense of hope and confidence to address the problem at hand. I find this especially helpful with children. If a child is having academic problems at school, the family, teachers, and child may not notice that the child is excelling in an extracurricular activity such as karate, soccer, or piano. Often noticing these areas of accomplishment makes it easier for all involved to find hope for improving the situation.

  Identifying abilities may also give clients or therapists creative ideas about how to solve a current problem. For example, I worked with a recovering alcoholic who hated the idea of writing but often spoke of how music inspired her. By drawing on this strength, we developed the idea of creating a special "sobriety mix" of favorite songs to help maintain sobriety and prevent relapse, an activity that had deep significance and inspiration for her.

- **Personal Qualities:** Ironically, the best place to find personal qualities is within the presenting problem or complaint. What brings clients to see a therapist is usually the flip side of a strength. For example, if a person complains about worrying too much, that person is equally likely to be a diligent and productive worker. Persons who argue with a spouse or child are more likely to speak up for themselves and are generally invested in the relationship in which they are arguing. In virtually all cases, the knife cuts both ways: each liability contains within it a strength in another context. Conversely, a strength in one context is often a problem in another. Here is a list of common problems and their related strengths.

PROBLEMS AND RELATED STRENGTHS

PROBLEM	POSSIBLE ASSOCIATED STRENGTH
Depression	• Is aware of what others think and feel • Is connected to others and/or desires connection • Has dreams and hopes • Has had the courage to take action to realize dreams • Has a realistic assessment of self/others (according to recent research; Seligman, 2004)
Anxiety	• Pays attention to details • Desires to perform well • Is careful and thoughtful about actions • Is able to plan for the future and anticipate potential obstacles
Arguing	• Stands up for self and/or beliefs • Fights injustice • Wants the relationship to work • Has hope for better things for others/self
Anger	• Is in touch with feelings and thoughts • Stands up against injustice • Believes in fairness • Is able to sense his/her boundaries and when they are crossed
Overwhelmed	• Is concerned about others' needs • Is thoughtful • Is able to see the big picture • Sets goals and pursues them

Identifying strengths relies heavily on the therapist's viewing skills. A skilled therapist is able to see the strengths that are the flip side of the presenting problem while still remaining aware of the problem.

Relational or Social Strengths and Resources

Family, friends, professionals, teachers, coworkers, bosses, neighbors, church members, salespeople, and numerous others in a person's life can be part of a social support network that helps the client in physical, emotional, and spiritual ways:

- **Physical** support includes people who may help with running errands, picking up the children, or doing tasks around the house.

- **Emotional** support may take the form of listening or helping resolve relational problems.

- **Community** support includes friendships and acceptance provided by any community and is almost always there in some form for a person who may be feeling marginalized because of culture, sexual orientation, language, religion, or similar factors. These communities are critical for coping with the stress of marginalization.

Simply naming, recognizing, and appreciating that there is support can immediately increase a client's sense of hope and reduce feelings of loneliness.

Spiritual Resources

Increasingly, family therapists are becoming aware of how clients' spiritual resources can be used to address their problems (Walsh, 2003). For this reason, therapists should become familiar with the major religious traditions in their community, such as Protestantism, Catholicism, Judaism, Islam, New Age religions, and Native American practices.

Spirituality can be defined as how a person conceptualizes his/her relationship to the universe, life, or God (or however he/she constructs that which is larger than the self). Everyone has some form of spirituality, or a belief in how the universe operates; see Bateson (1972, 1979/2002) and Gergen (1999).

SPIRITUALITY

The rules of "how life should go" always inform (a) what the person perceives to be a problem, (b) how a person feels about it, and (c) what that person believes can "realistically" be done about it, all of which a therapist wants to know to develop an effective therapeutic plan.

Questions for Assessing Spirituality

A therapist can use some of the following questions to assess a client's spirituality, whether traditional or nontraditional:

- Do you believe there is a god or some form of intelligence that organizes the universe? If so, what types of things does that being or force have control over?

- If there is not a god, by what rules does the universe operate? Why do things happen? Or is life entirely random?

- What is the purpose and/or meaning of human existence? How does this understanding inform how a person should approach life?

- Is there any reason to be kind to others? To one's self?

- What is the ideal versus the realistic way to approach life?

- Why do "bad" things happen to "good" people?

- Do you believe things happen for a reason? If so, what reason?

- Do you belong to a religious community or spiritual circle of friends that provides spiritual support, inspiration, and/or guidance in some way?

With the answers to these questions, therapists can create a map of the client's world that they can use to develop conversations and interventions that are deeply meaningful and a good "fit" for the client. An accurate understanding of a client's "map of life" reveals what logic and actions will motivate the client to make changes, providing therapists with invaluable resources. Often many clients from traditional religious backgrounds and New Age groups believe that "things happen for a reason." These clients can use this one belief to radically and quickly transform how they feel, think, and respond to difficult situations. For example, a recent client of mine who was feeling depressed after being unexpectedly fired experienced a rapid improvement in mood when she began to see the situation as a sign from the divine that she needed to pursue an old career dream she had been putting off for years; this belief allowed her to mobilize her energy and hope to start moving in a positive direction.

Family Structure and Interaction Patterns

The hallmark of systemic assessment is assessing family structure and interaction patterns. There are many ways to do this, the easiest being to break things into bite-size pieces by separately assessing the couple and parent-child subsystems, the smaller units of the family (Minuchin, 1974; Minuchin & Fishman, 1981).

When assessing the couple or marital subsystem, the therapist may choose to assess the most relevant subsystem:

An adult client's current relationship
An adult client's past or most recent relationship
A child or adult client's parents' relationship

Similarly, when assessing the parental subsystem, the therapist may choose to assess the following:

An adult's relationship with his/her child
An adult's relationship with his/her parent
A child's relationship with his/her parent

Whenever possible, it is preferable to assess both couple and family subsystems. For example, when treating an adult who does not have children, it is tempting to think that one does not need to assess the parental subsystem. However, often when the adult's relationship to his/her parents is assessed, patterns, themes, and insights emerge that can help address a problem in the client's work or personal life.

Couple Subsystem
Couple Boundaries: Internal and External

Most commonly associated with structural family therapy (Chapter 10), *boundaries* are the rules for negotiating interpersonal closeness and distance (Minuchin, 1974). Boundaries exist *internally* within the family and *externally* with those outside the nuclear family. These rules are generally unspoken and unfold as two people interact over time, each defining when, where, and how he/she prefers to relate to the other. With couples, these rules are often highly complex and difficult to track. Boundaries can be clear, diffuse, or rigid; all boundaries are strongly influenced by culture.

- **Clear Boundaries and Cultural Variance:** Clear boundaries refer to a range of possible ways that couples can negotiate a healthy balance between closeness (we-ness) and separation (individuality). Cultural factors shape how much closeness or separation is preferred. Collectivist cultures tend toward greater degrees of closeness, whereas individualistic cultures tend to value greater independence. The best way to determine whether a couple's boundaries are clear is to determine whether symptoms have developed in the individual, couple, or family. If they have, boundaries are probably too diffuse or too rigid. Most people who come in for therapy have reached a point where boundaries that may have worked in one context are no longer working. For relationships to weather the test of time, couples must constantly renegotiate their boundaries (rules for relating) to adjust to each person's evolving needs. The more flexible couples are in negotiating these rules, the more successful they will be in adjusting to life transitions and setbacks.

- **Diffuse Boundaries and Enmeshed Relationships:** When couples begin to overvalue togetherness at the expense of respecting each other's individuality, their boundaries become *diffuse* and the relationship becomes *enmeshed* (note: technically boundaries are not enmeshed; they are diffuse). In these relationships, partners may feel that they are being suffocated, that they lack freedom, or that they are not cared for enough. Often partners in these relationships feel threatened whenever the other disagrees or does not affirm them, resulting in an intense tug-of-war to convince the other to agree with them. Couples with diffuse boundaries may also have diffuse boundaries with their children, families of origin, and/or friends, with the result that these outside others becoming overly involved in one or both of the partners' lives (e.g., parents, friends, or children become involved in couple's arguments).

- **Rigid Boundaries and Disengaged Relationships:** When couples privilege independence over togetherness, their boundaries can become *rigid* and the relationship *disengaged*. In these relationships, partners may not allow the other to influence them, often value a career more than the relationship, and frequently have minimal emotional connection. These couples may have a pattern of keeping others at a distance or may compensate by having diffuse boundaries with children, friends, family, or an outside love interest (e.g., an emotional or physical affair). Often difficult to accurately assess, the key indicator of rigid boundaries is whether they are creating problems individually or for the partnership.

QUESTIONS FOR ASSESSING COUPLE BOUNDARIES

Here are some sample questions to think about while working with an individual or couple to assess boundaries:

- Does the couple have clear boundaries that are distinct from their parenting and family-of-origin relationships?
- Does the couple spend time alone not talking about the children?
- Do they report an active sex and romantic life?
- Do they still feel a sense of connection apart from being parents?
- Does one or both experience anxiety or frustration when there is a difference of opinion?
- Is one hurt or angry if the other has a different opinion or perspective on a problem?
- Do they use "we" or "I" more often when speaking? Is there a balance?
- Does each have a set of personal friends and activities separate from the family and partnership?
- How much energy do these get in relation to the couple relationship?
- What gets priority in their schedules? Children? Work? Personal activities? Couple time?

Problem Interaction Patterns

One of the hallmarks of family therapy is the ability to assess the family's interaction patterns around the presenting problem. This ability is central to the Mental Research Institute (MRI) approach (see Chapter 9; Watzlawick et al., 1974), strategic therapy (Haley, 1976), and the Milan approach (see Chapter 9; Selvini Palazzoli, Boscolo, Cecchin, & Prata, 1978) and is featured prominently in Satir's communication approach (see Chapter 11; Satir, Banmen, Gerber, & Gomori, 1991) and Whitaker's symbolic-experiential therapy (see Chapter 11; Whitaker & Bumberry, 1988). In interactional assessment, the therapist traces reciprocal relational patterns: how person A responds to person B and vice versa. Because more than one person is involved (persons C, D, E, etc.) in families or larger groups, patterns are complex.

Whether the client reports an individual symptom or relational problem, the therapist begins by assuming that it is embedded in the larger system and that the symptoms help maintain the system's homeostasis or sense of normalcy (even if the behavior is not considered normal by the members of the system). A therapist can assess these patterns using a series of questions, first by identifying the emergence of the problem and then tracing each person's emotional and/or behavioral responses to others until "normalcy" or homeostasis is achieved again. The process looks something like this:

ASSESSING INTERACTION PATTERNS

Client describes how the problem begins:

Example: Wife says she asks husband for help; he says, "yes" but "forgets" to follow through.

The therapist inquires about the wife's next actions and the husband's response:

Example: Wife says she gets mad at her husband and tells him that he failed her yet again; the husband explains that he has been very stressed at work and forgot because he is feeling so overwhelmed.

The therapist continues to trace this exchange in terms of how each responded to the other until they return to "normal" or homeostasis:

Example: Wife responds to husband's explanation by saying she's also stressed and that he is making it worse; he responds by saying that she is too demanding and perfectionistic; she responds by saying he is lazy; this continues until he finally agrees that he will try harder next time and she accepts the apology.

The therapist also inquires about how significant others in the system respond to the problem situation:

Example: Did the children and/or others overhear the conversation and respond to the couple's tension? Does either one share the scenario with a confidant? How does that person's response affect the cycle?

The therapist continues assessing the interaction pattern until it is clear that the entire family has returned to its sense of "normalcy."

Complementary Patterns

Complementary patterns characterize most couple relationships to a certain degree. *Complementary* in this case refers to each person taking on opposite or complementary roles, which range from functional to problematic. For example, a complementary relationship of introvert/extrovert can exist in a balanced and well-functioning relationship as well as in an out-of-balance, problematic relationship; the difference is in the rigidity of the pattern. Classic examples of complementary roles that often become problematic include pursuer/distancer, emotional/logical, overfunctioner/underfunctioner, friendly parent/strict parent, and so forth. Gottman (1999) indicated that the female-pursue (demand) and male-withdraw pattern existed to some extent in the majority of marriages he studied. However, in distressed marriages, this pattern becomes exaggerated and begins to be viewed as innate personality traits. Assessing for these patterns can help therapists intervene in couples' interactions. In most cases, couples readily identify their complementary roles in their complaints about the relationship: "he's too strict with the kids"; "she always emotionally overreacts"; "I have to do it all the time"; "she never wants sex." These broad, sweeping descriptions of the other suggest a likely problematic complementary pattern.

Satir's Communication Stances

Virginia Satir (Chapter 11; Satir et al., 1991) developed an approach for assessing communication patterns based on five communication stances: placating, blaming, superreasonable, irrelevant, and congruent, with the congruent stance being the model for healthy communication. The first four stances are *survival stances*, which people first develop as children when they are confronted with difficult situations, such as an angry parent, peer pressure, or the threat of rejection. Without the emotional and cognitive capacities to skillfully balance their own needs and wants (*self*), the *other*'s needs and wants, and what is appropriate to the *context*, children attend to one or two of these areas and neglect the rest. For example, a child who uses *placating* may quickly learn that by appeasing parents and friends she is able to keep people from being angry at her and get what she wants most: acceptance. Conversely, a child who copes by *blaming* may learn that by always fighting for his rights he is more likely to get adults to give him what he wants. Alternatively, a child who uses a *superreasonable* stance may find that when she always follows the contextual rules—home, school, church, societal rules, etc.—regardless of what she or others may feel, her world stays organized and stable. Lastly, a child who uses the *irrelevant* stance may learn that by always joking around, changing the subject, and being a little "off the wall," he is able to gain approval by being entertaining and/or keep people distracted enough to not be a problem to him. The survival stances, unfortunately, are unbalanced and do not work well in the long term. The following table shows how the different stances recognize the three elements of self, other, and context.

SATIR'S COMMUNICATION STANCES

STYLE	RECOGNIZES	IGNORES
Congruent	Self, other, context	None
Placator	Other, context	Self
Blamer	Self, context	Other
Superreasonable	Context	Self, other
Irrelevant	None	Self, other, context

To someone unfamiliar with these communication styles, they may initially seem simplistic and without significant clinical merit. However, the brief process of assessing these styles provides therapists with excellent information about how best to communicate with clients in session and how to design interventions. The following are some clinical implications.

- **Placator:** When working with people who use the placating stance, therapists are more successful when they use less directive therapy methods, such as multiple-choice questions and open-ended reflections, that ask clients to voice their opinion and take a stand, which is often quite painful and scary for placators. With clients who tend toward placating, therapists carefully avoid giving opinions (or even the slightest hint that they may have an opinion) or offering too much personal information. Clients will often use this type of information to know what parts of themselves to hide and what parts to foreground to gain therapist approval. Never underestimate placators; they are skilled in the art of people pleasing and regularly lie to make the therapist feel good about how therapy is progressing (Gehart & Lyle, 2001). Not until the client regularly and openly disagrees with the therapist has rapport been fully established with a client who tends toward the placating stance.

- **Blamer:** When working with those who frequently use the blaming stance, therapists strive to increase clients' awareness of others' thoughts and feelings and help them learn how to communicate their personal perspectives in a way that is respectful of others. Often therapists are more effective when they confront blamers directly and boldly. Counter to what one might expect, this approach typically strengthens the therapeutic relationship with a person who uses the blaming stance. Most people who use blaming lose respect for "wimpy" (think "placating") therapists who do not speak their minds honestly and directly, a skill a blamer has mastered. They generally prefer more upfront and direct communication than is generally tolerated in polite society.

- **Superreasonable:** When working with superreasonable clients, logic and rules reign supreme. To communicate effectively, therapists must identify and refer to the context these clients use to make meaning and inform their action, which may be perceived societal rules, religious norms, professional expectations, or even an idiosyncratic set of personal rules for living. The goal is to help these clients value their own internal, subjective realities and those of others.

- **Irrelevant:** The irrelevant type creates a unique challenge for therapists because there are no prepackaged "grips" of self, other, or context on which the therapist can rely. The therapist needs to find the unique anchors of the client's reality with which to connect. Often the first step is to make the therapeutic relationship a place of utmost safety for the client so that there is less need to distract. As treatment progresses, the therapist works to increase the client's ability to recognize thoughts and feelings of self and others as well as acknowledge the demands of context. Progress may be slower than with other communication stances.

Gottman's Divorce Indicators

John Gottman (see Chapter 13; Gottman, 1999) has researched couples and their communication patterns for over 30 years. His experience has given him the ability to predict divorce with 97.5% accuracy by assessing five key variables: the "Four Horsemen"—criticism, defensiveness, contempt, and stonewalling—and effective repair attempts. His extensive research provides therapists with a unique system for assessing couple functioning.

The Four Horsemen of the Apocalypse

In Gottman's research on divorce predictors, he found that negative interactions were not equally corrosive (e.g., expression of anger). Four specific interactions were more significant than others in predicting divorce; he has named these the *Four Horsemen of the Apocalypse*. The presence of these four factors predicts divorce with 85% accuracy.

- **Criticism:** Statement implying that something is globally wrong with the partner rather than stating dissatisfaction with a single, particular event (e.g., "always" or "never" statements; broad characterizations about the other's personality).

- **Defensiveness:** Statement or action to ward off perceived attack or criticism from partner: "I'm innocent."

- **Contempt:** Any statement or gesture that puts oneself on a higher level than one's partner, typically involving mockery, eye rolls, and contemptuous facial expressions. This is the most corrosive of the horsemen and is virtually nonexistent in happy marriages. *Contempt is the best single predictor of divorce.*

- **Stonewalling:** An action in which the listener withdraws from interaction, either physically leaving the room or refusing to continue the conversation.

Therapists assess for the horsemen by considering what the client says, in session interactions, and through written assessments (Gottman, 1999). The presence of the horsemen should not cause automatic alarm; happily married couples regularly engage in criticism, defensiveness, and stonewalling. However, the frequency of these behaviors is different with happy couples, as is their ability to successfully repair the interactions. Thus, therapists need to assess the frequency as well as the presence. Successful couples maintain a *ratio of 5 positive interactions for every 1 negative interaction* during conflict. Couples heading for divorce will have fewer than 5 positives for every negative and often will be closer to 1:1 positive to negative, or even more negative than positive interactions. The following are some of the interactions that therapists need to assess for frequency:

- **Failed Repair Attempt:** A repair attempt is any verbal or nonverbal attempt on the part of either partner to de-escalate conflict. It can include humor, apologies, touch, or compromise. A "failed" repair attempt means that the other partner rejected the attempt and continued the conflictual interaction. Distressed couples more frequently make repair attempts, and they are rejected more frequently.

- **Rejection of Influence:** Often one partner rejects the other's influence (e.g., suggestions, input). Husbands rejecting their wives' influence predicts divorce with 80% accuracy; the reverse is not true for women.

- **Harsh Startup:** This phrase refers to how problem issues are raised: with positive affect (soft startup) or negative affect (harsh startup). Harsh startup by the wife is associated with greater marital instability and higher rates of divorce; the reverse is not true for men.

When working with couples, therapists can keep Gottman's divorce indicators in mind to identify the severity of distress and determine how best to proceed.

Parental Subsystem

Parental and Sibling Subsystem Boundaries

As with the couple, the boundaries of the parental subsystem need to be assessed. The therapist must look at the parental subsystem, the sibling subsystem, and the special interest subsystem.

- **Parental Subsystem:** The parental subsystem most often involves two biological parents but can also include stepparents, grandparents, or older siblings. When a parental subsystem functions well, parents living in the same household can be consistent with rules and consequences; when parents are separated or divorced, rules and consequences do not need to be consistent (Visher & Visher, 1979). If grandparents are involved, their authority and roles should be clear and not interfere with the parents' effectiveness in setting rules and consequences.

  In addition, therapists need to assess the balance of roles within the parental system. Raser (1999) describes the parenting relationship as comprising *business roles* (setting rules, socializing) and *personal roles* (warmth, fun, caring, play). Typically, a parent is better at one than the other, which often leads to problematic polarization between the parents. Ideally, both parents are able to balance *within themselves* the business and personal sides of parenting, and both parents can then set an effective hierarchy as well as maintain a close emotional bond. Assessing this single dimension alone can provide therapists with a razor-sharp point of focus for treatment, often resulting in rapid improvements.

  The first step in assessing the parental subsystem is to determine who is in it and whether they are undermining each other in setting rules and consequences. Next, to determine whether each is able to balance the business and personal sides of parenting, therapists ask whether the kids follow instructions from each parent (see Hierarchy Between Child and Parents) and whether both parents have an emotional connection to each child (see Emotional Boundaries with Children).

- **Sibling Subsystem:** The sibling subsystem includes the children in the family. In blended families, these systems often include children who may or may not live in the same house, but this can also be the case in nuclear families, especially when there is a large age difference between children. Although the sibling subsystem is typically less problematic than the parental or marital subsystem, therapists can assess the relations between siblings for tension, conflict, jealousy, and/or hierarchy issues. Usually there is a complementary relationship in the form of good kid/bad kid.

- **Special Interest Subsystems:** Some families develop subsystems around special interests, such as music, sports, or gender. In many cultures, strong subsystems are built along gender lines. Women and girls engage in behaviors such as cooking, shopping, and childcare; and men have their activities, such as sports and repair work. Although typically not the primary source of conflict or dysfunction, these special interest subsystems can play an important role in family dynamics and often offer possibilities for resolving issues and conflict in unique ways. For example, if a father is heavily disciplining his teenage son for poor grades and has let the personal side of the parenting relationship dwindle over time and the family has a tradition of strong gender subsystems, the father and son may find fun ways to rebuild their personal relationship by watching sports, building cars, or working on a project together.

Family Life Cycle Stages

When assessing families, it is helpful to identify their stage in the life cycle (Carter & McGoldrick, 1999). Each stage is associated with specific developmental tasks; symptoms arise when families are having difficulty mastering these tasks:

- **Leaving Home, the Single Adult:** Accepting emotional and financial responsibility for oneself

- **Marriage:** Committing to a new system; realigning boundaries with family and friends

- **Families with Young Children:** Adjusting marriage to make space for children; joining in child-rearing tasks; realigning boundaries with parents and grandparents

- **Families with Adolescent Children:** Adjusting parental boundaries to increase freedom and responsibility for adolescents; refocusing on marriage and career life

- **Launching Children:** Renegotiating the marital subsystem; developing adult-to-adult relationships with children; coping with aging parents

- **Family in Later Life:** Accepting the shift of generational roles; coping with loss of abilities; middle generation takes more central role; creating space for wisdom of the elderly

Hierarchy Between Child and Parents

A key area in assessing parent and child relationships is hierarchy, a structural family concept (see Chapter 10). When assessing parental hierarchy, therapists must ask themselves: Is the parent-child hierarchy developmentally and culturally appropriate? If the hierarchy is appropriate, the child usually has few behavioral problems. If the child is exhibiting symptoms or there are problems in the parent-child relationship, there is usually some problem in the hierarchical structure: either an excessive (authoritarian) or insufficient (permissive) parental hierarchy given the family's current sociocultural context(s). Immigrant families, because they usually have two different sets of cultural norms for parental hierarchy (the traditional and the current cultural context), have difficulty finding a balance between authoritarian and permissive hierarchies.

Assessing hierarchy is critical because it tells the therapist where and how to intervene. If therapists assess only the symptoms, they may make inappropriate interventions. For example, though children diagnosed with ADD have similar symptoms—hyperactivity, defiance, failing to follow through on parents' requests— these same symptoms can occur in two dramatically different family structures: either too much or too little parental hierarchy. When the parental hierarchy is too rigid, the therapist works with the parents to develop a stronger personal relationship with the child and set developmentally and culturally appropriate expectations. If there is not enough parental hierarchy, the therapist helps parents become more consistent with consequences and set limits and rules. Thus the same set of symptoms can require very different interventions.

Emotional Boundaries with Children

Therapists assess the emotional connection between parents and children using the same principles that were used for evaluating couple boundaries. Clear emotional boundaries are evidenced by a clear sense of connection along with respect for each person's need for independence; as children get older, parents must continually adjust their boundaries to allow for greater individuality. *Enmeshed parental boundaries* often result in strong, emotional reactivity to the other, including arguments and defiance. With *disengaged parental boundaries,* the parent is disinterested in the child as a person and focuses on managing the child's behavior rather than developing a strong personal connection.

Problem Interaction Patterns

The same principles used to assess the problem interaction patterns with couples are used to assess patterns in parent-child relationships. For example:

ASSESSING PARENT-CHILD RELATIONSHIPS

Client describes how the problem begins:

Example: Mother gets a call from the school saying her son is failing a class.

The therapist inquires about the mother's next actions and the son's response:

Example: Mother lectures son and sets an extensive punishment; the child argues and says she is being unfair. Mother says, "Wait until I tell your dad."

The therapist continues to trace this exchange in terms of how each responded to the other until they return to normal:

Example: Mother responds to son's accusations of her being unfair by adding more consequences and punishments.

The therapist also inquires about how significant others in the family system respond to the problem situation:

Example: How did the father participate? What does the younger sister do while this is going on? What effects does this have in the marital relationship?

The therapist continues assessing the interaction pattern until it is clear that the entire family has returned to a sense of "normalcy."

Triangles and Coalitions

Problem systems are identified in most systemic family therapy approaches. Triangles (Kerr & Bowen, 1988), covert coalitions (Minuchin & Fishman, 1981), and cross-generational coalitions (Minuchin & Fishman, 1981) all refer to a similar process: tension between two people is resolved by drawing in a third person (or forth, a "tetrad"; Whitaker & Keith, 1981) to stabilize the original dyad. Many therapists include inanimate objects or other processes as potential "thirds" in the triangulation process. In this situation, some*thing* else is used to manage the tension in the dyad, such as drinking, drug use, work, or hobbies, which are used to help one or both partners soothe their internal stress at the expense of the relationship.

Therapists assess for triangles and problematic subsystems in several ways:

- Clients overtly describe another party as playing a role in their tension; in these cases the clients are aware of the process at some level.
- When clients describe the problem or conflict situation, another person plays the role of confidant or takes the side of one of the partners (e.g., one person has a friend or another family member who takes his/her side against the other).
- After being unable to get a need met in the primary dyad, a person finds what he/she is not getting in another person (e.g., a mother seeks emotional closeness from a child rather than from a husband).
- When therapy is inexplicably "stuck," there is often a triangle at work that distracts one or both parties from resolving critical issues (e.g., an affair, substance abuse, a friend who undermines agreements made in therapy, etc.).

Identifying triangles early in the assessment process enables therapists to intervene more successfully and quickly in a complex set of family dynamics.

Communication Stances

Using the same five stances that are used for assessing couples—congruent, placator, blamer, superreasonable, and irrelevant—therapists can assess communication patterns within the larger family system. Parents may or may not have the same stance toward the larger family that they have toward each other as a couple.

Systemic Hypothesis

After assessing family structure and interaction patterns, therapists develop a working hypothesis about the problem, a potential role the symptom may be playing in maintaining the family homeostasis (see Chapter 9; Selvini Palazolli et al., 1978). A classic example is that a child's symptom (e.g., tantrums, running away, school failure, eating disorder) (a) creates a common problem that forces the couple to cooperate, work together, and stay together, and/or (b) distracts one or more parents from an ailing marriage. Obviously, a child is rarely thinking, "Gee, I think I'll act out to keep mom and dad together," and a parent isn't thinking, "I'll just obsessively overfocus on the children to distract me from my pathetic marriage." Instead, the symptoms naturally emerge to fill "gaps" or systemic needs to maintain a sense of balance without anyone consciously cooking up a plan.

The following strategies are used for developing hypotheses:

- **Client Language and Metaphors:** The MRI team often described the entire homeostatic pattern using client language (Watzlawick et al., 1974). For example, if the family were sports enthusiasts, they would describe the interaction pattern using the metaphor of a game in which person A has to play defense (withdraw) when person B plays offense (pursues).

- **Positive Connotation:** The Milan team made it a rule to emphasize the positive and helpful effects of the symptom in the family (Selvini Palazzoli et al., 1978). For example, they would praise a child who was sacrificing personal success to give his mother someone to care for so she felt useful.

- **Love and Power:** Strategic therapists developed hypotheses around love and power. For example, they might hypothesize that the seemingly helpless person's role (e.g., as depressed, compliant, sexually uninterested) had the hidden dimension of giving the person power (through influencing others' behavior) that she could not acquire by other means.

Intergenerational Patterns

Assessing for intergenerational patterns is easiest when using a genogram (McGoldrick, Gerson, & Petry, 2008), which provides a visual map of these patterns. Therapists can create comprehensive genograms, which map numerous intergenerational patterns, or problem-specific genograms, which focus on patterns related to the presenting problem and how family members have dealt with similar problems across generations (e.g., how other couples have dealt with marital tension). The following patterns are frequently included in genograms:

• Substance and alcohol abuse and dependence
• Sexual, physical, and emotional abuse
• Personal qualities and/or family roles; complementary roles (e.g., black sheep, rebellious one, overachiever/underachiever, etc.)
• Physical and mental health issues (e.g., diabetes, cancer, depression, psychosis, etc.)
• Historical incidents of the presenting problem, either with the same people or how other generations and family members have managed this problem

Previous Solutions and Unique Outcomes
Previous Solutions That DID NOT Work

When assessing solutions, therapists need to assess two kinds: those that have worked and those that have not. The MRI group (Watzlawick et al., 1974) and cognitive-behavioral therapists (Baucom & Epstein, 1990) are best known for assessing what has not worked, although they use these in different ways when they intervene. With most clients, it is generally easy to assess failed previous solutions.

QUESTIONS FOR ASSESSING SOLUTIONS THAT DID NOT WORK

The therapist may begin by asking a straightforward question:

What have you tried to solve this problem?

Most clients respond with a list of things that have not worked. If they need more prompting therapists may ask:

I am guessing you have tried to solve this problem (address this issue) on your own and that some things were not as successful as you had hoped. What have you tried that did not work?

Previous Solutions That DID Work/Unique Outcomes

Solution-focused therapists (de Shazer, 1988; O'Hanlon & Weiner-Davis, 1989) assess for previous solutions that *did* work, a process that is similar to identifying *unique outcomes* to the dominant problem story in narrative therapy (Freedman & Combs, 1996; White & Epston, 1990). Assessing previous solutions and unique outcomes is difficult because most clients are less aware of when the problem is not a problem and how they have kept things from getting worse. Some of the questions therapists ask are the following:

> **QUESTIONS FOR ASSESSING SOLUTIONS
> AND UNIQUE OUTCOMES**
>
> - What keeps this problem from being worse than it is right now?
> - Is there any solution you have tried that worked for a while? Or made things slightly better?
> - Are there times or places when the problem is less of a problem or not a problem?
> - Have you ever been able to respond to the problem so that it is less of a problem or less severe?
> - Does this problem occur in all places with all people, or is it better in certain contexts?

These questions generally require more thought and reflection from the client and more follow-up questions from the therapist. Their answers often provide invaluable clues on how best to proceed and intervene in therapy.

Narratives and Social Discourses

Narratives and social discourses are the larger contexts in which the client's problem occurs. They can be divided into dominant discourses, identity narratives, and local and preferred discourses.

Dominant Discourses

Assessing the *dominant social discourses* in which a client's problems are embedded often creates a new and broader perspective on a client's situation (Freedman & Combs, 1996; White & Epston, 1990). I frequently find that this broader perspective helps me to feel more freedom and possibility, increasing my emotional attunement to clients and allowing me to be more creative in my work. For example, when I view a client's reported "anxiety" as part of a larger discourse in which the client feel powerless, such as being a sexual minority, I begin to see the anxiety as part of this larger social dance. I also see how it is possible for this person to give less "faith," weight, or credence to the dominant discourse and generate new stories about what is "normal" sexual behavior and what is not. By discussing the difficulty in concretely defining what is "normal" sexual behavior and what is not, the client and I can begin to explore the truths that this person has experienced. We join in an exploratory process that offers new ways for the client to understand the anxiety as well as his/her identity.

Common dominant discourses or broader narratives that inform clients' lives include the following:

- Culture, race, ethnicity, immigration
- Gender, sexual orientation, sexual preferences
- Family-of-origin experiences, such as alcoholism, sexual abuse, adoption, etc.
- Stories of divorce, death, and loss of significant relationships
- Wealth, poverty, power, fame
- Small-town, urban, regional discourses
- Health, illness, body image, etc.

Identity Narratives

When clients come for therapy, the problem discourse has usually become a significant part of their *identity narrative*, the story they tell themselves about who they are. For example, a child having problems in school may begin to think, "I am stupid," and his mother may also be feeling, "I have failed as a mother" because of her child's academic performance. Obviously, these negative sweeping judgments of a person's value or ability need to be addressed in therapy. Assessing them early in the process helps the therapist understand how to engage and motivate each person.

Local and Preferred Discourses

Local discourses are the stories that occur at the local (as opposed to the dominant societal) level (Anderson, 1997). These narratives often are built on personal beliefs and unique interpretations that contradict or significantly modify dominant discourses. Although it is theoretically possible for local discourses to contribute to the problem (e.g., having more oppressive versions of dominant discourses), they are usually a significant source of motivation, energy, and hope in addressing problems. Most often, local discourses are a person's "personal truth" that he/she has been hiding or is ashamed of because of anticipated disapproval from others. They can be common subculture values, such as a preference for certain religious or sexual practices, or they can be unique to the individual, such as wanting to sell everything and travel the world. Local discourses are often the source of *preferred discourses* in narrative therapy (Freedman & Combs, 1996), the versions of one's life and identity that serve as the goal in narrative therapy.

The Genogram

Genograms are often included with case conceptualizations in family therapy (see Chapter 12). Traditionally an intergenerational assessment instrument (McGoldrick et al., 2008), genograms have also been adapted for use with other models (Hardy & Laszloffy, 1995; Kuehl, 1995; Rubalcava & Waldman, 2004) and are regularly used by all therapists to conceptualize family dynamics.

V. Genogram

Construct a family genogram and include all relevant information, including:

- ages, birth/death dates
- names
- relational patterns
- occupations
- medical history
- psychiatric disorders
- abuse history

Also include a couple of adjectives for persons frequently discussed in session (these should describe personal qualities and/or relational patterns, e.g., quiet, family caretaker, emotionally distant, perfectionist, helpless, etc.). The genogram should be attached to the report.

As this box shows, genograms generally include the following types of information: ages, birth and death dates, names, relational pattern, occupations, medical history, psychiatric disorders, and abuse history. Including two to three adjectives for persons frequently discussed in the session (describing personal qualities and/or relational patterns, e.g., quiet, family caretaker, emotionally distant, perfectionist, helpless, etc.) helps create a complete sense of the family and people involved. See McGoldrick et al. (2008) for comprehensive instructions on using a genogram. The following figure depicts the symbols commonly used in creating a genogram.

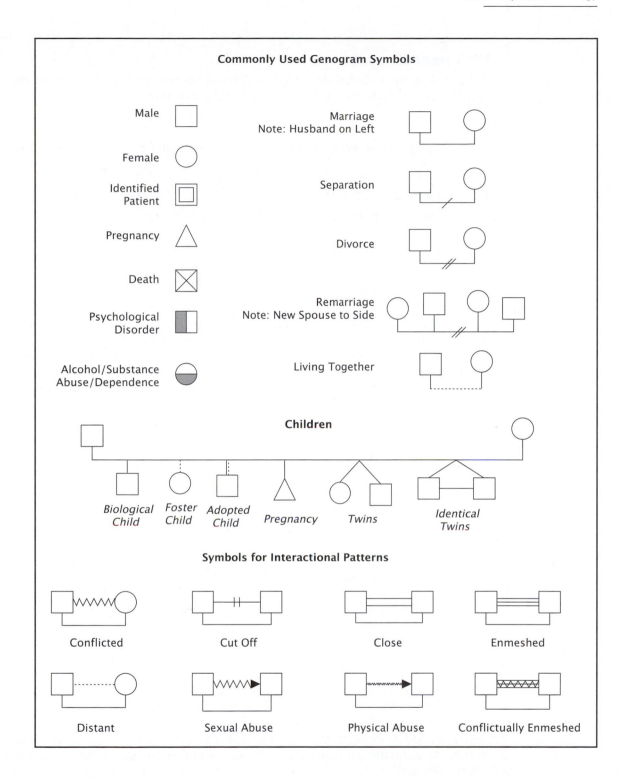

Client Perspectives

Finally, therapists should reflect on areas of client agreement and disagreement with a case conceptualization. Although it is often not clinically appropriate to hand the entire case conceptualization over to a client, discussing the key findings is. Which descriptions seem accurate from the client's perspective? Which do not? Would the client be surprised to hear any of this? If there is a significant disagreement between the client's and therapist's perspective, the therapist needs to consider how he/she will navigate this difference and remain open to the possibility that the assessment is not accurate.

VI. Client Perspectives

Areas of Agreement: Based on what the client(s) has(ve) said, what parts of the above assessment do they agree with or are likely to agree with?

_____

Areas of Disagreement: What parts do they disagree with or are likely to disagree with? Why?

_____

How do you plan to respectfully work with areas of disagreement?

_____

Considering the client perspective is particularly important when the client differs from the therapist in age, cultural background, gender, sexual orientation, or socioeconomic status, in which case the therapist may be less likely to fully understand the client's context. Conversely, many therapists have even more trouble with clients who are similar to them because they assume they know more than they do or that they already know the answer to the situation. Whether clients are similar or different, therapists need to carefully consider their perspectives when conceptualizing treatment.

Case Conceptualization, Diversity, and Sameness

Just in case you were beginning to feel that you finally understood something about case conceptualization, let me throw a wrench or two into the mix: diversity and sameness. The problem with case conceptualization and assessments in general (this applies to the next several chapters as well) is that unfortunately there are no objective standards against which a person can be measured for "clear boundaries," "healthy hierarchies," or "clear communication." Healthy, emotionally engaged boundaries look quite different in a Mexican-American family and an Asian-American family. In fact, problematic boundaries in a Mexican-American family (e.g., cool, disengaged) may look *more like* healthy boundaries (e.g., quietly respectful) than problem boundaries (e.g., overly involved) in Asian-American families. Thus, therapists cannot rely simply on objective descriptions of behavior in assessment. They must consider the broader culture norms, which may include *more than one* set of ethnic norms as well as local neighborhood cultures, school contexts, sexual orientation subcultures, religious communities, and so forth. Although you will undoubtedly take a course on cultural issues and will read that professional codes of ethics require respecting diversity, it takes working with a diverse range of families and a willingness to learn from them to cultivate a meaningful sense of cultural sensitivity. I believe this to be a lifelong journey.

Ironically, I have found that new therapists in training today sometimes have the most difficulty accepting diversity in clients from within their *same* culture of origin. The more similar clients are to us, the more we expect them to share our values and behavioral norms and the lower our tolerance of difference. For example, middle-class Caucasian therapists often expect middle-class Caucasian clients to have particular values regarding emotional expression, marital arrangements, extended family, and parent-child relationships and may be quick to encourage particular systems of values—namely, their own. Thus, whether working with someone very similar or very different than yourself, you need to *slowly* assess and evaluate, always considering clients' broader sociocultural context and norms. Therapists who excel in conceptualization and assessment approach these tasks with profound humility and a continual willingness to learn.

Ethical Considerations

Before you run off to start applying the concepts in this chapter (and those that follow) to evaluate your clients, friends, family, neighbors, and self, I need to caution you about the ethical parameters of family therapy. Professional organizations—such as the American Association for Marriage and Family Therapy, the American Counseling Association, the American Psychological Association, the International Association of Marriage and Family Counselors, and the National Association of Social Workers—all have codes of ethics that their members follow. Thankfully, there is general agreement on key issues. Although ethical and legal issues can only be adequately addressed in a separate textbook, I will quickly review some of the more applicable guidelines:

- **Confidentiality:** Client information is confidential and privileged, meaning that it cannot be shared with outside others unless written releases or state law permits; if you are using real clients for classroom exercises, you must take steps to remove any and all identifying information before turning in your work.

- **Diversity:** Therapists adapt assessment and treatment approaches to be respectful of and appropriately adapted for client diversity, including ethnicity, age, gender, socioeconomic status, physical and mental ability, sexual orientation, religious beliefs, and language.

- **Scope of Competence:** Therapists practice only within their scope of competence, areas in which they have been adequately trained; in areas of growth they are supervised. If you are using this book in a class setting, your instructor is your supervisor.

- **Dual Relationships:** Therapists avoid dual relationships with clients, meaning they should avoid working with people they know from other contexts (although this varies from country to country). Thus, I recommend you avoid trying to casually "assess," "treat," or otherwise make sense of your family and friends using the ideas in books such as this (as tempting as it is sometimes).

- **Defining the Client:** When initiating therapy with individuals, couples, or families, the therapist carefully identifies who the client is (the individual, couple, or family system) and discusses how confidential information will be handled between clients.

- **Child Rights to Confidentiality:** A particularly difficult issue when working with children and families is children's rights to privacy and confidentiality versus the parents' right to information about their children. Each state has different laws, with progressive states allowing children or teens with serious disorders to seek treatment without the knowledge of their parents (the therapist needs to justify potential harm) and conservative states allowing parents full access to children's treatment information.

- **Personal Concerns:** When therapists become aware of personal concerns that may affect their ability to interact, assess, or intervene with a client, they seek personal psychotherapy, supervision, or some other way to resolve the problem. Most training programs and many state legislatures strongly encourage therapists in training to seek their own personal therapy.

- **Mandated Reporting:** Most states have detailed laws that require therapists to report suspected child abuse and neglect, elder abuse and neglect, dependent adult abuse, serious suicidal threats, homicidal threats, and threats to personal property. Additionally, ethical standards encourage therapists to take steps to prevent self-harming behaviors and domestic violence, which involve serious life-threatening issues not typically addressed by state laws.

ONLINE RESOURCES

American Association for Marriage and Family Therapy Code of Ethics
www.aamft.org

American Counseling Association Code of Ethics
www.counseling.org

American Psychological Association Code of Ethics
www.apa.org

Family History Maker: U.S. Department of Health and Human Services
www.hhs.gov/familyhistory/

Genogram Maker: Genogram software
www.genogram.org

International Association for Marriage and Family Counseling Code of Ethics
www.iamfc.com

National Association of Social Workers Code of Ethics
www.socialworkers.org

REFERENCES

Anderson, H. (1997). *Conversations, language, and possibilities.* New York: Basic.

Anderson, H., & Gehart, D. R. (Eds.). (2006). *Collaborative therapy: Relationships and conversations that make a difference.* New York: Brunner-Routledge.

Bateson, G. (1972). *Steps to an ecology of mind.* New York: Ballantine.

Bateson, G. (1979/2002). *Mind and nature: A necessary unity.* Cresskill, NJ: Hampton.

Baucom, D. H., & Epstein, N. (1990). *Cognitive-behavioral marital therapy.* New York: Brunner/Mazel.

Carter, B., & McGoldrick, M. (1999). *The expanded family life cycle: Individuals, families, and social perspectives* (3rd ed.). New York: Allyn and Bacon.

de Shazer, S. (1988). *Clues: Investigating solutions in brief therapy.* New York: Norton.

Freedman, J., & Combs, G. (1996). *Narrative therapy: The social contruction of preferred realities.* New York: Norton.

Gehart, D. R., & Lyle, R. R. (2001). Client experience of gender in therapeutic relationships: An interpretive ethnography. *Family Process, 40,* 443–458.

Gergen, K. J. (1999). *An invitation to social construction.* Thousand Oaks, CA: Sage.

Gottman, J. M. (1999). *The marriage clinic: A scientifically based marital therapy.* New York: Norton.

Haley, J. (1976). *Problem-solving therapy: New strategies for effective family therapy.* San Francisco: Jossey-Bass.

Hardy, K. V., & Laszloffy, T. A. (1995). The cultural genogram: Key to training culturally competent family therapists. *Journal of Marital and Family Therapy, 21,* 227–237.

Keeney, B. P. (1983). *Aesthetics of change.* New York: Guilford.

Kerr, M., & Bowen, M. (1988). *Family evaluation.* New York: Norton.

Kuehl, B. P. (1995). The solution-oriented genogram: A collaborative approach. *Journal of Marital and Family Therapy, 21,* 239–250.

Lambert, M. J., & Ogles, B. M. (2004). The efficacy and effectiveness of psychotherapy. In M. J. Lambert (Ed.), *Bergin and Garfield's handbook of psychotherapy and behavior change* (5th ed., pp. 139–193). New York: Wiley.

McGoldrick, M., Gerson, R., & Petry, S. (2008). *Genograms: Assessment and intervention* (3rd ed.). New York: Norton.

Miller, S. D., Duncan, B. L., & Hubble, M. (1997). *Escape from Babel: Toward a unifying language for psychotherapy practice.* New York: Norton.

Minuchin, S. (1974). *Families and family therapy.* Cambridge, MA: Harvard University Press.

Minuchin, S., & Fishman, H. C. (1981). *Family therapy techniques.* Cambridge, MA: Harvard University Press.

O'Hanlon, W. H., & Weiner-Davis, M. (1989). *In search of solutions: A new direction in psychotherapy.* New York: Norton.

Raser, J. (1999). *Raising children you can live with: A guide for frustrated parents* (2nd ed.). Houston: Bayou.

Rubalcava, L. A., & Waldman, K. M. (2004). Working with intercultural couples: An intersubjective-constructivist perspective. *Progress in Self Psychology, 20,* 127–149.

Satir, V., Banmen, J., Gerber, J., & Gomori, M. (1991). *The Satir model: Family therapy and beyond.* Palo Alto, CA: Science and Behavior Books.

Seligman, M. (2004). *Authentic happiness: Using the new positive psychology to realize your potential for lasting fulfillment.* New York: Free Press.

Selvini Palazzoli, M., Boscolo, L., Cecchin, G., & Prata, G. (1978). *Paradox and counter-paradox.* New York: Jason Aronson.

Visher, E., & Visher, J. (1979). *Stepfamilies: A guide to working with stepparents and step-children.* New York: Brunner/Mazel.

Walsh, F. (Ed.). (2003). *Spiritual resources in family therapy.* New York: Guilford.

Watzlawick, P., Weakland, J., & Fisch, R. (1974). *Change: Principles of problem formation and problem resolution.* New York: Norton.

Whitaker, C. A., & Bumberry, W. M. (1988). *Dancing with the family: A symbolic experiential approach.* New York: Brunner/Mazel.

Whitaker, C. A., & Keith, D. V. (1981). Symbolic-experiential family therapy. In A. S. Gurman & D. P. Kniskern (Eds.), *Handbook of family therapy* (pp. 187–224). New York: Brunner/Mazel.

White, M., & Epston, D. (1990). *Narrative means to therapeutic ends.* New York: Norton.

CASE CONCEPTUALIZATION FORM

Therapist: _____   **Client/Case #:** _____   **Date:** _____

I. Introduction to Client and Significant Others *(Include age, ethnicity, occupation, grade, relevant identifiers, etc.). Put an * next to persons in session and/or IP for identified patient.*

AF† or _____ : _____

AM or _____ : _____

CF or _____ : _____

CM or _____ : _____

II. Presenting Concern

Client's/Family's Descriptions of Problem(s):

AF or _____ : _____

AM or _____ : _____

CF or _____ : _____

CM or _____ : _____

Broader System Problem Descriptions (description of problem from referring party, teachers, relatives, legal system, etc.):

_____ : _____

_____ : _____

III. Background Information

Recent Background (recent life changes, precipitating events, first symptoms, stressors, etc.):

_____

Related Historical Background (family history, related issues, past abuse, trauma, previous counseling, medical/mental health history, etc.):

_____

IV. Systemic Assessment

Client/Relational Strengths

Personal/individual: _____

Relational/social: _____

---

† *Abbreviations:* AF: Adult Female; AM: Adult Male; CF#: Child Female with age, e.g., CF15; CM#: Child Male with age; IP: Identified Patient; Hx: History; Ex: Explanation or Example; NA: Not Applicable.

Spiritual: _____

Family Structure and Interaction Patterns

Couple Subsystem (to be assessed): ☐ Personal current ☐ Personal past ☐ Parents'

Couple Boundaries: ☐ Clear ☐ Enmeshed ☐ Disengaged ☐ Other: _____

Rules for closeness/distance: _____

Couple Problem Interaction Pattern (A ⇄ B):

Start of tension: _____

Conflict/symptom escalation: _____

Return to "normal"/homeostasis: _____

Couple Complementary Patterns: ☐ Pursuer/distancer ☐ Over/under functioner

☐ Emotional/logical ☐ Good/bad parent ☐ Other: _____

Describe: _____

Satir's Communication Stances:
AF: ☐ Congruent ☐ Placator ☐ Blamer ☐ Superreasonable ☐ Irrelevant
AM: ☐ Congruent ☐ Placator ☐ Blamer ☐ Superreasonable ☐ Irrelevant

Describe dynamic: _____

Gottman's Divorce Indicators:

Criticism: ☐ AF ☐ AM Ex: _____

Defensiveness: ☐ AF ☐ AM Ex: _____

Contempt: ☐ AF ☐ AM Ex: _____

Stonewalling: ☐ AF ☐ AM Ex: _____

Failed repair attempts: ☐ AF ☐ AM Ex: _____

Not accept influence: ☐ AF ☐ AM Ex: _____

Harsh startup: ☐ AF ☐ AM Ex: _____

Parental Subsystem: ☐ Family of procreation ☐ Family of origin

Membership in Family Subsystems: Parental: ☐ AF ☐ AM ☐ Other: _____
Is parental subsystem distinct from couple subsystem? ☐ Yes ☐ No ☐ NA (divorce)

Sibling subsystem: _____

Special interest: _____

(continued)

(continued)

IV. Systemic Assessment

Family Structure and Interaction Patterns

Family Life Cycle Stage:

☐ Single adult ☐ Marriage ☐ Family with young children

☐ Family with adolescent children ☐ Launching children ☐ Later life

Describe struggles with mastering developmental tasks in one of these stages:

_____

Hierarchy Between Child/Parents:

AF: ☐ Effective ☐ Insufficient (permissive) ☐ Excessive (authoritarian) ☐ Inconsistent

AM: ☐ Effective ☐ Insufficient (permissive) ☐ Excessive (authoritarian) ☐ Inconsistent

Ex: _____

Emotional Boundaries with Children:

AF: ☐ Clear/balanced ☐ Enmeshed (reactive) ☐ Disengaged (disinterested)

    ☐ Other: _____

AM: ☐ Clear/balanced ☐ Enmeshed (reactive) ☐ Disengaged (disinterested)

    ☐ Other: _____

Ex: _____

Problem Interaction Pattern (A ⇄ B):

Start of tension: _____

Conflict/symptom escalation: _____

Return to "normal"/homeostasis: _____

Triangles/Coalitions:

☐ AF and C _____ against AM: Ex: _____

☐ AM and C _____ against AF: Ex: _____

☐ Other: Ex: _____

Communication Stances:

AF or _____ : ☐ Congruent ☐ Placator ☐ Blamer ☐ Superreasonable ☐ Irrelevant

AM or _____ : ☐ Congruent ☐ Placator ☐ Blamer ☐ Superreasonable ☐ Irrelevant

CF or _____ : ☐ Congruent ☐ Placator ☐ Blamer ☐ Superreasonable ☐ Irrelevant

CM or _____ : ☐ Congruent ☐ Placator ☐ Blamer ☐ Superreasonable ☐ Irrelevant

Ex: _____

Hypothesis (Describe possible role or function of symptom in maintaining family homeostasis):

_____

Intergenerational Patterns

Substance/alcohol abuse: ☐ NA ☐ Hx: _____

Sexual/physical/emotional abuse: ☐ NA ☐ Hx: _____

Parent/child relations: ☐ NA ☐ Hx: _____

Physical/mental disorders: ☐ NA ☐ Hx: _____

Historical incidents of presenting problem: ☐ NA ☐ Hx: _____

Family strengths: _____

Previous Solutions and Unique Outcomes

Solutions that DIDN'T work: _____

Solutions that DID work: _____

Narratives, Dominant Discourses, and Diversity
Dominant Discourses informing definition of problem:

Cultural, ethnic, SES, etc.: _____

Gender, sex orientation, etc.: _____

Other social influences: _____

Identity Narratives that have developed around problem for AF, AM, and/or CM/F:

_____

Local or Preferred Discourses: _____

Other Influential Discourses: _____

V. Genogram

Construct a family genogram and include all relevant information, including:

- ages, birth/death dates
- names
- relational patterns
- occupations
- medical history
- psychiatric disorders
- abuse history

Also include a couple of adjectives for persons frequently discussed in session (these should describe personal qualities and/or relational patterns, e.g., quiet, family caretaker, emotionally distant, perfectionist, helpless, etc.). Genogram should be attached to report.

(continued)

(continued)

VI. Client Perspectives

Areas of Agreement: Based on what the client(s) has(ve) said, what parts of the above assessment do they agree with or are likely to agree with?

_____

Areas of Disagreement: What parts do they disagree with or are likely to disagree with? Why?_

_____

How do you plan to respectfully work with areas of disagreement?

_____

CASE CONCEPTUALIZATION SCORING RUBRIC

The following scoring rubric describes the differences between exemplary, adequate, and deficient case conceptualizations. By closely attending to these requirements, you can hone in on what your instructors and supervisors are looking for when they grade your work.

Case Conceptualization Scoring Rubric

Date: _____

Therapist/Intern: _____

Evaluator/Instructor: _____

Level of Clinical Training:

☐ Preclinical training; coursework only

☐ 0–12 months   ☐ 12–24 months   ☐ 2+ years

Rating Scale

5 = Exceptional: Skills and understanding significantly beyond developmental level

4 = Outstanding: Strong mastery of skills and thorough understanding of concepts

3 = Mastered Basic Skills at Developmental Level: Understanding of concepts/skills evident

2 = Developing: Minor conceptual and skill errors; in process of developing

1 = Deficits: Significant remediation needed; deficits in knowledge/skills

NA = Not Applicable: Unable to measure with given data (do not use to indicate deficit)

	5	4	3	2	1	COMP	SCORE
Introduction	Sophisticated intro that identifies client, age, ethnicity, occupation, grade, etc. Descriptions clearly set context for understanding problem.	Detailed intro that identifies client, age, ethnicity, occupation, grade, etc. Descriptions useful for understanding problem.	Identifies client, age, ethnicity, occupation, grade, etc.	Missing 1–2 identifiers.	Missing, incorrect, or significant problem with identifiers and/or significant involved parties.	2.3.7	☐ NA
Presenting Concern	Description of problem provides sophisticated description of all stakeholders' views; word choice conveys empathy with each perspective; sophisticated conceptualization, choice of stakeholders.	Description of problem provides detailed description of all stakeholders' views; word choice conveys empathy with most perspectives; clear conceptualization.	Includes clear description of problem for each person and key stakeholders.	Minor problems or lack of clarity with problem descriptions; missing stakeholders.	Significant problems with problem descriptions; missing key perspectives; incorrect characterization.	2.3.9	☐ NA
Background Information	Includes sophisticated summary of recent and past events. Selection of information conveys insightful, thorough conceptualization.	Includes detailed summary of recent and past events. Selection of information conveys thoughtful conceptualization.	Includes clear summary of key recent and past events. Provides clear overview.	Insufficient, minimal, or missing background information. Basic information there but no clear development of conceptualization.	Significant information missing; unable to identify significant events.	2.3.7	☐ NA

(continued)

(continued)

	5	4	3	2	1	COMP	SCORE
Client/Relational Strengths	Sophisticated description of individual, relational, and spiritual strengths, resources, resiliency. Creative, insightful choices; clear clinical relevance.	Detailed description of individual, relational, and spiritual strengths, resources, resiliency. Highlights meaningful strengths.	Clear description of individual, relational, and spiritual strengths, resources, resiliency.	Underdeveloped description of strengths. Difficulty identifying clear strengths.	Significant problems identifying clinically relevant strengths (e.g., poor choice, insufficient number, etc.).	2.3.8	☐ NA
Couple Boundaries	Sophisticated characterization of couple boundary; insightful articulation of relational rules.	Detailed characterization of couple boundary; clear articulation of meaningful relational rules.	Clear characterization of couple boundary; articulates basic relational rules.	Inaccurate or unsupported description of boundaries; vague description of rules.	Incorrect, poor characterization of boundaries; problems with rule description.	1.1.1 2.2.3	☐ NA
Problem Interaction Pattern	Sophisticated, insightful description of interaction behavioral sequence; no evidence of bias; sophisticated description of homeostasis.	Detailed description of interaction behavioral sequence; no evidence of bias; detailed homeostasis description.	Clear description of interaction behavioral sequence; no evidence of bias; basic homeostatic pattern described.	Vague, unclear description of interaction pattern, homeostasis; may have some bias in description.	Significant problems with interaction pattern description; misidentified phases; clear bias.	1.1.1 2.2.3	☐ NA
Complementary Patterns	Sophisticated, insightful description of complementary patterns; clearly linked to presenting problem.	Detailed description of complementary patterns; linked to presenting problem.	Clear description of key complementary patterns.	Minor problems conceptualizing complementary patterns.	Significant problems identifying complementary roles, dynamics.	1.1.1 2.2.3	☐ NA
Communication Stances	Sophisticated, insightful description of communication stances; linked to problem dynamics; all significant persons in client's life included.	Detailed description of communication stances; linked to problem dynamics; most significant persons in client's life included.	Clear description of communication stances for all persons in therapy.	Misidentified stances for 1 or more persons.	Misidentified stances for 2 or more; failed to include all persons in therapy.	1.1.1 2.2.3	☐ NA

	Sophisticated	Detailed	Clear	Minor problems	Significant problems		
Divorce Indicators	Sophisticated, insightful description of divorce indicators; clearly understands divorce research.	Detailed description of divorce indicators; clearly understands divorce research.	Clear description of divorce indicators; understands divorce research.	Minor problems with 1–2 areas of divorce description.	Significant problems with 2 or more areas of divorce assessment.	2.1.1 6.3.2	☐ NA
Parental Subsystem	Sophisticated, insightful description of subsystems, membership, and their interactions; relates to problem formation.	Detailed description of subsystems, membership, and their interactions. Enhances understanding of general family dynamics.	Clear description of subsystems, membership, and their interactions.	Minor problems with description of subsystems, membership, and their interactions.	Significant problems identifying subsystems, membership, and how relate to problem.	1.1.1 2.2.3	☐ NA
Hierarchy Between Child/ Parents	Sophisticated, insightful description of parental hierarchy, ability to set rules, limits, consequences. Provides excellent example to support.	Detailed description of parental hierarchy, ability to set rules, limits, consequences. Provides meaningful notes to support.	Accurate description of parental hierarchy, ability to set rules, limits, consequences. Provides meaningful notes to support.	Minor problems with description of parental hierarchy.	Significant problems assessing hierarchy; unable to identify key family dynamics.	1.1.1 2.1.1 2.2.3	☐ NA
Emotional Boundaries with Children	Sophisticated, insightful description of emotional connection between parents and children. Provides excellent example to support.	Detailed description of emotional connection between parents and children with example.	Accurate description of emotional connection between parents and children. Basic notes or example provided.	Minor problems with description of emotional connection between parents and children.	Significant problems assessing emotional connection between parents and children; unable to identify key dynamics.	1.1.1 2.1.1 2.2.3	☐ NA
Problem Interaction Pattern	Sophisticated, insightful description of interaction behavioral sequence; no evidence of bias; sophisticated description of homeostasis.	Detailed description of interaction behavioral sequence; no evidence of bias; detailed homeostasis description.	Clear description of interaction behavioral sequence; no evidence of bias; basic homeostatic pattern described.	Vague, unclear description of interaction pattern, homeostasis; may have some bias in description.	Significant problems with interaction pattern description; misidentifies phases; clear bias.	1.1.1 2.2.3	☐ NA

(continued)

(continued)

	5	4	3	2	1	COMP	SCORE
Triangles/ Coalitions	Sophisticated, insightful description of covert alliances, triangles; able to clearly articulate their relation to problem.	Detailed description of covert alliances, triangles; able to relate to problem.	Clear description of covert alliances, triangles.	Minor problems with description of triangles	Significant problems with description of triangles; missed key dynamics.	1.1.1 2.2.3	☐ NA
Communication Stances	Sophisticated, insightful description of communication stances; linked to problem dynamics; all significant persons in client's life included.	Detailed description of communication stances; linked to problem dynamics; most significant persons in client's life included.	Clear description of communication stances for all persons in therapy.	Misidentified stances for 1 or more persons.	Misidentified stances for 2 or more; failed to include all persons in therapy.	1.1.1 2.2.3	☐ NA
Hypothesis	Sophisticated, unique systemic hypothesis regarding relational patterns, presenting problem. Includes all members; addresses key dynamics.	Detailed systemic hypothesis regarding relational patterns, presenting problem. Addresses key dynamics.	Clear, basic systemic hypothesis regarding relational patterns, presenting problem.	Vague or unclear hypothesis; dynamics not clearly addressed or certain dynamics ignored.	Significant problems with hypothesis; blaming or one-sided.	2.2.3	☐ NA
Intergenerational Patterns	Sophisticated, insightful tracking of intergenerational patterns, incl. substance abuse, sexual/phys abuse, mental health issues. 3+ generational patterns included.	Detailed tracking of intergenerational patterns, incl. substance abuse, sexual/phys abuse, mental health issues. At least 1–3 generational pattern included.	Clear description of key intergenerational patterns, incl. substance abuse, sexual/phys abuse, mental health issues.	Vague or incomplete description of intergenerational patterns, incl. substance abuse, sexual/phys abuse, mental health issues. No significant patterns missing.	One or more key intergenerational patterns not addressed and/or appears to not have fully assessed intergenerational issues.	2.3.6 2.3.7	☐ NA
Previous Solutions and Unique Outcomes	Sophisticated, insightful identification of solutions that did and did not work; clear implications for intervention.	Detailed description of solutions that did and did not work.	Clear, basic description of solutions that did and did not work.	Vague or unhelpful description of previous solutions.	Poor example of previous solutions; confusing what worked and what didn't.	2.3.8	☐ NA

Narrative Observations; Larger System	Sophisticated, insightful identification of dominant discourses (social, family, other) and effects on identities and problem; demonstrates sophisticated understanding of diversity issues and how they impact problem.	Detailed description of dominant discourses (social, family, other) and effects on identities and problem; demonstrates meaingful understanding of diversity issues and how they impact problem.	Clear, basic description of dominant discourses (social, family, other) and effects on identities and problem; demonstrates general understanding of diversity issues and how they impact problem.	Vague, unclear description of dominant discourses (social, family, other) and effects on identities and problem; does not demonstrate clear understanding of diversity issues and how they impact problem.	Misses impact of key dominant discourses and/or diversity issues.	1.2.1	☐ NA
Genogram	Comprehensive, sophisticated genogram with all relevant information, including ages, names, relational patterns, occupations, medical history, psychiatric disorders, abuse history; provides unique insight to presenting problem. No format errors.	Detailed genogram with most relevant information, including ages, names, relational patterns, occupations, medical history, psychiatric disorders, abuse history; provides useful background to presenting problem. 1–2 format errors.	Basic genogram with key relevant information, including ages, names, relational patterns, occupations, medical history, psychiatric disorders, abuse history. Minor format errors.	Genogram missing some key information; several format errors. Does not provide sufficient background to presenting problem.	Missing significant information and/or family members; several and/or significant format errors; does not provide useful clinical information.	2.3.6	☐ NA
Client Perspectives	Sophisticated and insightful identification of areas of agreement, disagreement; able to identify subtle, clinically relevant areas of potential difference; creative yet realistic plan for addressing differences.	Detailed identification of areas of agreement, disagreement; able to identify at least one specific area of difference; realistic plan for addressing differences.	Able to identify general areas of agreement, disagreement; realistic plan for addressing differences.	Minor problems identifying areas of agreement and disagreement; may be vague or miss issues; vague or problematic plan for addressing differences.	Significant problems identifying client perspective and areas of agreement, disagreement, strategies to manage. Does not demonstrate understanding of key client perspectives.	2.3.9	☐ NA

(continued)

(continued)

	5	4	3	2	1	COMP	SCORE
Overall Conceptualization: Quality of Assessment	Overall report systematically integrates available information to develop sophisticated, clinically relevant conceptualization; all assessment areas are consistent, developing a clear depiction of systemic functioning. Provides well-articulated focus for treatment.	Overall report systematically integrates available information to develop a clinically relevant conceptualization; most assessment areas are consistent, developing a clear depiction of systemic functioning. Provides clear focus for treatment.	Overall report integrates available information to develop a clinically relevant conceptualization; majority of assessment areas are consistent, developing a clear depiction of systemic functioning. Provides general focus for treatment.	Minor problems with integration and consistency across areas of assessment. Does not provide a single, clear focus for treatment.	Significant problems with integrating areas of assessment; numerous inconsistencies; no clear focus of treatment.	2.2.2	☐ NA
Additional Competency (Optional)							☐ NA
Additional Competency (Optional)							☐ NA
Comments:							

©2007. Diane R. Gehart, Ph.D

Clinical Assessment

Step 2: Identifying Oases and Obstacles

After completing a case conceptualization, you have a good sense of the "big picture" as it relates to the client and the problem and are probably feeling ready to set out on your therapeutic journey. But before you do, there is another type of assessment that will help you avoid obstacles and identify rest stops: clinical assessment. Clinical assessment focuses more on the psychological and health dynamics of clients, allowing you to have a better sense of how to more effectively partner with them as you start off on your journey. Although oftentimes assessment may not turn up information that causes you to radically shift direction from your case conceptualization, sometimes it does—and when it does, you will be very glad you spent the time to ask.

Clinical Assessment Overview

Mental health professionals from all disciplines—psychology, psychiatry, psychiatric nursing, counseling, family therapy, and social work—share a common set of standards related to clinical assessment:

- Monitoring for client safety
- Monitoring for medical and psychiatric conditions that warrant medical attention outside the therapist's scope of practice
- Performing a mental status exam and making a diagnosis
- Case management, including referrals to necessary social services

Although these basic skills are required of all mental health practitioners, therapists generally have significant freedom in choosing *how* they perform these tasks: through structured or unstructured interview methods, written or verbal assessments, or standardized or original instruments. The best method depends on the clinical setting and client characteristics. Although considered standard practice, therapists should be mindful that clinical assessment and diagnosis have both benefits and potential liabilities.

Benefits of Clinical Assessment and Diagnosis

Clinical assessment and diagnosis help therapists (a) identify potential courses of treatment, (b) decide how best to keep clients and the public safe, and (c) determine the need for referrals and additional services. For some clients, a diagnosis is helpful, even liberating. For example, many survivors of sexual abuse are relieved to hear that the symptoms they are experiencing—hypervigilance, nightmares, and flashbacks—are part of a larger syndrome, posttraumatic stress disorder, and that this condition has a good prognosis. Similarly, distinguishing between a learning disorder and attention deficit disorder can be helpful to parents and teachers. In many cases, diagnosis is a helpful first step in conceptualizing treatment.

Potential Dangers of Clinical Assessment and Diagnosis

The safety and treatment benefits of clinical assessment and diagnosis are readily apparent. So how could they possibly be dangerous? Like most things in life, these procedures are double-edged swords. One of the most obvious difficulties is that in practice an *objective* clinical mental health assessment is impossible. One thing always stands in the way: the therapist!

Inescapable Cultural Lenses

Each therapist views a client through a unique lens. As a therapist, your lens is your culture, values, history, beliefs, and norms. These are generally things that make us who we are, and they cannot be cast aside by simply telling yourself to be "neutral." In fact, most family models are based on the premise that it is impossible to be neutral and objective. For example, systemically oriented therapists, such as those using MRI and Milan Therapies, conceptualize the therapeutic system as a *second-order cybernetic system,* which refers to the dynamic of observer (therapist) and observed (client) (Keeney, 1983). Because therapists are part of the system they are trying to observe, they significantly influence its behavior. Moreover, any words they use to describe the client come from their worldview or epistemology/ontology, not the client's. Therapists' descriptions of clients reveal more about the *therapist* than about the client: clinical assessment reveals what the therapist and the broader mental health culture value as "good," "healthy," and "valuable" enough to focus on.

Postmodern family therapists are also keenly aware of the lenses therapists bring to the therapy encounter. Two "horizons of meaning" or worldviews meet when therapist and client talk (Gadamer, 1975). Because therapists cannot step out of their cultures, beliefs, personalities, histories, or theoretical training and be neutral and unbiased, they must always interpret the client from where they are standing, their particular horizon of meaning. For example, a therapist raised in a rural, conservative community will have a different interpretation of an inner-city teen's story than will a therapist living in a diverse, urban community, with neither being necessarily more "accurate" than the other. The "nearness" of the urban therapist does not ensure greater accuracy because the therapist may have *more* biases from repeat encounters with this type of client; the rural therapist may be more "objective" or more biased, depending on how aware the therapist is of his/her own *horizon of meaning,* the position from which one interprets the other.

Thus therapists' ability to become aware of their lenses and horizons for meaning increases their ability to see the other person more clearly and with less bias. When beginning the journey of becoming a therapist, everyone is very limited in the awareness of the lenses through which they view others. Part of the goal of training is to help awaken therapists to see the lenses through which they view the world.

Training also provides new therapists with an entirely new set of lenses that take the form of theories of health and normalcy. These can also be problematic, especially when working with people who are different from the "norm," such as cultural, sexual, or other minority clients. Clinical assessment is one of the most dangerous places to practice if one is not keenly aware of one's lenses because the client gives little feedback about its accuracy.

During therapy, of course, the inappropriateness of a therapeutic technique is often immediately obvious because the client will refuse to participate or in some way signal that he/she does not like the idea—the major exception being a client who wants to please the therapist. Similarly, if one's case conceptualization is incorrect, the client will not progress and/or new information will come to light that helps the therapist refine the conceptualization. Case conceptualization is a process of hypothesizing, gathering feedback from the family through interactions, and then refining the hypothesis based on this information. However, when doing clinical assessment, it is easier to get off course.

Family, culture, social class, and other variables also determine what "truth" is. If therapists follow the medical model, which assumes that they can accurately determine the truth, they are less likely to continually question and refine diagnoses and mental status reports. The model is predicated on the assumption that it is easy to distinguish between normal and abnormal behaviors, which is more difficult in the psychological than in the physical realm. For example, behaviors such as drinking, talking, emoting, eating, worrying, or seeing ghosts have different meanings and norms depending on one's family, culture, and social class. Thus, although therapists may seem to begin with a clear set of norms for mental health, when they fully attend to the client's broader social context, it becomes much less clear where normal ends and abnormal begins.

Understanding Diagnostic Labels

Although therapists need to diagnose in most treatment environments, in many cases *diagnosis may not be the most useful means of conceptualizing treatment or the therapist's relationship to clients.* In both systemic and postmodern therapies, diagnosis is not considered the most helpful concept around which to develop treatment. Instead, diagnostic and psychiatric descriptions are *one* of several descriptions of the problem.

Systemic Perspectives on Diagnosis

From a systemic perspective, a diagnosis describes the behaviors that a person has adopted to maintain balance in his/her current web of relationships; given a different set of circumstances, it is possible and even likely that the person will have a different set of behaviors, thoughts, and feelings. Thus a diagnosis is not viewed as an illness or inherently individual phenomenon, as it is in the traditional medical model. This does not mean that neurological changes have not occurred or that medication is unnecessary. Physiology interacts with the environment in an interdependent, mutually reinforcing system: when depression is part of maintaining a system's balance, the depressed person is likely to develop physiological symptoms of depression.

Postmodern Perspectives on Diagnosis

Postmodern therapists are skeptical of diagnoses because these become labels that clients use to inform their identity, often silencing their strengths, resiliencies, and capabilities (Gergen, Anderson, & Hoffman, 1996). Once they are given a diagnostic label, clients tend to interpret future behaviors and events through this lens, creating a self-fulfilling prophecy. For example, when a child is diagnosed with ADHD, parents, teachers, and the child tend to develop telescopic vision, focusing their attention on the child's hyperactivity and attention deficit and missing exceptions to the label as well as other elements of the child's identity, such as the fact that the child mentors a younger sibling, has a musical talent, or cares about the family.

A General Family Therapy Approach to Diagnosis

Although some differences exist between postmodern and systemic perspectives on mental health diagnosis, there is general agreement that diagnosis can focus on what is *least* likely to help the therapist effectively treat the client. When therapists focus on psychiatric symptoms and codes of classifications, they are less likely to bring about change using the models that are most closely associated with family therapy. However, this does not mean that family therapists should avoid diagnosis and the medical model altogether. Instead, they should find the proper place for diagnosis, which family therapists would say is "one voice among many."

Whether working from systemic or postmodern approaches, most family therapists value multiple descriptions of problems. For example, in Milan and MRI systemic approaches, each family member's description of the problem is used to construct the hypotheses about the family dynamics (Selvini Palazzoli, Boscolo, Cecchin, & Prata, 1978; Watzlawick, Weakland, & Fisch, 1974). Similarly, in collaborative therapy, multiple, contradictory descriptions of the problem are allowed to coexist to encourage the generation of new possibilities and understandings (Anderson, 1997). Thus each description of the problem is considered one of many possible "truths" that depend on webs of relationships and social discourse; it does not stand on its own. For example, even though a person may meet the diagnostic criteria for major depressive disorder at a given time based on one or more persons' description of the problem, this diagnosis does not carry the same fixed or essential truth that it would in traditional psychiatry. Instead, family therapists recognize that the symptoms, feelings, and behaviors that qualify a person for this diagnosis are subject to change based on the meanings generated by the person's relationships.

The importance of the diagnosis also varies from client to client rather than always being considered more important than other perspectives. Diagnosis is one voice in the conversation, a description that clients and therapists are free to question, try on, and refine. Therapists, outside professionals, or clients may introduce medical studies and knowledge into the conversation, but they never use medical knowledge to silence the voices and unique experiences of clients or therapists that may or may not be in alignment with this particular form of knowledge. In some cases, the diagnosis that fits early in treatment rapidly loses its meaning. At other times, clients use diagnostic descriptions to move forward with their goals, hopes, and dreams. The therapist's task is to be flexible in allowing a wide range of possible in-session uses for diagnosis with each client rather than insisting on the same diagnostic label based on the therapist's philosophy.

Parity and Nonparity Diagnoses

The Paul Wellstone and Pete Domenici Mental Health Parity and Addiction Equity Act was passed as part of the Economic Stabilization Act of 2008. This act requires that insurance companies reimburse for mental health and substance abuse disorders the same as for any other physiological disorders, meaning that they must cover mental issues as part of their health plans. Prior to the bill's passage, approximately 30 states had mental health parity laws. These laws, which tend to be more comprehensive than the federal act passed in 2008, often distinguish between parity diagnoses and nonparity diagnoses. When a client is diagnosed with a *parity* mental health diagnosis, insurance plans must reimburse the same as they would for physiological disorders; significantly, this implies that the number of sessions cannot be artificially limited, as was the practice with HMO-type plans, and co-pays must be the same as those for physiological disorders. Parity diagnoses typically include severe mental health disorders and must be the *primary Axis I diagnoses* in order for insurance co-pays and reimbursement policies to apply. These severe disorders usually include the following:

- Anorexia and bulimia
- Bipolar disorder

- Major depressive disorder
- Obsessive-compulsive disorder
- Panic disorder
- Pervasive-developmental disorder
- Schizoaffective disorder
- Schizophrenia
- Any mental health disorder in children (including adjustment disorders)

The Recovery Model and Diagnosis

An international movement, the Recovery Model, is quickly reshaping how government-funded agencies view diagnosis and mental illness (Fisher & Chamberlin, 2004; Onken, Craig, Ridgway, Ralph, & Cook, 2007; Repper & Perkins, 2006). With its origins in consumer self-help in the 1930s, the Recovery Movement captured the attention of rehabilitation and substance abuse professionals in the 1990s and mental health policymakers since 2000, and it has been formally adopted by most First World countries. In the United States, the 2002 New Freedom Commission on Mental Health proposed transforming the national mental health system using a paradigm of recovery, and in 2004 the U.S. Department of Health and Human Services launched a nationwide recovery campaign (Fisher & Chamberlin, 2004; U.S. Department of Health and Human Services, 2004). In 2008, the California Marriage and Family Therapy (MFT) licensing board revised the MFT educational curriculum to include the Recovery Model for preparing family therapists to work in today's public mental health system. So what is the Recovery Model, and why is it so popular?

In the 1990s, the World Health Organization released research findings from a cross-national study on recovery from severe mental illness that revealed surprising results: 28% of patients diagnosed with severe mental illness (e.g., schizophrenia, bipolar disorder, substance abuse) made a *full recovery*, and 52% reported a *social recovery* (e.g., were able to return to work, had satisfying family relationships, stayed out of jail, etc.; Ralph, 2000). Similarly, Jaakko Seikkula's (2002) and his colleagues' (Haarakangas, Seikkula, Alakare, & Aaltonen, 2007) open dialogue approach to treating clients with psychotic symptoms, a collaborative therapy approach with similar principles to the Recovery Model (see Chapter 15), has even more impressive outcomes: 83% of first-episode psychosis patients returning to work and 77% with no remaining psychotic symptoms after two years of treatment. These findings do not fit with medical model assumptions that the genetic and biological predispositions of severe mental illness preclude meaningful recovery (Ramon, Healy, & Renouf, 2007). Thus the Recovery Model is about helping clients lead rich, meaningful lives rather than simply reducing symptoms related to a mental health diagnosis, a perspective that resonates with family therapy and its historically uneasy relationship with the medical model and its emphasis on pathology.

The U.S. Department of Health and Human Services (2004) defines recovery as "a journey of healing and transformation enabling a person with a mental health problem to live a meaningful life in a community of his or her choice while striving to achieve his or her full potential" (p. 2). The Recovery Model uses a *social* model of disability rather than a medical model; thus, it de-emphasizes diagnostic labeling and emphasizes *psychosocial functioning*, the hallmark of family therapy approaches. The "National Consensus Statement on Mental Health Recovery" includes *10 Fundamental Components of Recovery* (U.S. Department of Health and Human Services, 2004):

- **Self-Direction:** Consumers (clients) exercise choice over their treatment and path to recovery.

- **Individualized and Person-Centered:** Paths to recovery are individualized based on a person's unique strengths, resiliencies, preferences, experiences, and cultural background.

- **Empowerment:** Consumers have the authority to choose from a range of options and participate in decision making; professional relationships encourage decision making and assertiveness.

- **Holistic:** Recovery encompasses all aspects of life: mind, body, spirit, and community.

- **Nonlinear:** Recovery is not a step-by-step process but an ongoing process that includes growth and setbacks.

- **Strengths-Based:** Recovery focuses on valuing and building upon strengths, resiliencies, and abilities.

- **Peer Support:** Consumers are encouraged to engage with other consumers in pursuing recovery.

- **Respect:** For recovery to occur, consumers need to experience respect from professionals, their communities, and other systems.

- **Responsibility:** Consumers are personally responsible for their recovery and self-care.

- **Hope:** Recovery requires a belief in the self and a willingness to persevere through difficulty.

These elements play leading roles in many family therapy theories, most notably postmodern approaches (Chapters 14 and 15) such as solution-based therapies (emphasis on client strengths, empowerment, and hope), collaborative therapy (views "client as the expert"; individualized, client-directed treatment), and narrative therapy (seeing people as separate from problems; dealing with social stigma, peer support). The Recovery Movement's approach to harnessing clients' strengths to help them fashion meaningful lives while reducing the expert role of the therapist fits with many family therapy approaches to working with clients diagnosed with severe mental illness. Although diagnosis still has its place, both family therapy models and the Recovery Model assume that diagnosis is not the most beneficial driving force of treatment; instead the client's motivation for a quality life directs the course of treatment.

Family Therapy Approach to Clinical Assessment
Diagnostic Interview and Mental Status Exam

In formal clinical environments, therapists are usually asked to conduct a structured diagnostic interview with clients, most frequently called a mental status exam (MSE). Based on the medical model, these exams require a more hierarchical, detached therapeutic relationship than that found in most family therapies. This shift is often confusing for both clients and therapists and can interfere with later interventions that require a more empathetic or egalitarian therapeutic relationship. Ideally, family therapists develop strategies for conducting a mental status exam that preserve the type of therapeutic alliance they intend to use throughout treatment.

Family Therapy Approaches to Clinical Assessment

Numerous case conceptualization techniques from family therapy methods lend themselves to clinical assessment while still preserving a strong therapeutic alliance characterized by nonjudgment and empathy. Broadly speaking, there are two approaches to clinical assessment: systemic and postmodern.

Systemic Approach to the MSE

A systemic approach to assessing a client's mental status and making a diagnosis uses a combination of two common systemic techniques: (a) problem assessment (Watzlawick, Weakland, & Fisch, 1974) and (b) circular questions (Selvini Palazzoli, Boscolo, Cecchin, & Prata, 1978).

As introduced in Chapter 2, *problem assessment* involves tracing interactions from initial homeostasis to escalation of symptoms (the positive feedback loop) until the system returns to normal or homeostasis. This assessment describes the following:

1. The initial homeostasis: what was going on before the problem occurred
2. The trigger that started an escalation in the system
3. The first person's behavioral response
4. The second (and additional) person's behavioral response to the first person
5. The first person's response to the second person
6. The back-and-forth interactions that occur between people until the symptoms dissipate and some sort of "normalcy" or "homeostasis" is restored

Therapists can use variants on *circular questions* to inquire about each person's symptoms at each stage of the cycle:

SYSTEMIC CLINICAL ASSESSMENT QUESTIONS

- Describe your mood during each phase of the cycle of events. Describe the mood of others during each phase. How do these compare?

- Does this cycle affect your sleeping or eating patterns? How does this compare to "normal" times?

- During this cycle, do you experience any unusual thoughts or experiences, such as feeling a sense of panic, seeing things other people do not, feeling disconnected from yourself or the situation, or engaging in repetitive behaviors or thoughts? Do these sorts of things happen outside the problem cycle of events?

- Do you ever use alcohol, drugs, or other things to help manage your feelings when things feel out of control? Does anyone else?

- At any time do you have thoughts of hurting yourself or others? Have you had these thoughts in the past? Are these feelings stronger or weaker during the escalation of events?

- Have you ever inflicted physical pain on yourself to manage emotions? Have you thought about it? When are these thoughts the strongest? The weakest?

- Have you or anyone else involved in this cycle used physical violence or emotional abuse? Is it worse or better during the problem cycle you describe?

- Did you experience any childhood abuse: sexual, physical, emotional, or neglect? Do you think these experiences are affecting the current problem cycle of behaviors?

- Have you experienced physical or sexual assault or abuse as an adult? Do you think these experiences are affecting the current problem cycle of behaviors?

- Are there any medical or physical issues that might be affecting the problem cycle you describe?

Postmodern Approach to the MSE

A mental status exam from a postmodern perspective involves honoring a client's description and perception of the problem. Narrative therapists can easily adapt the technique of mapping the influence of problems and persons (White & Epston, 1990; see Chapter 15) to collect information for a mental status exam and make a diagnosis. Mapping the influence of the problem involves the following:

1. Mapping the effect of the problem on persons in the areas of individual, relational, social, and spiritual functioning
2. Mapping the effect of persons on problems in the areas of individual, relational, social, and spiritual functioning

Therapists can ask the following questions to gather the information necessary for a diagnosis:

POSTMODERN APPROACH TO CLINICAL ASSESSMENT

Mapping the Effects of the Problem

- How does the problem affect you and others who are involved? Are there changes in:
  - Mood
  - Eating and sleeping
  - Feelings of panic, worry, or obsessive thinking
  - Seeing or hearing what others do not
  - Drinking or drug use
  - Thoughts of harming oneself or others
  - Cutting or other self-harming behaviors
  - Violent behaviors by self or others
- Is there a history of sexual, physical, or emotional abuse in childhood or adulthood that may be affecting the situation?
- How does the problem affect your relationships at home, work, school, extended family, or social circle?
- How does the problem affect your participation in social activities?
- How does the problem affect your spiritual life or beliefs?

Mapping the Effects of Persons

- How have you been able to affect the life of the problem, meaning keeping the things you just mentioned from getting worse?
- Are there times when you were able to not allow the problem to completely change your mood, thoughts, eating, sleeping, drinking, or other areas of functioning?
- Are there times when you were able to protect your relationships from being influenced by the problem?
- Are there times when you were able to continue with your normal social life despite the problem?
- Are there ways you have been able to maintain your sense of spirituality with the problem present?

Written Assessment Options

In addition to using in-session dialogue, therapists can gather additional information on paper. Written assessment takes two common forms:

1. Formal assessment instruments (e.g., Beck Depression Inventory, symptom inventories)
2. Informal assessments and self-reported client histories (e.g., initial intake forms)

Formal Written Assessments

Formal written assessments have been standardized to help therapists obtain a more objective assessment of client functioning. These instruments are generally considered more accurate than informal assessments because they have been carefully developed through research. Formal written assessments are especially useful in the following situations:

- The client demonstrates more severe and/or multiple symptoms.
- The therapist needs to make a differential diagnosis.
- The client is not responding to treatment as well as hoped.
- The client fits the demographic profile of a formal assessment instrument (most are insufficiently normed for diverse populations).

Pros and Cons

The advantages and disadvantages of this kind of assessment are shown in the following table:

PROS AND CONS OF FORMAL ASSESSMENTS

PROS	CONS
Likely to be more accurate than informal measures	Expensive; most require a fee for each application plus time to administer
Able to gather information in more objective manner	More time intensive
Able to compare with national norms	No clear link to improved outcomes
Helpful with more severe pathology	In most cases, do not change informal assessment and diagnosis
	May not fit or support therapist's theoretical support

Formal Assessment Options

Therapists have hundreds of options for formal clinical assessment. Because of cost considerations, most use only what is supplied to them at their place of employment. Some of the more common assessments include the following:

- **Minnesota Multiphasic Personality Inventory (MMPI-2):** The MMPI is the most frequently used clinical assessment instrument for diagnosing moderate to severe pathology. It contains 567 true-false items and takes 1–2 hours to complete; there are adult and adolescent versions. The MMPI is most frequently used in hospital settings and forensic psychology. More information can be found at www.pearsonassessments.com.

- **Beck Depression Inventory (BDI) and related inventories:** The BDI is a 21-item self-assessment inventory that assesses a client's level of depression for people 13 years and older. Because it is quick and easy to administer, it is one of the more frequently used tests. Beck also has several other similar inventories for assessing anxiety, suicidality, hopelessness, and obsessive-compulsiveness. More information can be found at www.harcourtassessment.com.

- **Michigan Alcoholic Screening Test (MAST):** The MAST is a 22-item self-report instrument to screen for problem drinking. Much like the Beck, the instrument is quick and easy to administer. The test is available for free download at www.ncadd-sfv.org/symptoms/mast_test.html.

- **Outcome Questionnaire:** The Outcome Questionnaire comes in adult and youth versions with 10-, 30-, or 45-item versions, with the longer versions providing more detailed assessments of mental health symptoms. Because of its brevity, it is popular in outpatient settings. More information can be found at www.oqmeasures.com.

- **Symptom Checklist 90:** The Symptom Checklist is a 90-item test that assesses for mental health symptoms and their intensity (mild, moderate, severe). It is designed for individuals 13 years and older and requires 12–15 minutes to complete. More information can be found at www.pearsonassessments.com tests/scl90r.htm.

Informal Written Assessments: "Intake Forms"

In virtually all professional therapy settings, clients are asked to complete a written assessment, such as the Client Information Form (see example at the end of this chapter). These forms are considered informal because they are not standardized. Nonetheless, some clients reveal information on them that they do not reveal in session (Gottman, 1999). The opposite can also be true, and less may be revealed in writing; clients differ in what feels safer. If possible, these forms should be made available to clients before the initial session via a website or mailed to clients so that they have time to thoroughly read through them, gather information, and complete the forms. Therapists are more likely to get accurate information if clients can complete the forms at home, especially if they have to supply detailed information such as medications and dosages.

Pros and Cons

As with formal assessments, informal assessments have advantages and disadvantages:

PROS AND CONS OF INFORMAL ASSESSMENTS

PROS	CONS
Inexpensive	No national norms
Minimal time required	Effectiveness largely determined by therapist's skill
In most outpatient cases are sufficient for effective treatment	May not capture more subtle clinical issues
Likely to be more appropriate with diverse clients than standardized instruments	Depend on client's honesty and memory for accuracy
Easily adapted to therapist's theoretical approach	

Common Information

Informal assessments usually gather the following information:

- Name, address, phone numbers, birthdates, occupations, grade in school
- List of symptoms and concerns
- List of goals for therapy and social/personal resources
- Prior psychological treatment for individual and family
- History of suicidal and homicidal ideation for individual and family
- List of medical conditions and medications for individual and family
- History of sexual, physical, emotional abuse, including domestic violence and assault for individual and family
- Alcohol and drug use history for individual and family
- Legal, work, and/or other social problems for individual and family

Example of a Clinical Assessment Form

In this chapter, clinical assessment includes elements common to most outpatient clinical assessments: client identifiers, presenting problem, mental status, diagnosis (including medication information), risk assessment, case management (including prognosis), and evaluation of assessment. The following is an example of a clinical assessment form.

CLINICAL ASSESSMENT

Client ID # (do not use name):	Ethnicity(ies):	Primary Language: ☐ Eng ☐ Span ☐ Other: _____

List all participants/significant others: Put a [★] for Identified Patient; [✓] for sig. others who **WILL** attend; [✕] for sig. others who will **NOT** attend.

Adult: Age: Profession/Employer	**Child: Age: School/Grade**
[ ] AM†: _____	[ ] CM: _____
[ ] AF: _____	[ ] CF: _____
[ ] AF/M #2: _____	[ ] CF/M #2: _____

Presenting Problem

Complete for children

☐ Depression/hopelessness	☐ Couple concern	☐ School failure/decline performance
☐ Anxiety/worry	☐ Parent/child conflict	
☐ Anger issues	☐ Partner violence/abuse	☐ Truancy/runaway
☐ Loss/grief	☐ Divorce adjustment	☐ Fighting w/peers
☐ Suicidal thoughts/attempts	☐ Remarriage adjustment	☐ Hyperactivity
☐ Sexual abuse/rape	☐ Sexuality/intimacy concerns	☐ Wetting/soiling clothing
☐ Alcohol/drug use	☐ Major life changes	☐ Child abuse/neglect
☐ Eating problems/disorders	☐ Legal issues/probation	☐ Isolation/withdrawal
☐ Job problems/unemployeds	☐ Other: _____	☐ Other: _____

---

† *Abbreviations:* AF: Adult Female; AM: Adult Male; CF#: Child Female with age, e.g., CF12; CM#: Child Male with age; Dx: Diagnosis; IP: Identified Patient; Hx: History; GAF: Global Assessment of Functioning; GARF: Global Assessment of Relational Functioning; NA: Not Applicable.

(continued)

(continued)

Mental Status for IP		
Interpersonal issues	☐ NA	☐ Conflict ☐ Enmeshment ☐ Isolation/avoidance ☐ Emotional disengagement ☐ Poor social skills ☐ Couple problems ☐ Prob w/friends ☐ Prob at work ☐ Overly shy ☐ Egocentricity ☐ Diff establish/maintain relationship ☐ Other: _____
Mood	☐ NA	☐ Depressed/sad ☐ Hopeless ☐ Fearful ☐ Anxious ☐ Angry ☐ Irritable ☐ Manic ☐ Other: _____
Affect	☐ NA	☐ Constricted ☐ Blunt ☐ Flat ☐ Labile ☐ Dramatic ☐ Other: _____
Sleep	☐ NA	☐ Hypersomnia ☐ Insomnia ☐ Disrupted ☐ Nightmares ☐ Other: _____
Eating	☐ NA	☐ Increase ☐ Decrease ☐ Anorectic restriction ☐ Binging ☐ Purging ☐ Body image ☐ Other: _____
Anxiety symptoms	☐ NA	☐ Chronic worry ☐ Panic attacks ☐ Dissociation ☐ Phobias ☐ Obsessions ☐ Compulsions ☐ Other: _____
Trauma symptoms	☐ NA	☐ Acute ☐ Chronic ☐ Hypervigilance ☐ Dreams/nightmares ☐ Dissociation ☐ Emotional numbness ☐ Other: _____
Psychotic symptoms	☐ NA	☐ Hallucinations ☐ Delusions ☐ Paranoia ☐ Loose associations ☐ Other: _____
Motor activity/ speech	☐ NA	☐ Low energy ☐ Restless/hyperactive ☐ Agitated ☐ Inattentive ☐ Impulsive ☐ Pressured speech ☐ Slow speech ☐ Other: _____
Thought	☐ NA	☐ Poor concentration/attention ☐ Denial ☐ Self-blame ☐ Other-blame ☐ Ruminative ☐ Tangential ☐ Illogical ☐ Concrete ☐ Poor insight ☐ Impaired decision making ☐ Disoriented ☐ Slow processing ☐ Other: _____
Socio-Legal	☐ NA	☐ Disregards rules ☐ Defiant ☐ Stealing ☐ Lying ☐ Tantrums ☐ Arrest/incarceration ☐ Initiates fights ☐ Other: _____
Other symptoms	☐ NA	

Diagnosis for IP

Contextual Factors considered in making Dx: ☐ Age ☐ Gender ☐ Family dynamics ☐ Culture ☐ Language ☐ Religion ☐ Economic ☐ Immigration ☐ Sexual orientation ☐ Trauma ☐ Dual dx/comorbid ☐ Addiction ☐ Cognitive ability

□ Other: _____

Describe impact of identified factors: _____

Axis I Primary: _____ Secondary: _____ **Axis II:** _____ **Axis III:** _____ **Axis IV:** □ Problems with primary support group □ Problems related to social environment/school □ Educational problems □ Occupational problems □ Housing problems □ Economic problems □ Problems with accessing health care services □ Problems related to interactions with the legal system □ Other psychosocial problems **Axis V:** GAF _____ GARF _____	**List DSM symptoms for Axis I Dx (include frequency and duration for each). Client meets _____ of _____ criteria for Axis I Primary Dx.** 1. _____ 2. _____ 3. _____ 4. _____ 5. _____ 6. _____
Have medical causes been ruled out? □ Yes □ No □ In process **Has patient been referred for psychiatric/ medical eval?** □ Yes □ No **Has patient agreed with referral?** □ Yes □ No □ NA List psychometric instruments or consults used for assessment: □ None or _____	**Medications (psychiatric & medical) Dose /Start Date** □ None prescribed 1. _____ / _____ mg; _____ 2. _____ / _____ mg; _____ 3. _____ / _____ mg; _____ Client response to diagnosis: □ Agree □ Somewhat agree □ Disagree □ Not informed for following reason: _____

Medical Necessity (*Check all that apply*): □ Significant impairment □ Probability of significant impairment
□ Probably developmental arrest
Areas of impairment: □ Daily activities □ Social relationships □ Health □ Work/school
□ Living arrangement □ Other: _____

Risk Assessment

Suicidality	**Homicidality**
□ No indication	□ No indication
□ Denies	□ Denies
□ Active ideation	□ Active ideation
□ Passive ideation	□ Passive ideation
□ Intent without plan	□ Intent without means
□ Intent with means	□ Intent with means
□ Ideation past yr	□ Ideation past yr
□ Attempt past yr	□ Violence past yr
□ Family/peer hx of completed suicide	□ Hx assault/temper
	□ Cruelty to animals

(*continued*)

(continued)

Hx Substance Abuse	Sexual & Physical Abuse and Other Risk Factors
Alcohol:	☐ Current child w abuse hx:
☐ No indication	☐ Sexual ☐ Physical ☐ Emotional ☐ Neglect
☐ Denies	☐ Adult w childhood abuse:
☐ Past	☐ Sexual ☐ Physical ☐ Emotional ☐ Neglect
☐ Current	☐ Adult w abuse/assault in adulthood:
Freq/Amt: _____	☐ Sexual ☐ Physical ☐ Current
	☐ History of perpetrating abuse:
Drugs:	☐ Sexual ☐ Physical
☐ No indication	☐ Elder/dependent adult abuse/neglect
☐ Denies	☐ Anorexia/bulimia/other eating disorder
☐ Past	☐ Cutting or other self-harm:
☐ Current	☐ Current
Drugs: _____	☐ Past Method: _____
Freq/Amt: _____	☐ Criminal/legal hx: _____
☐ Current alc/sub abuse by family/ significant other	☐ None reported

Indicators of Safety: ☐ At least one outside person who provides strong support ☐ Able to cite specific reasons to live, not harm self/other ☐ Hopeful ☐ Has future goals ☐ Willing to dispose of dangerous items ☐ Willing to reduce contact with people who make situation worse ☐ Willing to implement safety plan, safety interventions ☐ Developing set of alternatives to self/other harm ☐ Sustained period of safety: ☐ Other: _____

Safety Plan includes: ☐ Verbal no harm contract ☐ Written no harm contract ☐ Emergency contact card ☐ Emergency therapist/agency number ☐ Medication management ☐ Specific plan for contacting friends/ support persons during crisis ☐ Specific plan of where to go during crisis ☐ Specific self-calming tasks to reduce risk before reach crisis level (e.g., journaling, exercising, etc.) ☐ Specific daily/weekly activities to reduce stressors ☐ Other: _____

Legal/Ethical Action Taken: ☐ NA Explain: _____

Case Management

Date	Modalities:	Is client involved in mental health or other medical treatment elsewhere?
1st visit: _____	☐ Individual adult	☐ No
Last visit: _____	☐ Individual child	☐ Yes:
Session Freq:	☐ Couple	
☐ Once week ☐ Every other week ☐ Other: _____	☐ Family ☐ Group:	
Expected Length of Treatment:		**If Child/Adolescent:** Is family involved?
_____		☐ Yes ☐ No

Patient Referrals and Professional Contacts

Has contact been made with social worker?

☐ Yes ☐ No: explain: _____ ☐ NA

Has client been referred for physical assessment?

☐ Yes ☐ No evidence for need

Has client been referred for psychiatric assessment?

☐ Yes; cl agree ☐ Yes, cl disagree ☐ Not rec.

Has contact been made with treating physicians or other professionals?
☐ Yes ☐ No ☐ NA

Has client been referred for social/legal services?
☐ Job/training ☐ Welfare/food/housing ☐ Victim services
☐ Legal aid ☐ Medical ☐ Other: _____ ☐ NA

Anticipated forensic/legal processes related to treatment:
☐ No ☐ Yes _____

Has client been referred for group or other support services?
☐ Yes ☐ No ☐ NA

Client social support network includes:
☐ Supportive family ☐ Supportive partner ☐ Friends ☐ Religious/spiritual organization ☐ Supportive work/social group ☐ Other: _____

Anticipated effects treatment will have on others in support system (parents, children, siblings, significant others, etc.):

_____

Is there anything else client will need to be successful?

_____

Client Sense of Hope: Little 1--------------------10 High

Expected Outcome and Prognosis
☐ Return to normal functioning
☐ Expect improvement, anticipate less than normal functioning
☐ Maintain current status/prevent deterioration

Evaluation of Assessment/Client Perspective
How was assessment method adapted to client needs?

_____

Age, culture, ability level, and other diversity issues adjusted for by:

_____

Systemic/family dynamics considered in following ways:

_____

Describe actual or potential areas of client-therapist agreement/disagreement related to the above assessment:

_____

Completing a Clinical Assessment

Identifying Information

Generally, a client number is used instead of a name to maximize client confidentiality. Abbreviations are used to refer to the client and significant others:

AF: Adult Female
AM: Adult Male
CF: Child Female
CM: Child Male

These abbreviations can be followed by each person's age. Other important identifiers are profession or grade in school, ethnicities, and languages spoken. These provide a basic introduction to the client.

Presenting Problem

Presenting problems include what clients identify as the initial problems when they enter therapy, including the primary reason they are seeking treatment (e.g., a child's behavior problem) as well as secondary issues they may more casually mention (e.g., marital tension). The list of presenting problems provides a quick overview of the client's and/or family's current difficulties.

Mental Status Exam

A mental status exam is used to develop a comprehensive overview of clients' mental health functioning to support diagnoses. Designed for family therapists, it begins with interpersonal issues to focus attention on the *scope of practice*—what the law allows a licensed family therapist to do. The law allows therapists to help people with interpersonal functioning. Family therapists should always include something in this category to ensure they are practicing within their scope of practice. The final section of this chapter defines the common terms used in a mental status exam.

Diagnosis

Although this book cannot teach the full diagnosis process, this section is included to provide an introduction for those new to the process and a review for those already familiar.

The Five-Axis System

Mental health practitioners use a five-axis system for diagnosis:

- **Axis I:** Clinical disorders that are the focus of treatment, including developmental and learning disorders; may include primary plus additional diagnoses

- **Axis II:** Underlying or pervasive conditions, including personality disorders, defensive mechanisms, and mental retardation

- **Axis III:** Medical conditions and disorders (indicate if by "client report" or if diagnosed by another medical professional)

- **Axis IV:** Psychosocial stressors and environmental conditions that may be contributing to condition and/or its treatment, such as:
  - Economic or housing problems
  - Problems accessing health care
  - Legal situations
  - Social, school, and/or occupational issues

- **Axis V:** Global Assessment of Function (GAF) score: a score from 0 to 100 indicating the level of functioning:
  - 70 and above: Indicates adaptive coping, with higher scores indicating greater mental health
  - 60–69: Mild symptoms; *most third-party payers require that a client's level of functioning be 69 or below to be a reimbursable medical expense (hint: therapists generally diagnose lower than this when a client is starting outpatient treatment)*
  - 50–59: Moderate symptoms
  - 40–49: Severe symptoms
  - 39 and below: Significant impairment that generally requires hospitalization and intensive treatment

GARF: Global Assessment of Relational Functioning

On Axis V, practitioners can also record other indicators of functioning, such as the GARF scale, which is commonly used by family therapists to assess relational functioning and may or may not correlate with the GAF score. The *Diagnostic and*

Statistical Manual (DSM) includes a detailed description of the GARF and other scales for psychosocial functioning (American Psychiatric Association, 1994).

Contextual Factors

Before making a diagnosis, therapists should consider contextual factors, such as age, ethnicity, family dynamics, language, religion, economic issues, sexual orientation, trauma history, addictions, and cognitive ability. For example, often a woman from a culture that values emotional expression and who has a history of trauma will present with histrionic features that are more a function of cultural communication than an actual personality disorder; these symptoms generally dissipate as trauma is treated. Taking such issues into consideration improves the accuracy of diagnosis.

Making a Diagnosis

When making a diagnosis, clinicians consult the *DSM,* or *Diagnostic and Statistical Manual;* each diagnosis requires that a certain number of criteria be met, and these criteria should be reflected in the mental status exam. In addition, medical causes, trauma, and substance abuse should be ruled out. Depending on the diagnosis, therapists may want to refer out for an evaluation for medication; diagnoses with symptoms that typically warrant referral include depression, anxiety, mania, psychosis, trauma, disordered eating, alcohol and substance abuse, and sleep disorders.

Medical Necessity

Most third-party payers require that therapists document that the condition meets the criteria for medical necessity and that there is significant impairment in functioning, a high probability of significant impairment, and/or probable developmental arrest in children. Areas of impairment may include the following:

- Daily activities (e.g., getting out of bed, feeding self, chores)
- Social relationships (e.g., maintaining satisfying marriage, friendships)
- Health (e.g., maintaining physical health)
- Work and school (e.g., able to maintain employment, complete school tasks)
- Living arrangement (e.g., having a place to live)

Risk Management

Therapists also assess for crisis and danger in clinical assessment, including a client's potential for suicide, homicide, substance abuse (past, present, or by others), and sexual or physical abuse history. If a client has any indicators of potential problems in these areas, therapists should assess for indicators of safety, generate a safety plan, and document the legal actions taken.

Suicidality and Homicidality

Clients who present with depression and hostility for others should be assessed for suicidal and/or homicidal intentions. Each state has different laws governing when and how a therapist can take action to protect clients, the public, and property from danger. In most states, therapists must take some form of action to protect clients who have a clear plan and intent for killing themselves or others; when there is no clear plan or intent, therapists are still ethically bound to create safety plans in case the situation escalates. The following are various indicators of degrees of danger:

- **No indication:** No verbal, nonverbal, or situational indications of danger.

- **Denial:** Client was asked and denies suicidal and/or homicidal intent.

- **Passive Ideation:** Client "would like to be dead" or "have the other person gone" but denies any plan or willingness to kill self or another.

- **Active Ideation:** Client thinks about killing self or others.

- **Attempt:** Client has attempted to kill self or another at any point; a significant risk factor.

- **Family History:** A family history of suicide is another significant risk factor.

Substance Abuse

The therapist can use pen-and-paper tests such as the MAST (see previous discussion) as well as verbal and written self-reports to assess for alcohol and substance abuse. Because often these issues are not fully revealed early in treatment, therapists should routinely and frequently inquire about substance and alcohol use throughout treatment, especially when they see lack of progress.

Child Abuse

Four types of child abuse are generally outlined in state child abuse laws:

- **Sexual Abuse:** Inappropriate sexual contact with a minor by an adult or another minor; may or may not be consensual (defined by state laws).

- **Physical Abuse:** Hitting, beating, kicking, or otherwise inflicting bodily harm by hand, with an object, and/or other means (e.g., locking child in enclosed space); includes most forms of spanking in many states.

- **Emotional Abuse:** Inflicting severe psychological harm, such as fear of death, physical intimidation, and intense rejection and disapproval.

- **Neglect:** Failing to provide for basic physical needs, such as sufficient food, clothing, shelter, and medicine.

In most states all forms of child abuse except emotional abuse legally require a child abuse report to state authorities (e.g., child protective services, sheriff, police).

Elder and Dependent Adult Abuse

Most states have laws for reporting elder and dependent adult abuse and neglect, which includes the categories for child abuse as well as *financial abuse:* illegal or unauthorized use of a person's property, money, or pension.

Other Risk Factors

- **Anorexia, Bulimia, and Other Eating Disorders:** Eating disorders are some of the most dangerous mental health disorders; anorexia is frequently cited as having the highest fatality rate of any mental health diagnosis. These disorders almost always require coordinated care with a medical professional.

- **Cutting and Self-Harm:** Cutting, burning, and other forms of self-harm are used to cope with emotional pain; therapists need to interview clients to determine if there is suicidal intent or if the self-harm is intended for another purpose, such as relieving emotional pain.

- **Criminal or Legal History:** Criminal or legal history is helpful in assessing the potential for harm and danger.

Indicators of Safety

In addition to assessing for danger, therapists should assess for the potential for safety: what factors are in place to keep the client safe? The balance of these two potentials helps therapists determine the overall level of crisis. The following indicators suggest safety:

Indicators of Safety

- At least one outside support person
- Is able to cite reasons to live and/or not harm others (e.g., "I couldn't do it because of my kids")

- Hope; goals for future
- Is willing to dispose of dangerous items (e.g., gun)
- Agrees to reduce contact with people who make the situation worse
- Agrees to safety plan and develops an alternative to harming self or other

Safety Plans

Safety plans should be developed for any situation in which potential risk is identified, such as passive suicidal ideation, history of cutting, and history of abuse. These plans should be tailored to each client's individual needs using combinations of the following components as well as unique elements for each client:

Safety Plan Components

- Verbal or written agreement or contract to not harm themselves or others
- A card with emergency contact numbers for local hotlines, supportive friends, therapist's emergency contact number, etc.
- Working with medical professionals who prescribe medication to reduce crisis potential
- Specific action plan as to who to call and what to do if a crisis begins to arise
- Identifying tasks to calm self, such as journaling and exercising, at low levels of precrisis stress
- Specific daily or weekly activities to reduce overall level of stress and triggers for crisis

Scaling for Safety

I have developed scaling for safety, a variation of solution-oriented scaling questions (O'Hanlon & Weiner-Davis, 1989), to help stabilize crisis situations with clients who are dealing with severe depression, suicidal ideation, cutting, eating disorders, substance abuse, and violence. Using a white board, I have clients define both emotionally and behaviorally a "1" when things are good, a "5" when things are neutral or okay, and a "10" for the crisis point of a dangerous activity. I then have them describe emotions and behaviors for each point on the scale (or if there is limited time, from 5 to 9), looking for the point at which they are relatively able to take action, generally a 7. Then we develop a realistic safety plan for what to do when they reach a 7, detailing what the clients will do, whom they will call, and so forth. If clients engage in the dangerous behavior after the plan is in place, it should be revised to take action at a lower level on the scale. For most clients, this is specific and realistic enough to prevent them from getting close to the crisis behavior.

The following form can be used for this technique:

SCALING FOR SAFETY FORM

	BEHAVIORS AND ACTIONS	THOUGHTS AND FEELINGS
10: Crisis/Dangerous Act Occurs		
9		
8		
7		
6		

(continued)

SCALING FOR SAFETY FORM *(continued)*

	BEHAVIORS AND ACTIONS	**THOUGHTS AND FEELINGS**
5: Doing/Feeling OK		
4		
3		
2		
1: Feeling Great		

- Number at which I feel I still have enough control to easily enact safety plan: _____
- Top 5 warning signs that I have hit #_____.
- 5 things I can do when I hit #_____.

Commitment to Treatment

In cases involving suicide, Rudd, Mandrusiak, and Joiner (2006) recommend obtaining a commitment to treatment agreement rather than a no-harm contract, which although standard practice has no empirical support. In a no-harm contract, clients agree not to harm themselves and to contact emergency services when they feel in danger of doing so. In contrast, a commitment to treatment is an agreement between the client and therapist in which the client agrees to commit to the treatment process. The commitment involves three elements:

1. It identifies the roles, obligations, and expectations of both the therapist and the client in treatment.
2. The client promises to communicate openly about all aspects of treatment, including suicidal thoughts and plans.
3. The client promises to use agreed-upon emergency resources during a crisis that might threaten the client's ability to fulfill his/her commitment to treatment (e.g., a crisis during which the client contemplates suicide).

Rudd et al. (2006) believe that obtaining a commitment to treatment provides a more useful clinical intervention than a no-harm contract because it is a more hopeful and therapeutically useful framework for both client and therapist, clearly outlining each person's responsibilities and encouraging open communication. Rather than emphasizing *not* committing suicide, the focus is on *committing* to meaningfully participate in psychotherapy treatment.

Case Management

Case management is a collaborative process of working with clients to develop a comprehensive plan of care that takes into account the resources and services necessary to ensure a successful treatment outcome. Therapists rendering mental health services must develop treatment plans (see Chapter 4) that detail how they plan to address the client's presenting problems as part of standard practice. In addition, they need to "think outside of the therapy room" to coordinate care with other professionals, advocate for clients, and help clients identify and access necessary resources.

Common Case Management Activities

- Contacting and coordinating care with client's social workers
- Referring client for a medical assessment to rule out medical causes and/or exacerbating conditions

- Referring client for a psychiatric evaluation for diagnosis and/or prescription for psychotropic medication
- Contacting treating physician regarding mental health treatment
- Referring client for social services such as job training, welfare, housing, victim services, and legal assistance
- Referring client for legal and/or forensic services (e.g., custody evaluations)
- Referring client for group counseling and/or psychoeducational classes (e.g., parenting classes)
- Helping client connect with new or existing social supports, such as religious groups, friends, and family
- Considering the effects of treatment on significant others in the system (e.g., the effect of treating substance dependence on the family)
- Identifying any unique needs the client has to be successful (e.g., transportation, safe place to exercise, a computer)

Evaluation of Assessment

The final section of the clinical assessment encourages therapists to reflect on how they have adapted the assessment to fit the client's unique needs, including diversity factors, effects of treatment on the family system, and areas of client-therapist agreement and disagreement. Considering these factors helps therapists develop a plan that is likely to succeed and also helps identify potential pitfalls.

Communicating with Other Professionals
DSM-ese

Perhaps one of family therapy's most unique contributions to the field of mental health is the concept of learning to speak your client's language. Rooted in communications theory, family therapists from the beginning have emphasized the importance of delivering messages in a way that the audience can receive it. Originally, this insight was applied to clients and later to help therapists work with diverse clients from different backgrounds, age groups, and social classes. As the field has become more integrated into formalized mental health services, it has become increasingly important to learn how to speak with other medical and mental health practitioners. Therefore, family therapists must learn to speak the language of other professionals to effectively work with the larger system that is involved with the client's care.

When speaking to medical doctors and psychiatrists involved in a patient's care, therapists need to speak their language, or "DSM-ese," even if this is not the language they use to conceptualize the case. It is much like learning to speak a foreign language. In the beginning, therapists must clumsily translate from one language to another in their heads. With time and practice, they learn to actually think in the foreign language and speak more fluidly and eloquently, expressing more and more complex ideas. As with any foreign language, it often helps to "go abroad" and spend time living in an environment where the language is spoken: inpatient, intensive outpatient, county mental health, and similar settings.

DSM-ese is a technical language whose preferred vocabulary is found in its dictionary, the DSM-IV-TR (*Diagnostic and Statistical Manual, 4th Edition, Text Revision*). It is not hard to learn but can seem too dry and boring for most therapists. If you like the warm-fuzzy feel, you will need to shift gears to get into the mood, which should remind you of your math and science classes more than English and history. To speed up the process of learning how to speak DSM-ese, just memorize the following four principles:

- **Use DSM Symptom Language:** Rather than use vernacular descriptions of client symptoms, DSM-ese describes the symptoms that are the foundation for making diagnoses:
  - Panic attack (rather than "nervous breakdown")
  - Depressed mood (rather than "feeling down")
  - Irritability (rather than "feeling upset")

- **Use Behavioral Descriptions:** When symptoms can be described in more detail using behavioral description, the behavioral description should be added.
  - Yells at partner (rather than "gets angry")
  - Loss of interest in hobbies (rather than "doesn't care anymore")
  - Loses focus on homework after 15 minutes (rather than "doesn't pay attention")

- **Include Duration of Symptoms:**
  - Depressed mood for 3 months
  - Hypomanic episode for 3 days
  - Auditory hallucinations reported since age 14

- **Include Frequency of Symptoms:**
  - Tantrums 3–4 times per week for past year
  - Violent outburst every 1–2 months for past 3 years
  - Bingeing and vomiting 2 times per week for past 6 months

By simply using symptom and behavioral descriptors with frequency and duration, therapists can quickly achieve fluency in DSM-ese and improve their communication with other professionals. The following comprehensive list of the symptoms and mental status terms provides a good starting place for learning the language of clinical assessment.

Mental Status Terms

Interpersonal Issues

- *Conflict:* Frequent arguments and conflict with one or more person.
- *Enmeshment:* Boundaries with one or more persons are diffuse, not allowing for significant sense of independence (e.g., needing the other to always agree to feel okay; unable to tolerate differences with significant others; feelings easily hurt and/or easily feels rejected).
- *Isolation/Avoidance:* Avoids social contact to manage difficult feelings; reports actively isolating self or feeling isolated; reports few social contacts.
- *Emotional Disengagement:* Clients are in a relationship but lack meaningful emotional connection with one or more significant persons in their life.

Common Mood Descriptors

- *Mood Versus Affect:* Mood is how a person reports feeling inside; affect is the outer expression of emotion.
- *Depressed:* Feeling of sadness and unhappiness; "blue," "down."
- *Hopeless:* Feeling as though there is no possibility of a good future.
- *Fearful:* Concerns about a specific negative event happening.
- *Anxiety:* Generalized worry about unspecified or vague negative events happening.
- *Angry:* Feeling indignant or wronged about a specific happening.
- *Irritability:* Generalized feelings of anger or upset without a specific object of anger; angry reactions are easily triggered.
- *Manic:* Unusually energetic feelings of elation, euphoria, or irritability.

Common Affect Descriptors

- *Constricted or Restricted:* Emotional expression is restrained but emotions are evident.
- *Blunt or Blunted:* Emotional expression is severely restrained; little emotional reactivity.
- *Flat:* Associated with psychosis and severe pathology; emotional expression is virtually nonexistent.
- *Labile:* Mood vacillates frequently, rapidly, and abruptly.
- *Dramatic:* Expression of emotion is generally overdramatized.

Common Sleep Descriptors

- *Hypersomnia:* Sleeping more than usual.
- *Insomnia:* Unable to get usual amounts of sleep, due to difficulties falling or staying asleep.
- *Disrupted Sleep:* Sleep disturbed by nightmares, night terrors, or other issues.
- *Nightmares:* Dreams that frighten the dreamer; occur during REM sleep.
- *Night Terrors:* A general sense of panic or terror is experienced while sleeping without dream content; the sleeper generally cannot be roused during night terrors, although he/she may scream or act panicked; occur in slow-wave sleep, not REM.

Common Eating Descriptors

- *Anorectic Restriction:* Restrictive eating that characterizes anorexia.
- *Bingeing:* Episodes of uncontrolled overeating.
- *Purging:* Following a binge episode, an attempt to rid body of food by vomiting, overexercising, fasting, or laxative abuse.
- *Body Image Distortion:* Image of body, particularly related to weight, is grossly inconsistent with others' perception and medical weight norms.

Common Anxiety Descriptors

- *Anxiety:* Anticipation of danger, problems, or misfortune that creates uneasiness, tension, and/or somatic symptoms.
- *Chronic Worry:* A specific form of anxiety that involves dwelling on anticipated problems.
- *Panic Attacks:* Discrete periods of intense anxiety or terror that may be characterized by shortness of breath, pounding heart, sense of losing control, or sense of doom; may be unexpected or situationally bound.
- *Dissociation:* Disruption in integration of consciousness, memory, identity, and/or perception; may come on suddenly or gradually.
- *Phobias:* Persistent, irrational fears of specific objects or situations.
- *Obsessions:* Intrusive and recurrent thoughts, impulses, or images that cause marked distress.
- *Compulsions:* Repetitive behaviors or mental acts (counting, praying, etc.) that one is driven to perform to reduce some form of distress; generally the act is not realistically related to the distress.

Common Psychotic Descriptors

- *Hallucinations:* Sensory perceptions (sight, sound, touch, smell, or taste) that have no external stimuli; perceptions are experienced as real.
- *Delusions:* False beliefs based on an incorrect inference about external reality that is rigidly maintained despite substantial evidence to the contrary. May be bizarre (considered culturally implausible) or nonbizarre.

- *Paranoia:* Suspicion that one is being harassed or persecuted with little corroborating evidence; less severe than delusion.
- *Loose Associations:* Thought disorder characterized by frequent derailment from topic of conversation, jumping from thought to thought often triggered by a "loose" connection to a word or phrase.

Common Motor Activity Descriptors

- *Low Energy:* Little movement or energy behind movement.
- *Restless:* Excessive movement associated with emotional or physical discomfort.
- *Agitated:* Excessive activity associated with inner tension or frustration.
- *Hyperactive:* Excessive motor activity, such as fidgeting or moving about; not necessarily associated with tension or discomfort.

Common Thought Descriptors

- *Poor Concentration or Attention:* Unable to sustain the attention expected for the developmental level.
- *Denial:* Unable or refuses to acknowledge clearly evident problems that most others in the situation identify as problems.
- *Self-Blame:* Tendency to blame self for things that are outside of personal control and/or that others hold greater responsibility for.
- *Other-Blame:* Tendency to blame others for things that are primarily a personal responsibility.
- *Insightful:* Able to articulate insight into personal behaviors and emotions even if unable to behave consistently with insight.
- *Poor Insight:* Unusually great difficulty identifying one's own thoughts, feelings, and motivations.
- *Impaired Decision Making:* Pattern of making decisions that result in negative consequences for self and others.
- *Tangential:* Tendency to make comments that move conversation away from original topic to a tangentially or loosely related topic; typically done when discussing a difficult subject.

ONLINE RESOURCES

Beck Depression Inventory (BDI) and related inventories

    www.harcourtassessment.com

Michigan Alcoholic Screening Test (MAST)

    Test is available for free download at
    www.ncadd-sfv.org/symptoms/mast_test.html

Minnesota Multiphasic Personality Inventory (MMPI-2)

    www.pearsonassessments.com

National Consensus Statement on Recovery: US Department of Health and Human Services

    www.mentalhealth.samhsa.gov/publications/allpubs/sma05-4129

Outcome Questionnaire

    More information at www.oqmeasures.com

Symptom Checklist 90

    www.pearsonassessments.com tests/scl90r.htm

REFERENCES

American Psychiatric Association. (1994). *Diagnostic and statistical manual for mental disorders* (4th ed. Text Revision). Washington, DC: Author.

Anderson, H. (1997). *Conversations, language, and possibilities.* New York: Basic Books.

Fisher, D. B., & Chamberlin, J. (2004, March). Consumer-directed transformation to a recovery-based mental health system. Downloaded August 16, 2008 from www.mentalhealth.samhsa.gov/publications/allpubs/NMH05-0193/default.asp

Gadamer, H. (1975). *Truth and method.* New York: Seabury.

Gergen, K., Anderson, H., & Hoffman, L. (1996). Is diagnosis a disaster? A constructionist trialogue. In F. Kaslow (Ed.), *Relational diagnosis.* New York: Wiley.

Gottman, J. M. (1999). *The marriage clinic: A scientifically based marital therapy.* New York: Norton.

Haarakangas, K., Seikkula, J., Alakare, B., & Aaltonen, J. (2007). Open dialogue: An approach to psychotherapuetic treatment of psychosis in Northern Finland. In H. Anderson & D. Gehart (Eds.), *Collaborative therapy: Relationships and conversations that make a difference* (pp. 221–233). New York: Brunner/Routledge.

Keeney, B. P. (1983). *Aesthetics of change.* New York: Guilford.

O'Hanlon, W. H., & Weiner-Davis, M. (1989). *In search of solutions: A new direction in psychotherapy.* New York: Norton.

Onken, S. J., Craig, C., Ridgway, P., Ralph, R. O., & Cook, J. A. (2007). An analysis of the definitions and elements of recovery: A review of the literature. *Psychiatric Rehabilitation Journal, 31,* 9–22.

Ralph, R. (2000). *Review of the recovery literature: Synthesis of a sample recovery literature 2000.* National Association for State Mental Health Program Directors. Downloaded September 2, 2008 from www.bbs.ca.gov/pdf/mhsa/resource/recovery/recovery_oriented_resources.pdf

Ramon, S., Healy, B., & Renouf, N. (2007). Recovery from mental illness as an emergent concept and practice. *Australia and the UK International Journal of Social Psychiatry, 53*(2), 108–122.

Repper, J., & Perkins, R. (2006). *Social inclusion and recovery: A model for mental health practice.* Oxford, UK: Bailliere Tindall.

Rudd, M. D., Mandrusiak, M., & Joiner, T. E., Jr. (2006). The case against no-suicide contracts: Commitment to Treatment Statement as a practice alternative. *Journal of Clinical Psychology in Session, 62,* 243–251.

Seikkula, J. (2002). Open dialogues with good and poor outcomes for psychotic crises: Examples from families with violence. *Journal of Marital and Family Therapy, 28*(3), 263–274.

Selvini Palazzoli, M., Boscolo, L., Cecchin, G., & Prata, G. (1978). *Paradox and counterparadox.* New York: Jason Aronson.

U.S. Department of Health and Human Services. (2004). *National consensus statement on mental health recovery.* Downloaded August 26, 2008 from www.mentalhealth.samhsa.gov/publications/allpubs/sma05-4129

Watzlawick, P., Weakland, J., & Fisch, R. (1974). *Change: Principles of problem formation and problem resolution.* New York: Norton.

White, M., & Epston, D. (1990). *Narrative means to therapeutic ends.* New York: Norton.

SAMPLE CLIENT INFORMATION FORM

Welcome to our counseling center. We look forward to providing you with excellent and efficient counseling services. Please take a few minutes to fill out this form. The information will help us better understand your situation as well as how best to help you get your life back on track. Please note: the information is confidential and will not be released to anyone without your written permission.

Today's Date (Intake Date): _____

Type of services being sought *(Check all that apply):*
☐ Individual adult ☐ Individual child ☐ Marital/couple ☐ Family

Referral Source: ☐ School ☐ Another client ☐ Ad ☐ Friend/relative ☐ Court/probation ☐ Self ☐ Other

Name of person filling out application: _____

Address: _____

City: _____ Zip: _____

Home phone: _____ Messages: ☐ Okay machine ☐ Okay other resident ☐ Quiet

Mobile: _____ Messages: ☐ Okay machine ☐ Quiet

Work phone: _____ Messages: ☐ Okay ☐ Quiet

May we send material/information to your home? ☐ Yes ☐ No

Second Household (if applicable):

Name: _____

Address: _____

City: _____ Zip: _____

Home phone: _____ Messages: ☐ Okay machine ☐ Okay other resident ☐ Quiet

Mobile: _____ Messages: ☐ Okay machine ☐ Quiet

Work phone: _____ Messages: ☐ Okay ☐ Quiet

May we send material/information to your home? ☐ Yes ☐ No

Names of individuals living in the primary household (Please check those who are attending counseling): *C=Caucasian; L-C=Latino/Chicano; AfA=African-American; AsA=Asian-American; NA=Native American; O=Other*

☑	LAST, FIRST NAME	RELATION	BIRTH DATE	EMPLOYMENT/SCHOOL & GRADE	ETHNICITY
√		Self			C/L-C/AfA/AsA/NA/O

☑	Last, First Name	Relation	Birth date	Employment/School & Grade	Ethnicity
					C/L-C/AfA/AsA/NA/O
					C/L-C/AfA/AsA/NA/O
					C/L-C/AfA/AsA/NA/O
Additional Household Members/Second Household/Children Outside the Home					
					C/L-C/AfA/AsA/NA/O
					C/L-C/AfA/AsA/NA/O
					C/L-C/AfA/AsA/NA/O
					C/L-C/AfA/AsA/NA/O

Sources of Stress: What are the primary concerns that bring you here?

1. _____

2. _____

3. _____

What is the most important thing you think your counselor should know about these concerns?

_____

_____

_____

Personal and Family Strengths and Resources:

Please indicate the strengths that you and others in your family have (write in names below).

Strength/Resource	Self			
Is willing to come to therapy				
Gets along well with friends and most family members				
Sets goals and works toward them				
Has at least one close friend or support person				
Handles disappointment relatively well				

(continued)

(continued)

STRENGTH/RESOURCE	Self			
Manages anger productively				
Generally enjoys life and has favorite activities				
Generally feels good about self and decisions				
Has an activity or spiritual practice for coping with stress				

List the people, activities, groups, and hobbies that are supportive to you/your family:

_____

_____

Struggles: Is anyone in the family struggling with the following? √ **Check all that apply;** ○ **Circle primary concern**

Complete for Children

☐ Parent/child conflict ☐ Partner violence/abuse ☐ School failure
☐ Couple concerns ☐ Sexual abuse/rape ☐ Truancy runaway
☐ Anger issues ☐ Alcohol/drug concerns ☐ Fighting w/peers
☐ Depression/hopelessness ☐ Loss/grief ☐ Hyperactivity
☐ Anxiety/worry ☐ Legal issues ☐ Wetting/soiling clothing
☐ Communication problems ☐ Eating problems ☐ Isolation/withdrawal
☐ Divorce adjustment ☐ Sexuality/intimacy concerns ☐ Child abuse/neglect
☐ Remarriage adjustment ☐ Suicidal thoughts/attempts ☐ Other: _____
☐ Job problems/ unemployed ☐ Major life changes

Please let us know about your family's background:

Estimated yearly household income: *(Financial information is used to seek outside funding to keep counseling fees affordable)* ☐ Under $10,000 ☐ $10,000–$19,999 ☐ $20,000–$29,999 ☐ $30,000–$39,999 ☐ $40,000–$49,999 ☐ $50,000–$59,999 ☐ $60,000–$69,999 ☐ $70,000 and over
Religion: ☐ Catholic ☐ Protestant: _____ ☐ Jewish ☐ Mormon ☐ Jehovah's Witness ☐ Buddhist ☐ Muslim ☐ Other: _____ **Importance of religion to you/your family:** ☐ Not important ☐ Somewhat important ☐ Very important
Country of origin: ☐ USA ☐ Mexico ☐ Thailand ☐ Laos ☐ China ☐ Other: _____ **Parents' country of origin:** ☐ USA ☐ Mexico ☐ Thailand ☐ Laos ☐ China ☐ Other: _____

Primary language: ☐ English ☐ Spanish ☐ Hmong ☐ Laotian ☐ Chinese
☐ Other: _____
Secondary language: ☐ English ☐ Spanish ☐ Hmong ☐ Laotian ☐ Chinese
☐ Other: _____

Mental Health and Social History:

Has anyone in the family <u>attended therapy previously</u> or is <u>currently in treatment</u>?
☐ No ☐ Yes; if yes, please indicate:

Name	Type of problem/condition	Dates of treatment (if applicable)

Has anyone in the family had <u>emotional difficulties</u> (depression, anxiety, etc.) or <u>suicidal thoughts/attempts?</u>
☐ No ☐ Yes; if yes, please indicate:

Name	Type of problem/condition	Dates of treatment (if applicable)

Has anyone in the family been a *victim* or *perpetrator* of <u>child abuse</u> (physical, sexual, emotional, neglect), <u>domestic violence</u>, <u>rape</u> or other <u>violent act</u>?
☐ No ☐ Yes; if yes, please indicate:

Name	Description of abuse/trauma

Does/has any family member have/had trouble with <u>alcohol or other substances</u>?
☐ No ☐ Yes; if yes, please indicate:

Name	Substance used/frequency/amount

Has anyone in the family been involved with the <u>legal system</u> (probation, parole, jail, prison, DUI)?
☐ No ☐ Yes; if yes, please indicate:

Name	Reason	Outcome

(continued)

(continued)

Medical History:

Is anyone in the family being treated for a <u>medical problem</u>(s) and/or <u>disability</u>?

Name   Condition   Medication

_____

_____

_____

List physician(s) currently treating family members: _____

_____

What are your goals for counseling?

1. _____

2. _____

3. _____

Thank you for taking the time to complete this form! This information will help us understand your situation better and will allow us to assist you in reaching your goals as quickly as possible.

CLINICAL ASSESSMENT SCORING RUBRIC

The following scoring rubric describes the differences between exemplary, adequate, and deficient clinical assessment. By closely attending to these requirements, you can hone in on what your instructors and supervisors are looking for when they grade your work.

Clinical Assessment Scoring Rubric

Date: _____

Therapist/Intern: _____

Evaluator/Instructor: _____

Level of Clinical Training:

☐ Preclinical training; coursework only

☐ 0–12 months ☐ 12–24 months ☐ 2+ years

Rating Scale

5 = Exceptional: Skills and understanding significantly beyond developmental level

4 = Outstanding: Strong mastery of skills and thorough understanding of concepts

3 = Mastered Basic Skills at Developmental Level: Understanding of concepts/skills evident

2 = Developing: Minor conceptual and skill errors; in process of developing

1 = Deficits: Significant remediation needed; deficits in knowledge/skills

NA = Not Applicable: Unable to measure with given data (do not use to indicate deficit)

	5	4	3	2	1	COMP	SCORE
Identification of Client	Thoughtful identification of IP and all significant others in system; subtle ethnicity, language info; detailed info on age, professional info, school info; proper use of confidential notation.	Completed all info for IP and all significant others, including ethnicity, language, age, professional info, school info; proper use of confidential notation.	Basic IP identification, including confidential client ID, persons treated; proper use of confidential notation.	Minor mistakes and/or vague identification of client(s); did not identify IP; missing or unclear information.	Mistakes, inconsistencies with notation, identification of client; failed to protect client confidentiality.	1,3,2 1,5,3 5,3,2	☐ NA
Presenting Problem	Thoughtful identification of presenting problems; evidence of sophisticated assessment and insight into systemic dynamics; sensitive to individual, family, child, community, cultural factors.	Clear identification of presenting problems; evidence of thorough assessment and awareness of systemic dynamics; sensitive to individual, family, child, community, cultural factors.	Clearly identified presenting problem; demonstrates awareness of systemic dynamics and sensitivity to diversity issues.	Insufficient or inconsistent identification of presenting problem.	No clear presenting problem indicated; problem does not fit with rest of assessment and/or case conceptualization (if applicable).	1,3,1	
Mental Status Exam	Sophisticated, comprehensive assessment; accurate use of diagnostic terminology; assessed all areas; succinct, consistent depiction of mental status that clearly supports diagnosis.	Detailed, accurate use of diagnostic terminology; assessed all areas; develops clear, consistent depiction of mental status.	Accurate use of diagnostic terminology; assessed most areas; depiction of mental status supports diagnosis.	Insufficient information or inconsistencies in assessment; misunderstanding of terms.	Significant problems with assessment; key information missing; does not support diagnosis.	1,2,2 2,1,1	☐ NA

(continued)

(continued)

	5	4	3	2	1	COMP	SCORE
Diagnosis	Sophisticated 5 axis diagnosis with behavioral identification of all required indicators; all codes correct; subtle attention to culture, age, health, context, comorbid issues; excellent use of assessment instruments.	Detailed 5 axis diagnosis with identification of all indicators; codes correct; attention to culture, age, health, context, comorbid issues; proper use of assessment instruments.	Completed 5 axis diagnosis with sufficient justification; most codes correct; attention to culture, age, health, context, comorbid issues; use of assessment instruments as needed.	Missing or incomplete diagnosis or justification; problems with codes; insufficient attention to culture, age, health, context, comorbid issues.	Unsupportable diagnosis, insufficient justification; failed to take into account culture, age, health, context, comorbid issues.	2.1.2 2.1.5 2.1.6 2.3.1 2.3.4	☐ NA
Medical Issues and Medication Referrals	Sophisticated, thorough consideration of medical issues; includes detailed info for medication; referrals reflect sophisticated understanding of meds and possible medical issues.	Thoughtful consideration of medical issues and referrals; includes most of medication info; referrals reflect understanding of medications and possible medical issues.	Evidence that medications and medical issues were considered, most obvious referrals were made.	Evidence that proper referrals were made if necessary; incomplete medication info, client response info, etc.	Missed proper referrals for stated diagnosis.	2.2.5 3.1.3	☐ NA
Risk Assessment	Sophisticated risk assessment for harm to self, others; substance abuse; child, elder abuse; violence; evidence of comprehensive assessment and attention to all details; able to track multiple, related risks.	Thorough risk assessment for harm to self, others; substance abuse; child, elder abuse; violence; evidence of thorough assessment.	Completes risk assessment for all areas: suicide, homicide, substance abuse, and child, elder abuse.	Missing or incomplete assessment in 1 area and/or other minor problems.	Missing or incomplete assessment in 2 or more areas; fails to identify significant risk factors.	2.3.5	☐ NA

Legal/Ethical Action	Sophisticated, professional handling of potential and immediate crises; evidence of thoughtful ethical decision making; demonstrates understanding of laws, ethics; develops safety plans for potential and immediate risks; skillfully makes reports; takes all approp actions.	Proper handling of potential and immediate crises; approp ethical decision making; demonstrates understanding of laws, ethics; develops safety plans when required; makes needed reports; takes approp action.	Proper handling of immediate crises; approp ethical decision making; demonstrates understanding of laws, ethics; develops safety plans when required; makes needed reports; takes approp action.	Minor problems in taking required legal, ethical action; however, all laws and ethical codes are followed; all risks are essentially managed.	Significant problems handling legal or ethical action, including failing to take action when necessary or taking action when not legally allowed.	3.3.6 3.4.3 5.1.1 5.1.2 5.1.4 5.2.1 5.3.4 5.3.5 5.3.6	☐ NA
Case Management; Referrals	Sophisticated identification of referrals for all parties; all appropriate contacts made; subtle assessment of need for medical, psychiatric, support referral; professionally manages legal and forensic needs; subtle anticipation of effects on extra-therapeutic relationships.	Thoughtful identification of referrals for IP; has made key contacts; thoughtful assessment of need for medical, psychiatric, support referral; manages required legal and forensic needs; thoughtful anticipation of effects on extra-therapeutic relationships.	Identifies key referrals for IP; has made or in process of making contacts; makes standard medical, psychiatric referral; manages required legal and forensic needs; anticipation of effects on extra-therapeutic relationships.	Missing potentially helpful referral, contacts, support opportunities, legal issues, effects on extra-therapeutic relationships.	Missing critical referral and/ or contact; not accessing support network; unrealistic assessment of legal issues, effects on extra-therapeutic relationships.	1.2.3 2.2.4 3.5.2	☐ NA
Prognosis, Modalities, & Frequency	Prognosis, modality choices, and frequency demonstrate sophisticated understanding of behavioral disorders and relational dynamics; clearly follows from foregoing assessment.	Prognosis, modality choices, and frequency demonstrate realistic understanding of behavioral disorders and relational dynamics; supported in foregoing assessment.	Prognosis, modality choices, and frequency appropriate given foregoing assessment.	Prognosis unlikely given information in foregoing assessment. Modality choice and frequency not optimal given foregoing assessment.	Prognosis unrealistic given information in foregoing assessment. Modality choice and/or frequency not appropriate.	1.3.2 2.1.2	☐ NA

(continued)

(continued)

	5	4	3	2	1	COMP	SCORE
Evaluation/Client Perspective	Sophisticated, insightful evaluation of assessment; subtle responsiveness to age, culture, ability, and other diversity issues; subtle attention to systemic factors; sophisticated assessment of ability to account for systemic dynamics and client-therapist agreement on goals/dx.	Thoughtful evaluation of assessment; responsiveness to age, culture, ability, and other diversity issues; thoughtful attention to systemic factors; thoughtful assessment of ability to account for systemic dynamics and client-therapist agreement on goals/dx.	Addresses all areas of evaluation of assessment; attends to most prominent issues related to age, culture, ability, or other diversity issues; attention to systemic factors; assesses ability to account for systemic dynamics and client-therapist agreement on goals/dx.	Missing and/or vague evaluation of assessment; missing information on minor or more subtle issues.	Missing critical factors and/or significant trouble identifying key issues.	2.4.1 2.4.2 2.4.3 2.4.4	☐ NA
Additional Competency (Optional)							☐ NA
Additional Competency (Optional)							☐ NA
Comments:							

Abbreviations: IP = Identified Patient; dx = Diagnosis.

©2007. Diane R. Gehart, Ph.D.

Treatment Planning

Treatment + Plan = ???

It was the first day at my new training site, one of the best in town. During the orientation, my supervisor went over the clinical paperwork that we would need to complete: intake forms, assessments, and treatment plans. Although I had learned about gathering intake and assessment information in my diagnosis class, I had never actually seen a treatment plan. Using sophisticated etymological skills that all graduate students rely on—treatment + plan—I deduced that this document would somehow describe my plans for how to treat the client. But how?

Like many interns, I was too embarrassed to ask and kept my ignorance quiet. I decided that if I could find a sample, I could probably fake it and not have to risk looking ignorant in the eyes of my well-respected supervisor. Thankfully, I was assigned cases handled by previous interns that included this o-so-mysterious document. So, I gathered up as many files as I could and found an uncomfortable yet well-worn seat in a poorly lit corner assigned to interns and tried to crack the code. THAT is how I learned to do treatment plans: secretly and shamefully. Thankfully, because you have this book in your hands, you have the opportunity to learn this once secret art with more dignity—and without a backache.

Just in case you missed it, the moral of the above story is to talk with your supervisors—no matter how brilliant they may appear—and do not be afraid to ask what seems like a silly question. Trust me, the chair was not the hardest part of learning treatment planning on my own.

Step 3: Selecting a Path

After completing your case conceptualization and clinical assessment, you are ready to develop a plan for addressing the problems you have identified in these other two documents. Treatment plans are fun: they are filled with hopes and dreams. In creating them, you have tremendous freedom but also the burden of responsibility. Because numerous good plans can be developed for any one client, you may choose which theory and techniques are the best fit for a specific client, the specific problem, and the particular therapist-client relationship. As the therapist, you are responsible for shepherding an effective process and selecting a plan that is most likely to help the client; this plan should be based on clinical experience, current research, and standards of practice.

A Brief History of Mental Health Treatment Planning

The history of treatment planning in the field of marriage and family therapy is relatively short. The original theorists did not talk or write about treatment planning, and, in fact, if you search the literature you will find no form that would be accepted by a managed care company or county mental health agency for payment. If the approved approach to treatment planning did not come from the field of family therapy or even mental health more broadly, where did it come from? The short answer: the medical field.

Symptom-Based Treatment Plans

The type of treatment planning that most marriage and family therapists must complete to receive third-party payment and to maintain standard practice of care in the 21st century is derived from the medical model. Jongsma and his colleagues (Dattilio & Jongsma, 2000; Jongsma, Peterson, & Bruce, 2006; Jongsma, Peterson, McInnis, & Bruce, 2006; O'Leary, Heyman, & Jongsma, 1998) have developed the most extensive models. Called *symptom-based treatment plans,* these documents focus solely on clients' medical symptoms. Most publications on treatment planning use a similar symptom-based model (Johnson, 2004; Wiger, 2005). But although these plans are relevant to those in the medical community, they do not help therapists conceptualize treatment in the most useful ways.

For example, if a parent brings a child to therapy who is having tantrums and the therapist develops a plan around the presenting problem (e.g., "reduce child's tantrums to less than one per week") and proceeds to deal directly with the tantrums without thoroughly conceptualizing the case, treatment is less likely to be successful. A systemic assessment will typically reveal that marital and/or parenting issues are contributing to the presenting problem, and couples therapy that targets tension in the marriage may actually be the best way to reduce the child's tantrums. The danger of symptom-based treatment planning is that the therapist will underutilize theory, focus on symptoms, and forget to assess the larger picture. Arguably, a good therapist would not do this; however, today's workplace realities include (a) heavy caseloads, (b) pressure to complete diagnosis and treatment plans by the end of the first session, and (c) highly structured paperwork and payment systems, all of which make it hard for a therapist to do a good job. Thus, symptom-based treatment planning, although convenient, may not be the best choice for today's practice environments.

Theory-Based Treatment Plans

Theory-based treatment planning, described by Gehart and Tuttle (2003), uses theory to create more clinically relevant treatment plans than the symptom model offers. Berman (1997) developed a similar approach for traditional psychotherapies. Both models include goals that are informed by clinical theories. However, I found that new trainees confuse theory-based goals and interventions because they use the same language. Furthermore, it is difficult for most students to address diagnostic issues and clinical symptoms in these theory-based plans because the language of these two systems is radically different. The solution was to develop a new, "both/and" model, called the "clinical treatment plan," that draws from the best of theory-based and symptom-based treatment plans and adds elements of measurability.

Clinical Treatment Plans

Clinical treatment plans provide a straightforward, comprehensive overview of treatment. They include the following parts:

- **Introduction:** Defines who is being treated, if medications are being used, and what contextual factors were considered in creating a plan that is sensitive to client needs.

- **Therapeutic Tasks:** Describes treatment tasks that the therapist should perform at the initial, working, and closing phases of therapy. These tasks are informed by theory as well as ethical and legal requirements.

- **Client Goals:** Determines what goals are unique to each client and what behaviors, thoughts, feelings, or interactions will be either increased or decreased as a result of treatment. Client goals are derived from the assessment of the presenting problem and are stated in theory-specific language.

- **Interventions:** Describes, for each goal, two to three interventions for achieving this goal using the therapist's chosen theory.

- **Client Perspective:** Describes areas of client agreement and concern with the outlined plan.

Here is the general treatment plan format. In this form, *TT* refers to "therapeutic task," and *I* refers to "intervention."

TREATMENT PLAN

Therapist: _____   Client ID #: _____

Theory: _____

Primary Configuration: ☐ Individual ☐ Couple ☐ Family ☐ Group _____

Additional: ☐ Individual ☐ Couple ☐ Family ☐ Group: _____

Medication(s): ☐ NA ☐ _____

Contextual Factors considered in making plan: ☐ Age ☐ Gender ☐ Family dynamics

☐ Culture ☐ Language ☐ Religion ☐ Economic ☐ Immigration ☐ Sexual orientation

☐ Trauma ☐ Dual dx/comorbid ☐ Addiction ☐ Cognitive ability

☐ Other: _____

Describe how plan is adapted to contextual factors: _____
_____

I. Initial Phase of Treatment (First 1–3 Sessions)

I.A. Initial Therapeutic Tasks

Therapeutic Relationship

TT1: Develop therapeutic relationship with all members. Note: _____

I1: Intervention: _____

(continued)

(continued)

I. Initial Phase of Treatment (First 1–3 Sessions)

I.A. Initial Therapeutic Tasks

Assessment

TT2: Assess individual, system, and broader cultural dynamics. Note: _____

    I1: Intervention: _____

    I2: Intervention: _____

Goals

TT3: Define and obtain client agreement on treatment goals. Note: _____

    I1: Intervention: _____

Referrals and Crisis

TT4: Identify needed referrals, crisis issues, and other client needs. Note: _____

    I1: Intervention: _____

I.B. Initial Client Goals (1–2 Goals): Manage crisis issues and/or reduce most distressing symptoms.

Goal #1: ☐ Increase ☐ Decrease _____ (personal/relational dynamic) to reduce _____ (symptom).

Measure: Able to sustain _____ for period of _____ ☐ wks ☐ mos with no more than _____ mild episodes of _____ .

    I1: Intervention: _____

    I2: Intervention: _____

II. Working Phase of Treatment (Sessions 2+)

II.A. Working Therapeutic Tasks

Monitor Progress

TT1: Monitor progress toward goals. Note: _____

    I1: Intervention: _____

Monitor Relationship

TT2: Monitor quality of therapeutic alliance as therapy proceeds. Note: _____

    I1: Intervention: _____

II.B. Working Client Goals (2–3 Goals): Target individual and relational dynamics in case conceptualization using theoretical language (e.g., reduce enmeshment, increase differentiation, increase agency in relational narrative, etc.).

Goal #1: ☐ Increase ☐ Decrease _____ (personal/relational dynamic) to reduce _____ (symptom).

Measure: Able to sustain _____ for period of _____ ☐ wks ☐ mos with no more than _____ mild episodes of _____.

   I1: Intervention: _____

   I2: Intervention: _____

Goal #2: ☐ Increase ☐ Decrease _____ (personal/relational dynamic) to reduce _____ (symptom).

Measure: Able to sustain _____ for period of _____ ☐ wks ☐ mos with no more than _____ mild episodes of _____.

   I1: Intervention: _____

   I2: Intervention: _____

Goal #3: ☐ Increase ☐ Decrease _____ (personal/relational dynamic) to reduce _____ (symptom).

Measure: Able to sustain _____ for period of _____ ☐ wks ☐ mos with no more than _____ mild episodes of _____.

   I1: Intervention: _____

   I2: Intervention: _____

III. Closing Phase of Treatment (Last 2+ Weeks)

III.A. Closing Therapeutic Tasks

Termination Plan

   TT1: Develop aftercare plan and maintain gains. Note: _____

   I1: Intervention: _____

III.B. Closing Client Goals: Determined by theory's definition of health.

Goal #1: ☐ Increase ☐ Decrease _____ (personal/relational dynamic) to reduce _____ (symptom).

Measure: Able to sustain _____ for period of _____ ☐ wks ☐ mos with no more than _____ mild episodes of _____.

   I1: Intervention: _____

   I2: Intervention: _____

(continued)

(continued)

IV. Client Perspective

Has treatment plan been reviewed with client? ☐ Yes ☐ No; If no, explain: _____

_____

Describe areas of client agreement and concern: _____

©2007. Diane R. Gehart

Writing Useful Therapeutic Tasks

Therapeutic tasks are generally the easiest part of the treatment plan to develop because they are the most formulaic. Each theory has its own language and interventions for describing how to create a therapeutic relationship, and a good plan should reflect these differences. For example, a Bowen intergenerational therapist focuses on remaining nonreactive to clients, whereas a therapist using experiential family therapy has a more emotionally engaged approach to creating a therapeutic relationship.

Initial Phase

Perhaps not surprisingly, therapists have the most tasks in the initial phase of treatment because this is when they establish the foundation for therapy. Virtually all theories include four therapeutic tasks (TTs) early in therapy, as shown in the form already presented:

> TT1: Establish a therapeutic relationship
> TT2: Assess individual, family, and social dynamics
> TT3: Develop treatment goals
> TT4: Case management: refer for medical/psychiatric evaluation; connect with needed community resources; rule out substance abuse, violence, and medical issues

Although each theoretical approach has different ways to do these four things, the cross-theory similarities make it easy for therapists to conceptualize this early phase of treatment. If problems arise in treatment, therapists can be sure that one of these four initial tasks needs to be readdressed.

Working Phase

In the working phase, the primary task is to keep the ball rolling. As therapy progresses, therapists need to assess whether treatment is effective. Is the client making progress on the identified goals? If not, what might be the reason, and how can therapy be adjusted to accomplish those goals? Family therapists rarely cite "resistance" as a valid reason for lack of progress. Steve de Shazer (1984) declared the "death of resistance," implying that lack of progress cannot be blamed on the client. If initial interventions don't work, the therapist does not need to blame clients or himself/herself and instead should simply focus on figuring out what does work. Similarly, systemic therapists have consistently admonished that, if clients are not progressing, the therapist has not yet developed a useful working hypothesis or found a way to usefully deliver it to clients (Selvini Palazzoli, Boscolo, Cecchin, & Prata, 1978; Watzlawick, Weakland, & Fisch, 1974). In the systemic approach, each "failed" intervention tells the therapist what doesn't work and therefore provides clues as to what might work.

Closing Phase

Simply put, the primary task of the closing phase is for therapists to make themselves unnecessary in clients' lives. During this phase of therapy, therapists work with clients to develop aftercare plans that include identifying (a) what they did to make the changes they have made, (b) how they will maintain their success, and (c) how they will handle the next set of challenges in their lives. Each therapeutic model has different ways of doing this, but there is a cross-theoretical consistency as well as a consistent logic to this task that is useful in most therapeutic situations. When this phase is done well, clients leave therapy feeling better able to handle the inevitable problems that will continue to arise in their lives. As MRI therapist John Weakland reportedly stated, "Clients come in experiencing the same damn problem over and over. Therapy is successful when life is one damn problem after another" (as cited in Gehart & McCollum, 2007, p. 214).

Writing Useful Client Goals

I am going to tell you the truth: writing good client goals is a difficult task. The trick is that they can be written only after one has done a thorough case conceptualization and clinical assessment.

PREPARATORY STEPS TO WRITING USEFUL CLIENT GOALS

Step 1: Complete a thorough case conceptualization (Chapter 2) and clinical assessment (Chapter 3).

Step 2: Identify any crises or pressing issues that need to be managed early in treatment.

Step 3: Identify two to three themes from the case conceptualization and clinical assessment.

Step 4: Identify the long-term theoretical goals from the theory of choice.

The Basic Steps

Step 1: Case Conceptualization and Clinical Assessment

Therapists should use the forms in Chapters 2 and 3 to conduct a thorough assessment.

Step 2: Crises or Pressing Issues

In the clinical assessment, the therapist should have identified crisis issues such as the following:

- Suicidal or homicidal threats
- Potential, current, or past child, dependent adult, or elder abuse
- Current or past domestic or social violence
- Alcohol or substance abuse issues
- Need for an evaluation for medication or other medical issues that could impact treatment
- Eating disorders, self-mutilation, or other danger symptoms that need immediate attention
- Severe depressive, psychotic, or panic episodes or other serious symptoms that need to be stabilized for outpatient treatment

If any of these issues have been identified, they should be addressed in the Initial Client Goals section; if not, the therapist can include an early-stage goal that relates to the presenting problem.

Step 3: Themes from the Case Conceptualization and Clinical Assessment

After completing these two assessments, the therapist steps back and asks the following questions:

- What two to three key patterns emerged in the case conceptualization?
- How do these fit with the clinical assessment?
- What theory do I want to use, and how would it describe these key themes?

Step 4: Long-Term Goals

Some theories, such as structural therapy (Chapter 10), experiential therapies (Chapter 11), and the Bowen intergenerational therapy (Chapter 12), have theoretically defined long-term goals, such as clear interpersonal boundaries, differentiation, or self-actualization. When using such therapeutic models, therapists begin with larger goals in mind and design the middle-phase goals to prepare clients for the closing-phase goals.

The Goal-Writing Process

The hardest part is always writing the goal. There are no clear rules for every situation because each client is unique. However, goal writing has three basic components:

GUIDELINES FOR WRITING USEFUL GOALS

1. **Start with a Key Concept or Assessment Area from the Theory of Choice:** Start with "increase" or "decrease" followed by a description using language from the chosen theory about what is going to change.

2. **Link to Symptoms:** Describe what symptoms will be addressed by changing the personal or relational dynamic.

3. **Use the Client's Name:** Using a name (or equivalent confidential notation) ensures that it is a unique goal rather than a formulaic one.

Anatomy of a Client Goal

"Increase/Decrease" + [individual/relational dynamic] + "to reduce/increase" + [symptom/behavior]

Part A   Part B

Part A gives the therapist a clear focus of treatment that fits with the theory of choice. Part B clearly links the changes in symptoms to the focus of treatment stated in A.

Examples

- *Increase* effectiveness of parental hierarchy between AF and CF *to reduce* frequency of CF's tantrums per week (structural therapy)
- *Reduce and interrupt* pursuer-distancer pattern between AF and AM *to reduce* AF's sense of hopelessness and AM's irritability (systemic therapy)
- *Increase* frequency of social interaction and re-engagement in music and sports hobbies *to increase* periods of positive mood (solution-focused therapy)

Each part has a different function. Part A is most useful to therapists for conceptualizing treatment; Part B is most useful to third-party payers who require a medical model assessment. When therapists write goals that address both A and B, they allow themselves maximum freedom and flexibility to work in their preferred way while also answering the needs of third-party payers.

Initial Phase

During the initial phase of therapy—in most cases the first one to three sessions—client goals generally involve stabilizing crisis symptoms, such as suicidal and homicidal thinking, severe depressive or panic episodes, and poor eating and sleeping patterns; managing child, dependent adult, and elder abuse issues; addressing substance and alcohol abuse issues; and stopping self-harming behaviors such as cutting.

In addition to stabilizing crisis issues, some theories have specific clinical goals that should be addressed in the initial phases. For example, solution-based therapists begin working on clinical symptoms in the first session by setting small, measurable goals toward desired behaviors as well as increasing clients' level of hope (O'Hanlon & Weiner-Davis, 1989).

Working Phase

Working-phase goals address the dynamics that create and/or sustain the symptoms and problems for which clients came to therapy. These are the goals that most interest third-party payers. The secret to writing good working-phase goals is framing them *in the theoretical language* used for conceptualization and then linking this language to the psychiatric symptoms. Using theoretical language enables therapists to document a coherent treatment using their preferred language of conceptualization rather than language that is geared for those prescribing medication.

For example, when a client is diagnosed with depression, many therapists include a goal such as "reduce depressed mood." Let's not kid ourselves: a person does not need a master's degree and thousands of hours of training to come up with such a goal. This medical-model, symptom-based goal does not provide clues as to what the therapist will actually do. Furthermore, all documentation for the case will need to monitor the client's level of depression each week. In contrast, a clinical client goal should address the theoretical conceptualization that will guide the reduction of depression. For example:

- **Structural Therapy:** Reduce enmeshment with children and increase parental hierarchy to reduce episodes of depressed mood.

- **Satir's Communication Approach:** Reduce placating behaviors in marriage and at work to increase congruent communication and positive mood.

- **Narrative Therapy:** Reduce influence of family and societal evaluations of self-worth to increase sense of autonomy and reduce depressed mood.

Each of these goals addresses a client's depressed mood and provides a clear clinical conceptualization and sense of direction, being much more useful to therapists than the medical goal of "reduce depressed mood."

Closing Phase

Closing-phase client goals address (a) larger, more global issues that clients bring to therapy and/or (b) move the client toward greater "health" as defined by the therapist's theoretical perspective. As an example of the former type, clients may present with one issue, perhaps marital discord, and then later in therapy want to address their parenting issues. Similarly, often clients may present with depression or anxiety and in the later phase want to address relationship issues or an unresolved issue with their family of origin. A couple may present with several pressing issues, such as conflict and sexual concerns to be treated in the working phase, and in the later phase want to examine more global issues, such as redefining their identities and relational agreements.

The second type of client goal is driven by the therapist's agenda. Some approaches, such as Bowen intergenerational, humanistic, and structural therapies, have clearly defined theories of health that therapists work toward. Other approaches, such as systemic and solution-focused therapies, have less clearly defined long-term goals and theories. Closing-phase goals often include an agenda item that clients may not have verbalized. For example, differentiation, a long-term goal that is embedded in the theory of Bowenian intergenerational therapy, is too theoretical for clients to present.

Writing Useful Interventions

The final element of treatment plans is including interventions to support each therapeutic task or client goal. Once treatment has been conceptualized and therapeutic tasks and client goals have been identified, identifying useful interventions is generally quite easy. The interventions should come from the therapist's chosen theory and be specific to the client. The following points are guidelines for writing interventions:

GUIDELINES FOR WRITING INTERVENTIONS

- **Use Specific Interventions from Chosen Theory:** Interventions should be clearly derived from the theory used to conceptualize therapeutic tasks and client goals. If an intervention from another theory is integrated, the modifications should be clearly spelled out. For example, genograms can be adapted to solution-focused therapy (Kuehl, 1995).

- **Make Interventions Specific to Client:** Use confidential notation (e.g., AF for adult female and AM for adult male) to make the goal as specific and clear as possible: for example, "Sculpt AF's pattern of pursuing and AM's tendency to withdraw."

- **Include Exact Language When Possible:** Whenever possible, therapists should use the exact question or language they will use to deliver the intervention; for example, "On a scale of 1 to 10, how would you rate your current level of satisfaction in the marriage?"

Client Perspectives

Finally, therapists need to ask themselves, or better yet, their clients, "What do my clients think of this plan?"

- Are these the things the client wants to change?
- Are these interventions and activities that my client would be willing to try?
- Do the goals and interventions "fit" with my client's personality, cultural background, age, gender, values, educational level, cognitive level, and lifestyle?
- Are there areas where the client and I have different ideas about what might be the source of the problem?
- Will we be starting where my client wants to start or where there is the most immediate distress?
- Does the plan make sense to my client?

Considering the client's perspective is crucial to designing an effective plan. Therapists should discuss the plan directly with clients and ensure that there is a shared understanding about the goals, strategies for change, and outcomes. Many agencies have moved to having clients sign the treatment plan to ensure agreement. However, to avoid overwhelming the client with too much jargon, the therapist should probably include only the Client Goals from the treatment plan.

Do Plans Make a Difference?

Of course, therapy rarely goes according to plan. Life happens; new problems arise; original problems lose their importance; new stressors change the playing field. But that does not make plans useless. Treatment plans help therapists in numerous ways:

- They help therapists think through which dynamics need to be changed and how.
- They provide therapists with a clear understanding of the client situation so that they can quickly and skillfully address new crisis issues or stressors.
- They give therapists a sense of confidence and clarity of thought that make it easier to respond to new issues.
- They ground therapists in their theory and in their understanding of how their theory relates to clinical symptoms.

All this is to say, do not be surprised when therapy does not go according to plan: instead, expect it. And know that the time you took to create a treatment plan makes you much better able to respond to the unplanned.

ONLINE RESOURCES

Symptom-Based Treatment Planners

www.jongsma.com

Theory-Based Treatment Planning

www.cengage.com/brookscole/ (search for "treatment plan")

REFERENCES

Berman, P. S. (1997). *Case conceptualization and treatment planning.* Thousand Oaks, CA: Sage.

Datillio, F. M., & Jongsma, A. E. (2000). *The family therapy treatment planner.* New York: Wiley.

de Shazer, S. (1984). The death of resistance. *Family Process, 23,* 11–17.

Gehart, D., & McCollum, E. (2007). Engaging suffering: Towards a mindful re-visioning of marriage and family therapy practice. *Journal of Marital and Family Therapy, 33,* 214–226.

Gehart, D. R., & Tuttle, A. R. (2003). *Theory-based treatment planning for marriage and family therapists: Integrating theory and practice.* Pacific Grove, CA: Brooks/Cole.

Johnson, S. L. (2004). *Therapist's guide to clinical intervention: The 1-2-3's of treatment planning* (2nd ed.). San Diego, CA: Academic Press.

Jongsma, A. E., Peterson, L. M., & Bruce, T. J. (2006). *The complete adult psychotherapy treatment planner* (4th ed.). New York: Wiley.

Jongsma, A. E., Peterson, L. M., McInnis, W. P., & Bruce, T. J. (2006). *The child psychotherapy treatment planner* (4th ed.). New York: Wiley.

Kuehl, B. P. (1995). The solution-oriented genogram: A collaborative approach. *Journal of Marital and Family Therapy, 21,* 239–250.

O'Hanlon, W. H., & Weiner-Davis, M. (1989). *In search of solutions: A new direction in psychotherapy.* New York: Norton.

O'Leary, K. D., Heyman, R. E., & Jongsma, A. E. (1998). *The couples psychotherapy treatment planner.* New York: Wiley.

Selvini Palazzoli, M., Boscolo, L., Cecchin, G., & Prata, G. (1978). *Paradox and counterparadox.* New York: Jason Aronson.

Watzlawick, P., Weakland, J., & Fisch, R. (1974). *Change: Principles of problem formation and problem resolution.* New York: Norton.

Wiger, D. E. (2005). *The psychotherapy documentation primer* (2nd ed.). New York: Wiley.

TREATMENT PLAN SCORING RUBRIC

The following scoring rubric describes the differences between exemplary, adequate, and deficient treatment plans. By closely attending to these requirements, you can hone in on what your instructors and supervisors are looking for when they grade your work.

Treatment Plan Scoring Rubric

Date: _____

Therapist/Intern: _____

Evaluator/Instructor: _____

Level of Clinical Training:

☐ Preclinical training; coursework only

☐ 0–12 months ☐ 12–24 months ☐ 2+ years

Rating Scale

5 = **Exceptional:** Skills and understanding significantly beyond developmental level

4 = **Outstanding:** Strong mastery of skills and thorough understanding of concepts

3 = **Mastered Basic Skills at Developmental Level:** Understanding of concepts/skills evident

2 = **Developing:** Minor conceptual and skill errors; in process of developing

1 = **Deficits:** Significant remediation needed; deficits in knowledge/skills

NA = **Not Applicable:** Unable to measure with given data (do not use to indicate deficit)

	5	4	3	2	1	COMP	SCORE
Choice of Theory and Configuration	Choice of theory and configuration demonstrates sophisticated understanding of research and modalities for presenting problem; thoughtful choice for age, culture, ability, values, etc.; choice demonstrates subtle knowledge of strengths, risks of model.	Choice of theory and configuration demonstrates thoughtful understanding of research and modalities for presenting problem; good choice for age, culture, ability, values, etc.; choice demonstrates knowledge of strengths, risks of model.	Choice of theory and configuration demonstrates understanding of general research and modalities for presenting problem; appropriate choice for age, culture, ability, values, etc.; choice demonstrates general knowledge of strengths, risks of model.	Choices neither particularly appropriate nor inappropriate given research and modality options; no particular attention to age, culture, ability, values, etc.	Inappropriate choice of theory and/or configuration given problem, research, age, culture, ability, values, etc.	1.3.2 3.1.1 4.1.1 4.1.2 4.3.1 6.1.1 6.3.2	☐ NA
Initial TTs: Relationship	Sophisticated understanding of theory's specific form of therapeutic relationship; relates directly to specifics of case; facilitates involvement of appropriate parties	Thoughtful understanding of theory's form of therapeutic relationship; relates to case; facilitates involvement of appropriate parties.	Captures general spirit of theory's form of therapeutic relationship; relates generally to case; facilitates involvement of appropriate parties.	Minor theoretical inconsistencies related to therapeutic relationship and/or no specific application to case; problems attending to client involvement.	Significant problems or theoretical inconsistencies addressing therapeutic relationship.	1.3.3 1.3.6	☐ NA

(continued)

(continued)

	5	4	3	2	1	COMP	SCORE
Initial TTs: Assess	Sophisticated use of theory-specific assessment; uniquely applied to case; sophisticated systemic interviewing; proposed assessments appropriate for age, culture, education, etc.; approp choice of assessment instruments for systems and mental health.	Thoughtful use of theory-specific assessment; directly applied to case; detailed systemic interviewing; proposed assessments appropriate for age, culture, education, etc.; approp choice of assessment instruments for systems and mental health.	Appropriate use of theory-specific assessment; generally applies to case; appropriate systemic interviewing; proposed assessments appropriate for age, culture, education, etc.; approp choice of assessment instruments for systems and mental health.	Minor problems or theoretical inconsistencies with proposed assessments.	Significant problems with proposed assessment; insensitive to age, culture, education, etc.	2.1.4 2.3.2 2.3.3	☐ NA
Initial TTs: Goals	Sophisticated and theoretically consistent approach to developing goals using systemic perspective; demonstrates refined understanding of treating comorbid disorders if applicable; treatment structured to meet unique client/family needs. Subtle attention to diversity.	Thoughtful and theoretically consistent approach to developing goals; demonstrates understanding of treating comorbid disorders if applicable; treatment structured to meet specific client/family needs. Attention to diversity.	Theoretically consistent approach to developing goals; demonstrates understanding of treating comorbid disorders if applicable; treatment structured to meet client/family needs. Attention to diversity.	Approach to setting goals not consistent with theory and/or neglects comorbid issues; treatment could be better tailored to fit client needs.	Inappropriate approach to setting goals; neglects significant comorbid issues.	2.1.3 3.3.4	☐ NA
Initial TTs: Crises	Sophisticated assessment of subtle and major crises and ethical issues, including abuse, substance use, medical issues, threats of harm. Subtle evaluation of risk level.	Thoughtful assessment of minor and major crises and ethical issues, including abuse, substance use, medical issues, threats of harm. Thoughtful evaluation of risk level.	Assessment of major crises and ethical issues, including abuse, substance use, medical issues, threats of harm. Attention to evaluation of risk level.	Minor or potential crises or issues missed; no distinction of level of risk.	Significant crises or issues missed; no distinction of level of risk.	3.3.6 3.4.3	☐ NA

Initial TTs: Referrals	Unusually resourceful and thorough referrals that demonstrate understanding of health care system; assists and advocates for clients in obtaining care; thoughtful referrals to recovery services as needed.	Thoughtful referrals that demonstrate understanding of health care system; assists and advocates for clients in obtaining care; referrals to recovery services as needed.	Appropriate standard referrals that demonstrate basic understanding of health care system; assists and advocates for clients in obtaining care; referrals to recovery services as needed.	Vague referrals and/or does not demonstrate understanding of health care system. Missing a practical but not a life- or health-threatening referral (e.g., legal referrals).	Missing necessary referrals and does not demonstrate understanding of health care system.	1.1.3 3.1.4 3.3.8 3.5.1 □ NA
Initial CGs	Sophisticated, well-chosen initial goals that address specific, immediate client needs; goals clearly prioritized based on research, treatment model, and client needs. Unique to client.	Well-chosen initial goals that address immediate client needs; goals prioritized based on research, treatment model, and client needs. Specific to client.	Appropriate initial goals that address immediate client needs; goals prioritized based on research, treatment model, and client needs.	Minor problems with initial goals; may not be prioritized correctly or specific enough.	Initial goals inappropriate; misses immediate issues.	3.3.2 □ NA
Initial Interventions	Sophisticated choice of interventions; theory-specific and tailored to client; specific interventions to maintain alliance; considers impact on early process.	Thoughtful choice of interventions; theory-specific; clear interventions to maintain alliance; considers impact on early process.	Appropriate choice of interventions; considers impact on early treatment process; interventions to maintain alliance.	Minor problems or vague interventions for early process and/or therapeutic alliance.	Significant problems with initial interventions; theoretically inappropriate or poor fit for client.	4.2.1 □ NA
Working TTs	Sophisticated understanding of therapeutic tasks in working phase that strategically manage progression of therapy to goals.	Thoughtful understanding of therapeutic tasks in working phase that clearly manage progression of therapy to goals.	Appropriate understanding of therapeutic tasks in working phase that help manage progression of therapy to goals.	Minor problems with understanding therapeutic tasks; vague management of progression toward goals.	Significant problems with understanding therapeutic tasks; does not sufficiently manage progression toward goals.	3.3.5 □ NA

(continued)

(continued)

	5	4	3	2	1	COMP	SCORE
Working CGs	Easily measured goals that clearly target major and minor assessed problems and address all systemic issues in CC and symptoms in CA; goals consistent with theory and applied to specific client; goals within scope of competence and practice; goals clearly reflect understanding of content vs. process; goals developed with client.	Measurable goals that target major and minor assessed problems and address systemic issues in CC and symptoms in CA; goals consistent with theory and applied to client; goals within scope of competence and practice; goals reflect understanding of content vs. process; goals developed with client.	Clear goals that target major assessed problems and address systemic issues in CC and symptoms in CA; largely theoretically consistent; goals within scope of competence and practice; goals reflect basic understanding of content vs. process; goals developed with client.	Vague goals and/or theoretically inconsistent yet appropriate goals. No clear distinction between content and process. No evidence of collaboration with client.	Inappropriate goals and/or unclear goals; goals outside scope of competence or practice.	1.4.1 3.3.1 4.2.2 5.3.7	☐ NA
Working Interventions	Sophisticated interventions that support goal achievement; theory-specific and tailored to client; clear and realistic plan of how to conduct sessions; interventions include specific examples of reframing, reflexive questions, generating solutions, empowering clients, psychoed as approp; involve all family members as approp.	Thoughtful interventions that support goal achievement; theory-specific and applied to client; clear plan of how to conduct sessions; interventions include examples of reframing, reflexive questions, generating solutions, empowering clients, psychoed as approp; involve all family members as approp.	Appropriate interventions that largely fit with goal; consistent with theory; plan for how to conduct sessions; interventions, including reframing, reflexive questions, generating solutions, empowering clients, psychoed as approp; involve all family members as approp.	Suggested interventions do not support stated goal; theoretically inconsistent; vague examples of specific interventions.	Poor choice of intervention given stated goals. Poor description of intervention.	2.3.2 3.3.3 4.2.1 4.3.3 4.3.4 4.3.5 4.3.6 4.3.8 4.3.9	☐ NA
Closing TTs	Sophisticated and detailed approach to termination and aftercare plans; theory specific and tailored to fit unique client needs; modifies plan to fit goals as needed; evaluates client outcomes and need to continue.	Thoughtful approach to termination and aftercare plans; theory and client specific; modifies plan to fit goals as needed; evaluates client outcomes and need to continue.	Appropriate termination and aftercare plans; broadly reflects theory and client needs; modifies plan to fit goals as needed; evaluates client outcomes and need to continue.	Minor problems with closing plan; unrealistic or inappropriately adapted for client. Problems with evaluation of outcomes.	Significant problems with closing plan; unrealistic or inappropriately adapted for client. Poor evaluation of outcomes.	3.3.9 4.4.5	☐ NA

Closing CGs	Uniquely constructive approach to termination; sophisticated and uniquely tailored application of model's theory of health in closing goals.	Highly constructive approach to termination; thoughtful and specific application of model's theory of health in closing goals.	Constructive approach to termination; appropriate application of model's theory of health in closing goals.	Minor problems with closing goals; does not attend to theory's model of health.	Significant problems with closing goals; inappropriate or unrealistic.	4.3.11 ☐NA
Closing Interventions	Sophisticated interventions that support goal achievement; theory-specific and tailored to client; clear and realistic plan of how to conduct sessions; interventions include specific examples of reframing, reflexive questions, generating solutions, empowering clients, psychoed as approp; involves all family members as approp.	Thoughtful interventions that support goal achievement; theory-specific and applied to client; clear plan of how to conduct sessions; interventions include examples of reframing, reflexive questions, generating solutions, empowering clients, psychoed as approp; involves all family members as approp.	Appropriate interventions that largely fit with goal; consistent with theory; plan for how to conduct sessions; interventions, including reframing, reflexive questions, generating solutions, empowering clients, psychoed as approp; involves all family members as approp.	Suggested interventions do not support stated goal; theoretically inconsistent; vague examples of specific interventions.	Poor choice of intervention given stated goals. Poor description of intervention.	3.3.3 4.2.1 4.3.3 4.3.4 4.3.5 4.3.6 4.3.8 4.3.9 ☐NA
Overall Understanding of Theory and Technique	Sophisticated understanding of theories and techniques of individual, couple, family, and group psychotherapy; interventions highly consistent with theory and cultural/context factors; rationale for interventions clearly evident.	Thoughtful understanding of theories and techniques of individual, couple, family, and group psychotherapy; interventions consistent with theory and cultural/context factors; clear rationale for interventions.	Basic understanding of theories and techniques of individual, couple, family, and group psychotherapy; interventions generally consistent with theory and cultural/context factors; rationale for interventions.	Some problems with understanding of theories and techniques; interventions often not consistent with theory; vague rationale for interventions.	Significant problems with understanding of theories and techniques; interventions generally not consistent with theory; poor rationale for interventions.	1.1.2 4.4.1 4.5.3 ☐NA

(continued)

(continued)

	5	4	3	2	1	COMP	SCORE
Overall Plan	All details of plan in accordance with practice setting, legal and professional requirements; demonstrates sophisticated understanding of risks, benefits of treatment.	Entire plan in accordance with practice setting, legal and professional requirements; demonstrates thoughtful understanding of risks, benefits of treatment.	General plan in accordance with practice setting, legal and professional requirements; demonstrates appropriate understanding of risks, benefits of treatment.	Minor problems with plan's compliance with practice, legal, and/or professional requirements; does not clearly demonstrate understanding of risks, benefits of treatment.	Significant problems with plan's compliance with practice, legal, and/or professional requirements; does not demonstrate understanding of risks, benefits of treatment.	1.1.4 3.5.3	☐ NA
Client Perspective	Sophisticated and insightful description of areas of agreement and disagreement; significant insight into how client views process.	Detailed description of areas of agreement and disagreement; notable insight into how client views process.	Identifies meaningful areas of agreement and disagreement.	Minor problems identifying areas of agreement and disagreement; little evidence of considering client perspective.	Significant problems identifying areas of agreement and disagreement; no evidence of considering client perspective.	3.2.1	☐ NA
Additional Competency (Optional)							☐ NA
Additional Competency (Optional)							☐ NA
Comments:							

Abbreviations: TT = Therapeutic Task; CG = Client Goal; CC = Case Conceptualization; CA = Clinical Assessment.   ©2007. Diane R. Gehart, Ph.D.

Evaluating Progress in Therapy

Step 4: Evaluating Progress

Critics tease therapists on numerous fronts: we make people lie on couches, repeatedly ask, "How does that make you feel?," encourage omphaloskepsis (the technical term for navel gazing), and often lead crazier lives than our clients. There may or may not be much truth in any of these accusations. But there is one question that therapists need to take seriously: Do I make a difference?

Increasingly, insurance companies, state legislators, and other third-party payers are asking therapists to evaluate progress (Lambert & Hawkins, 2004). This is a daunting task, especially when compared to evaluation in other medical professions. It is relatively easy to determine whether a surgery was successful, physical therapy made a difference, or a medication is working because these are physical things that can be measured with a fair degree of reliability. But when therapists are asked to measure whether depression is getting better, anxiety is less, or a person is worrying less, measurement becomes trickier. If we could x-ray a person's mind or psyche and get an objective measure of levels of mood, that might help. If we could control for all the factors that contribute to a person's feelings and behaviors—including relationship ups and downs, work stress, news headlines, physical illness, and weather—that would also give us a clearer sense of whether we are helping. If we could factor out the biases of our own personalities, histories, and moods, that might also give us a clearer picture. Because these factors are difficult to pinpoint, therapists need to be more creative and thoughtful when measuring progress.

Due to the subtlety of what is being measured, assessing client progress—the fourth step of competent therapy—requires strategy and thought. Therapists have two general options for measuring progress: (a) nonstandardized measures, the client's and therapist's subjective reports of progress; and (b) standardized measures, which track specific psychological variables.

Nonstandardized Evaluations

Nonstandardized evaluations of progress are simply verbal or written descriptions by either the client or the therapist. In either case, the evaluation should be included in the written documentation for the client (his/her "file"). Increasingly, third-party payers require client evaluations of their progress in addition to therapist descriptions. Many insurance companies have shifted from having therapists complete treatment plans and assessments to having clients complete progress checklists to assess if therapy is warranted and effective. Although some research suggests that clients' assessment of their level of functioning is useful, such self-reports are generally considered less reliable than standardized measures.

Pros and Cons

Nonstandardized evaluations have both advantages and disadvantages.

Advantages of Nonstandardized Evaluations

- Financial costs are minimal.
- They can be done every session.
- Including client and therapist perspectives creates greater validity.
- They are easily adapted for diverse clients (see Chapter 2).
- When used weekly, they provide feedback on what is not working so that the therapist can adjust the treatment plan.

Disadvantages of Nonstandardized Evaluations

- They are not as reliable or valid as standardized measures.
- They are difficult to use with children if parents are not there to help provide information (although this is an even bigger problem with standardized instruments).
- They are more difficult to use with persons with severe pathology and/or with those who are unable to accurately recall events between sessions.
- With certain couples or families, data should be collected on paper to get assessments that are not influenced by the comments of other members.

Strategies

There are several easy ways to gather this information:

- Ask clients to assess their progress since the last meeting. The therapist can ask about changes in specific symptoms or progress toward goals (how often were you depressed, how often did you have a panic attack, how often did you binge?).
- Ask clients to rate their own change using solution-focused scaling questions (Chapter 14; Berg & de Shazer, 1993).

Therapists can document both the clients' and their own assessment of progress (a) in a narrative style (using phrases or sentences) or (b) by using a scale.

Examples of Narrative Descriptions

- Client reports an increase in depressive episodes over the week (5 out of 7 days).
- Clients report a decrease in conflict over the week; only one major argument.
- Client reports no change in difficulty sleeping in past week (1–2 hours to fall asleep).

Examples of Scaling

Client Report: Improve _____ No change _____ Worse _____
Therapist Observation: Improve _____ No change _____ Worse _____
Scaling: Worst things have been 1 _____ 5 _____ 10 Goal achievement

Standardized Evaluations

Standardized measures of progress are generally considered more accurate than nonstandardized measures. These evaluations involve pen-and-paper or electronic questionnaires that are completed by clients and/or significant others. They have been tested for reliability and validity and allow therapists to more carefully track changes and compare a single client with a group norm, which is most meaningful when the client is similar to the comparative group (e.g., in level of functioning, culture, age).

The common problem with these evaluations is that each person has unique frames of reference and situations that make it difficult to interpret the scores. Generally, the more diverse the clientele, the more difficult it is to accurately interpret scores. For example, I once had a trainee work with a Chinese immigrant (sessions were in Mandarin), and she used a standardized instrument to collect initial symptoms and symptoms at the end of the semester three months later. Although the client appeared to have made significant progress, the instrument indicated that she had gotten *worse*. When the student followed up with the client about whether things were significantly worse, the client stated that she had minimized the reporting of symptoms initially because she did not trust the therapist and was uncomfortable admitting to certain problems. After she had developed a good rapport with the therapist, she felt free to more accurately answer the questions, which is consistent with her cultural values of saving face. The moral of the story is that standardized forms only work if clients are able to "play by the rules" by answering questions the way the authors intended. Clearly, therapists need to proceed with caution when trying to interpret standardized forms, and they must talk with clients when the results are unexpected.

Pros and Cons

As with nonstandardized evaluations, standardized measures have both advantages and disadvantages.

Advantages of Standardized Evaluations

- They are considered more reliable and valid.
- The therapist is better able to make cross-client comparisons.
- The therapist is better able to make comparisons across time.

Disadvantages of Standardized Evaluations

- Almost all standardized forms must be purchased; some require a fee for each administration of the instrument, which can quickly become expensive.
- They may require more therapist time and/or equipment and resources (e.g., computers, copies).
- They require more client time, and clients may be reluctant to give this time without a motivating explanation.
- Not all measures are standardized for diverse populations and/or available in the client's primary language.

Effects on the Therapeutic Relationship

Using questionnaires always impacts the therapeutic relationship because it places the therapist in a more hierarchical position. Therefore, therapists need to be thoughtful about how they present formal assessments and help clients make sense of the therapeutic relationship when they do use these measures.

Real-World Options for Standardized Evaluations of Progress

In the ideal world (or obsession-compulsive fantasy, depending on your perspective) described by academics, theoreticians, and researchers, therapists would have clients complete the most reliable and valid assessments at regular intervals over the course of therapy. This is great in theory—that is, until you factor in the fact that reliability and validity are generally correlated with the *length* of the instrument (Lambert & Hawkins, 2004; Miller, Duncan, Brown, Sparks, & Claud, 2003), and for those who work in typical clinical settings—community agencies and private practices—the reality is that neither clients nor clinicians are enthusiastic about completing lengthy questionnaires. Short and sweet is the reality with most clients and therapists. Thankfully, therapists have an increasing number of shorter options.

Guidelines for Standardized Measures in Everyday Practice

The following are guidelines for using standardized measures in everyday practice:

- **First Session:** Because there is evidence that most change occurs early in therapy, the initial measures of symptoms and functioning should occur in the first session (Lambert & Hawkins, 2004).

- **5 Minutes or Less:** Lambert and Hawkins (2004) recommend instruments that take no longer than 5 minutes to complete.

- **Regular (Weekly or Monthly) Intervals:** Although pre- and post-test measures are straightforward in research studies, defining "post" in real-world practice is difficult because clients may drop out rather than announce their intention to end treatment—and rarely agree to return to complete the post-test. Therefore, therapists should develop a regular interval for measuring client progress in clinical settings. Depending on the instrument and setting, weekly, monthly, or quarterly evaluations may be appropriate.

- **Before the Session:** It does not take much time to learn that asking clients to complete a questionnaire before the session is generally much more successful than afterwards, when clients are often in a rush to leave. When used before, questionnaires help develop an agenda for the session.

- **Framing the Measurement:** If the therapist conveys the message that the measurement is helpful to treatment, most clients will be willing to spend 5 minutes to improve their treatment outcomes. Lambert and Hawkins (2004) recommend comparing it to a medical doctor getting blood pressure or vital signs at the beginning of each visit: this information helps the doctor or therapist be more useful to the client.

Ultra-Brief Measures

Marriage and family therapists have several options for measuring both clinical and relational functioning with instruments that are *ultra brief*, requiring as little as 1 minute to complete, or *brief*, requiring less than 10 minutes to complete. Ultra-brief measures include the Outcome Rating Scale (ORS) and the Session Rating Scale (SRS).

Outcome Rating Scale (ORS)

Miller et al. (2003) developed the Outcome Rating Scale as an ultra-brief version of the Outcome Questionnaire (discussed under Brief Measures) in response to client and therapist complaints that even 45 questions were too much. It was designed by clinicians for clinicians and is the most clinician-friendly of the outcome measures. The ORS is composed of only four visual analog scales that take less than a minute to complete, making it ideal for weekly use and highly economical: it is free via the Internet, with photocopying the only remaining cost. The scale measures four areas of functioning:

- **Individually** (personal well-being)
- **Interpersonally** (family and close relationships)
- **Socially** (work, school, friendship)
- **Overall** (general sense of well-being)

Outcome Rating Scale (ORS)

Name _____ Age (Yrs):____
ID# _____ Sex: M / F
Session # ____ Date: _____

Looking back over the last week, including today, help us understand how you have been feeling by rating how well you have been doing in the following areas of your life, where marks to the left represent low levels and marks to the right indicate high levels.

Individually:
(Personal well-being)

I----Examination Copy Only----I

Interpersonally:
(Family, close relationships)

I----Examination Copy Only----I

Socially:
(Work, School, Friendships)

I----Examination Copy Only----I

Overall:
(General sense of well-being)

I----Examination Copy Only----I

Institute for the Study of Therapeutic Change

---

www.talkingcure.com

© 2000, Scott D. Miller and Barry L. Duncan

Two versions for children are also available: the Child Outcome Rating Scale, which includes a similar scale to the adult version, and the Young Child Outcome Rating Scale, which uses happy, neutral, and unhappy faces to measure how the child is feeling (Duncan, Miller, Sparks, Claud, Reynolds, Brown, & Johnson, 2003). Scoring is simple: a ruler is used to measure how far on the 10-cm scale the client scored, and cut-off scores are used to address potential problems.

The ORS has high internal consistency (0.93) and test-retest reliability (0.84) and moderate concurrent validity with the OQ-45.2 (0.59; Miller et al., 2003). Given its ultra-brief format, it is not as sensitive as other outcome measures, such as the OQ-45.2, but it is sensitive enough to measure change in clinical settings, which is the primary aim of the everyday practitioner. The ORS's greatest strength is its feasibility for regular and consistent use in real-world practice settings. When therapists were trained in using either the ORS or OQ-45.2 for outcome measures, 86% were still using the ORS after one year compared to only 25% who were using the 45-item OQ-45.2 (Miller et al., 2003), a dramatic difference.

Session Rating Scale (SRS)

Also developed by Duncan et al. (2003), the Session Rating Scale, Version 3.0 (SRS V3.0), is typically used with the ORS. Whereas the ORS is given at the beginning of the session, the SRS is used at the end of the session to measure the therapeutic alliance, which is consistently found to be one of the best predictors of positive outcome (Orlinsky, Rønnestad, & Willutzki, 2004). Client ratings of alliance are better predictors of outcome than therapist ratings of alliance (Batchelor & Horvath, 1999). In a study conducted by Whipple, Lambert, Vermeersch, Smart, Nielsen, & Hawkins (2003), therapists who had access to both alliance and outcome information were twice as likely to achieve clinically significant change than those who did not.

Like the ORS, the SRS consists of only four analog scales:

- **Relationship:** Does the client feel heard, understood, and respected?
- **Goals and Topics:** Does the client feel that the session focused on what he/she wanted to work on?
- **Approach or Method:** Was the therapist's approach a good fit?
- **Overall:** Was the session helpful ("right") for the client?

As with the ORS, two versions for children are also available: the Child Session Rating Scale (CSRS), which includes a similar scale to the adult version, and the Young Child Session Rating Scale (YCSRS), which uses happy, neutral, and unhappy faces to measure how the child is feeling (Duncan et al., 2003). Scoring is simple: a ruler is used to measure how far on the 10-cm scale the client scored, and cut-off scores are used to address potential problems. Research has identified a very high cut-off score for this instrument, meaning that when clients start indicating there are minor problems with alliance, therapists need to swiftly address these issues to ensure positive outcome. This scale can be particularly helpful for newer therapists wanting to create a strong alliance.

The SRS has good internal consistency (0.88) and a test-retest reliability of 0.64, which is comparable to other alliance measures (Duncan et al., 2003). The concurrent validity of the measure when compared to similar measures is 0.48, providing evidence that a similar construct is being measured. The greatest strength of the SRS, as of the ORS, is its feasibility and user-friendliness. It is used by 96% of clinicians who are introduced to it, compared to only 29% of clinicians using the 12-item Working Alliance Inventory.

Brief Measures

Brief measures are assessment instruments that require less than 10 minutes to complete. Two of the more common ones are the Outcome Questionnaire (OQ) and the Symptom Check List (SCL).

Session Rating Scale (SRS V.3.0)

Name _____ Age (Yrs):_____
ID# _____ Sex: M / F
Session # _____ Date: _____

Please rate today's session by placing a hash mark on the line nearest to the description that best fits your experience.

Relationship:

I did not feel heard, understood, and respected   I----Examination Copy Only----I   I felt heard, understood, and respected

Goals and Topics:

We did *not* work on or talk about what I wanted to work on and talk about   I----Examination Copy Only----I   We worked on and talked about what I wanted to work on and talk about

Approach or Method:

The therapist's approach is not a good fit for me.   I----Examination Copy Only----I   The therapist's approach is a good fit for me.

Overall:

There was something missing in the session today   I----Examination Copy Only----I   Overall, today's session was right for me

Institute for the Study of Therapeutic Change

www.talkingcure.com

© 2002, Scott D. Miller, Barry L. Duncan, & Lynn Johnson

Outcome Questionnaire (OQ-45.2)

The Outcome Questionnaire (OQ-45.2) was designed to measure outcome in clinical settings (Lambert, Hansen, Umphress, Lunnen, Okiishi, Burlingame, Huefner, & Reisinger, 1996). The questionnaire has a total of 45 items, takes less than 5 minutes to complete, and includes three subscales:

1. Symptom Distress (clinical, mental health symptoms)
2. Interpersonal Relationships
3. Social Role Performance.

There is also a youth version, the Youth Outcome Questionnaire (YOQ), that can be completed by parents, and a Youth Outcome Questionnaire Self Report (YOQ-SR) for youth from 12 to 18. Briefer, single-scale (only a global score), 30-item versions are available for the OQ and YOQ, and a 10-item version is also available for the OQ. These measures are affordable and easy to administer, score, and interpret, with the briefer versions being more practical for frequent measurement.

The OQ-45.2 has good test-retest reliability (0.66–0.86) and internal consistency (0.7–0.9; Lambert & Hawkins, 2004). Its minor weakness is that the subscales are highly correlated with one another, meaning that they may not be measuring unique constructs. Most of the research on its validity and reliability has been conducted on the summary score, and clinicians are encouraged to use this as the primary measure of progress (Lambert & Hawkins, 2004). Here are some sample questions used on this questionnaire.

SAMPLE QUESTIONS FROM THE OUTCOME QUESTIONNAIRE

	NEVER	RARELY	SOMETIMES	FREQUENTLY	ALMOST ALWAYS
1. I get along well with others	☐	☐	☐	☐	☐
2. I tire quickly	☐	☐	☐	☐	☐
3. I feel no interest in things	☐	☐	☐	☐	☐
4. I feel stressed at work/ school	☐	☐	☐	☐	☐
5. I blame myself for things	☐	☐	☐	☐	☐
6. I feel irritated	☐	☐	☐	☐	☐
18. I feel lonely	☐	☐	☐	☐	☐
19. I have frequent arguments	☐	☐	☐	☐	☐
20. I feel loved and wanted	☐	☐	☐	☐	☐
21. I enjoy my spare time	☐	☐	☐	☐	☐
22. I have difficulty concentrating	☐	☐	☐	☐	☐
23. I feel hopeless about the future	☐	☐	☐	☐	☐
24. I like myself	☐	☐	☐	☐	☐

Developed by Michael J. Lambert, Ph.D. and Gary M. Burlingame, Ph.D. For more information contact:
OQ Measures LLC © Copyright, 2005

Symptom Check List (SCL-90-R) and Brief Symptom Inventory (BSI)

The Symptom Check List is a 90-item test that assesses for mental health symptoms and their intensity (mild, moderate, severe). It is designed for individuals 13 years and older and requires 12 to 15 minutes to complete. The Brief Symptom Inventory (BSI) is based on the SCL but is, as the name indicates, briefer. The BSI has 53 items, is designed for individuals 13 years and older, and takes 8 to 10 minutes to complete. Both measures have nine symptom subscales and three global indices:

Subscales

- Somatization
- Obsessive-Compulsive
- Interpersonal Sensitivity
- Depression

- Anxiety
- Hostility
- Phobic Anxiety
- Paranoid Ideation
- Psychoticism

Global Indices

- Global Severity Index: overall psychological distress
- Positive Symptom Distress Index (PSDI): intensity of symptoms
- Positive Symptom Total (PST): number of self-reported symptoms

Ultra-brief 6- and 10-item versions that correlate to the overall distress scores have also been developed (Rosen, Drescher, Moos, Finney, Murphy, & Gusman, 2000), and are more feasible options for everyday practice. The SCL-90-R has good test-retest validity, ranging from 0.63 to 0.86 for online versions and 0.68 to 0.84 for pen-and-paper versions (Derogatis & Fitzpatrick, 2004; Vallejo, Jordán, Díaz, Comeche, & Ortega, 2007). The internal consistency coefficients are also good, ranging from 0.70 to 0.90.

Final Thoughts on Outcome

Therapists are assessing client progress more closely and precisely than in the past. Although assessment involves additional paperwork and time, numerous quick and effective options are available that integrate easily in today's practice environment. Therapist attitude is critical to the success and usefulness of an assessment system. If therapists believe in it, they communicate this to clients and the assessments become a unique resource for helping clients achieve their goals. When therapists see assessment as burdensome or unnecessary, it becomes a lifeless bureaucratic task of little use to anyone.

ONLINE RESOURCES

Outcome Rating Scale and Session Rating Scale
> **Free download at www.talkingcure.com**
> **Direct link for assessment forms: www.talkingcure.com/bookstore.asp?id=106**

Outcome Questionnaire 45
> **For purchase at www.oqmeasures.com**

Symptom Checklist 90
> **For purchase at www.pearsonassessments.com/tests/scl90r.htm**

REFERENCES

Batchelor, A., & Horvath, A. (1999). The therapeutic relationship. In M. A. Hubble, B. L. Duncan, & S. D. Miller (Eds.), *The heart and soul of change* (pp. 133–178). Washington, DC: APA Press.

Berg, I., & de Shazer, S. (1993). Making numbers talk: Language in therapy. In S. Friedman (Ed.), *The new language of change: Constructive collaborative in psychotherapy.* New York: Guilford.

Derogatis, L. R., & Fitzpatrick, M. (2004). The SCL-90-R, the Brief Symptom Inventory, and the BSI-81. In M. E. Murish (Ed.), *The use of psychological testing for treatment planning and outcome.* New York: Routledge.

Duncan, B. L., Miller, S. D., Sparks, J. A., Claud, D. A., Reynolds, L. R., Brown, J., & Johnson, L. D. (2003). *Journal of Brief Therapy, 3*, 3–12.

Lambert, M. J., Hansen, N. B., Umphress, V. J., Lunnen, K., Okiishi, J., Burlingame, G. M., Huefner, J. C., & Reisinger, C. W. (1996). *Administration and scoring manual for the Outcome Questionnaire (OQ-45.2).* Wilmington, DE: American Professional Credentialing Services.

Lambert, M. J., & Hawkins, E. J. (2004). Measuring outcome in professional practice: Considerations in selecting and using brief outcome instruments. *Professional Psychology: Research and Practice, 35*, 492–499.

Miller, S. D., Duncan, B. L., Brown, J., Sparks, J. A., & Claud, D. A. (2003). The Outcome Rating Scale: A preliminary study of the reliability, validity, and feasibility of a brief visual analog measure. *Journal of Brief Therapy, 2*, 91–100.

Miller, S. D., Duncan, B. L., & Hubble, M. A. (2004). Beyond integration: The triumph of outcome over process in clinical practice. *Psychotherapy in Australia, 10*(2), 2–19.

Orlinsky, D. E., Rønnestad, M. H., & Willutzki, U. (2004). Fifty years of process-outcome research: Continuity and change. In M. J. Lambert (Ed.), *Bergin and Garfield's handbook of psychotherapy and behavior change* (5th ed., pp. 307–393). New York: Wiley.

Rosen, C. S., Drescher, K. D., Moos, R. H., Finney, J. W., Murphy, R. T., & Gusman, F. (2000). Six- and ten-item indexes of psychological distress based on the Symptom Checklist-90. *Assessment, 7*, 103–111.

Vallejo, M. A., Jordán, C. M., Díaz, M. I., Comeche, M. I., & Ortega, J. (2007). Psychological assessment via the internet: A reliability and validity study of online (vs paper-and-pencil) versions of the General Health Questionnaire-28 (GHQ-28) and the Symptoms Check-List-90-Revised (SCL-90-R). *Journal of Medical Internet Research, 10*, 2.

Whipple, J. L., Lambert, M. J., Vermeersch, D. A., Smart, D. W., Nielsen, S. L., & Hawkins, E. J. (2003). Improving the effects of psychotherapy: The use of early identification of treatment and problem strategies in routine practice. *Journal of Counseling Psychology, 50*, 59–68.

Document It: Progress Notes

Step 5: Documenting It: A Profession Behind Closed Doors

Here's a fact that frightens many: the majority of therapists practicing today have never had another professional observe them conducting a session with a live-in-the-flesh client (Jordan, 1999). Rather than live supervision, what usually happens is case consultation, meaning that therapists report to their supervisor what was said, what happened, and what they did (Jordan, 1999). The more that interested outsiders—especially third-party payers—learn about how therapists are trained, the more they start to wonder what goes on behind closed doors. As health costs keep rising, third-party payers increasingly demand to know what therapists are doing and whether it makes a difference.

Thankfully, rather than bugging our offices or hiring spies, third-party payers have decided that the most practical means of tracking what happens in closed therapy sessions is to require therapists to leave a detailed paper trail in the form of case or progress notes, which is the final step to competent therapy. Progress notes are therapists' primary means of showing that they are rendering professional care that conforms to legal and ethical guidelines. The therapist's opinion, supervisor's judgment, and even the client's enthusiastic exclamation that "that was a helpful session", unless written down, do not mean much to third-party payers: the information documented in the progress note is what counts when determining whether therapy has conformed to standard practice. Additionally, case notes are critical when things get dicey; professionally kept progress notes are therapists' primary means of protecting against lawsuits and complaints.

However, if you take a walk down the halls of most community and public mental health agencies, you will hear grumbling about paperwork: "there's too much" and "it's a waste of time." This may be true, at least in part. However, if there is a clinical document therapists should not grumble about, it is progress notes. These are therapists' greatest sources of protection, and thanks to recent legislation, there is more clarity than ever about what should be in them.

Two Different Animals: Progress Notes Versus Psychotherapy Notes

In 2003, the U.S. Department of Health and Human Services began enforcing a new set of medical documentation guidelines outlined in HIPAA (Health Insurance Portability and Accountability Act; USDHHS, 2003). Along with solving other health care issues such as portability of health care insurance coverage, HIPAA regulations included new privacy standards for medical documentation. Most significantly for therapists—and startling to those who had been practicing for years—was the new distinction between two sets of clinical documents: *progress notes* and *psychotherapy notes* (Halloway, 2003). Formerly, keeping two sets of notes was somewhere between unethical and illegal, depending on how you handled requests for information. However, to increase patient privacy, the new HIPAA legislation sanctioned the practice of keeping two different kinds of documents:

PROGRESS NOTES AND PSYCHOTHERAPY NOTES

- **Progress Notes:** These are the "official" medical file, the formal medical record that is shared with other medical professionals, clients (upon written request), and/or in response to subpoenas. Third-party payers generally have detailed requirements for the content of these notes.

- **Psychotherapy Notes:** These are the property of the therapist (or person who created them) and remain separate from the formal medical file *if they are kept separately* (in a separate physical file). These records may include personal impressions, analyses of the client, hypotheses, and so forth. They have a much greater protection under HIPAA legislation (if kept separately) and are rarely, if ever, disclosed to an outside third party. There are no standards for what information should be placed in these records because their purpose is to help therapists think through, plan, and reflect on client progress.

Progress Notes

Because psychotherapy notes are kept separate and private and have few guidelines, therapists' primary concern is with progress notes, which constitute the formal medical file. HIPAA regulations encourage psychotherapists to minimize the potentially damaging information kept in progress notes because they are likely to be shared with other professionals, courts, and other parties. The goal is to *maximize client privacy* while simultaneously *documenting competent treatment that conforms to professional standards of care.* Rather than names, conversation topics, or the personal content of a client's life or the therapeutic conversation, third-party payers prefer detailed information about (a) the frequency and duration of symptoms and (b) the specific interventions used to treat these symptoms. Such notes increase client privacy by *not* including potentially damaging information, such as fantasies of an affair, details about family interactions, and names of colleagues and friends.

Crisis situations are the most notable exception to this general principle of minimal private information. When stabilizing a suicidal, self-harming, abused, or homicidal client, therapists must include detailed information about the assessment of safety, the safety plan (including the names and roles of people who are part of the plan), and specific actions taken to ensure safety and conform with legal requirements. When stabilizing a crisis situation, a therapist gains additional "insurance" by documenting prudent, professional care in this high-risk legal situation and also provides other health care professionals with the information they need to treat the client.

Progress Note Ingredients

HIPAA guidelines and third-party payers provide guidance on what to include in a progress note, thus increasing uniformity in the field. These common ingredients include the following:

- Client case number, not a name (to protect client confidentiality)
- Date, time, and length of session
- Who attended the session
- Provider's original signature (not initials) with professional license status or degree
- Client progress, including improvement or worsening of symptoms (with frequency and/or duration)
- Interventions used and client response
- Plan for future sessions; modification to treatment plan
- Assessment for crisis issues and description of how they are managed

Progress Note Options

The necessary ingredients for progress notes are generally agreed upon. However, just like any list of ingredients, there are many ways to combine them to serve up different dishes. Translated into the world of progress notes, this means that there is more than one right way to do a progress note. Many therapists choose to conform to HIPAA by adapting pre-HIPAA forms to the new standards; others use formats they create or that an agency has developed. Although one might assume that HIPAA regulations have unified progress note formats, my annual trips to agencies around town indicate that there are probably more types of progress notes than ice cream flavors at your local Baskin-Robbins™. The most common are DAP and SOAP notes.

DAP Notes

Developed in response to early managed care requirements, DAP (Data, Assessment, Plan) notes are one of the more common formats for progress notes (Wiger, 2005). They include the following:

- **Data:** What happened in session, interventions, clinical observations, test results, symptom diagnosis, stressors.

- **Assessment:** Assessment of symptoms, outcome of current session and overall course of therapy, treatment plan goals and objectives being met, areas needing more work, areas of progress.

- **Plan:** Homework, interventions for next session, timing of next sessions, changes to treatment plan. Some therapists use *P* for progress and emphasize any progress that was made.

Although there is a general outline, DAP notes can be interpreted in numerous ways, and each practitioner or agency often develops a unique style, emphasizing different information in each section.

SOAP Notes

Another widespread format for progress notes is SOAP (Subjective, Objective, Assessment, Plan) notes (Wiger, 2005). Many medical professionals, including general practice doctors, chiropractors, and occupational therapists use them. Because SOAP notes were originally designed for documenting treatment of physical conditions, they are often awkward when applied to mental health. Therefore, as with DAP notes, the interpretation of each section can vary significantly across practitioners and agencies. SOAP notes include the following:

- **Subjective Observations:** Description of client's narrative and/or reported symptoms; some mental health practitioners have adapted the *S* to mean "situation," referring to the concerns and problems the client brought to sessions

- **Objective Observations:** Therapists' observations, test results, findings from physical examination, vital signs

- **Assessment:** Summary of symptoms, assessment, and diagnosis; differential diagnosis considerations

- **Plan:** Plan to treat listed symptoms, including instructions and medications given to client

The All-Purpose HIPAA Form for Progress Notes

Unfortunately, neither DAP nor SOAP notes may be particularly helpful to new therapists. The following form was developed to address the most common requirements of private insurance and public agencies in a format that is easy to follow.

PROGRESS NOTES

Progress Notes for Client # _____

Date: _____ **Time:** ___:___ am/pm **Session Length:** ☐ 50 min. or ☐ _____

Present: ☐ AM ☐ AF ☐ CM ☐ CF ☐ _____
Billing Code: ☐ 90801 (Assess) ☐ 90806 (Insight-50 min) ☐ 90847 (Family-50 min)

☐ Other _____

Symptoms(s)	Dur/Freq Since Last Visit	Progress: Setback------Initial------Goal
1.		-5----------1----------5----------10
2.		-5----------1----------5----------10
3.		-5----------1----------5----------10

Explanatory Notes: _____

_____

_____

Interventions/HW: _____

Client Response/Feedback: _____

_____

Abbreviation: HW = Homework.

Plan: ☐ Continue with treatment plan; plan for next session: _____

☐ Modify plan: _____

Next session: Date: _____ Time: ___:___ am/pm

Crisis Issues: ☐ Denies suicide/homicide/abuse/crisis ☐ Crisis assessed/addressed: _____

_____

_____, _____ _____

Therapist signature   License/intern status   Date

◇◇

Case Consultation/Supervision Notes: _____

Collateral Contacts: Date: _____ Time: _____ Name: _____

Notes: _____

☐ Written release on file: ☐ Sent ☐ Received ☐ In court docs ☐ Other: _____

_____, _____ _____

Therapist signature   License/intern status   Date

_____, _____ _____

Supervisor signature   License   Date

©2007. Diane R. Gehart

Completing a Progress Notes Form

Client Number

To protect confidentiality, client names should never be put on file labels or progress notes. If a note accidentally slips out of a binder at Starbucks (this has happened), it should be impossible to identify the client. Actually, notes should never leave the building, and therapists should never leave the building after seeing clients until they have completed their progress notes.

Date, Time, and Session Length

Each note should begin with the date of the session, the time the session started, and the length of the session.

Persons Present

Because more than one person may be in therapy, therapists should indicate who was there. I recommend the following notation system, the same as that cited in Chapter 3:

AF: Adult Female
AM: Adult Male
CF#: Child Female plus age (e.g., CF8 = eight-year-old girl)
CM#: Child Male plus age (e.g., CM8 = eight-year-old boy)

If these abbreviations are used throughout the note, supervisors who read the notes will know who's who without using names.

CPT Billing Codes

Insurance companies use CPT (Current Procedural Terminology) codes, which have been established and updated by the American Medical Association to identify what type of service was provided. The CPT codes most commonly used by therapists are as follows:

- **90801:** Diagnostic interview (generally used for the first session)
- **90804:** 20–30 minutes of individual insight-oriented psychotherapy
- **90810:** 20–30 minutes of individual interactive psychotherapy (e.g., play therapy, music therapy)
- **90806:** 50 minutes of individual insight-oriented psychotherapy
- **90812:** 50 minutes of individual interactive psychotherapy (e.g., play therapy, music therapy)
- **90846:** 50 minutes of family psychotherapy (client not present)
- **90847:** 50 minutes of family psychotherapy (client present)
- **90857:** group therapy

Most county mental health agencies have their own set of billing codes. Although they are often not standardized within the same state, they generally use categories similar to the CPT codes.

Symptoms and Progress

Each week, therapists document the *duration, frequency,* and *severity* of symptoms. Here are some examples:

- "Client reports mild depressed mood most days (or 5 out of 7 days)."
- "Client reports 1 panic attack the past week, moderate severity."
- "Client reports decreased conflict with parents; 2 arguments past week."

The 1–10 scale can also be used to visually track progress and setbacks.

Interventions

Progress notes should clearly identify which interventions the therapist used to help the client address the problems identified in the treatment plan. Here it is best to use theory-specific language:

- "Used solution-focused scaling to identify steps to reduce depression over next week."
- "Used enactments to practice alternatives to conflict."
- "Created genogram to increase insight related to family drinking patterns."

Therapists should avoid statements such as

"Discussed work stress" (not a therapeutic intervention)
"Talked about fears" (how does this distinguish you from a bartender or hairstylist?)

Client Response

Increasingly, therapists document how clients responded to treatment, that is, what did and did not work:

- "Client receptive to reframe related to work issues; less receptive to reframe of pattern related to relationship."
- "Client actively engaged in enactment; optimistic could work at home."
- "Client expressed enthusiasm about mindfulness exercises."

Plan

This section describes the agenda for the next session and/or thoughts about modifying the treatment plan; for example:

- "Will bring in parents to next session."
- "Follow up on journal assignment."
- "Continue to assess for self-harm."

Crisis Issues

Therapists document any crisis issues that arose in session and any issues they followed up from prior sessions. If there have been crisis issues, such as cutting or suicidal ideation, therapists should continue noting *in writing* that they checked on these issues during subsequent sessions. If a crisis issue was detected, therapists must clearly detail (a) the assessment process and the data used to support conclusions, and (b) the specific actions taken to ensure the safety of the client and/or public. Documenting crisis situations requires much more detailed and specific information than documenting general progress and interventions. Here are some examples:

- "Client reported suspected abuse to child in family; reported child hit with belt on more than one occasion; report called in to CPS at 7:15 pm; taken by Christine K.; full report placed in file."
- "Client reported passive suicidal ideation: "wish I were dead"; denied plan or intent: "I would never do it because of my kids"; developed safety plan of 3 names to call; went over emergency contact for therapist."
- "Client reported cutting twice this week; developed safety plan in which the client agreed to use scaling-for-safety to develop alternative action at level 7; client readily agreed to plan."
- "Client denies cutting this week; no new cuts on wrists evident."

Consultation and Supervision

When obtaining supervision, peer consultation, or legal consultation (from a lawyer), therapists should document recommendations and/or information, especially regarding ethical and legal issues.

Collateral Contacts

Whenever you contact another professional or family member regarding a client, such as a teacher, physician, psychiatrist, social worker, parent, and so forth, the contact needs to be documented, noting that a release of information is on file.

Signature

Finally, therapists must (a) sign the progress notes by hand (no initials) and (b) indicate their license status. If a therapist is unlicensed, his/her supervisor typically also signs the progress notes.

A Time and Place for Progress Notes

The proper time for writing progress notes is simple: *immediately following the session.* Because therapists conduct 45- to 50-minute sessions, progress notes can be written in the 10 to 15 minutes between sessions. If this is not possible, therapists must complete progress notes before leaving at the end of the day. Anything else gets you into a gray ethical area because a session is hard to remember with the same level of detail a day or two later—no matter how good your memory is. Trust me, I've tried it once or twice, and it does not work; therefore, I recommend you put daily progress notes in your "religious practice" category: they get done every time on time for fear of eternal damnation or worse—the wrath of an ethics review board.

In addition, there is only one place for progress notes: a locked file cabinet. Like all medical professionals, therapists are required to keep client files and progress notes securely locked when not in immediate use—in some cases, under two sets of locks (e.g., in a locked file cabinet in a locked room). Digital files require high levels of computer security, outlined in the HIPAA policy (USDHHS, 2003). Moreover, *any piece of paper that has identifying client information,* such as phone message pads or calendars, must also be locked when not in use. In most states, therapists must keep records for seven years past the age of majority (adulthood), after which time they may be destroyed (e.g., shredded). The upside of these security requirements is that they keep your desk clean, and, for many, the ritual act of shredding has the therapeutic benefit of releasing pent-up stress and frustration.

Final Note on Notes

Progress notes are the heart of clinical documentation, and in many ways the most important documents we produce because they provide the clearest record of what happens behind closed doors. They are the only place where we can document that we conducted ourselves as professionals, rendering appropriate and necessary medical services. Because they are the documents most likely to be viewed by outsiders should papers be released or subpoenaed, we must ensure that these notes protect us as well as our clients' privacy. The art of writing progress notes is one of the most important clinical skills to master. Thankfully, we get ample opportunity to practice.

ONLINE RESOURCES

HIPAA Guidelines

www.hhs.gov/ocr/hipaa

CPT Codes from the AMA

www.ama-assn.org

REFERENCES

Halloway, J. D. (2003). More protections for patients and psychologists under HIPAA. *Monitor on Psychology, 34*(2), 22.

Jordan, K. (1999). Live supervision for beginning therapists in practicum: Crucial for quality counseling and avoiding litigation. *Family Therapy, 26*(2), 81–86.

U.S. Department of Health and Human Services (USDHHS). (2003). *Summary of HIPAA privacy rule.* Washington, DC: Author. Retrieved December 2, 2007, from www.hhs.gov/ocr/hipaa

Wiger, D. E. (2005). *The psychotherapy documentation primer* (2nd ed.). New York: Wiley.

PROGRESS NOTE SCORING RUBRIC

The following scoring rubric describes the differences between exemplary, adequate, and deficient progress notes. By closely attending to these requirements, you can hone in on what your instructors and supervisors are looking for when they grade your work.

Progress Note Scoring Rubric

Date: _____

Therapist/Intern: _____

Evaluator/Instructor: _____

Level of Clinical Training:

☐ Preclinical training; coursework only

☐ 0–12 months ☐ 12–24 months ☐ 2+ years

Rating Scale

5 = **Exceptional**: Skills and understanding significantly beyond developmental level

4 = **Outstanding**: Strong mastery of skills and thorough understanding of concepts

3 = **Mastered Basic Skills at Developmental Level**: Understanding of concepts/skills evident

2 = **Developing**: Minor conceptual and skill errors; in process of developing

1 = **Deficits**: Significant remediation needed; deficits in knowledge/skills

NA = **Not Applicable**: Unable to measure with given data (do not use to indicate deficit)

	5	4	3	2	1	COMP	SCORE
Basic Record Keeping	Confidential notation used; includes ages and other distinguishing info; sophisticated and clear tracking of clients using notation; correct billing code.	Confidential notation used; includes ages and other key info; clients easy to track using notation; correct billing code.	Confidential notation used throughout; clients distinguishable using notation; correct billing code.	Minor errors or omissions with confidential notation and billing; minor confusion using notation.	Fails to maintain confidentiality or use notation that clearly identifies clients who attended session; incorrect/missing billing code.	1-5.3 3.1.2 5.5.4	☐ NA
Symptoms	Specific DSM symptoms cited; detailed frequency, duration, progress; sophisticated linking of symptoms to systemic dynamics, interventions, and all other aspects of note.	Specific DSM symptoms with frequency and/ or duration cited; progress included; links symptoms to interventions.	Symptoms with frequency and/or duration; progress included.	Minor problems; vague or inaccurate descriptors; missing key frequency, duration, or progress info; contradicts other aspects of note.	Significant problems; inaccurate or inconsistent in symptoms and described treatment. Missing meaningful frequency, duration, progress.	5.5.1	☐ NA
Progress Toward Goals	Detailed documentation of progress; explanations for progress, setbacks, and need to continue include sophisticated integration of symptoms and systems dynamics.	Clear documentation of progress; explanations for progress, setbacks, and need to continue include some integration of symptoms and systems dynamics.	Includes appropriate explanation for progress, setbacks, and/or need to continue.	Minor problems; vague description of progress, setbacks, and/or need to continue.	Significant problems; not included or inconsistent with rest of note.	3.4.1 4.4.3 4.4.5	☐ NA

(continued)

(continued)

	5	4	3	2	1	COMP	SCORE
Interventions	Sophisticated choice of interventions/HW consistent with symptoms; uniquely sensitive to age, culture, education, etc.; develops effective solutions with clients.	Well-chosen interventions or HW; sensitive to client age, culture, education, etc.; develops effective solution with clients.	Appropriate choice of interventions; appropriate for client age, culture, education, etc.; begins moving client in useful direction.	Intervention not clearly related to presenting problem or symptoms; would be more effective if diversity issues more carefully considered.	Inappropriate choice of intervention for client problem, symptom, or unique needs.	4.3.2 4.3.6	☐ NA
Integrate Client Feedback	Sensitive to client response; creative integration of feedback into treatment; clear use of feedback to evaluate ability to deliver interventions.	Clear description of client response; clear description of how used to inform plan.	Includes basic description of client response and description of how treatment was adjusted.	Includes client response but not clear how treatment adjusted to negative response.	No mention of client response.	1.3.7 3.2.1 4.4.2 4.4.4	☐ NA
Plan	Thoughtful adjustment of plan based on client response to treatment; modification demonstrates sensitivity to client needs, diversity issues.	Specific adjustment of plan based on client response to treatment; modification demonstrates awareness of client needs, diversity issues.	Basic indication that client needs, diversity issues considered in planning.	No specific indication that client needs, diversity issues are guiding treatment.	Failure to identify significant need to adjust treatment to meet client needs, diversity issues.	3.4.2 4.3.10	☐ NA
Crisis Management	Clear evidence of ability to identify ethical issues, dilemmas, ethical decision making; sophisticated management of crisis, legal, ethical issues; sophisticated safety plan; mandated reporting handled smoothly.	Evidence of ability to identify ethical issues, dilemmas, ethical decision making; proper management of crisis, legal, ethical issues; clear safety plan; mandated reporting handled well.	No evidence that a crisis issue was missed. If crisis identified, basic information covered meeting legal and ethical requirements.	Misses minor information related to identifying and/or reporting of crisis issue.	Failure to identify or properly manage legal, ethical, or crisis issue.	2.3.5 5.1.4 5.2.1 5.2.2 5.3.1 5.3.4 5.3.5 5.3.6	☐ NA

							NA
Legal Issues	Progress notes consistently timely; in exact accordance with legal, ethical requirements.	Progress notes timely; in clear accordance with legal and ethical requirements.	Progress notes timely; meet basic legal and ethical requirements.	Progress notes untimely and/or missing minor ethical requirements.	Fails to meet legal or ethical requirements; untimely.	1.5.2 1.5.3	☐ NA
Case Consultation/ Supervision	Proactive use of consultation, supervision, esp for legal, ethical issues; specific integration of feedback into treatment; insightful attention to personal issues that affect tx.	Clear use of consultation, supervision, esp for legal, ethical issues; integrates feedback into treatment; thoughtful attention to personal issues that affect tx.	Seeks supervision for basic legal, ethical issues; integrate into treatment; attends to significant personal issues.	Reactive rather than proactive approach to supervision; misses opportunities to use supervision; little insight into personal issues.	Fails to seek supervision when needed or fails to implement feedback; unable to attend to how personal issues affect treatment.	2.5.1 4.3.12 5.2.3 5.2.4 5.5.2	☐ NA
Collateral Contacts	Thoughtful and sensitive collaborative work with other stakeholders; obtains all consents; clearly respects multiple perspectives of all involved.	Works collaboratively with other stakeholders; obtains all consents; respectful of multiple perspectives.	Follows through on required collateral contacts; obtains legally required consents; respect for multiple perspectives.	Misses opportunities to make collateral contacts; appears to have some biases.	Fails to make needed collateral contacts; fails to obtain needed consent; clear bias demonstrated.	1.3.8 3.3.7 4.5.1	☐ NA
Additional Competency (Optional)							☐ NA
Additional Competency (Optional)							☐ NA
Comments							

Abbreviations: HW = Homework; tx = Treatment.

CHAPTER

7

Understanding the Role of Theory in Therapy

Eeny-Meeney-Miney-Moe and Other Strategies for Choosing a Theory

What theory should I use? Which is the best? Which is the best for me? Do I have to pick a theory? What if I like them all? Can't I just be eclectic? These are some of the first questions students ask as they begin to study family therapy theories. The answers are more complex than one would imagine, leaving honest supervisors no option but to respond with maddening "both/and" or "yes-and-no" answers (trust me, supervisors do not do this just to torture students for recreation and sport—it really is an honest answer).

Over the years, the role of theory in psychotherapy has gained less rather than more clarity. Initially, the general recommendation was to select and train in one theory, which became a therapist's primary identity. However, in practice, mixing, matching, and integrating theories has been an increasingly popular and justified practice in the field (Miller, Duncan, & Hubble, 2004). Some—but not all—of the confusion surrounding the implementation of theory can be clarified by identifying common factors.

Common Factors

Many of the questions on the role of theory have been spurred by what is commonly referred to as the "common factors debate" (Sprenkle, Davis, & Lebow, 2009; Blow, Sprenkle, & Davis, 2007; Sprenkle & Blow, 2004). Common factors proponents contend that the effectiveness of therapy has more to do with the key elements found in all theories than with the unique components of a specific theory. To simplify the argument even further: the similarities matter more than the differences. This position is supported by meta-analyses (research on several research studies) of outcome studies in the field: when research studies control for confounding variables (such as therapist loyalty, comparison group, or measures of outcome), there is little evidence to support the superiority of one theory over another, both in psychotherapy more broadly (Lambert, 1992; Wampold, 2001) and in family therapy specifically (Shadish & Baldwin, 2002).

Within the common factors community, some (Miller, Duncan, and Hubble, 1997) emphasize the common factors while minimizing the role of theory, whereas others take a more moderate approach (Sprenkle & Blow, 2004), maintaining that theories are still important because they are the vehicles through which therapists deliver the common factors and because specific models may have an added benefit in certain contexts. Sprenkle and Blow (2004) point out that the common factors approach does not require therapists to relinquish therapeutic models but instead to understand their purpose differently. Rather than providing the "answer" to the client's problems, common factor proponents propose that using a structured treatment inspires confidence from clients in the therapeutic process, allowing therapists to coherently actualize common factors. From this perspective, a therapeutic model is better understood as a tool that increases therapist effectiveness rather than the "one and only true path" that resolves the client's problem.

Lambert's Common Factors Model

The most frequently cited common factors model is grounded in the work of Michael Lambert (1992). After reviewing outcome studies in psychotherapy, Lambert estimated that outcome variance (the degree to which change is attributed to a specific variable) could be attributed to four factors:

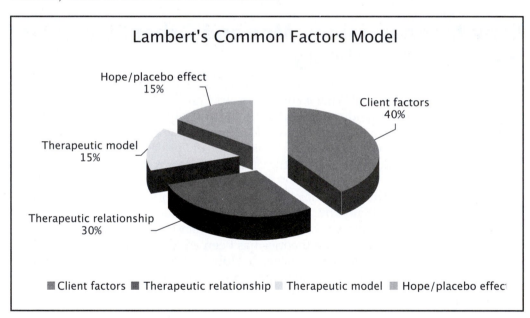

LAMBERT'S COMMON FACTORS MODEL

- **Client Factors:** An estimated 40%; includes client motivation and resources
- **Therapeutic Relationship:** An estimated 30%; the quality of the therapeutic relationship as the *client* evaluates it
- **Therapeutic Model:** An estimated 15%; the therapist's specific model for treatment and the techniques used
- **Hope and the Placebo Effect:** An estimated 15%; the client's level of hope and belief that therapy will help

Often these percentages are cited as facts, but although they are well-informed estimates based on a careful analysis of existing research, the numbers were not generated through an actual research study. They should be considered general trends in the research that inspires therapists to critically reconsider how they can help clients rather than exact percentages.

Wampold's Common Factors Model

Wampold (2001), who conducted a meta-analysis similar to Lambert's but compared only studies that included two or more actual therapy models (rather than comparing a model to the generic "treatment as usual" or a no-treatment control group), presents evidence for the following:

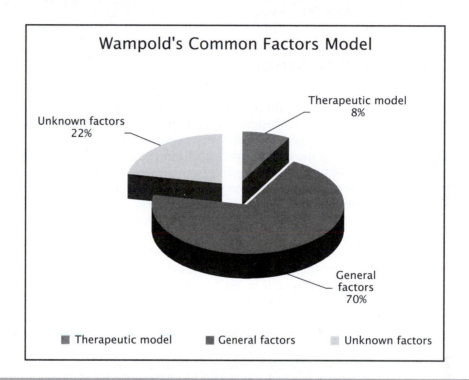

WAMPOLD'S COMMON FACTOR MODEL

- **Therapeutic Model:** 8%; the unique contributions of a specific theory (compare with 15% in Lambert's model)
- **General Factors:** 70%; therapeutic alliance, expectancy, hope
- **Unknown Factors:** 22%; variance that is not related to known variables

Wampold's research further underscores that common elements across theories contribute more to positive therapeutic outcomes than the unique elements of a specific theory. Thus research across theories continually indicates that general or common factors have the greatest impact on outcome; although this result may be due to the limits of research (Sprenkle & Blow, 2004) or other factors, it is the best information to date on the subject.

Client Factors

Lambert's (1992) research, which has been made most accessible to clinicians in the work of Miller, Duncan, and Hubble (1997), emphasizes the importance of activating client resources, such as by encouraging clients to create and use support networks and increasing client motivation and engagement in the therapeutic process. Tallman and Bohart (1999) propose that most theories work equally well because of the client's ability to adapt and utilize whatever techniques and insights the therapist may offer, the therapeutic process effectively becoming a Rorschach (ink blot test) that the client uses to create change.

Miller, Duncan, and Hubble (1997) describe two general categories of client factors:

1. *Client characteristics* include the client's motivation to change, attitude about therapy and change, commitment to change, personal strengths and resources (cognitive, emotional, social, financial, spiritual), and duration of complaints.
2. *Extra-therapeutic factors* include social support, community involvement, and fortuitous life events.

Therapeutic Relationship

In both Lambert's and Wampold's research, the quality of the therapeutic relationship appears to be more important than the specific model in predicting outcome, a finding that is consistent with much of the traditional wisdom in the field. In an effective relationship, the therapist accommodates to the client's level of motivation, works toward the client's goals, and demonstrates a genuine, nonjudgmental attitude. A particularly interesting—and humbling—finding is that the client's evaluation of the relationship is more strongly correlated with positive outcome than the therapist's evaluation (Miller, Duncan, & Hubble, 1997).

Despite the clear and consistent evidence for the importance of the therapeutic relationship, most outcome studies, especially those on evidence-based therapies, try to control for and factor out the impact of the therapist on treatment, thereby obscuring the role of the therapist in effective treatment (Blow, Sprenkle, & Davis, 2007). Perhaps this is done because it is hard to fully operationalize and measure the therapeutic relationship, or perhaps because researchers want a more scientific-sounding explanation (the treatment did it, not the relationship). Whatever the reason, the research literature seems to undervalue and underestimate the importance of the therapeutic relationship. However, common factors research redirects therapists' attention to this important component. Therapists wanting to closely attend to relationship variables can use measures such as the Session Rating Scale (in Chapter 5) to monitor the relationship on a weekly basis.

Therapeutic Model: Theory-Specific Factors

Theory-specific factors are what the therapist says and does to facilitate change while following his/her therapeutic model. These factors are what therapists and third-party payers consider important. However, as Lambert's research and estimations indicate, technique may not be as important as is typically assumed, actually being only half as important as the therapeutic relationship. However, it is still an influential factor over which therapists have significant control.

Hope and the Placebo Effect: Expectancy

Hope and expectancy, or the *placebo* effect, refer to clients' belief that therapy will help them resolve their problem. Lambert's (1992) emphasis on this factor heightens therapists' awareness of an often-neglected aspect of the therapeutic process, at least in the research literature (Blow, Sprenkle, & Davis, 2007). With this awareness, therapists can more consciously work to instill hope, which is particularly critical in the initial sessions.

Diversity and the Common Factors

Common factors can be particularly useful when working with diverse clients—whether culturally, sexually, linguistically, or in ability—because diversity always implies unique client resources and challenges, particularly for the therapeutic relationship, choice of approach, and strategies for instilling hope. For example, although gay, lesbian, bisexual, and transgendered clients are often ostracized in the general community, many have extensive informal and formal social support networks; the same is true of many ethnic groups and disabled or chronically ill people. Thus the societal challenge is partially offset by unique resources. Therapists can help clients leverage these resources to better manage the often daunting challenges of being different from the majority.

Similarly, with diverse clients the task of creating a therapeutic relationship in which the client feels accepted rather than judged requires more mindfulness and thoughtfulness because the therapist may not be aware of all the dynamics and traditions of these groups. Education on local diverse communities is of course necessary, but humility and admitting that you do not know the answer is often more important because it cultivates respect and openness (Anderson, 1997). When therapists proceed with curiosity and a willingness to learn, they often discover distinct and effective means for instilling hope from within the client's culture and primary community, further strengthening the therapeutic relationship.

Do We Still Need Theory?

The natural question that follows from the common factors debate is: Do we still need theory? As noted by Sprenkle and Blow (2004), some therapists lean toward the "dodo bird verdict," suggesting that theory matters very little. The more moderate stance of Sprenkle and Blow (2004) emphasizes that "the models are important because they are the vehicles through which the common factors do their work" (p. 126).

Following this moderate position, theory still plays a critical role for new and seasoned clinicians, but not the role one might initially expect it to play. Rather than providing a system to help clients alleviate their symptoms and resolve their problems, a theory is a *tool* that helps the therapist help the client. *Thus theory may be most relevant for the therapist—not the client.*

Theory gives therapists a system for interpreting the information they get about clients so that they can say and do things that will be useful. It also helps therapists know how best to relate and respond to clients. Without theory, it is easy to get lost in a sea of information, emotion, and challenging behaviors. Theory gives therapists a systematic way of dealing with the wide range of difficulties clients bring. Thus, choosing a theory involves identifying a theory that makes sense to the therapist and is useful to the therapist in navigating the "wild ride" that is psychotherapy. That said, future research may identify specific circumstances in which certain models work better for certain clients (Sprenkle & Blow, 2004).

Show Me Proof: Evidence-Based Therapies

If you are not confused enough, there is yet another thread in the theory debate that is pulling therapists in the apparently opposite direction from the common factors research: empirically supported treatments, generally referred to as "evidenced-based therapies." These therapeutic models, which were developed through research and randomized trials (Sprenkle, 2002), should not be confused with evidence-based *practice* (EBP), which although sounding quite similar, refers to a different practice: using "evidence" and research to make clinical decisions (Patterson, Miller, Carnes, & Wilson, 2004).

When therapists, licensing boards, or funding institutions refer to therapy models as "evidence-based," they are generally referring to a set of standards that a 1993 task force of the American Psychological Association (APA) established for what was initially called *empirically validated treatments (EVTs)* and later called *empirically supported treatments (ESTs)*, the change underscoring that a treatment is always in the process of being further studied and refined (American Psychological Association, 1993; Chambless et al., 1996). The APA established several categories for describing empirically supported therapies, and others have developed similar categories.

Empirically Supported Treatments and Their Kin

Empirically Supported Treatment Criteria

Empirically supported treatments (ESTs) meet the following criteria (Chambless & Hollon, 1998; Sprenkle, 2002):

- Subjects are randomly assigned to treatment groups.
- In addition to the group that receives the treatment being studied, there must also be *one* of the following:
  - A no-treatment control (usually subjects are on a waiting list)
  - An alternative treatment (for comparison; may be an unspecified approach: "treatment as usual")
  - A placebo treatment
- Treatment is significantly better than the no-treatment control and at least equally as effective as an established alternative.
- Treatment is based on a written treatment manual with specific criteria for including or excluding clients.
- A specific population with a specific problem is identified.
- Researchers use reliable and valid outcome measures with appropriate statistical measures.

Pros and Cons

The advantages of ESTs are the following:

1. They have greater scientific support.
2. They have written manuals to guide treatment and are highly structured.
3. They target a specific population with a specific problem.

The disadvantages of ESTs are these:

1. They have limited applicability because they target a specific and therefore limited population.
2. They are expensive: therapists need highly specific training in the model and also need to be trained in a number of models to function effectively in most work environments.

Criteria for Additional Forms of Evidence-Based Treatments

In addition to the criteria for empirically supported treatments, criteria have been set for other evidence-based treatments:

- **Efficacious Treatments:** These treatments must meet the requirements for EBTs and in addition must undergo two independent investigations (studies conducted by someone who is not closely involved in the development of the treatment or invested in its outcome) (Chambless & Hollon, 1998; Sprenkle, 2002).

- **Efficacious and Specific Treatments:** These treatments must meet the criteria for efficacious treatments and in addition must be superior to alternative treatments in at least two independent studies (Chambless & Hollon, 1998; Sprenkle, 2002).

- **Meta-Analytically Supported Treatments (MASTs):** A meta-analysis is a quantitative research method that combines results from multiple studies, generally by examining the effect size, or the outcome variance attributed to the treatment. Using meta-analytic studies, Shadish and Baldwin (2002) developed the following criteria for MASTs to broaden the type of research that can be used to establish efficacy while maintaining rigorous scientific standards:

  - Effect sizes from more than one study of the treatment must be combined meta-analytically.
  - All studies must be randomized comparisons of the treatment to a no-treatment control group.
  - Meta-analysis must indicate a statistically significant effect size and a significant test.
  - Meta-analysis must use sound methods (e.g., aggregating effect sizes).

Real-World Applications of ESTs and MASTs

In 2002, Shadish and Baldwin identified 24 family therapy theories that fit the criteria for a MAST, whereas only 5 met the criteria for an EST. This difference existed primarily because ESTs require (a) a written treatment manual and (b) a narrowly defined population with a specific problem, whereas MASTs allow for other forms of training and more general populations to demonstrate efficacy. The findings of the APA's 2005 follow-up report on ESTs highlight the necessity for more broadly defined standards for evidence-based treatments such as MASTs (Woody, Weisz, & McLean, 2005). This survey indicated that although a higher percentage of ESTs were taught in the classroom, clinical training in ESTs dropped significantly from 1993 to 2003. When asked to identify the reasons, supervisors cited "uncertainty about how to conceptualize training in ESTs, lack of time, shortage of trained supervisors, inappropriateness of established ESTs for a given population, and philosophical opposition" (p. 9). Arguably, all but perhaps the last of these obstacles are clearly linked to the exact things that make ESTs unique: written treatment manuals and a narrowly defined population. Thus, although promising, ESTs have significant practical limitations at this time.

Evidence-Based Practice (EBP)

More commonly used in the medical field, *evidence-based practice* (EBP) uses research findings to inform clinical decisions for the care of individual clients. Patterson et al. (2004) describe five steps in employing EBPs:

Step 1: Develop an answerable question to focus the search for information: e.g., What treatments are most effective for teens who cut to relieve emotional pain?

Step 2: Search the literature for the best empirical evidence to answer the question: e.g., search digital databases such as PsychInfo and scholar.google.com using the keywords *adolescents, self-harm*, and *treatment*.

Step 3: Evaluate the validity, impact, and applicability of the research to determine its usefulness in this case: e.g., Is the study randomized? Were there comparison groups? What was the treatment effect size? Were the findings clinically relevant?

Step 4: Determine whether the research findings are applicable to the current client's situation: e.g., What are the potential benefits and risks of applying these findings with this client? Do I need to consider any diversity factors, such as age, ethnicity, class, or family system?

Step 5: After implementing the EBP, evaluate the effectiveness in this client's individual case: e.g., How did the client respond? Were there signs of improvement, no change, or worsening?

In comparison to ESTs, EBP is a practical and practice-friendly approach to using research to enhance family therapy.

Research in Perspective

Therapists need to keep the evidence-based therapy movement in perspective. Almost all research indicates that any therapy is better than no treatment at all: that is one of the major ideas behind the common factors movement (Miller, Duncan, & Hubble, 1997; Sprenkle & Blow, 2004). The evidence-based therapy approach refines what we know and aims to develop better and more specific therapies; however, this does not mean that nothing in the field has ever been researched or studied before. A more fair and realistic assessment is that family therapy and mental health therapies have an established history of meaningful research and our ability to do research more precisely continually increases. Research courses have been part of family therapy curricula from the beginning and are increasingly valued and expanded. A research orientation is not new; however, our ability to conduct more meticulous and useful studies is improving.

Perhaps it is useful to reflect on the broader picture. More than in many other mental health disciplines, family therapy theories were developed through observational research (Moon, Dillon, & Sprenkle, 1990). Teams of therapists observed sessions through one-way mirrors, developed hypotheses about what might work, tested these hypotheses, and then refined them as they went along. Rather than trying to prove a theory, these therapist-researchers were using outcomes to inform the development of a new frontier in mental health: working with couples and families. This type of research is rigorous in a different dimension than ESTs; namely, it can be usefully applied in everyday work settings by persons with standard training. According to Shadish and Baldwin (2002), many family therapy approaches that draw from this tradition fit the criteria for MASTs: these treatments worked for decades and have been refined and designed to target specific populations in the evidence-based approaches.

How to Choose: Dating Versus Marrying

Much like parents' advice to their teenage children, in the first few years I recommend that you casually "date" a theory before you decide to settle down. I am always surprised by new therapists who feel this tremendous pressure to find the "perfect" or "right" theory for them immediately—much like teenagers who are convinced that their first love will be their lifelong partner: it's possible, just not the most common scenario. You might want to "play the field" for a while to learn what is out there and what works best for you.

Fortunately, theory-dating generally ends better than romantic dating. After dating a theory, you are almost always forever enriched with new skills and knowledge, which is only sometimes true in the romantic realm. Additionally, the break-up part is almost always gentler. Thus, you can decide to try out a new theory every semester of your training or every year or so in your practice. After dating even two or three, your skill set and knowledge base will have significantly grown. You will have also learned more about who you are and your style as a therapist. At that point, you may find that it is time to settle down with one more than the others. When that happens, you are ready to define your philosophy.

Defining Your Philosophy

Once you have spent a few years dating, you may find that you are ready to settle down with one theory. Just as in love, there should be an engagement period during which you clearly define your commitment and get to know your new partner—and family of origin—more intimately. In the case of theory-dating, this involves pursuing advanced training in your theory of choice, usually by going to intensive seminars or working with a supervisor who specializes in your theory. Just as in marriage, in which a commitment to one person entails a commitment to an entire family, once you decide to commit to a theory, you are also committing to the broader philosophy that is the theory's foundation. I believe therapists who are clear about their philosophy of what it means to be human (ontology) and how people learn and change (epistemology) are best positioned to handle the variety of problems with which skilled therapists must learn to work. If you only master the techniques (system of doing), then you are less well prepared for handling the variety of issues that highly competent therapists must master.

Although there are many ways to define philosophical foundations of family therapies, I find it simplest to begin by considering four major categories: modernist, humanistic, systemic, and postmodern, each having its own approach to defining truth, reality, the therapeutic relationship, and the therapist's role in the change process. The following table summarizes their differences.

OVERVIEW OF PHILOSOPHICAL SCHOOLS

	MODERNIST	**HUMANISTIC**	**SYSTEMIC**	**POSTMODERN**
Truth	Objective truth	Subjective truth	Contextual truth	Multiple, coexisting truths
Reality	Objective; observable	Subjective; individually accessible	Contextual; emerges through systemic interactions; no one person has unilateral control	Co-constructed through language and social interaction; occurs at individual, relational, and societal levels
Therapeutic Relationship	Therapist as expert; hierarchical	Therapist as empathetic other	Therapist as participant in therapeutic system	Therapist as nonexpert; co-constructor of meaning
Therapist's Role in Change Process	Teaching and guiding clients in better ways of being and interacting	Creating a context that supports natural self-actualization process	"Perturbing" system, allowing system to reorganize itself; no direct control of system	Facilitating a dialogue in which client constructs new meanings and interpretations

Modernism

Modernism is founded on logical-positivist assumptions of an external, knowable "Truth." In modernist approaches, the therapist assumes an unequivocal role as expert, as in common in individual and family forms of cognitive-behavioral and psychodynamic therapies (see Chapter 13; e.g., Dattilio & Padesky, 1990; Ellis, 1994; Sharff & Sharff, 1987).

MODERNIST ASSUMPTIONS

- The therapist is an expert who assumes the primary responsibility for identifying pathology, problems, and goals, often assuming the role of teacher or mentor.
- Theory and research are the primary sources of information for identifying problems and diagnosing.
- The therapist uses theory and research to select treatment approaches; clients are expected to adapt to the selected treatment.

Two family therapy schools fit this category: psychodynamic and cognitive-behavioral therapies. Although broadly grounded in modernist assumptions about knowledge, each theory has its own unique position on the primary source of truth, the means through which it is best identified, and how best to define the therapeutic relationship.

MODERNIST THERAPIES

	PSYCHODYNAMIC THERAPIES	COGNITIVE-BEHAVIORAL THERAPIES
Primary Source of Objective Truth	Therapist's analysis of client dynamics based on theory	Measurable, external variables
Means of Identifying Truth	"Reality check"; comparing client experience against external perceptions, events, etc.	Scientific experimentation; therapist's definition of "reality" and/or social norms (identified through research)
Therapeutic Relationship	Hierarchical; therapist indirectly leads client toward goals	Educational; therapist is straightforward in directing client toward goals

Humanism

Humanistic therapies (Chapter 11) are founded on a phenomenological philosophy that prioritizes the individual's subjective truth. They include Carl Rogers's (1951) client-centered therapy, Fritz Perl's gestalt therapy (Passons, 1975), Virginia Satir's (1972) communication approach, Carl Whitaker's symbolic-experiential therapy (Whitaker & Keith, 1981), and Sue Johnson's emotionally focused therapy (Johnson, 2004).

HUMANISTIC ASSUMPTIONS

- By nature, humans are essentially good.
- All people naturally tend toward growth and strive for self-actualization, a process of becoming authentically human.
- The primary focus of treatment is the subjective, internal world of clients.
- Therapeutic interventions target emotions with the goal of promoting catharsis, the release of repressed emotions.
- A supportive, nurturing environment promotes therapeutic change.

The work of Virginia Satir and Carl Whitaker most clearly illustrates this philosophical stance, which in family therapy is always combined with a systemic perspective that accounts for the effect of family dynamics on an individual's emotional inner life. Although Satir's and Whitaker's approaches are based on the same philosophical traditions, their therapeutic approaches have dramatically different styles and assumptions, including the best ways to address self-actualization, change, confrontation, and the therapist's use of self (referring to how therapists use their personhood in session).

HUMANISTIC THERAPIES

	SATIR'S COMMUNICATION APPROACH	WHITAKER'S SYMBOLIC-EXPERIENTIAL APPROACH
Means of Promoting Self-Actualization	Emotionally safe and nurturing environment	Affective confrontation; "perturbing" the system
Change	Structured experiential exercises; role modeling	In vivo interactions with the therapist
Style of Confrontation	Gentle, educational	Direct, affective
"Authentic" Use of Self	Genuine caring for the client	Unedited and honest sharing of emotions and thoughts

Systemic Therapy

Rather than a formal philosophical school, systemic therapies are grounded in *general systems theory,* which stresses that living systems are open systems, connected with and embedded within other systems (von Bertalanffy, 1968), and *cybernetic systems theory,* which emphasizes a system's ability to self-correct to maintain homeostasis (Bateson, 1972). The latter is more influential in the development of specific therapeutic models, such as the Mental Research Institute's brief, problem-focused approach (Watzlawick, Weakland, & Fisch, 1974), strategic therapy (Haley, 1976; Madanes, 1981), and the Milan team's systemic approach (Boscolo, Cecchin, Hoffman, & Penn, 1987). Systems theories emphasize *contextual* truth, truth generated through repeated interpersonal interactions that set a "norm" and rules for behavior.

SYSTEMIC ASSUMPTIONS

- One cannot *not* communicate; all behavior is a form of communication.
- An individual's behavior and symptoms always make sense in the person's broader relational contexts.
- All behaviors, including unwanted symptoms, serve a purpose within the system, allowing the system to maintain or regain its homeostasis or feeling of "normalcy."
- No one individual unilaterally controls behavior in a system; thus no one person can be blamed for problems in a couple or family relationship; instead, problematic behavior is viewed as emerging from the interactions between members of the system.
- Therapeutic change involves alternating the interaction patterns within the system.

Within the field of systemic family therapy, Bateson's (1972) distinction between first-order and second-order cybernetics had significant impact on how therapists worked with families. With *first-order cybernetics,* the therapist is an objective, neutral observer describing the family as an outsider. Such therapy relies on assessment instruments and the therapist's perception of the family system. *Second-order cybernetic* theory applies the rules of first-order cybernetics on itself, positing that the therapist cannot be an objective, outside observer but instead creates a new system with the family: the observer-observed or therapist-family system. This second-order system is subject to the same dynamics as the first, including the drive to maintain homeostasis and rules for relating that are mutually reinforced. Second-order cybernetic theory maintains that whatever the therapist observes in the family reveals more about the therapist's values and priorities than about the family's because any description exposes what the therapist pays attention to and what the therapist ignores or misses. Second-order cybernetics laid the foundation for the transition to postmodern therapy, specifically constructivism in the MRI and Milan schools (Watzlawick, 1984).

In general, all systems therapists are influenced by both first- and second-order cybernetic theory. In practice, therapists generally emphasize one level of systems analysis or another. Broadly speaking, strategic and structural therapies were based on first-order theory and the MRI and Milan approaches gravitated toward second-order and later constructivist approaches.

- *First-order cybernetic approaches* lean toward the modernist tendency to find a more objective form of truth. Therapists who practice systemic therapies with a first-order orientation use more assessment instruments of family functioning and rely heavily on the therapist's perception of the system to guide practice.

- *Second-order cybernetic approaches* lean more toward a postmodern approach to truth (see next section). Their focus is on how the therapist and client co-construct a second-order system, which has its own unique set of rules for establishing truth.

SYSTEMIC THEORIES

	FIRST-ORDER CYBERNETICS	SECOND-ORDER CYBERNETICS
Level(s) of Analysis	Family system	Family system (level 1) and therapist-family system (level 2)
Target of Interventions	Correcting interactional sequences	"Perturbing" or interrupting interactional sequences
Therapist's Role	Tends to appear as a knowledgeable expert	Co-creator of therapeutic system
Focus of Assessment	Behavioral sequences	Meaning-making systems (epistemology)

Postmodern Therapy

Postmodern therapies are based on the premise that objective truth can never be fully known because it must always pass through subjective and intersubjective filters.

POSTMODERN ASSUMPTIONS

- The human mind does not have access to an outside reality independent of human interpretation; objectivity is not humanly possible.
- All knowledge and truth are culturally, historically, and relationally bound and therefore intersubjective: constructed within and between people.

- What a person experiences as "real" and believes to be "true" is shaped primarily through language and relationships.
- Language and the words used to describe one's experiences significantly affect how one's identity is shaped and experienced.
- The identification of a "problem" is a social process that occurs through language, both at the immediate local level and at the broader societal level.
- Therapy is a process of co-constructing new realities related to the client's personal identity and relationship with the problem.

Within family therapy, three schools of postmodernism are particularly influential (Anderson, 1997; Hoffman, 2002; Watzlawick, 1984):

- **Constructivism:** Constructivists focus on the construction of meaning within the individual organism, on how information is received and interpreted.

- **Social Constructionism:** Social constructionists focus on how people co-create meaning in relationships. They emphasize how truth is generated at the local (immediate) relational level.

- **Structuralism and Poststructuralism:** Structuralists and poststructuralists focus on analyzing how meanings are produced and reproduced within a culture through various practices and discourses.

POSTMODERN PHILOSOPHICAL FOUNDATIONS

	CONSTRUCTIVISM	**SOCIAL CONSTRUCTIONISM**	**STRUCTURALISM AND POSTSTRUCTURALISM**
Level of Reality Construction	Individual organism	Local relationship	Societal, political
Associated Theories	Later MRI and Milan theories	Collaborative therapy; reflecting teams	Narrative therapy; feminist and culturally informed therapies
Focus of Interventions	Recasting interpretations with new language	Dialogues that highlight multiple meanings and interpretations	Deconstruction and questioning of dominant discourses (popular knowledge)
Therapist's Role	Facilitate alternative interpretations	Noninterventional; facilitate dialogical process	Help identify external and historical influences

Dancing with Others Once You Marry

Once you commit yourself to a theory and philosophical stance, it ironically becomes much easier to dance with others. As you master one theoretical approach and deepen your understanding of the philosophical assumptions underlying it, you are able to understand other theories at a greater depth. This is perhaps where the common factors come in. There are similar principles that seem to be at play in all theories, and the more intimate you are with one theory the better able you are to identify these factors in others. It is also the case that you can see more clearly the subtle differences in outcome from philosophical assumptions, word choices, and interventions that differ across theories.

As therapists become more aware of the set of philosophical assumptions underlying their theory, whichever school that might be, they learn to skillfully adapt and integrate ideas from other approaches in a way that is philosophically consistent with their own approach. When a therapist is "eclectic" or "integrative" in a way that is not grounded in a single philosophical set of assumptions, that therapist is going to confuse his/her clients. One week the therapist might use a modernist approach and is an expert who has answers and knows the best way to approach the problem. The next week the therapist might try to use a postmodern approach in which the client is expected to be the expert and participate more as an equal. The following week the therapist might then shift to systemic ideas that emphasize the importance of context in defining the problem. As you might well imagine, a client working with this therapist is going to be very confused because each week the *client is required to relate differently to the therapist and to assume a different level of participation.* The therapist is also sending contradictory messages as to what is the measuring stick for "truth," progress, and direction. However, if the therapist is able to keep the philosophical assumptions consistent throughout therapy—what is our measuring stick for truth? what are our roles?—then the therapist can adapt concepts and techniques from other approaches without sending conflicting messages to the client, thus effectively incorporating a wider range of practices within a coherent approach to therapy.

ONLINE RESOURCES

Talking Cure.com
Information on the common factors.

www.talkingcure.com

Empirically Supported Treatment Documents
Links to APA documents on ESTs.

www.apa.org/divisions/div12/journals.html

REFERENCES

American Psychological Association. (1993, October). *Task force on promotion and dissemination of psychological procedures: A report adopted by the Division 12 Board.* Retrieved August 24, 2008, from www.apa.org/divisions/div12/journals.html

Anderson, H. (1997). *Conversations, language, and possibilities: A postmodern approach to therapy.* New York: Basic Books.

Bateson, G. (1972). *Steps to an ecology of mind.* San Francisco: Chandler.

Blow, A. J., Sprenkle, D. H., & Davis, S. D. (2007). Is who delivers the treatment more important than the treatment itself? *Journal of Marital and Family Therapy, 33,* 298–317.

Boscolo, L., Cecchin, G., Hoffman, L., & Penn, P. (1987). *Milan systemic family therapy.* New York: Basic Books.

Chambless, D. L., & Hollon, S. D. (1998). Defining empirically supported therapies. *Journal of Consulting and Clinical Psychology, 66,* 7–18.

Chambless, D. L., Sanderson, W. C., Shoham, V., Johnson, S. B., Pope, K. S., Crits-Christoph, P., Baker, M., Johnson, B., Woody, S. R., Sue, S., Beutler, L., Williams, D. A., & McCurry, S. (1996.). An update on empirically validated treatments. *Clinical Psychologist, 49*(2), 5–18. Available from www.apa.org/divisions/div12/journals.html

Dattilio, F. M., & Padesky, C. A. (1990). *Cognitive therapy with couples.* Sarasota, FL: Professional Resources Exchange.

Ellis, A. (1994). *Reason and emotion in therapy* (rev. ed.). New York: Kensington.

Haley, J. (1976). *Problem-solving therapy: New strategies for effective family therapy.* San Francisco: Jossey-Bass.

Hoffman, L. (2002). *Family therapy: An intimate history.* New York: Norton.

Johnson, S. M. (2004). *The practice of emotionally focused marital therapy: Creating connection* (2nd ed.). New York: Brunner/Routledge.

Lambert, M. (1992). Psychotherapy outcome research: Implications for integrative and eclectic therapists. In J. C. Norcross & M. R. Goldfried (Eds.), *Handbook of psychotherapy integration* (pp. 94–129). New York: Wiley.

Madanes, C. (1981). *Strategic family therapy.* San Francisco: Jossey-Bass.

Miller, S. D., Duncan, B. L., & Hubble, M. (1997). *Escape from Babel: Toward a unifying language for psychotherapy practice.* New York: Norton.

Miller, S. D., Duncan, B. L., & Hubble, M. A. (2004). Beyond integration: The triumph of outcome over process in clinical practice. *Psychotherapy in Australia, 10*(2), 2–19.

Moon, S. M., Dillon, D. R., & Sprenkle, D. H. (1990). Family therapy and qualitative research. *Journal of Marital and Family Therapy, 16,* 357–373.

Passons, W. R. (1975). *Gestalt therapies in counseling.* New York: Holt, Rinehart, & Winston.

Patterson, J. E., Miller, R. B., Carnes, S., & Wilson, S. (2004). Evidence-based practice for marriage and family therapies. *Journal of Marital and Family Therapy, 30,* 183–195.

Rogers, C. (1951). *Client-centered therapy.* Boston: Houghton Mifflin.

Satir, V. (1972). *Peoplemaking.* Palo Alto, CA: Science and Behavior Books.

Scharff, D., & Scharff, J. S. (1987). *Object relations family therapy.* New York: Jason Aronson.

Shadish, W. R., & Baldwin, S. A. (2002). Meta-analysis of MFT interventions. In D. H. Sprenkle (Ed.), *Effectiveness research in marriage and family therapy* (pp. 339–370). Alexandria, VA: American Association for Marriage and Family Therapy.

Sprenkle, D. H. (Ed.). (2002). Editor's introduction. In D. H. Sprenkle (Ed.), *Effectiveness research in marriage and family therapy* (pp. 9–25). Alexandria, VA: American Association for Marriage and Family Therapy.

Sprenkle, D. H., & Blow, A. J. (2004). Common factors and our sacred models. *Journal of Marital and Family Therapy, 30,* 113–129.

Sprenkle, D. H., Davis, S. D., & Lebow, J. (2009). *Beyond our sacred models: Common factors in couple, family, and relational psychotherapy.* New York: Guilford.

Tallman, K., & Bohart, A. C. (1999). The client as a common factor: Clients as self-healers. In M. A. Hubble, B. L. Duncan, & S. D. Miller (Eds.), *The heart and soul of change: What works in therapy* (pp. 91–131). Washington, DC: American Psychological Association.

von Bertalanffy, L. (1968). *General system theory: Foundations, development, applications* (rev. ed.). New York: George Braziller.

Wampold, B. E. (2001). *The great psychotherapy debate: Models, methods, and findings.* Mahwah, NJ: Erlbaum.

Watzlawick, P. (1984). *The invented reality: How do we know what we believe we know? Contributions to constructivism.* New York: Norton.

Watzlawick, P., Weakland, J., & Fisch, R. (1974). *Change: Principles of problem formation and problem resolution.* New York: Norton.

Whitaker, C. A., & Keith, D. V. (1981). Symbolic-experiential family therapy. In A. S. Gurman & D. P. Kniskern (Eds.), *Handbook of family therapy* (pp. 187–224). New York: Brunner/Mazel.

Woody, S. R., Weisz, J., & McLean, C. (2005). Empirically supported treatments: 10 years later. *Clinical Psychologist, 58,* 5–11.

Philosophical Foundations of Family Therapy Theories

Lay of the Land

Before exploring the various models of family therapy, I want to briefly introduce you to their philosophical foundations. The two closely related philosophical traditions that inform family therapy approaches are *systems theory* and *social constructionism*, a particular strand of postmodernism. To some degree or another, all schools of family therapy have been influenced by these two theories, with traditional therapies drawing more heavily from systemic theory and more recent ones from social constructionist theory.

Systemically Influenced Family Therapies and Theories

- **Systemic and Strategic Theories:** Mental Research Institute (MRI), Milan, and strategic therapies (Chapter 9)
- **Structural Family Therapy** (Chapter 10)
- **Experiential Family Therapy Theories:** Satir's growth model, symbolic–experiential therapy, and emotionally focused couples therapy (Chapter 11)
- **Intergenerational Theories:** Bowen's intergenerational and psychoanalytic therapies (Chapter 12)
- **Cognitive-Behavioral Family Therapies** (Chapter 13)
- **Early Solution-Based Therapies** (Chapter 14)

Social Constructionist Family Therapies

- **Later Solution-Based Therapies** (Chapter 14)
- **Narrative Therapy** (Chapter 15)
- **Collaborative Therapy** (Chapter 15)

Systemic Foundations
Rumor Has It: The People and Their Stories

The Macy Conferences

Not so long ago (1940) in a place not so far away (New York), Josiah Macy (of Macy's department store fame) assembled an unexpected configuration of scholars and researchers to discuss how groups of things operate to form a system (Segal, 1991). This series of conferences in the early 1940s, the Macy Conferences, gave birth to *general systems theory* and *cybernetic systems theory*, which describe how biological, social, and mechanical systems operate. Rather than being developed by a single person, these ideas emerged from interactive dialogue and shared research that involved numerous cutting-edge experts and scholars. Their theories led to a new approach to psychotherapy—family therapy—which is not simply a modality (i.e., working with a family versus an individual) but a unique philosophical view of human behavior.

Systemic Theorists

"The concepts that constitute Communication or Interactional [Systems] Theory emerged not from any one individual, but, rather were the product of the interaction between the members of what has become known as the Palo Alto Group [the Bateson Team]."—Weakland, 1988, p. 58

Gregory Bateson

Gregory Bateson, who participated in the Macy Conferences with his then wife Margaret Mead, was a British anthropologist who explored cybernetic theory by studying intertribal interactions in New Guinea and Bali (Bateson, 1972, 1979, 1991; Mental Research Institute, 2002). Bateson's elegant and thoughtful articulations of cybernetic theory influenced numerous disciplines, including communications, anthropology, and family therapy. As part of his research on human communications, he assembled what was later known as the *Bateson Group*: Don Jackson, Jay Haley, William Fry, and John Weakland. For 10 years, he studied communication in families with members diagnosed with schizophrenia, provided consultation on cybernetic theory, and introduced team members to the trance work of Milton Erickson. The result was the *double-bind theory of schizophrenia* (Bateson, 1972), which reconceptualized psychotic behavior as an attempt to meaningfully respond in a family system characterized by double-bind communications. Bateson's prior anthropological research helped the team view problematic human behavior as a function of larger social systems rather than being purely intrapsychic.

Heinz von Foerster

Another participant of the Macy Conferences, Heinz von Foerster was born in Austria and originally studied physics before developing his theories on cybernetic systems, second-order cybernetics, and radical constructivism, a postmodern theory that describes how an individual constructs his/her reality (Mental Research Institute, 2002). His work also contributed to the philosophical foundation for systemic therapies.

Milton Erickson

Trained in medicine as a psychiatrist, Erickson was a master therapist, well known for his brief, rapid, and creative interventions and considered by many to be the father of modern hypnosis (Erickson & Keeney, 2006; Mental Research Institute, 2002). The early MRI team consulted with Erickson as they developed their brief approach to family therapy. Erickson's clinical innovations, brief approach, and emphasis on possibilities are reflected in their therapies. Erickson's work was also highly influential in the development of solution-based therapies (Chapter 14).

Bradford Keeney

A family therapist, Keeney studied with Bateson in exploring the implications of cybernetics of cybernetics, or second-order cybernetics, which acknowledges the role of the observer (e.g., the therapist) on what is observed (Keeney, 1983, 1985).

In his more recent anthropological work he has studied shamanism and the cybernetic (i.e., wholistic) worldviews of native cultures, most notably the Kalahari Bushmen (Keeney, 1994, 1997, 1998, 2000a, 2000b, 2001a, 2001b, 2002a, 2002b, 2003). He has also used concepts from improvisational theater to develop *improvisational therapy* (Keeney, 1990) and, with his colleague Wendell Ray, has also developed *resource-focused therapy*, a strength-focused, systemic approach (Ray & Keeney, 1994).

Systemic Assumptions

General Systems and Cybernetic Systems Theories

Systems theory has its origin in the cross-disciplinary study that began at the Macy Conferences, which were attended by rocket scientists building self-guided missiles, anthropologists studying intertribal interactions in Bali, and ecologists studying the interactions between species. These researchers discovered that, whether studying mechanical parts, social groups, or animals, they were noticing that systems operated using the same basic principles, which von Bertalanffy (1968) developed into *general systems theory.* Closely related but more focused on social systems was the *cybernetic systems theory* articulated by Gregory Bateson (1972), which has had the most influence on the field of family therapy.

Homeostasis and Self-Correction

The term *cybernetic* means "steersman" in Greek, which hints at the functional principles of cybernetic systems: they are *self-correcting*, and therefore able to "steer" their own course, in contrast to a computer, for example, which needs an outside entity to steer it (Bateson, 1972). What does a cybernetic system steer toward? *Homeostasis.* Homeostasis, in the case of families, refers to the unique set of behavioral, emotional, and interactional norms that create stability for the family or other social group. Despite what the name might imply, homeostasis is not static but *dynamic.* Much like a gymnast constantly moving to maintain her balance on a beam, systems must be constantly in flux to maintain stability. In all living systems, it takes work to maintain balance, whether in mood, habits, weight, or overall health. The key to maintaining stability is the ability to self-correct, which requires feedback.

Negative and Positive Feedback

You can pretty much guarantee that *negative* and *positive feedback* will be on any multiple-choice test about family therapy. Why? Because the disciplinary use of the terms are the opposite of their colloquial use. So, remember, the negative and positive feedback questions are always *trick questions*—that is, if you haven't studied. Here's how to remember it:

NEGATIVE VERSUS POSITIVE FEEDBACK

Negative Feedback: No new information to steersman = the waters are the same = homeostasis.

Positive Feedback: Yes, new information is coming to the steersman = the waters are choppy, moving faster, colder = something is *changing*.

Negative feedback is "more of the same" feedback, meaning there is no new news or change (Bateson, 1972; Watzlawick, Bavelas, & Jackson, 1967). In contrast, like "positive test results" in medicine, positive feedback is news that things are not within expected parameters, which may be experienced as a problem or a crisis, depending on the situation. The problem or change could be due to what is generally considered bad news (death of a loved one, a fight with a spouse, a problem at work) or good news (graduation from college and needing to find a job, getting married and starting a new household, moving to a new city for a job). Both good and bad news can create positive feedback loops, which result in one of two options: (a) return to former homeostasis, or (b) create a new homeostasis.

In most cases, a system initially responds to positive feedback by trying to get back to its former homeostasis as quickly as possible. After a fight, most couples quickly want to make up and "get back to normal." After a death, most talk about how getting back to normal will take a while, depending on how significant the deceased person was. However, sometimes it is not possible to get back to the "old normal," and a new normal needs to be created. The new norm or homeostasis is also referred to as "second-order change."

First- and Second-Order Change

Second-order change describes when a system restructures its homeostasis in response to positive feedback and the rules that govern the system fundamentally shift (Watzlawick, Weakland, & Fisch, 1974). *First-order change* refers to when the system returns to its previous homeostasis after positive feedback. In first-order change, the roles can reverse (e.g., a former distancer could start pursuing), but the underlying family structure and rules for relating stay essentially the same: someone is pursuing someone. This type of first-order shift is frequent in the early stages of couples therapy when partners shift between being the pursuer and the distancer. For example, if in the beginning the woman was asking for more closeness from her husband and he was asking for more space, as therapy progresses they may shift roles. Although the problem may appear solved, functionally there has been no shift in the rules that regulate intimacy in the relationship; the partners have just changed roles, so it looks and feels different. A second-order shift with this couple would involve reducing the overall pursuer-distancer pattern and increasing each person's ability to tolerate more togetherness and more distance.

It is also important to remember that second-order change is not always necessary in therapy, depending on the client's situation. In therapy, first-order solutions make logical sense; second-order solutions seem odd and illogical because they are introducing new rules into the system. Here's a clinical confession: in actual practice the distinction between first- and second-order change is often difficult to discern. I sometimes like to say, "That was 1.5-order change." Perhaps that is because most of us change in small shifts. However, the concept of first- and second-order change enables the therapist to ask whether roles have merely shifted or whether there has been a fundamental change in the ability to negotiate more intense intimacy and tolerate greater independence.

"One Cannot Not Communicate"

The early work of the Bateson team resulted in Watzlawick et al.'s (1967) classic text, *Pragmatics of Human Communication*, in which they proposed the following axiom: "One cannot not communicate." In addition to blatantly ignoring high school English teachers' rules about double negatives, this axiom seems to contradict the most common problem presented by couples and families: "We can't (or don't) communicate." So, where did this claim come from? The Bateson team learned from their research with schizophrenic family members that even schizophrenic attempts to not communicate (e.g., nonsense, immobile states, etc.) still sent a message, often communicating a desire to not communicate. Since all behavior is a form of communication and it is impossible to not be engaged in some form of behavior (at least while we are alive), it follows that we are always communicating. As we all know, silence speaks volumes, as does nonsense, withdrawal, or a frozen pose; thus even the most creative attempts to not communicate send a message. More commonly, the claim "we just can't communicate" means that one person doesn't like what the other has to say and that the two are unable to reach agreement, at which point it is helpful to examine the anatomy of the communicated messages—namely, the report and command aspects of communication.

Communication: Report and Command (Metacommunication)

Each communication has two components—*report* (content) and *command* (relationship)—that help therapists conceptualize communication and, more importantly, miscommunication. The report is the content: the literal meaning of the statement. The command is the *metacommunication,* or the communication about how to interpret the communication (Watzlawick et al., 1967). The command aspect always *defines the relationship* between two people. For example, the same piece of advice (content), such as "You might want to wear sunscreen today," can be accompanied by a command that defines either a peer-peer relationship or a one-up/one-down relationship. This is where miscommunication, double-bind communication, and arguments come in.

ELEMENTS OF A COMMUNICATED MESSAGE

Communicated message = **Report:** Data, information (primarily verbal)
+ **Command:** Defining relationship (primarily nonverbal)

The concept of report and command helps explain why couples, families, friends, coworkers, and basically any two humans can have elaborate, drawn-out arguments over taking out trash, toilet seat lids, cat litter, toothpaste, and the recalled order of events at last night's party. These arguments, although appearing to be over "little things," are really about *how the relationship is being defined* in relation to the little things; thus they are about a big thing, namely, how to define each person's role in the relationship.

When arguing over trash and cat litter, couples are usually disagreeing with each other's message at the command (relationship) level, not the content. It often helps to move the discussion directly to the metacommunication level, communicating about the command aspect of the communication, which in the case of household chores may include power dynamics or perceived caring. By directly discussing the metacommunication aspects (e.g., when the wife tells her husband to take out the trash, he feels that she is treating him like a child), the couple can clarify these relational issues, at which point the content issues are usually quickly resolved. Since every communication, verbal or nonverbal, has both report and command functions, the process of "getting meta" is infinite, because the partners can then talk about the metacommunication (command) aspect of the first metacommunication.

Psychoeducation note: Although psychoeducation is not a traditional systemic technique, spending a minute or so teaching clients about this issue can help some clients better understand what is going on in their arguments if it fits with your theoretical orientation.

Double Binds

Double-bind theory goes back to the Bateson Group's (Jackson, Haley, Fry, and Weakland) earliest research on families with a member diagnosed with schizophrenia (Bateson, 1972). Watzlawick et al. (1967) identify the following ingredients of a double-bind communication:

1. Two people are in an *intense relationship* that has high survival value, such as a familial relation, a friendship, a religious affiliation, a doctor-patient relationship, a therapist-client relationship, or a relationship between an individual and his/her social group.

2. Within this relationship a message is given that is structured with (a) a primary injunction (e.g., a request or order) and (b) a simultaneous secondary injunction that contradicts the first, usually at the metacommunication level.

3. The receiver of the contradictory injunctions has the sense that he/she *cannot escape* or step outside the cognitive frame of the contradictions, either by metacommunicating (e.g., commenting on the contradiction) or by withdrawing, without threatening the relationship. The receiver is made to feel "bad" or "mad" for even suggesting there is a discrepancy.

Common examples are the commands "love me" or "be genuine," in which one person orders another to have spontaneous and authentic feelings. In their research, the MRI team noticed that this type of communication characterized families who had a member diagnosed with schizophrenia. A common exchange in these families was a mother who gave her child a cold, distant hug (command aspect communicates distance) and then said, "Why are you never happy to see me?" (report aspect suggests closeness). No matter how the child responds, the mother can prove him/her wrong. Thus the "logical" response is a *nonresponse* or *nonsense response*, which characterizes schizophrenic behavior, such as word salad (spoken words that have no real meaning), loose associations (tangentially relating words or topics), or catatonic behavior (rigid, repetitive behavior that has no interactive meaning).

Although the double-bind theory does not account entirely for how schizophrenia develops or who develops it, it is still useful for clinicians working with families that get stuck—whether or not there is a member diagnosed with schizophrenia. Common examples of double binds in families that present for therapy are the following:

- Someone asks a partner or child to spontaneously "show love" in a specific manner (bring flowers, do chores), but when the person shows love in the way requested, the partner or parent says, "That does not count because I had to ask you to do it." This becomes a double-bind situation with no way for the person to show genuine feeling.

- A very strict parent makes all the child's decisions but says, "I trust you to make good decisions." When the child tries to comment on the incongruency, the parent reverts to "But I *do* trust you."

Identifying the double bind is the therapist's first step at intervening in these destructive patterns.

Symmetrical and Complementary Relationships

Originating in Bateson's (1972) anthropological work, the distinction between symmetrical and complementary relationships is frequently used to understand family interactions. In *symmetrical* relationships, the parties have "symmetrical" or evenly distributed abilities and roles in the system: an equal relationship (Watzlawick et al., 1967). Conflict in symmetrical systems generally takes the form of two equals fighting until there is a winner: each is viewed and experienced as a relative equal and the outcome is not predictable. In family relationships, symmetrical dynamics are often seen in couples and similar-aged siblings.

In contrast, in *complementary* relationships each party has a distinct role that balances or complements the other, often resulting in a form of hierarchy. Conflict in these relationships is less frequent because there are clearly defined, separate roles. Complementary dynamics often become a problem with couples when their roles become exaggerated or rigid. Examples of common complementary dynamics include pursuer/distancer, emotional/logical, visionary/planner, and easygoing/organized. These dynamics can provide a counterbalance that is enjoyable and helpful, especially early in the relationship; however, often these roles become exaggerated and rigid, creating a feeling of "stuckness." By the time clients present for therapy, often appear to be deeply ingrained personality traits rather than roles that each person has taken on as part of the systemic dance. The family therapist's task is to see these rigid complementary roles as part of the larger system rather than as fixed personality structures. It is then much easier to have hope for change and to be creative in making change.

The Family as a System

The defining feature of systemic approaches is viewing the family as a system, an entity in itself, with the whole greater than the sum of its parts (Watzlawick et al., 1967). What does this really mean? Systemic therapists view the interactional patterns of the family as a sort of "mind" or organism that is not controlled by any single member or outside entity, such as a therapist. This view results in several startling propositions:

- **No Single Person Orchestrates the Interactional Patterns.** The rules that govern family interactions are not consciously constructed like the U.S. Constitution; instead they emerge through an organic process of interaction, feedback (reaction), and correction until a norm or homeostasis is formed. In fact, many of the arguments early in a relationship serve as feedback to shape the emerging relationship's homeostatic norms. In most cases, this whole process occurs with minimal metacommunication about how the relational rules are being formed.

- **All Behavior Makes Sense in Context.** Because all behavior is a form of communication, it makes sense in the context in which it is expressed, within the rules of that particular system. Thus, even the seemingly nonsensical communication of schizophrenia makes sense in the larger family system.

- **No Single Person Can Be Blamed for Family Distress.** Because no one consciously creates the rules but instead the patterns are mutually negotiated through ongoing interactions, it follows that no single person can be fully to blame for family problems. Although individuals do have moral and ethical obligations in cases of abuse, the interactions "make sense" within the broader relational context and rules.

- **Personal Characteristics Are Dependent on the System.** Although a member may display certain characteristics or tendencies, these are not inherent personality characteristics that exist independent of the system; rather, they emerge from the interactional patterns in the system. Thus, even when a family reports, "Suzie has always been like this" (e.g., angry, helpful, forgetful), the therapist takes this to be a statement more about the rules (possible rigidity) of the system than a truth about Suzie.

Epistemology

"The proposition 'I see you' or 'You see me' is a proposition which contains within it what I am calling 'epistemology.' It contains within it assumptions about how we get information, what sort of stuff information is, and so forth . . . certain propositions about the nature of knowing and the nature of the universe in which we live and how we know about it."—Bateson, 1972, p. 478

Bateson's ideas about epistemology are foundational to all systemic family therapies. In the strict philosophical sense, *epistemology* is the study of knowledge and the process of knowing. From his cybernetic investigations, Bateson concluded that most of the propositions humans assume to be true are erroneous; they *appear* true because they capture one dimension of an interactional sequence, but they rarely include the broader awareness of how observer and observed reciprocally reinforce and impact each other. Thus a wife's complaint that her husband is cold and indifferent does not take into account how their ongoing series of interactions have impacted each of their behaviors and frames for interpretation. Family therapists pay careful attention to the family's epistemology, the operating premises that underlie their actions and cognitions (Keeney, 1983).

Second-Order Cybernetics

A later distinction in systemic literature, *second-order cybernetics* (see Chapter 7) refers to applying systemic principles to the observing system, such as to the therapy system (therapist observing the family system). In the process of observing another system, a new observer-observed system is created: a second-order (or second-level) system. The therapist can no longer assume to be a neutral, unbiased observer, but is rather an active participant in creating what is observed.

The co-creation process happens in several different ways. First, a therapist's descriptions reveals *more about the therapist* than about the family in that any description reflects what information the therapist deems most valuable and useful. Second, *how* a therapist interacts with or treats a family significantly impacts the actions and attitudes of the family while in the therapist's presence. A therapist who engages a family in a detached, professional manner will elicit different behaviors than one who uses a playful, low-key style. Which is more "real"? Neither, or more accurately, both. Each response is a "natural, honest" response for the family system *in the context* of a particular professional. Therapists who maintain an awareness of second-order cybernetic principles remain continually attuned to how their behavior is shaping that of the client and how their descriptions of clients reflect their own values. This attention to the co-creation of the therapist-client reality became the focus of social constructionist therapists.

Social Constructionist Foundations

Social constructionist philosophy is a particular strand of postmodern philosophy, which has influenced a wide range of disciplines, including art, theater, music, architecture, literature studies, cultural studies, and philosophy. Because their systemic foundations had already conceptualized reality from a relational perspective, family therapists were the first mental health professionals to embrace postmodern philosophy. Of the various postmodern schools—constructivist, social constructionist, structuralist and poststructuralist (see Chapter 7)—social constructionism has been the most influential in the development of new psychotherapy models, such as solution-focused, collaborative, and narrative therapies (see Chapters 14 and 15).

Systems Theory and Social Constructionism: Similarities and Differences

The move from a systemic view (particularly the second-order cybernetic perspective) to a social constructionist perspective can be seen as a natural evolution and continuation of systemic concepts, which describe how social interactions shape a person's experience of reality. Although the vocabulary and metaphors change, the *emphasis on relationships and the relational construction of reality does not.* The earliest writings in family therapy explored how people construct their lived reality through interpersonal relations (Bateson, 1972; Fisch, Weakland, & Segal, 1982; Jackson, 1952, 1955; Watzlawick, 1977, 1978, 1984; Weakland, 1951), laying the foundation for postmodern approaches. In fact, many of the original approaches that began systemically, such as Milan therapy and the MRI approach (see Chapter 9), over time evolved to a more constructionist form. Thus systemic and postmodern therapies have more shared views than differences, especially when compared with other nonrelational psychotherapies.

Systemic and social constructionist theories share the following assumptions:

- A person's lived reality is relationally constructed.
- Personal identity and an individual's symptoms are related to the social systems of which they are a part.

- Changing one's language and description of a problem alters how it is experienced.
- Truth can only be determined within relational contexts; an objective, outsider perspective is impossible.

Despite these and other similarities, there are notable differences that can be traced to a shift in metaphor. Systems theory uses a *systems* metaphor: a family is a system, a group of individuals who coordinate meaning and their understanding of the world. Social constructionist therapies use a *textual* metaphor: people narrate their lives to create meaning using the social discourses available to them. In addition, social constructionist therapies emphasize the role of the therapist in the co-construction of the client's reality, much like systemic therapists' attention to second-order cybernetic dynamics, resulting in a different approach to relating to clients and their problems. Furthermore, constructionist therapists use clients' language and stories differently than systemic therapies to create interventions.

Social Constructionist and Related Theorists

Kenneth Gergen

A social psychologist, Ken Gergen first introduced social constructionist ideas to the mental health professions in his 1985 article in *American Psychologist.* His work has laid the foundation for the development of social constructionist therapy approaches, most notably collaborative therapy (Anderson, 1997; Anderson & Gehart, 2007; Anderson & Goolishian, 1992) and to a lesser degree narrative therapy (Freedman & Combs, 1996; White & Epston, 1990). His work has included detailed applications of social constructionism to psychological and social issues (Gergen, 1999, 2001) and to postmodern ethics (McNamee & Gergen, 1999). His most recent work is on positive aging (Gergen & Gergen, 2007).

Sheila McNamee

Working with Gergen, Sheila McNamee, a communications theorist, has been a leader in translating social constructionist ideas to therapy (McNamee & Gergen, 1992), including an in-depth exploration of ethical issues (McNamee & Gergen, 1999). She has also been at the forefront of developing social constructionist pedagogy (McNamee, 2007).

John Shotter

John Shotter's social constructionist work focuses on how people coordinate *joint action* through shared meanings and understanding (Shotter, 1993). His work emphasizes the ethics of mutual accountability in social relationships (Shotter, 1984).

Michel Foucault

Rejecting philosophical labels such as a *postmodernist, structuralist,* or *poststructuralist,* Michel Foucault (1972, 1979, 1980) was a prolific social critic and philosopher who described how power and knowledge shape individual realities in a given society. A significant influence on Michael White's narrative therapy (see Chapter 15), Foucault's work introduces the political and social justice ramifications of language and power in therapy.

Ludvig Wittgenstein

An Austrian philosopher, Wittgenstein's philosophy of language (1973) is highly influential in postmodern therapies, notably solution-focused brief therapy and collaborative therapy (Chapters 14 and 15). He describes language as inextricably woven into the fabric of life and argues that language cannot be meaningfully removed from its everyday use, as it commonly is in philosophical and theoretical discussions.

Mikhail Bakhtin

A Russian critic and philosopher, Bakhtin worked on dialogue and concepts of identity, emphasizing that the self is *unfinalizable* (can never be fully known) and that self and other are inextricably intertwined (Baxter & Montgomery, 1996).

Postmodern Assumptions

Skeptical of Objective Reality: "Whatever Exists Is Mute"

Postmodernists are skeptical about the possibility of identifying an *objective reality*, such as *x* is a healthy behavior and *y* is not (Gergen, 1985). They describe reality as "mute" (Gergen, 1998), meaning that events and things in life do not come with prepackaged meanings, such as marriage is good, fat is ugly, and cars are bad. Instead, meaning is constructed by communities of people.

Reality Is Constructed

Postmodernists view all "truths" and "realities" as *constructed* (you will notice and perhaps be irritated by the frequent use of quote marks to emphasize that a concept is a construction, not a truth). Language and consciousness are necessary to develop meanings and to determine the value of an object or thing (Gergen, 1985; Watzlawick, 1984). Different postmodern schools emphasize and analyze different levels of reality construction; however, they principally recognize that the construction of reality is a complex process that involves all of these levels:

- **Linguistic Level—Poststructuralism and Philosophy of Language:** Focuses on how words shape our reality rather than being a reflection of it, a premise shared by all forms of postmodern thinking.

- **Personal Level—Constructivism:** Focuses on how reality is constructed within an individual organism; most closely associated with later developments of MRI and Milan therapies (Watzlawick, 1984).

- **Relational Level—Social Constructionism:** Focuses on how reality is created in immediate relationships (Gergen, 1985, 1999, 2001); most closely associated with collaborative therapy.

- **Societal Level—Critical Theory:** Focuses on how reality is constructed at the larger, societal level; most closely associated with narrative therapy, which draws heavily on the work of Michel Foucault (1972, 1979, 1980).

Reality Is Constructed Through Language

Postmodernists generally agree that reality is constructed primarily through language. Language is not neutral: words have real effects in our lives (Gergen, 1985). Most importantly for therapeutic purposes, words are the primary medium for (a) fashioning our identities, and (b) identifying what is a problem and what is not (Anderson, 1997; Gergen, 2001). For example, a person can interpret the same set of events (e.g., losing one's cool) as "having a bad day" or "being a bad person," each having dramatically different implications for identity and the definition of the problem. This level of reality construction, used in all postmodern therapies, is emphasized by poststructuralists and constructivists.

Reality Is Negotiated Through Relationships

The meanings we attribute to life experiences are not developed alone but in relationships, with immediate friends and family and more broadly with society and the subcultures of which we are a part (Gergen, 1985). The meaning a person gives to a particular behavior, hair cut, job, family relation, sex act, or religious view is always embedded in a web of "local" (immediate) relationships as well as the larger societal dialogue about the particular issue. Thus how a person views premarital sex, lying, or disciplining children develops through and within the multiple layers of outer dialogues. Postmodern therapists help clients untangle the dialogues around problems so that clients can determine those with which they choose to affiliate. This level of reality construction is emphasized in theories that emphasize social constructionism and critical theory.

Shared Meanings Coordinate Social Action

Shared meanings and values are needed to coordinate social action, or more simply, get along with others (Gergen, 2001; Shotter, 1993). Without agreed-upon meanings on what is polite and what is rude or what is good and what is bad, it would be impossible for humans to live together—there would be total chaos. Instead, groups of people coordinate meanings and values: we call this *culture.*

Tradition, Culture, and Oppression

We cannot make sense of our lives outside of tradition or culture, which refers to not only ethnicity and nationality but any small or large group that has a set of norms. Cultural traditions create a framework for (a) making meaning of our individual lives and (b) successfully coordinating our actions with others. Culture provides a set of values that its members can use to interpret their lives, knowing whether they are living a "good" life. In addition, culture provides a framework for safely and effectively interacting with others, allowing for the shared meanings necessary for marriage, family life, commerce, recreation, and religion. However, selecting certain goods and values over others inevitably labels certain behaviors and qualities as bad and undesirable. If a culture values productivity, it views taking time to relax negatively; if a culture values family, it de-emphasizes individuality. Thus *all cultures are by their very nature oppressive* (Gergen, 1998), because—by definition—they must identify certain behaviors as acceptable and others as unacceptable. The degree to which a culture is oppressive is directly correlated with its ability to be reflexive.

Reflexivity and Humanity

Any given culture remains *humane* to the extent that it is *reflexive,* able to examine its effects on others and to question and doubt its values and meanings (Gergen, 1998). Within any group of people, there are some people for whom the dominant cultural norms fit and others for whom they do not. The extent to which a culture listens and responds to the minority voices within it is the extent to which that culture maintains its humanity, growing and expanding to reduce the oppressive forces that are inescapable if humans are to live with one another.

Social Constructionism, Postmodernism, and Diversity

Postmodern philosophy, with its suspiciousness about singular "truths," has profoundly affected most current therapies because it heightens awareness of diversity issues. Postmodernists challenge the concept that norms cannot be fairly established because these norms are created by one group within the society and do not fairly capture the lived experience of others in that society and even less so the reality of other groups or cultures. This is readily seen with gender, socioeconomic status, age, culture, religion, and other factors. Postmodernism proposes that the behaviors, thoughts, and feelings of a white, middle-aged, Protestant male from the Northeast cannot be assumed to be the same as those of an adolescent son of Southeast Asian immigrants who are semimigrant farmers in California's Central Valley. They both have their own reality and truth and their respective norms and definitions of the good life; therapists must meet each with this fact in mind.

Philosophical Wrap-Up

This chapter has briefly reviewed some the key philosophical concepts that inform the various approaches to family therapy that you will be reading about in the following chapters. Each approach has found unique ways to use these philosophical concepts. Thus the same concepts have different practical expressions in the various theories. Nonetheless, they provide connecting threads that can be traced from one theory to the next, resulting in an undeniable kinship.

ONLINE RESOURCES

Ken Gergen's Web Page

www.swarthmore.edu/SocSci/kgergen1/web/page.phtml?st=home&id=home

Mental Research Institute

www.mri.org

John Shotter's Web Page

www.pubpages.unh.edu/~jds/

The Taos Institute
Explores social constructionist practices in a wide range of disciplines.

www.taosinstitute.org

REFERENCES

Anderson, H. (1997). *Conversations, language, and possibilities: A postmodern approach to therapy.* New York: Basic Books.

Anderson, H., & Gehart, D. (Eds.). (2007). *Collaborative therapy: Relationships and conversations that make a difference.* New York: Brunner/Routledge.

Anderson, H., & Goolishian, H. (1992). The client is the expert: A not-knowing approach to therapy. In S. McNamee & K. J. Gergen (Eds.), *Therapy as social construction* (pp. 25–39). Newbury Park, CA: Sage.

Bateson, G. (1972). *Steps to an ecology of mind.* San Francisco: Chandler.

Bateson, G. (1979). *Mind and nature: A necessary unity.* New York: Dutton.

Bateson, G. (1991). *A sacred unity: Further steps to an ecology of mind.* New York: Harper/Collins.

Baxter, L. A., & Montgomery, B. M. (1996). *Relating: Dialogues and dialectics.* New York: Guilford.

Erickson, B. A., & Keeney, B. (Eds). (2006). *Milton Erickson, M.D.: An American healer.* Sedona, AZ: Leete Island Books.

Fisch, R., Weakland, J., & Segal, L. (1982). *The tactics of change: Doing therapy briefly.* New York: Jossey-Bass.

Foucault, M. (1972). *The archeology of knowledge* (A. Sheridan-Smith, trans.). New York: Harper & Row.

Foucault, M. (1979). *Discipline and punish: The birth of the prison.* Middlesex: Peregrine Books.

Foucault, M. (1980). *Power/knowledge: Selected interviews and other writings.* New York: Pantheon Books.

Freedman, J., & Combs, G. (1996). *Narrative therapy: The social construction of preferred realities.* New York: Norton.

Gergen, K. J. (1985). The social constructionist movement in modern psychology. *American Psychologist, 40,* 266–275.

Gergen, K. J. (1998, January). *Introduction to social constructionism.* Workshop presented at the Texas Association for Marriage and Family Therapy Annual Conference, Dallas, TX.

Gergen, K. (1999). *An invitation to social construction.* Newbury Park, CA: Sage.

Gergen, K. (2001). *Social construction in context.* Newbury Park, CA: Sage.

Gergen, M., & Gergen, K. (2007). Collaboration without end: The case of the Positive Psychology Newsletter. In H. Anderson & D. Gehart (Eds.), *Collaborative therapy: Relationships and conversations that make a difference* (pp. 391–402). Brunner/Routledge.

Jackson, D. (1952, June). The relationship of the referring physician to the psychiatrist. *California Medicine, 76* (6), 391–394.

Jackson, D. (1955). Therapist personality in the therapy of ambulatory schizophrenics. *Archives of Neurology and Psychiatry, 74,* 292–299.

Keeney, B. (1983*). Aesthetics of change.* New York: Guilford.

Keeney, B. (1985*). Mind in therapy: Constructing systematic family therapies.* Basic Books.

Keeney, B. (1990). *Improvisational therapy: A practical guide for creative clinical strategies.* New York: Guilford.

Keeney, B. (1994). *Shaking out the spirits: A psychotherapist's entry into the healing mysteries of global shamanism.* Barrytown, NY: Station Hill.

Keeney, B. (1997). *Everyday soul: Awakening the spirit in daily life.* New York: Riverhead Books.

Keeney, B. (1998). *The energy break: Recharge your life with autokinetics.* New York: Golden Books.

Keeney B. (2000a). *Gary Holy Bull: Lakota Yuwipi man.* Stony Creek, CT: Leete's Island Books.

Keeney, B. (2000b). *Kalahari Bushmen.* Stony Creek, CT: Leete's Island Books.

Keeney, B. (2001a). *Vusamazulu Credo Mutwa: Zulu High Sanusi.* Stony Creek, CT: Leete's Island Books.

Keeney, B. (2001b). *Walking Thunder: Diné medicine woman.* Stony Creek, CT: Leete's Island Books.

Keeney B. (2002a). *Ikuko Osumi: Japanese master of Seiki Jutsu.* Stony Creek, CT: Leete's Island Books.

Keeney, B. (2002b). *Shakers of St. Vincent.* Stony Creek, CT: Leete's Island Books.

Keeney, B. (2003). *Ropes to god.* Stony Creek, CT: Leete's Island Books.

McNamee, S. (2007). Relational practices in education: Teaching as conversation. In H. Anderson & D. Gehart (Eds.), *Collaborative therapy: Relationships and conversations that make a difference* (pp. 313–336). New York: Brunner/Routledge.

McNamee, S., & Gergen, K. J. (Eds.). (1992). *Therapy as social construction.* Newbury Park, CA: Sage.

McNamee, S., & Gergen, K. J. (1999). *Relational responsibility: Resources for sustainable dialogue.* Newbury Park, CA: Sage.

Mental Research Institute. (2002). *On the shoulder of giants.* Palo Alto, CA: Author.

Ray, W. A., & Keeney, B. (1994*). Resource focused therapy.* Karnac Books.

Segal, L. (1991). Brief therapy: The MRI approach. In A. S. Gurman & D. P. Knishern (Eds.), *Handbook of family therapy* (pp. 171–199). New York: Brunner/Mazel.

Shotter, J. (1984). *Social accountability and selfhood.* Oxford: Blackwell.

Shotter, J. (1993). *Conversational realities: Constructing life through language.* Thousand Oaks, CA: Sage.

von Bertalanffy, L. (1968). *General system theory: Foundations, development, applications.* New York: George Braziller.

Watzlawick, P. (1977). *How real is real?: Confusion, disinformation, communication.* New York: Random House.

Watzlawick, P. (1978/1993). *The language of change: Elements of therapeutic conversation.* New York: Norton.

Watzlawick, P. (Ed.). (1984). *The invented reality: How do we know what we believe we know?* New York: Norton.

Watzlawick, P., Bavelas, J. B., & Jackson, D. D. (1967). *Pragmatics of human communication: A study of interactional patterns, pathologies, and paradoxes.* New York: Norton.

Watzlawick, P., Weakland, J., & Fisch, R. (1974). *Change: Principles of problem formation and problem resolution.* New York: Norton.

Weakland, J. (1951). Method in cultural anthropology. *Philosophy of Science, 18,* 55.

Weakland, J. (1988, June 10). Personal interview with Wendel A. Ray. Mental Research Institute, Palo Alto, CA.

White, M., & Epston, D. (1990). *Narrative means to therapeutic ends.* New York: Norton.

Wittgenstein, L. (1973). *Philosophical investigations* (3rd ed.; G. E. M. Anscombe, trans.). New York: Prentice Hall.

Systemic and Strategic Therapies

"Through time, you learn how to look at a system and appreciate it for what it is. Never expect the system to be different. It's important for the therapist and for the trainee to train themselves to see the system, to be interested in it, to appreciate this kind of a system without wanting to change it."
—Boscolo, Cecchin, Hoffman, & Penn, 1987, p. 152

Lay of the Land

Chapter 8 outlined the systemic foundations of various kinds of therapy, especially the contributions of the Bateson Group. This chapter discusses these therapies in more detail. Three teams of therapists developed what are broadly considered systemic or strategic theories:

- **Mental Research Institute (MRI; a.k.a. The Palo Alto Group):** After the Bateson team concluded their groundbreaking research on family dynamics with schizophrenia, Richard Fisch and Don Jackson worked together to found the Mental Research Institute, which has since served as the most influential training center in family therapy, inspiring Jay Haley's strategic work (which he conceptualized prior to the MRI approach), the Milan team's systemic approach, Virginia Satir's human growth model (see Chapter 11), and solution-focused brief therapy (see Chapter 14). The Brief Therapy Project at the MRI was designed to find the quickest possible resolution to client complaints, typically relying on action-based interventions (Watzlawick & Weakland, 1977; Watzlawick, Weakland, & Fisch, 1974; Weakland & Ray, 1995).

- **Milan Systemic Therapy:** After joining together to further Selvini Palazzoli's work with families who have anorectic or schizophrenic children, Mara Selvini Palazzoli, Gianfranco Cecchin, Giuliana Prata, and Luigi Boscolo formed the Milan team. Early in their work, they studied at the MRI and returned to Italy to design a therapeutic model that embodied the cybernetic systems theory of Gregory Bateson (1972, 1979; see Chapter 8). This model is called Milan systemic therapy, or long-term brief therapy. Milan therapists closely attend to how client language shapes family dynamics (Selvini Palazzoli, Cecchin, Prata, & Boscolo, 1978).

- **Strategic Therapy:** One of the original associates at the MRI, Jay Haley developed his own form of systemic therapy with his then wife, Cloe Madanes. Their approach focuses on the use of power and, in their later work, love in family systems (Haley, 1976).

In a Nutshell: The Least You Need to Know

Using what most therapists consider the classic family therapy method, systemic family therapists conceptualize the symptoms of individuals within the larger network of their family and social systems while maintaining a nonblaming, nonpathologizing stance toward all members of the family. Systemic therapies are based on *general systems* and *cybernetic systems theories,* which propose that families are living systems characterized by certain principles, including *homeostasis,* the tendency to maintain a particular range of behaviors and norms, and *self-correction,* the ability to identify when the system has gone too far from its homeostatic norm and then to self-correct to maintain balance (see Chapter 8). Systemic therapists rarely attempt linear, logical solutions to "educate" a family on better ways to communicate—this is almost never successful—but instead tap into the systemic dynamics to effect change. They introduce small, innocuous, yet highly meaningful alterations to the family's interactions, allowing the family to naturally reorganize in response to the new information. Because this method effects change quickly, systemic therapies were the original *brief therapies.*

The Juice: Significant Contributions to the Field

If you remember anything from this chapter, it should be these ideas:

Systemic Reframing: Juice from MRI

Reframing is a central technique that is found in most forms of systemic family therapy, such as structural therapy (see Chapter 10) and experiential family therapy (see Chapter 11). The MRI team approached reframing from a constructivist position that is summarized in the following propositions (Watzlawick et al., 1974):

1. We experience the world through our categorizations of objects, people, and events ("If my husband does not bring flowers or offer other romantic gestures, he does not really love me").
2. Once an object, person, or event is categorized, it is very difficult to see it as part of another category ("Our relationship must be in trouble if he has stopped being romantic").
3. Reframing uses the same "fact" that supports one categorization to support another categorization; once a person sees things using this second perspective, it is difficult to see the original situation in the same way (e.g., "My husband's drop in romance may mean that he has become more comfortable and authentic in the relationship rather than playing courting games; it could be a sign of deepening commitment").

The basic component of a reframe is finding an alternative yet equally plausible explanation (categorization) for the same set of facts. Of course, the key is identifying the client's current worldview and finding an equally viable frame for the problem behavior from the *client's perspective.* Reframing in systemic family therapies typically involves considering the role of the symptom in the broader relational system, often highlighting how it helps maintain balance (homeostasis) in the relationship. Unlike in cognitive-behavioral therapies, clients are not expected to literally believe or adopt the proposed reframe; instead, it is hoped that the reframe will be *"news that makes a difference,"* allowing clients to generate useful understandings. For example, with certain couples it makes sense to reframe their arguments as a way to build passion and maintain connection in their relationship. Such a reframe is offered to a couple without expectation that it will have a specific effect, because the system is considered a unique entity that will make its own meaning. If the couple does not find the reframe helpful, perhaps not responding or disagreeing with it, the therapist uses this information to better understand their worldview and then identify other potentials for reframing the problem.

Circular Questions: Juice from Milan

Regardless of which therapeutic model one chooses to practice, circular questions are perhaps one of the most useful techniques when working with more than one person in the room. Such questions help (a) assess and (b) make overt the overall dynamics and interactive patterns in the system, thereby reframing the problem for all participants without the therapist having to verbally provide a reframe, as already described in Systemic Reframing (Selvini Palazzoli et al., 1978; Selvini Palazzoli, Boscolo, Cecchin, & Prata, 1980). For example, I once had a family come to me complaining about a child's "anger problem." After they described the child's "problem" behavior, I inquired about how the rest of the family responded to the child's anger. The mother reported that she responded by getting frustrated and often yelled, and the father sharply corrected the child. As they listened to themselves describe their responses, both conceded that they responded to his anger with anger, and also noted that the younger sister disappeared into another room or somehow disengaged because of the intensity. As the parents began to look at their half of the interaction pattern, it became clear that anger was highly "contagious" for the three of them while it evoked anxiety in the daughter. These questions allowed the family to view their "son's anger problem" in the context of the broader interaction pattern, thus opening new options for relating.

Specific forms of circular questions (Cecchin, 1987) include the following:

- **Behavioral Sequence Questions:** Therapists use these questions to trace the entire sequence of behaviors that constitute the problem: "After John got mad, what did mom do? What did dad do? What did his sister do?" And after the response, "what did John do next?" The therapist follows the sequence of interactions until homeostasis is restored (you may recognize this from assessing the "problem interaction pattern" in the case conceptualization described in Chapter 2).

- **Behavioral Difference Questions:** Therapists use behavioral difference questions when clients start labeling people and assuming that a particular behavior is part of a person's inherent personality. For example, if a child claims, "My mom's a nag," the therapist would ask, "What does she do that makes her a nag?" The description of problem behavior, "tells me to do things," is then compared with others: "How does your dad ask you to do things? Your teacher? How do *you* ask others to do things?"

- **Comparison and Ranking Questions:** Comparison and ranking questions are useful for reducing labeling and other rigid descriptions in the family: "Who is the most upset when Jackie has an episode? Who is the least affected? Who is the most helpful during these times? The least helpful?"

- **Before-and-After Questions:** When a specific event has occurred, before-and-after questions can be useful in assessing how the event affected the family dynamics: "Did you and your mother fight more or less after your dad got sick?"

- **Hypothetical Circular Questions:** Hypothetical questions are used to offer a scenario and have family members describe how each is likely to respond: "If mom were suddenly placed in the hospital, who would be the most likely person at her bedside? The least likely?"

Directives: Juice from Strategic Therapy

Directives are the most basic of strategic techniques (Madanes, 1991); however, they are also the most frequently misunderstood by new therapists. In essence, directives are directions for the family to complete a specific task, usually between sessions but sometimes within the session. The tasks are rarely "logical" or linear solutions to the problem; instead they somehow "perturb" the system's interaction patterns to create new interactions (Haley, 1987). Thus, if a couple are arguing, the therapist will *not* ask them to set the timer so that each person speaks for 5 minutes followed by the other summarizing or responding for the next 5 minutes. That would be a logical or linear directive such as those found in cognitive-behavioral family therapy (Chapter 13). Nor will the therapist ask the couple to simply stop or learn a communication technique; the assumption is that if they could do this, they would have already done so. Instead, the therapist asks them to argue but to change one or two key elements, such as the place, timing, or turn-taking style. A directive may be to have their "normal" argument while fully clothed in the bathtub or to have it after rearranging furniture to simulate a courtroom.

Directives get people out of their ruts with the *smallest change possible.* When these directives work, clients generally experience a simultaneous shift in emotions, insight, and behavior. I like to compare it to a chocolate-vanilla swirl soft serve ice cream: the changes are perfectly synchronized and come fully integrated together. From the clients' perspective, directives jolt them awake from their usual life patterns, and generally the clients know exactly how to shift themselves to make the necessary changes. Unlike insight in traditional psychodynamic therapy, directives create visceral "ah-ha" moments because clients are in the midst of the action that needs to change. It is a bit like sudden enlightenment in the Zen tradition—hence, I like to think of systemic therapists as the Zen Masters and Mistresses of the field.

Rumor Has It: The People and Their Stories

The Clinical MRI Team

Don Jackson

A brilliant clinician and founder of the MRI in 1958, Jackson was a principal figure in family therapy, especially in the development of concepts such as family homeostasis, family rules, relational quid pro quo, conjoint therapy, interactional theory, and, along with others at MRI, the double-bind theory (MRI, 2002; Watzlawick, Bavelas, & Jackson, 1967); he also was one of the first to question the myth of normality (Jackson, 1967).

John Weakland

Originally trained as a chemical engineer, Weakland joined the Bateson Group and helped to articulate the application of communication theory, emphasizing the importance of basing theory on concrete and observable behaviors rather than inferences or constructs, which are not observable (MRI, 2002). Along with Haley, Weakland integrated Erickson's work at the MRI with the Brief Therapy Project.

Richard Fisch

After initially proposing the creation of the MRI, Richard Fisch was appointed by Jackson to be the director of the new Brief Therapy Project, which was inspired by Erickson's brief hypnotic work; the goal was to develop a highly teachable form of brief psychotherapy (Watzlawick et al., 1974). Thus Fisch spearheaded the development of the therapy model for which the MRI is most famous, studying how to influence others with words and indirect influence (Fisch & Schlanger, 1999; Fisch, Weakland, & Segal, 1982; MRI, 2002).

Paul Watzlawick

Born in Austria, Paul Watzlawick was a communications theorist who co-founded the Brief Therapy Center at the MRI with Weakland and Fisch, with a goal of developing an ultra-brief approach to therapy (Watzlawick, 1977, 1978/1993, 1984, 1990). In his later writings, Watzlawick explored implications of radical constructivism for therapy and human communication in cleverly titled books such as *How Real Is Real?* (1977), *The Invented Reality* (1984), *Ultra Solutions: How to Fail Most Successfully* (1988), and *The Situation Is Hopeless but Not Serious: The Pursuit of Unhappiness* (1993).

Art Bodin

One of the founding members of the Brief Therapy Project at the MRI, Art Bodin has continued his research on families, developing the Relationship Conflict Inventory (RCI) and the Teasing and Bullying Survey (TABS) as well as helping found the American Psychological Association's Division of Family Psychology.

William Fry

A member of Gregory Bateson's original team studying paradoxical communication, Bill Fry continued research on the interactional elements of humor and nonverbal communication (MRI, 2002).

Jules Riskin

The only surviving member of the original clinical staff at MRI, Jules Riskin developed one of the first methodologies for studying family interaction and conducted the first study of the normal family process, a decade before others in the field recognized the importance of such a project (MRI, 2002).

Wendel Ray

Former director and senior research fellow at the MRI, Wendel Ray has been instrumental in ushering systemic therapies into the 21st century, working with Bradford Keeney (Chapter 8) to develop *resource-focused therapy,* a strength-based systems therapy (Ray & Keeney, 1994); with Milan team colleagues to further develop systemic concepts, such as *irreverence, cybernetics of prejudices,* and *eccentricity* (Cecchin, Lane, & Ray, 1992); and with colleagues at the MRI on theoretical and archival work (Weakland & Ray, 1995). He also serves as the Hammond Endowed Professor of Education and Professor of Family Systems Theory at the University of Louisiana at Monroe.

Barbara Anger-Diaz and Karin Schlanger

Barbara Anger-Diaz and Karin Schlanger train therapists in brief therapy with Latino families; training and therapy are conducted in Spanish at the Latino Brief Therapy and Training Center at the MRI.

Giorgio Nardone

Working closely with Watzlawick in his later works (Nardone & Watzlawick, 1993), Giorgio Nardone founded the Centro di Terapia Strategica in Arezzo, Italy, and the Brief Strategic and Systemic World Network. Founded in 2003, the latter brings together strategic and systemic therapy practitioners from around the world.

The Milan Team

The Milan team included *Mara Selvini Palazzoli, Gianfranco Cecchin, Luigi Boscolo,* and *Guiliana Prata* and was founded in 1967 by Selvini Palazzoli, who was studying anorexia in Italy at the time (Campbell, Draper, & Crutchley, 1991). They met weekly without pay, seeing families and studying the work of Bateson and the MRI group and frequently inviting Watzlawick for consultations. The team developed a unique approach that focused on meaning and ritual. In 1979, the team separated along interest and gender lines: Selvini Palazzoli and Prata, primarily researchers, wanted to continue their investigation into treating families with psychotic members, while Cecchin and Boscolo worked together on clinical and training applications. The later work of Selvini Palazzoli and Prata centered on the *invariant prescription* (discussed later in this chapter), while Cecchin and Boscolo explored Keeney's *second-order cybernetics* (1983) and related works, attending to language and the construction of meaning through multiple descriptors and eventually moving toward a more postmodern, social constructionist stance (see Chapter 15). Lynn Hoffman and Peggy Penn, featured in Chapter 15, worked closely with Boscolo and Cecchin.

Strategic Therapists

Jay Haley and Cloe Madanes

Jay Haley, one of the original members of the Bateson Team, student of Milton Erickson, and co-founder of the Brief Therapy Project at MRI, developed his own systemic approach, strategic therapy (Haley, 1963, 1973, 1976, 1980, 1981, 1984, 1987, 1996; Haley & Richeport-Haley, 2007; MRI, 2002). He and his wife, Cloe Madanes (1981, 1990, 1991, 1993), founded the Family Therapy Institute in Washington, D.C. Their approach is based on the concepts of hierarchy, power, and love, and uses *directives* for interventions.

Eileen Bobrow

Eileen Bobrow founded and directs the Strategic Family Therapy and Training Center at the Mental Research Institute, which prior to her arrival focused primarily on the Brief Therapy Model developed at the MRI.

Jim Keim

A research fellow at the MRI, Jim Keim (1998) uses strategic therapy to work with families with oppositional-defiant and conduct-disordered children.

The Big Picture: Overview of Treatment

Systemic and strategic therapies focus solely on resolving the presenting problem, with the therapist imposing no other goals or agendas. Therapists see the presenting problem not as an individual problem but a relational one, specifically an *interactional* one (Cecchin, 1987; Haley, 1987). Neither an individual nor a relationship is considered "dysfunctional"; instead, the problem is viewed as part of the interactional sequence of behaviors that have emerged through repeated exchanges, with no one person to blame.

The early stages of all three approaches involve getting a clear, behavioral description of the interaction sequence surrounding the problem, beginning with the initial exchange prior to the escalation of symptoms and ending with the interaction sequence that returns the system to homeostasis. Once the therapist has identified the interactional behavioral patterns and meanings associated with the problem, he/she uses one of many potential interventions to *interrupt* this sequence—not correct it. Much the way a school of fish cannot be shepherded but only interrupted and allowed to regroup, systemic and strategic therapists do not try to linearly instruct clients in preferred behaviors, because it rarely if ever works (Haley, 1987). Instead, they interrupt the problem sequence of behaviors, allowing the family to reconfigure itself around the new information that has been introduced to the system. For example, if a parent and child complain of frequent arguments, the therapist does not try to educate them in better communication. Instead, the therapist interrupts the sequence by reframing the child's defiance as a veiled attempt to remain close to the parent because the child fears the transition to college, or the therapist may ask parent and child to ritualize the process with hats symbolizing their positions. For example, in the case study at the end of this chapter, the therapist working with Alba, a 16-year-old who started drinking and smoking pot after her parents separated, reframes her acting-out behaviors as attempts to bring the parents together over a common goal and to distract the family from the pain of the father's affair; the therapist does not believe Alba does this consciously or intentionally but rather is following the "pull" of the system to restore family homeostasis.

Usually the therapist gives the family a task or reframe before they leave the session, with instructions to either complete the task or reflect on the new interpretation presented by the therapist. The next week, the therapist follows up on the prior week and then designs another task or reframe based on the response to the prior week's intervention. This process continues only as long as is necessary to resolve the presenting problem; then therapy is terminated. To recap, the general flow of systemic or strategic therapies is as follows:

THE PROCESS OF SYSTEMIC AND STRATEGIC THERAPY

- **Assess the Interactional Sequence and Associated Meanings:** The therapist identifies the interactional behavior sequences that constitute the problem, including the actions and reactions of everyone in the system and the associated meanings.

- **Intervene by Interrupting the Interactional Sequence:** Using a reframing technique or a task, the therapist interrupts the sequence (avoids trying to fix or repair the sequence), allowing the family to reorganize itself in response to the perturbation. *The differences between MRI, strategic, and Milan therapies are primarily seen in the preferred method of interrupting the interactional sequence.*

- **Evaluate Outcome and Client Response:** After the intervention, the therapist assesses the family's response and uses this information to design the next intervention.

- **Interrupt the New Pattern:** Then the therapist interrupts the new pattern with another intervention. This continues—interrupt behavioral sequence, allow family to reorganize and respond, and intervene again—until the problem is resolved.

Making Connection: The Therapeutic Relationship

Respecting and Trusting the System

Systemic therapists respect the family as a system, as an entity that has its unique epistemology, or way of knowing and understanding the world. They have a deep, abiding trust that the system can reorganize itself without the therapist forcing change. Instead, the therapist provides opportunities for the family to reorganize itself. The symptoms are never seen as indicators of individual pathology but rather as the byproduct of family interactional sequences that have served a purpose.

Adapting to Client Language and Viewpoint

In the first meeting, the therapist tries to establish a positive, trusting relationship with the client (Nardone & Watzlawick, 1993; Watzlawick et al., 1974). One approach is to adapt to the clients' language, communicative style, and worldview, speaking logically with clients who focus on reason and more intensely with clients who have a more emotional manner of expression. First and foremost, the therapist respectfully engages with the client's representational framework or epistemology, including beliefs, values, and language. This is the inverse of traditional psychoanalysis, in which the patient must adapt to the language and viewpoint of the therapist.

Neutrality

In 1978 (Selvini Palazzoli et al.; Selvini Palazzoli et al., 1980), the Milan team first described their therapeutic stance as one of *neutrality*, which has been one of the most misunderstood concepts related to their work (Boscolo et al., 1987). For the Milan team, neutrality connoted not only nonpartiality toward particular family members or problem descriptions but also multipartiality, the willingness to honor all perspectives.

In one sense, neutrality refers to the *pragmatic effect* the therapist has on the family, not the therapist's own feelings (Cecchin, 1987). Thus if, at the end of the session, the family cannot identify which "side" the therapist took, then the therapist has had the effect of being neutral. However, during the session, the therapist often appears to take a side by asking questions that align with a certain person's view of the problem; the therapist must counterbalance this by asking questions that align with each of the other perspectives so that at the end the therapist is viewed as neutral.

Neutrality also implies not becoming attached to particular meanings, descriptions, or outcomes (Boscolo et al., 1987). The Milan team carefully avoided buying into any one description of the problem, *including their own.* Neutrality extended to their own hypotheses and ideas about the family, and they avoided "falling in love" with their own ideas. Later, Cecchin, Lane, and Ray (1992) characterized this form of neutrality as a form of *irreverence* (discussed in next section) that allows for broad maneuverability. When therapists do not rigidly adhere to a particular problem description, they can see more possibilities for intervention rather than focus on the single solution that fits with their preferred hypothesis.

Irreverence

The concept of irreverence was not highlighted until later in the literature (Cecchin, Lane, & Ray, 1992), but—when properly understood—it clearly captures the therapist's relationship to the *problem* (not the client). The magic of this approach is derived from the therapist's irreverent relationship with problems.

What is there to be irreverent about? Systemic therapists are irreverent regarding the "catastrophic" appearance of problems. They do not give in to the appearance that a person has a "personality flaw," "illness," "unresolved childhood issue," or other deep, troubling problem, even though problems appear that way, especially to those who live them. But the systemic therapist knows that appearances are deceiving because problems are intimately connected with the relational and broader social context. In a different context, a person's problem behaviors would be different. The context and problem are always influencing each other. The art of irreverence is to not honor the problem as a mighty foe and assume it has more power than it does. Its power is entirely dependent on its context. With experience, the therapist is able to see through the appearance of a "big, horrible" problem and instead see that the person, problem, and context form a fluid dance—and experience teaches that by changing only a few steps in the dance, the problem shifts, diminishes, and eventually disappears.

Irreverence is felt in the therapist's confidence and unpanicked response to problem issues. It is driven not by disrespect but *fearlessness.* Whatever problem the client brings—whether the loss of a child or a teen's drama of the week—the therapist remains fearless, maintaining a deep sense of calm and faith in systemic processes, knowing that the problems are never as insurmountable as they appear and that systems are inherently self-correcting. Irreverence does not imply lack of empathy or sensitivity. Instead, it allows the therapist to maintain an openness, creativity, and flexibility to provide maximum benefit to the client. In this chapter's case study, the therapist's irreverence toward 16-year-old Alba's decision to start drinking and smoking pot after her parents separated, keeps the therapist from being overly panicked about the acting-out behaviors and enables her and the whole family to focus on the issue: Alba's sense of betrayal and loss. By not overreacting to the drinking and drugs—but not ignoring them either—the therapist gives them less power and creates space for more critical issues.

Maneuverability

Maneuverability refers to the therapist's freedom to use personal judgment in defining the therapeutic relationship (Nardone & Watzlawick, 1993; Segal, 1991; Watzlawick et al., 1974). Therapists may choose to maintain an expert position or a one-down stance (see next section), depending on what would be most helpful to the family. Similarly, the therapist may be more distant or emotionally engaged, depending on the circumstances. Furthermore, the therapist may choose to be disliked by the client or be the "bad guy" in order to achieve the desired change in the family system, always attuned to whatever role might be most beneficial for the family.

The One-Down Stance or Helplessness

The one-down stance is used to increase clients' motivation, often paradoxically by claiming, "I'm not sure if I am able to handle such a problem" (Segal, 1991). This move is often helpful with clients who act as if their situation is hopeless; when the therapist instead takes the hopeless stance, the client is then motivated to find hope. Systemically this works because in most systems there is a counterbalance: if one person is hopeless, the other feels compelled to be hopeful to maintain a balance. This same dynamic is also observed between couples in crisis: generally one person will manage the crisis, allowing the other one to more fully feel the panic and trauma.

Beyond serving this paradoxical purpose, the one-down stance also expresses a certain attitude toward the family system. Systemic therapists view the system as an entity with its own rules and integrity that must be respected, much like a mountain climber must respect the awesome forces of nature or the sailor an ocean. Like a family system, nature and the ocean are not things the therapist can control; instead, there is a deep respect for their power and ways. Thus the one-down stance is a sincere and genuine position for a systemically-trained therapist.

Social Courtesy

Haley (1987) describes the initial stage of therapy as the social stage, a time during which the therapist engages in casual social conversation, about the weather or traffic, to make clients comfortable and reduce their sense of shame: "the model for this stage is the courtesy behavior one would use with guests in the home" (p. 15). Before discussing the problem, the therapist ensures that all members have been properly greeted. During this first social stage, the therapist is assessing interactions and mood (Haley & Richeport-Haley, 2007).

The Viewing: Case Conceptualization and Assessment

Focus on Interactions and Family Games

When systemic or strategic therapists view a family, they focus on the interaction patterns *between* people (Boscolo et al., 1987; Watzlawick et al., 1974). To illustrate this focus to new therapists, I have a "family of four" grab hold of a bright yellow rope to form a circle. Then I have them "dance" and move about in various patterns. Initially, the audience's eyes naturally focus on the movement of the dancers, our default, socialized habit of viewing interactions. I then have the family do the dance again, asking the audience to focus exclusively on the yellow rope and how it moves as it traces the interactional patterns of distance and closeness. This is a very gross and incomplete metaphor for how a systemic therapist looks at a family, but I think it helps get the point across: the focus is always on the yellow rope—the interaction—or what Milan therapists call the "game" (Boscolo et al., 1987). Often, English speakers think that the Milan term *family game* implies manipulation and ill intent, meanings the term may have in English. However, that is not the connotation of *game* in the systemic context, which focuses on the relational rules for how the family interacts, rules that are not consciously created but rather naturally emerge from the family interaction pattern.

Family interactions can be hard to detect, especially early in training. The trick is tracing the homeostatic dance (how A responds to B and B in turn responds to A). When observing a family interact, therapists can assess the dance patterns by focusing less on the content of the conversation and more on the metacommunication (see Chapter 8) and interactions (movement of the rope). For example, if a couple are arguing about how to discipline a defiant child, the therapist will not focus on solving the problem with the child but rather on how the parents communicate: Does each share opinions, thoughts, and feelings? How does each respond to the other's divergent opinion? What strategies does each use to convince the other? Does one person get the last word? By focusing on the interactional pattern or couple game for negotiating this type of problem, the therapist can identify where they are stuck.

In addition to observing actual interactions, it is often necessary to ask circular questions to assess the interactional sequence; these questions can be used with individuals, couples, or families. For example, with the couple having trouble with the defiant child, the therapist would ask: "What is happening just before the problem incident? What is each person saying and doing? How does the child respond? How does each parent and anyone else involved respond to the defiance? How does the child respond to this? How do the parents respond to the child next?" and so on, until family homeostasis is restored.

QUESTIONS FOR ASSESSING FAMILY INTERACTIONS

To develop a concrete description of the interactional pattern, Nardone and Watzlawick (1993, p. 30) recommend that therapists answer the following questions:

- What are the patient's usual, observable behavior patterns?
- How does the patient define the problem?
- How does the problem manifest itself?
- In whose company does the problem appear, worsen, disguise itself, or not appear?
- Where does it usually appear?
- In what situations?
- How often does the problem appear, and how serious is it?
- What has been done and is currently being done (by the patient alone or by others) to resolve the problem?
- Whom or what does the problem benefit?
- Who could be hurt by the disappearance of the problem?

"More of the Same" Solutions

When tracking interactional patterns, MRI therapists also focus on identifying *"more of the same" solutions*, that is, solutions that perpetuate the problem (Watzlawick et al., 1974). For example, if the parents always respond to a child's defiance with some form of lecture and verbal punishment, this would be a "more of the same" solution that is not working for the family. This "attempted solution" (i.e., verbal punishment) would be identified as the interactional behavior sequence that maintains the problem. After identifying the more-of-the-same behaviors and logic system (e.g., bad behavior is corrected with punishment), the therapist then identifies a behavior that represents a 180-degree shift in logic (e.g., cooperative behavior that is motivated by a strong emotional bond).

More-of-the-same solutions can further be described as mishandling the problem in one of three ways (Watzlawick et al., 1974):

- **Terrible Simplifications (Action Is Necessary but None Is Taken):** The client or family attempts to solve the problem by *denying* it: this solution is common with addictions, marital problems, and problematic family dynamics.

- **The Utopian Syndrome (Action Is Taken When It Is Not Necessary):** The client or family tries to change something that is either unchangeable or nonexistent: this solution is common with depression, anxiety, procrastination, perfectionism, and unrealistic demands on a relationship or a child.

- **Paradox (Action Is Taken at the Wrong Level):** Either a first-order solution is attempted for a problem that necessitates a second-order solution (e.g., parents are unable to adjust parenting techniques as child matures) or a second-order solution is attempted for a first-order problem (e.g., when people demand attitude or personality changes and are not content with behavioral changes). This solution is common with schizophrenia, relational impasses, domestic violence, and abuse.

The Tyranny of Linguistics

When assessing families, the Milan team paid particular attention to the family's word choices and expressions. They were mindful of how language, particularly descriptions of self and others, shape lived reality: they called this the "tyranny of linguistics" (Selvini Palazzoli et al., 1978). For example, the statements "I am depressed" or "he's an angry person" are global labels that create little space for noticing numerous moments throughout the day when other feelings and identities may be experienced. Instead, Milan therapists encourage descriptions of a person's *action*: times when I "do" depression or when he is "doing" anger. This subtle shift of words suddenly opens new opportunities for how people experience themselves while also allowing for descriptions of times when the depression is not as strong or a person is not angry.

For Milan therapists, positive labels, such as "intelligent" or "good," are as limiting and problematic as negative descriptors. Like negative descriptions, positive labels obscure the relational context that shapes them (Boscolo et al., 1987). Both positive and negative descriptors are avoided in favor of interactional behavioral descriptions.

Strategic Conceptualization

Madanes (1991) identifies six ways to think about a problem in strategic therapy; these dimensions can be used to conceptualize the role of a symptom in the family system or in an individual's broader social world. One or more of these is used, depending on the case.

- **Involuntary Versus Voluntary:** Clients generally present by viewing the problem as involuntary; strategic therapists instead view the symptoms as voluntary, with the exception of organic illness. For example, they see arguing, worrying, or being depressed as behaviors or solutions clients choose.

- **Helplessness Versus Power:** Although symptomatic people appear helpless, their symptoms also generate significant power, allowing them to make otherwise unreasonable demands, receive more care and attention, or excuse otherwise unacceptable behavior. For example, agoraphobia can be seen as an attempt to keep the family close.

- **Metaphorical Versus Literal:** Symptoms may be viewed as a metaphor for another problem sequence of behaviors in the system. For example, a child's defiance can be seen as a metaphor for the same defiance the husband feels but does not express toward the mother; or bingeing can be seen as a metaphor for rejecting the mother's attempt to overnurture the child.

- **Hierarchy Versus Equality:** Therapists may conceptualize the presenting problem as a demand for more or less hierarchy, depending on the family's set of circumstances. For example, caving in to a child's tantrums allows the child to be at the top of the power hierarchy.

- **Hostility Versus Love:** Many family interactions—rejecting a lover because one feels unworthy, disciplining a child, pursuing a partner for sex or communication—can be viewed as motivated by either hostility or love. Strategic therapists may use either interpretation, depending on the therapeutic situation. For example, a husband's constant pursuit for sex may be a sign of love and caring *or* a power move because he feels he has none, depending on the situation. Similarly, a wife's refusal of sex could be motivated by love for husband (e.g., only wanting sex when she really has feelings) or family (e.g., give's too much and is too tired) *or* a power move to gain control because she feels she has none.

Strategic Humanism

The latest developments in strategic therapy emphasize increasing the family's ability to love and nurture rather than dominate and control, which is consonant more generally with the evolution of the field of family therapy (Madanes, 1993). Thus case conceptualizations focus more on the family's unsuccessful attempts to show love rather than on their attempts to control one another. For example, Jim Keim's (1998) work with oppositional children aims to increase parental nurturing behaviors to help them re-establish a more effective hierarchy, highlighting that a nurturing parent can be as much of an authority as a disciplinarian; once some authority has been re-established in the nurturing realm, Keim instructs parents to begin enforcing behavioral rules.

The Observation Team

The hallmark of the art of systemic or strategic viewing has always been the *observation team.* Early in the development of these ideas, teams would sit behind a one-way mirror to observe the therapist working with the family. The team could see the systemic dance more rapidly and completely because the person in the room very quickly falls in sync with the family system and has a more difficult time seeing the entire dance. Anyone who has spent time behind a mirror and in front of it knows that you are always smarter behind it. The distance created by not being part of the interactional dance of the family increases one's ability to see the dance more clearly and quickly. Arguably the main reason family therapists still train with a mirror is to develop the ability to see the system's dynamics. This is not to say that a therapist in the room can't see the systemic dynamics; it is just harder and takes more practice.

Targeting Change: Goal Setting

Symptom-Free Interaction Patterns

Systemic therapists help the family to develop a new set of interaction patterns (i.e., homeostasis), a new game or dance that does not include symptoms (or any subsequent symptoms; Boscolo et al., 1987). Stated yet again, the goal is to create a family homeostasis that is problem-free—or at least does not involve facing the same problem over and over again (Watzlawick et al., 1974).

No Theory of Health

Unlike many earlier schools of therapy, such as psychodynamic or humanistic, systemic therapy does not have a predetermined definition of "healthy family functioning" that the therapist uses to define therapeutic goals. As already stated, therapists do not have a theory of health that defines how the family should look at the end of therapy. Instead, it is believed that the family system (not individual members) will reorganize itself from within to find a "functional," symptom-free interaction pattern in response to the *perturbations* or disruptions introduced by the therapist.

The Problem Is the Attempted Solution (MRI Therapy)

Goals in the MRI brief therapy approach are developed using the following four-step procedure (Watzlawick et al., 1974):

1. **Define the Problem:** Use concrete, behavioral terms to describe the actions and reactions of all involved. For example, "My son is always defiant" is not a well-defined problem; a preferred problem description is "When I ask my son to do something, he says 'no' and when I push further he starts yelling and cursing; that's when I give in."

2. **Identify Attempted Solutions:** The therapist may ask, "How have you attempted to deal with this problem?" and listens for patterns in the various attempted solutions (e.g., threats that are not carried out, negotiating with child).

3. **Describe the Desired Behavioral Change:** MRI therapists take great care to develop concrete, behavioral goals that meaningfully focus clients' and therapists' attention in useful directions. The goals must be realistic, specific, and time-limited.

   - **Realistic:** Therapists need to be careful to avoid utopian goals, such as "Every time I ask my son to do something, he will obey." Instead, the therapist helps the client develop the more realistic goal of "increasing the frequency that my son politely carries out my first request."
   - **Specific:** Goals describe clear behaviors and interactions rather than vague intentions, such as "communicate better." As Watzlawick says, "It is the vagueness of goals that make their attainment impossible" (Watzlawick et al., 1974, p. 112).
   - **Time Limited:** MRI brief therapists prefer to set a clear time limit for a specified goal, such as "within 4 weeks."

4. **Develop a Plan:** MRI therapists use two basic systemic principles:

   - The target of change is the *attempted solution*.
   - The tactic of change is to use the *client's own language* to speak directly to the client's view of reality.

Thus the plan is never linear or directive psychoeducation on how to "better communicate." Such plans and interventions are used in cognitive-behavioral therapy (see Chapter 13), not systemic therapy. In dramatic contrast, an MRI systemic approach targets the attempted solution rather than the presenting problem; again, this differs from solution-based therapies that target the preferred solution (see Chapter 14). Thus, rather than target a child's tantrums by teaching parents how to employ positive and negative reinforcement, systemic therapists identify the class of solutions used by the parents and develop an intervention that represents a 180-degree shift. If the parents respond by becoming embarrassed and giving in, the therapist designs an intervention in which the parents are emotionally unaffected and consistent in their consequences. On the other hand, if the parents typically respond with strict, harsh punishment, the therapist suggests an emotionally engaged and gentle approach.

Strategic Goals

"The main goal of therapy is to get people to behave differently and so to have different subjective experiences."—Haley, 1987, p. 56

Strategic therapy does not have a predefined set of long-term goals for individual or family functioning, other than to promote a change that alters people's subjective experiences (mood, thoughts, and behaviors). Madanes (1990, 1991) conceptualizes all problems brought to therapy as stemming from an existential dilemma between love and violence, because these two experiences tend to be closely correlated in human affairs. Thus the ultimate strategic goal is to help clients find ways to love without dominating, intruding upon, or harming the other. This goal may be achieved by doing the following (Madanes, 1991):

- Correcting the couple or family hierarchy (either increasing or decreasing it)
- Reducing intrusion or increasing engagement by changing a parent or partner's level of involvement
- Reuniting family members
- Changing who is helpful and how, including empowering children to be appropriately helpful
- Repenting for an injustice and forgiving
- Increasing the expression of compassion and unity

The Doing: Language-Based Interventions

Reframing and Circular Questions (see Juice)
The Hypothesizing Process (Milan Therapy)

"The construction of hypotheses is a continuous process, coevolving with the family's movement. The act of hypothesizing is best described using the concepts of cybernetic feedback loops, for as the family's response to the question modifies or alters one hypothesis, another is formed based on the specifics of that new feedback. This continuous process of hypothesis construction requires the therapist to reconceptualize constantly, both as an interviewer and team member."—Boscolo et al., 1987, p. 94

The process of generating a hypothesis, emphasized in the Milan approach, continues throughout therapy and generally has two phases:

1. **Hypothesizing for Conceptualization:** This is the behind-the-mirror process of developing and revising hypotheses that the therapist and team use to guide their "viewing" and provide an overall focus and direction for therapy.

2. **Hypothesizing as Intervention:** When the therapist and team believe it will benefit the family, the hypothesis they have been developing behind the mirror is shared verbally with the family as an in-session intervention.

As already discussed, a hypothesis usually defines the role of the symptom in maintaining the family's homeostasis (Boscolo et al., 1987). For example, a teen's delinquent behavior may serve to bring the parents closer together; without the child's "problem" behavior, the couple might experience other difficulties that would be more difficult for the family to manage. Hypotheses can also highlight how the family wants to simultaneously keep things the same and change, two counterbalancing forces. When therapists deliver hypotheses to the family, the purpose is to "create news of a difference" and shift how they think about the problem, thus creating new possibilities for change. Hypotheses need to be worded so that they are different from how the family is currently viewing the situation yet not too different so that they react against it. Instead, hypotheses need to be *plausible* in the family's current worldview (Watzlawick et al., 1974).

The Milan team identified three common types of hypotheses (Boscolo et al., 1987):

- **Hypotheses About Alliances:** These describe alliances and coalitions: who is on whose team.

- **Hypotheses About Myths and Premises:** These identify unrealistic or problematic myths and premises that are contributing to the problem (myths of the perfect marriage, ideal child, etc.).

- **Hypotheses That Analyze Communication:** These track problematic communication patterns, such as double binds.

Positive Connotation (Milan Reframe)

Milan therapists originally developed positive connotations to not contradict themselves when prescribing paradoxical interventions (Selvini Palazzoli et al., 1978). Therapists use positive connotation to respect both the family's fear of change and their request for change. They *interpret the behavior of* each member of the family positively, as having an underlying benevolent motivation (Boscolo et al., 1987). A common positive connotation is reframing a child's problematic behavior as a way to keep the parents together and reframing the parents' arguments about how to handle this behavior as a way to show their dedication to the family and each other. Perhaps the most important outcome of positive connotation is the effect it has on the therapist, enabling the therapist to view members of the system less judgmentally and with greater hope.

The Therapeutic Double Bind and Counterparadox (MRI and Milan, respectively)

The MRI therapeutic double bind is used to undo a double-bind message in a family or relationship; similarly, the Milan counterparadox is used to therapeutically respond to the paradoxes, or double binds, that families and couples create for themselves (Selvini Palazzoli et al., 1978; Watzlawick, Bavelas, & Jackson, 1967). The difference between a problem-generating double bind and a therapeutic double bind is simple: in the problem-generating form, no matter what you do, you are wrong; there is no escape. In a therapeutic double bind or counterparadox, no matter what you do, you do something different: something that moves you in a new direction.

A common double bind is when one party demands that the other show spontaneous displays of love and affection. For example, a wife may demand that her husband spontaneously express his love in more romantic ways: flowers, candlelight dinners, and gifts. If he does what she asks, she can say that he only did it because she asked and that it wasn't spontaneous; if he does not do anything romantic, then she can say he obviously doesn't care because he didn't follow through. Either way he loses. A therapeutic double bind would be to have him show his romantic side in any way *other than* the specific ways his wife demands. If he follows this directive literally, he will initiate new romantic behavior in the system; if he does not follow the instructions and instead chooses to use one of his wife's suggestions, then he is doing so *without the command* to do so. If you think it is tough to design such an intervention on your own, you are right—that is why the early family therapists preferred to work in teams. They could then more quickly assess the family's double binds and identify helpful therapeutic paradoxes.

Invariant Prescriptions (Milan Therapy)

One of the Selvini Palazzoli's earliest therapeutic innovations and the focus of her long-term research, the *invariant prescription* is just what it sounds like: an intervention that is not varied across families (Selvini Palazzoli, 1988). Used primarily with families whose children are labeled anorexic or schizophrenic, the intervention severs covert coalitions between a parent and a child. Parents are instructed to arrange to go on a date (or other outing) and to not tell the children where they are going or why. The desired effect is to create a secret between the parents, ending inappropriate coalitions by creating a clear boundary between the parents as a unified team and the symptomatic child. The child loses the status of being a special confidant of the one parent, lessening his/her emotional burden and resulting in fewer problem symptoms. Although originally designed for severe pathology such as anorexia and psychosis, this intervention is also effective with modern parents who overemphasize transparent and open communication with their children to the extent that the children use this information to "manipulate" them. The therapist in this chapter's case study uses a variation of this technique with 16-year-old Alba, who is acting out after her parents separate; the invariant prescription helps restore the parental alliance so that Alba does not feel the "systemic pull" to act out to get her parents to work together.

Dangers of Improvement (MRI and Strategic Therapy)

A technique used by MRI and strategic therapists, the *dangers of improvement* involves asking clients to identify potential problems that might arise if the problem were resolved (Segal, 1991). For example, if a child becomes more independent in doing homework and getting chores done, what will the mother and father do to feel that they are parenting their son? If a couple suddenly stop arguing, how will they keep the flame of passion alive in their relationship? If a person stops being depressed and starts socializing again, how will he protect his solitude and quiet time? These questions undermine unrealistic and utopian worldviews that not only created the current problem but are also likely to be the source of new problems to come.

Restraining, Going Slow

Restraining or the directive to *go slow* is another common systemic and strategic intervention that carries a paradoxical flavor (Segal, 1991). When therapists "restrain" or instruct clients to "go slow," they warn clients to avoid changing too fast and encourage them to take change slowly. This has a paradoxical effect similar to a therapeutic double bind in that if the client complies, change will happen and the client will be better prepared for the setbacks that characterize most attempts at change. On the other hand, if the client has a rebellious response, he/she will attempt to rebel against slowness by working harder toward desired change. In either case, the change process is supported and "immunized" against setbacks.

The Doing: Action-Oriented Interventions

Directives (MRI and Strategic Therapy)

Used in both strategic and MRI approaches, directives are behavioral tasks that the therapist gives to clients to alter their interaction patterns. Haley (1987) identifies two general types of directives: straightforward and indirect. *Straightforward directives* are used when the therapist has the power and influence to get people to do what is asked; *indirect directives* are used when the therapist has less authority in the eyes of the client. Indirect directives generally take the form of paradoxical or metaphorical tasks.

Technically, straightforward directives mean giving good advice, but Haley is quick to admonish against them: "Giving good advice means the therapist assumes that people have rational control of what they are doing. To be successful in the therapy business, it may be better to drop that idea" (Haley, 1987, p. 61). Therefore, most straightforward directives aim to change the way the family interacts by introducing *new action*. Often therapists are tempted to ask clients to stop doing something;

Haley warns against this also: "If the therapist tells someone to stop usual behavior, he must usually go to an extreme or get other family members to cooperate and change their behavior" (p. 60). Thus most strategic directives *resequence* interaction patterns by requesting *small behavioral or contextual changes*, such as having the *other* parent discipline a child who has broken house rules or asking a couple to add a 10-second pause between exchanges in a fight. These smaller changes are much easier to accomplish. The differences between straightforward and indirect directives are outlined in the following table.

THERAPEUTIC DIRECTIVES

	STRAIGHTFORWARD DIRECTIVES	INDIRECT DIRECTIVES
Type of Task	• Do something different: alter behavioral sequence • Stop a behavior (rarely used) • Good advice; psychoeducation (rarely if ever used)	• Paradoxical tasks • Metaphorical tasks
Type of Therapeutic Relationship	• Therapist has influence; well accepted as expert	• Therapist less well accepted as expert
Type of Problem	• Client able to feel control over small behaviors requested as part of task	• Client feels has very little control

Straightforward Directives

Haley maintained that "the best task is one that uses the presenting problem to make a structural change in the family" (Haley, 1987, p. 85). Designing straightforward directives involves several steps:

1. **Assess the Situation:** The therapist identifies the interaction sequence of behaviors that constitute the presenting problem; for example, the child comes home after curfew; the father angrily enforces a harsh punishment; the mother defends the child to the husband and does not enforce the punishment over the week.

2. **Target a Small Sequence Change:** The therapist finds one small behavioral change in the sequence that the family can reasonably make that would alter the problem sequence; for example, have the mother enforce the curfew; have the daughter propose a "fair" punishment for breaking curfew.

3. **Motivate the Family:** Haley (1987) emphasizes the importance of motivating the family *before* the task is issued. For straightforward tasks this is usually done by appealing to the shared goal: begin by first talking about how everyone wants the problem behavior to stop: "Everyone agrees that they want the arguing at home to stop."

3. **Give Precise, Doable Instructions for the Directive:** When describing the task, the therapist needs to be extremely precise—when, where, how, who, on which day of the week—while accounting for weekend changes in schedules, weekday home-making tasks, and special events during the week that the task is assigned. Tasks should be clearly *given* rather than suggested: "Next week, when Susan comes in late from curfew or breaks any other house rule, mom, I want you to enforce the consequences, and dad, you are not to be part of the discussion with Susan and your wife. If you need to discuss what happened, you will discuss it with your wife alone."

4. **Review the Task:** The therapist asks the family members to repeat their parts: "Just to review and make sure we all understand, can each of you tell me what you are going to do this week?"

5. **Request a Task Report:** The following week, the therapist asks the family how it went. Generally, one of three things happens: (a) they do it, (b) they don't do it, or (c) they partially do it (Haley, 1987). If clients complete the task, they are congratulated. If they have partially done the task, the therapist does not excuse them too quickly because that would send a message that undermines the therapist's authority. If they fail to attempt the task, Haley uses two responses, one nice and one not so nice. In the nice response, the therapist says, "I must have misunderstood you or your situation to ask that of you—otherwise you would have done it" (Haley, 1987, p. 71). In the not-so-nice approach, the therapist emphasizes that the family has missed an opportunity to make changes for their own good and that this is a failure and a loss for them (not that they disappointed the therapist); the therapist does not ask them to redo the task even if they say they want to. Instead, the therapist uses this experience to increase motivation for the next task.

Indirect Directives: Paradoxical Interventions (MRI, Milan, and Strategic Therapies)

Perhaps the most misunderstood of strategic and systemic interventions, *paradoxical intervention*, also called *symptom prescription*, involves instructing clients to engage in the problem behavior in some fashion, such as by assigning a couple to argue from 7:00 to 7:15 on Tuesday and Thursday. Symptom prescription and other paradoxical interventions are "paradoxical" because they do not follow linear logic—or at least at first blush. You will know when it is time to use one of these because when it is appropriate to use paradox it will not seem paradoxical—at least in the mind of the therapist—it will be the only logical, obvious action to take. Paradox makes sense with two general types of problems: (a) when making any other therapeutic changes disrupts the family's current level of stability or (b) when the problem seems "uncontrollable" from the client's perspective: I can't keep myself from worrying, nagging, eating, fighting, etc.

- **Paradox with Families That Avoid Change:** When family members stabilize around one member being the problem, they are often resistant to the therapist's attempts to change that perception because it may create more discomfort than they are currently experiencing; in these situations paradox can be useful (Haley, 1987). The therapist may restrain or caution against certain changes: "Perhaps you need to argue to keep your passion strong; if you stopped, things might get worse." Or the therapist might choose to paradoxically encourage relapse to prevent it (Haley, 1976). Paradoxical tasks are difficult to deliver because the therapist must communicate several messages at once:

  - I want to help you resolve your problem.
  - I am sincerely concerned about you.
  - I think you can be normal, but perhaps you cannot be.

  When paradox is successful, change is usually spontaneous.

- **Paradox with Uncontrollable Symptoms:** If clients have symptoms that they claim they absolutely cannot control, it makes sense to use *symptom prescription* as an intervention. Symptom prescription changes the *context* of the problem behavior. If the context changes, the *meaning* of the behavior must change. When the meaning changes, thoughts, feelings, and subsequent behaviors automatically change also. A common example is using paradox for worrying, which is particularly difficult to treat because it is a cognitive and emotional process that often has few associated behaviors. When clients are given the directive to set an egg timer and worry for 10 minutes at a particular time in the day, worrying radically changes from a vague, free-floating experience to a consciously chosen activity that they can voluntarily start and, most often quickly discover, can also stop at will. When the context is changed, the meaning and experience of worrying change, often creating significant movement on a symptom that seemed totally out of the client's control.

Indirect Directives: Metaphorical Tasks (Strategic Therapy)

Inspired by Milton Erickson's trance work and therapeutic style, the metaphoric task is used when it is not appropriate to explicitly address a problem (Haley, 1987). Haley believes that metaphors need to be acted on, not just talked about, to create change. Metaphoric tasks involve four stages:

1. The therapist identifies an area of the client's life with similar dynamics to an area the therapist wants to change (e.g., discussing adopting a pet with a child who has been adopted).
2. The therapist uses a story or conversation to discuss how adoption works (e.g., what happens when the dog gets sick).
3. The therapist takes a position about how things should change in the metaphoric area (e.g., child is ready to adopt first pet).
4. A task is usually assigned in the metaphoric area (e.g., child's parents are encouraged to help him adopt a pet).

Pretend Techniques (Strategic Therapy)

"Fake it 'til you make it" sums up the spirit of pretend techniques, used principally by strategic therapists. In these techniques, clients are asked to "pretend" they have achieved their goal for a designated period of time (from minutes to days) to help make their desired changes. When they fake a behavior, even for a short period of time, often there is a genuine change in perspective, feeling, or behaviors. For example, when a couple are asked to fake being in love for an evening, they often feel those genuine feelings return. Systemically, this technique works by triggering old, preferred interaction patterns that are already there or, if this is an entirely new behavior, by creating new interaction sequences that are now available within the system. In either case, brief periods of pretending introduce new interactional sequences, creating new options for behavioral, emotional, and cognitive change.

Ordeals (Strategic Therapy)

Inspired by the work of Milton Erickson, *ordeals* are often used in strategic therapy when the client feels helpless in controlling a symptom such as overeating, smoking, nail biting, and drinking. They are based on a simple premise: "If one makes it more difficult for a person to have a symptom than to give it up, the person will give up the symptom" (Haley, 1984, p. 5). Rather than try to develop linear, logical means for stopping the behavior (that would be a cognitive-behavioral approach), the strategic therapist allows the symptom with a twist: the client must complete another task, an "ordeal," first or afterwards.

The ordeal need not be directly related to the undesired activity but often carries a metaphoric relation to it. For example, if a person is trying to reduce his/her "emotional eating" to soothe difficult emotions, the ordeal would target the behavior and internal tension in either a linear or logical way (e.g., engage in a favorite hobby, write in a journal) or in an indirect or nonlogical way (e.g., perform a random act of kindness for a stranger or loved one, clean the house). In most cases, ordeal therapy is less about creating a horrific, unappealing ordeal to stop undesired behavior and more about shaking up or perturbing the systemic pattern so that new behavioral sequences can evolve. To return to the family dance metaphor, the ordeal isn't a behavioral deterrent or punishment as much as a new piece of furniture in the middle of the dance floor that forces the system to make changes to navigate around it. As the system adjusts to this rather small and innocuous twist, it must change to create new steps and is able to do so with less fear and resistance than if it were told to stop dancing its favorite (or at least best-rehearsed) dance.

Snapshot: Research and the Evidence Base

Quick Summary: Newer empirically supported approaches have excellent support.

Systemic therapy began as a research project: the Bateson team began by studying communication in families with members diagnosed with schizophrenia. The tradition of observational research has been integrated into required standard training in systemic and strategic models in the form of observation teams. Although there has been less systematic research on outcomes of specific models, such as strategic, Milan, or MRI, there is consistent and growing research on the effectiveness of systemic approaches in general (Shadish & Baldwin, 2002).

Numerous empirically supported treatments incorporate systemic and strategic therapies:

- **Brief Strategic Family Therapy** (structural ecosystemic therapy, structural eco-developmental preventive interventions; see Chapter 10 for detailed description; Szapocznik & Williams, 2000)

- **Ecosystemic Structural Therapy** (Lindblad-Goldberg, Dore, & Stern, 1998)

- **Multisystemic Family Therapy** (Henggeler, Schoenwald, Borduin, Rowland, & Cunningham, 1998; see section later in this chapter)

- **Multidimensional Family Therapy** (Liddle, Dakof, & Diamond, 1991)

These approaches are manualized treatments (have a detailed manual outlining treatment protocols for a specific population) for working with defiant, conduct-disordered, or substance-abusing youth and their families.

Clinical Spotlight: Multisystemic Therapy

Multisystemic therapy (MST) was developed in the 1970s to treat serious juvenile offenders (Multisystemic Therapy Services, 1998). A family-based treatment model, MST draws from strategic, structural, socio-ecological, and cognitive-behavioral therapy models. In addition, MST also places significant emphasis on the adolescent's and family's broader social network, removing offenders from problematic social networks, improving school and/or vocational performance, and developing a strong support network for the child and the family (Henggeler, 1998; Henggeler & Borduin, 1990; Multisystemic Therapy Services, 1998).

Goals

The overarching goals of MST include the following:

- Decrease antisocial behavior and other clinical problems
- Improve functioning in family relations
- Improve functioning in school and/or work contexts
- Minimize out-of-home placements, including incarceration, residential treatment, and hospitalization

Case Conceptualization

When conceptualizing treatment, MST therapists consider risks and protective factors in the following domains: individual, family, peer, school, and neighborhood and community (Multisystemic Therapy Services, 1998).

	RISKS	**PROTECTIVE FACTORS**
Individual	Positive attitude toward antisocial behavior, psychological symptoms, hostility, low intellectual functioning and verbal skills	Intelligence, eldest child, easygoing personality, prosocial values, problem-solving skills
Family	Lack of parental supervision, ineffective or inconsistent discipline, lack of emotional expression, conflict, parental difficulties	Connection to parents and family, supportive family, strong parental relationship
Peer	Association with socially deviant peers, poor relational skills, few prosocial friends	Connections with prosocial friends
School	Poor performance, little interest, little support	Committed to education, goals, acceptable performance
Neighborhood and Community	High family mobility, criminal subculture, disorganized	Involvement in religious or social organizations, strong support network

Principles of Intervention

1. **Finding the Fit:** The therapist assesses how the adolescent's problems systemically fit within the broader family, peer, school, and community culture.

2. **Focus on Positives and Strengths:** Therapeutic interactions emphasize strengths and potential strengths, in both the individual adolescent and the family.

3. **Increasing Responsibility:** Interventions aim to increase responsible behavior with all family members, promoting parental involvement and helping teens accept responsibility for their choices.

4. **Focus on the Present, on Action, and on Clarity:** Interventions are action oriented and present focused and target specific, easily defined problems that are easily tracked and measured, such as achieving a specific grade point average or adhering to curfew.

5. **Targeting Sequences:** Consistent with its systemic foundation, sequences of behaviors are the target of change; these sequences can be between family members or with peers and the larger social systems.

6. **Developmentally Appropriate:** Interventions are developmentally appropriate for youth, promoting step-by-step development of the competencies and skills needed for success as an adult.

7. **Continuous Effort:** Interventions, by design, require daily or weekly effort from the family.

8. **Evaluation and Accountability:** Rather than blame the family if an intervention does not work, MST continually assesses the effectiveness of interventions and adjusts as necessary to ensure success.

9. **Generalization:** Treatment is designed to help the adolescent and family generalize their skills and abilities to solve problems in other life area.

Snapshot: Working with Diverse Populations

Because systemic and strategic family therapies do not rely on a therapist-defined theory of health and normalcy, they can adapt to different cultural groups and sub-populations: "Since in strategic family therapy a specific therapeutic plan is designed for each problem, there are no contraindications in terms of patient selection and suitability" (Madanes, 1991, p. 396). The evidence-based therapies that draw heavily on systemic and strategic therapy, such as multisystemic therapy and brief strategic family therapy (see Chapter 10), have been used extensively with Hispanic and African-American families. Furthermore, these therapies aim to work from *within* the client's worldview; when this is successfully achieved, the therapist adapts the language and interventions to the client's values and beliefs. The case study that follows at the end of this chapter illustrates how a systemic approach can be used with a second-generation Catholic Mexican-American family whose teenage daughter has begun smoking pot and drinking.

ONLINE RESOURCES

Brief Strategic and Systemic World Network

www.bsst.org

Mental Research Institute

www.mri.org

Multisystemic Therapy

www.mstservices.com

Strategic Therapy: Jay Haley

www.jay-haley-on-therapy.com/html/strategic_therapy.html

Strategic Therapy: Cloe Madanes

www.cloemadanes.com

Strategic Therapy: Eileen Bobrow

www.briefstrategicfamilytherapy.com

Systemic Therapy: Wendel Ray

www.wendelray.com

REFERENCES

*Asterisk indicates recommended introductory readings.

*Bateson, G. (1972). *Steps to an ecology of mind.* San Francisco: Chandler.

Bateson, G. (1979). *Mind and nature: A necessary unity.* New York: Dutton.

*Boscolo, L., Cecchin, G., Hoffman, L., & Penn, P. (1987). *Milan systemic family therapy.* New York: Basic Books.

Campbell, D., Draper, R., & Crutchley, E. (1991). The Milan systemic approach to family therapy. In A. S. Gurman & D. P. Knishern (Eds.), *Handbook of family therapy* (pp. 325–362). New York: Brunner/Mazel.

*Cecchin, G. (1987). Hypothesizing, circularity, and neutrality revisited: An invitation to curiosity. *Family Process, 26*(4), 405–413.

Cecchin, G., Lane, G., & Ray, W. (1992). *Irreverence: A strategy for therapist survival.* London: Karnac.

Fisch, R., & Schlanger, K. (1999). *Brief therapy with intimidating clients.* New York: Jossey-Bass.

*Fisch, R., Weakland, J. & Segal, L. (1982). *The tactics of change: Doing therapy briefly.* New York: Jossey-Bass.

Haley, J. (1963). *Strategies of psychotherapy.* New York: Grune & Stratton.

Haley, J. (1973). *Uncommon therapy: The psychiatric techniques of Milton H. Erickson, M.D.* New York: Norton.

Haley, J. (1976). *Problem-solving therapy: New strategies for effective family therapy.* San Francisco: Jossey-Bass.

Haley, J. (1980). *Leaving home: The therapy of disturbed young people.* New York: McGraw-Hill.

Haley, J. (1981). *Reflections on therapy.* Chevy Chase, MD: The Family Therapy Institute of Washington, DC.

Haley, J. (1984). *Ordeal therapy.* San Francisco: Jossey-Bass.

*Haley, J. (1987). *Problem-solving therapy* (2nd ed.). San Francisco: Jossey-Bass.

Haley, J. (1996). *Learning and teaching therapy.* New York: Guilford.

Haley, J., & Richeport-Haley, M. (2007). *Directive family therapy.* New York: Hawthorne.

Henggeler, S. W. (1998). *Multisystemic therapy.* Charleston, NC: Targeted Publications Group. Downloaded May 2, 2008 from www.addictionrecov.org/paradigm/P_PR_W99/mutisys_therapy.html

Henggeler, S. W., & Borduin, C. M. (1990). *Family therapy and beyond: A multisystemic approach to treating the behavior problems of children and adolescents.* Pacific Grove, CA: Brooks/Cole.

Henggeler, S. W., Schoenwald, S. K., Borduin, C. M., Rowland, M. D., & Cunningham, P. B. (1998). *Multisystemic treatment of antisocial behavior in children and adolescents.* New York: Guilford.

Jackson, D. D. (1967). The myth of normality. *Medical Opinion and Review, 3,* 28–33.

*Keeney, B. (1983). *Aesthetics of change.* New York: Guilford.

Keim, J. (1998). Strategic family therapy. In E. Dattilio (Ed.), *Case studies in couple and family therapy* (pp. 132–157). New York: Guilford.

Liddle, H. A., Dakof, G. A., & Diamond, G. (1991). Adolescent substance abuse: Multidimensional family therapy in action. In E. Daufman & P. Kaufman (Eds.), *Family therapy of drug and alcohol abuse* (pp. 120–171). Boston: Allyn & Bacon.

Lindblad-Goldberg, M., Dore, M., & Stern, L. (1998). *Creating competence from chaos.* New York: Norton.

Madanes, C. (1981). *Strategic family therapy.* San Francisco: Jossey-Bass.

Madanes, C. (1990). *Sex, love, and violence: Strategies for transformation.* New York: Norton.

Madanes, C. (1991). Strategic family therapy. In A. S. Gurman & D. P. Knishern (Eds.), *Handbook of family therapy* (pp. 396–416). New York: Brunner/Mazel.

Madanes, C. (1993). Strategic humanism. *Journal of Systemic Therapies, 12*(4), 69–75.

Mental Research Institute. (2002). *On the shoulder of giants.* Palo Alto, CA: Author.

Multisystemic Therapy Services. (1998). *Multisytemic therapy.* Downloaded May 2, 2008, from www.mstservices.com/text/treatment.html

*Nardone, G., & Watzlawick, P. (1993). *The art of change: Strategic therapy and hypnotherapy without trance.* Jossey-Bass.

Ray, W. A., & Keeney, B. (1994). *Resource focused therapy.* Karnac Books.

Segal, L. (1991). Brief therapy: The MRI approach. In A. S. Gurman & D. P. Knishern (Eds.), *Handbook of family therapy* (pp. 171–199). New York: Brunner/Mazel.

Selvini Palazzoli, M. (Ed.). (1988). *The work of Mara Selvini Palazzoli.* New York: Jason Aronson.

*Selvini Palazzoli, M., Boscolo, L., Cecchin, G., & Prata, G. (1980). Hypothesizing-circularity-neutrality: Three guidelines for the conductor of the session. *Family Process, 19*(1), 3–12.

Selvini Palazzoli, M., Cecchin, G., Prata, G., & Boscolo, L. (1978). *Paradox and counter-paradox: A new model in the therapy of the family in schizophrenic transaction.* New York: Jason Aronson.

Shadish, W. R., & Baldwin, S. A. (2002). Meta-analysis of MFT interventions. In D. H. Sprenkle (Ed.), *Effectiveness research in marriage and family therapy* (pp. 339–370). Alexandria, VA: American Association for Marriage and Family Therapy.

Szapocznik, J., & Williams, R. A. (2000). Brief strategic family therapy: Twenty-five years of interplay among theory, research and practice in adolescent behavior problems and drug abuse. *Clinical Child and Family Psychology Review, 3*(2), 117–135.

Watzlawick, P. (1977). *How real is real? Confusion, disinformation, communication.* New York: Random House.

Watzlawick, P. (1978/1993). *The language of change: Elements of therapeutic conversation.* New York: Norton.

Watzlawick, P. (Ed.). (1984). *The invented reality: How do we know what we believe we know?* New York: Norton.

Watzlawick, P. (1988). *Ultra solutions: How to fail most successfully.* New York: Norton.

Watzlawick, P. (1990). *Munchhausen's pigtail or psychotherapy and "reality" essays and lectures.* New York: Norton.

Watzlawick, P. (1993*). The situation is hopeless but not serious: The pursuit of unhappiness.* New York: Norton.

Watzlawick, P., Bavelas, J. B., & Jackson, D. D. (1967). *Pragmatics of human communication: A study of interactional patterns, pathologies, and paradoxes.* New York: Norton.

Watzlawick, P., & Weakland, J. H. (1977). *The interactional view: Studies at the Mental Research Institute, Palo Alto, 1965–1974.* New York: Norton.

*Watzlawick, P., Weakland, J., & Fisch, R. (1974). *Change: Principles of problem formation and problem resolution.* New York: Norton.

Weakland, J., & Ray, W. (Eds.). (1995). *Propagations: Thirty years of influence from the Mental Research Institute.* Binghamton, NY: Haworth Press.

SYSTEMIC CASE STUDY

The Fernandez family has brought their daughter, Alba (16), to counseling because she has begun drinking and smoking pot on the weekends with a new group of friends. Up to this point, she had been a good student who was active in numerous school activities. Her parents separated six months ago after Alba's mother Irma discovered that her husband Tom was having an affair. When the affair was discovered, Tom refused to end the relationship. Irma kicked him out but is torn about following through with the divorce because she comes from a devout Catholic family who disapprove of divorce even under these circumstances. Alba's younger brother, Jesse (14), is an honor student who tries to stay out of the conflict between Alba and the parents.

After meeting with the family, a systemic family therapist developed the following case conceptualization.

Shaded Sections Emphasized in Systemic Planning and Intervention

CASE CONCEPTUALIZATION FORM

Therapist: Maria Sanchez, MFT Trainee   **Client/Case #:** 8101   **Date:** 6/24/08

I. Introduction to Client and Significant Others *(Include age, ethnicity, occupation, grade, relevant identifiers, etc.). Put an * next to persons in session and/or IP for identified patient.*

*AF†:   38, Mexican-American, department store clerk, Catholic

*AM: 36, son of immigrants from Mexico, insurance agent, Catholic

*CF: 16 (IP) 10th grade, active in multiple school activities (drama, sports, etc.)

*CM: 14 8th grade, honor student

II. Presenting Concern
Client's/Family's Descriptions of Problem(s):

AF: Couple separated six months ago due to AM's affair; AF's family very disapproving but AF refuses to stay married; primary concern is CF16's recent alcohol/drug use.

AM: Fell in love with another woman; feels bad about effects on family but is not sure what else to do; primary concern is the children and CF16's drug use.

CF: 16 Angry about parents' divorce; feels father abandoned family; sees "partying" as normal and she is entitled because of the stress her parents caused her.

CM: 14 Sees father as weak for affair and frustrated with mother's anxiety over religious issues. Disappointed in parents but copes by staying focused on school.

Broader System Problem Descriptions (description of problem from referring party, teachers, relatives, legal system, etc.):

AF family of origin: Views divorce from religious perspective and believes couples should work things out.

AM family of origin: Understanding of divorce given the distant marriage that AM parents have.

School counselor: Concerned that CF16 is starting down dangerous path in reaction to parents' separation.

III. Background Information
Recent Background (recent life changes, precipitating events, first symptoms, stressors, etc.):

Six months prior, the CF16 and CM14 were both excelling academically and socially, and they report things at home were relatively calm. However, six months ago, AF discovered AM was having an affair; AM refused to end it. AF asked him to leave and she stayed in the home with the children. They have filed for

† *Abbreviations:* AF: Adult Female; AM: Adult Male; CF#: Child Female with age, e.g., CF12: CM#: Child Male with age; Hx: History; Ex: Explanation or Example; NA: Not Applicable.

(continued)

III. Background Information *(continued)*

divorce but are not actively moving the process along. Both children were very surprised and disappointed in father. Parents bickered frequently but seemed to be committed in the relationship. Since the separation, CF16 started hanging out for longer hours with friends, getting connected with a crowd that regularly uses alcohol and pot and has periodic access to heroin and methamphetamines. CF regularly partakes in alcohol and pot but has only tried the harder drugs a couple of times. Since the separation, CM has been quieter than usual, focusing on his studies. Neither of the children is enthusiastic about seeing their father, often choosing to go with friends or engaging in school activities during their scheduled visits.

Related Historical Background (family history, related issues, past abuse, trauma, previous counseling, medical/mental health history, etc.):

The couple had sought marital counseling two years prior for their arguing; things improved for a while but later returned to about the same level of conflict. AF comes from a very religious family; her oldest brother is a Catholic priest and her younger brother is cut off from the family because he is in a same-sex relationship. AM's father was an alcoholic, as is his brother, which has resulted in numerous cut-offs and distant relationships in his family. The parents are concerned that CF16 may develop substance abuse issues that run on AM's side of the family.

IV. Systemic Assessment

Client/Relational Strengths

Personal/individual: CF16 is an active, socially skilled, intelligent young woman; she excels at most everything she attempts; CM14 is in honors classes and is a dedicated student with goals of becoming a doctor; AF has strong family and friend relationships that have kept her going during this difficult time; AM has proven himself a dedicated father even after his kids have been rejecting him; he understands their anger and is willing to work for their forgiveness.

Relational/social: The children have strong support networks that are helping them through this difficult time: CF16's school counselor is aware of what is going on. AF's sister has helped with childcare. AM's new girlfriend supports him and has stayed out of the family dynamics.

Spiritual: AF has a strong faith that she turns to for inspiration during this difficult time; AM also has a sense that "things happen for a reason," which he finds consoling.

Family Structure and Interaction Patterns

Couple Subsystem (to be assessed): ☒ Personal current ☐ Personal past ☐ Parents'

Couple Boundaries: ☐ Clear ☒ Enmeshed ☐ Disengaged ☐ Other: _____

Rules for closeness/distance: Historically enmeshed, the couple's boundary definition has only gotten more confusing with the separation, each having a more difficult time allowing the other to have unique opinions and feelings, especially about the children. Almost every interaction is charged with overpersonalization.

Couple Problem Interaction Pattern (A ⇆ B):

Start of tension: AM brings up how to proceed with divorce.

Conflict/symptom escalation: AF begins discussing practical matters but soon goes back to old, unresolved issues. AM becomes angry, making personal attacks on AF.

Return to "normal"/homeostasis: AM leaves and topic of divorce never resolved.

Couple Complementary Patterns: ☒ Pursuer/distancer ☐ Over/under functioner

☐ Emotional/logical ☐ Good/bad parent ☐ Other: _____

Ex: Historically, AF pursued AM for connection and engagement; similar dynamic during separation.

Satir Communication Stances:

AF: ☐ Congruent ☒ Placator ☐ Blamer ☐ Superreasonable ☐ Irrelevant

AM: ☐ Congruent ☐ Placator ☐ Blamer ☒ Superreasonable ☐ Irrelevant

Describe dynamic: Although AF is often angry with AM, she seeks peace and reconciliation at all costs. AM focuses on what's logical, with minimal attention to how people are feeling, a pattern common in his family of origin.

Gottman's Divorce Indicators:

Criticism: ☒ AF ☐ AM. Ex: AF "You never cared at all about our family and were always a philanderer."

Defensiveness: ☒ AF ☒ AM. Ex: AF "You never supported me; that's why I had to find companionship in another woman." AF "Don't blame me for your affair; I have had plenty of opportunities to cheat on you but didn't."

Contempt: ☐ AF ☐ AM. Ex: _____

Stonewalling: ☐ AF ☒ AM. Ex: AM would shut AF out when tensions arose.

Failed repair attempts: ☒ AF ☒ AM. Ex: Both reportedly did not accept repair efforts.

Not accept influence: ☐ AF ☒ AM. Ex: AF reports AM rarely valued her opinions and needs.

Harsh startup: ☒ AF ☐ AM. Ex: AF reports raising issues with husband harshly.

Parental Subsystem: ☒ Family of procreation ☐ Family of origin

Membership in Family Subsystems: Parental: ☒ AF ☒ AM. ☐ Other: _____

(continued)

IV. Systemic Assessment *(continued)*

Family Structure and Interaction Patterns

Is parental subsystem distinct from couple subsystem? ☐ Yes ☒ No ☐ NA (divorce)

Sibling subsystem: CF16 and CM14 get along fairly well but have become more distant as CF16 has begun drinking and smoking.

Special interest: _____

Family Life Cycle Stage:

☐ Single adult ☐ Marriage ☐ Family with young children
☒ Family with adolescent children ☐ Launching children ☐ Later life
Describe struggles with mastering developmental tasks in one of these stages:

Couple has had difficulty maintaining couple connection since having children. AF feels as though she has had primary responsibility for raising the children. AM feeling disconnected from family life.

Hierarchy Between Child/Parents:
AF: ☐ Effective ☒ Insufficient (permissive) ☐ Excessive (authoritarian) ☒ Inconsistent
AM: ☐ Effective ☐ Insufficient (permissive) ☒ Excessive (authoritarian) ☐ Inconsistent

Ex: AF has tended to be a lenient parent with moderate effectiveness. AM has always left the majority of daily parenting to AF, but when he does discipline, he is very directive, wanting the kids to "shape up" quickly.

Emotional Boundaries with Children:
AF: ☐ Clear/balanced ☒ Enmeshed (reactive) ☐ Disengaged (disinterested)
    ☐ Other: _____
AM: ☐ Clear/balanced ☐ Enmeshed (reactive) ☒ Disengaged (disinterested)
    ☐ Other: _____

Ex: AF can be highly reactive when kids do not follow rules and has taken CF16's drug use very personally. AM has always been a more detached father figure, which is even more exaggerated since the separation.

Problem Interaction Pattern (A ⇆ B):

Start of tension: CF16 gets caught drinking.

Conflict/symptom escalation: AF begins yelling and lecturing and sets a harsh punishment she does not follow through on. When AM hears, he tries having a long talk with CF16 about her choices, focusing on the detrimental effects on her future and ignoring her emotional reasons for "escaping."

Return to "normal"/homeostasis: Neither parent is effective, and CF16 repeats behavior the following weekend.

Triangles/Coalitions:

☒ AF and CF and CM against AM: Ex: AF, CF and CM have united against AM because of the affair; CF and CM hold AM responsible for parents' separation.

☐ AM and CF and CM against AF: Ex: _____

☐ Other: Ex: _____

Communication Stances:

AF or _____ : ☐ Congruent ☒ Placator ☐ Blamer ☐ Superreasonable ☐ Irrelevant

AM or _____ : ☐ Congruent ☐ Placator ☐ Blamer ☒ Superreasonable ☐ Irrelevant

CF or _____ : ☐ Congruent ☐ Placator ☒ Blamer ☐ Superreasonable ☐ Irrelevant

CM or _____ : ☐ Congruent ☐ Placator ☐ Blamer ☐ Superreasonable ☒ Irrelevant

Ex: Although AF tries to set limits, she rarely follows through; AM has difficulty connecting with children at an emotional level because he tends to "live in his head"; CF is currently taking a blaming stance, overly focused on her needs to the detriment of others; CM tries to avoid all conflict and emotional connection in the family, which has only gotten worse since the separation.

Hypothesis (Describe possible role or function of symptom in maintaining family homeostasis):

CF's extreme acting out serves the purpose of drawing the parents together to manage her; it also distracts all members of the family from the pain of the separation and disapproval (and potential cut off) from AF's family of origin.

Intergenerational Patterns

Substance/alcohol abuse: ☐ NA ☒ Hx: AM's father and brother abuse alcohol; CF has potential to develop same problem.

Sexual/physical/emotional abuse: ☐ NA ☐ Hx: _____

Parent/child relations: ☐ NA ☒ Hx: Cut-offs between parents and children on both sides of the family; AF's brother cut off from family due to sexual orientation.

Physical/mental disorders: ☐ NA ☒ Hx: AF father died of heart attack.

Historical incidents of presenting problem: ☐ NA ☒ Hx: No divorce on either side; alcohol abuse on father's side.

Family strengths: AF has strong religious tradition; AM's family supportive of his decision.

(continued)

IV. Systemic Assessment *(continued)*

Family Structure and Interaction Patterns

Previous Solutions and Unique Outcomes

Solutions that DIDN'T work: Parents lecturing CF has not reduced her drinking and drug use. AF setting harsh but unenforced consequences not working; stalling on moving forward with the divorce may not be as effective as hoped.

Solutions that DID work: CF reports choosing to not continue using harder drugs because she is afraid of them; although her grades have dropped, she is still passing; she has retained some friends who support healthier choices. CF reports using less the weekend the family went out of town.

Narratives, Dominant Discourses, and Diversity

Dominant Discourses informing definition of problem:

Cultural, ethnic, SES, etc.: AF's cultural, religious, and family background reinforce the idea that divorce is a sin, which is creating significant internal struggle for her because a part of her believes it is unwise to remain in a relationship with a man who will not leave his mistress. This view seems to increase the stress of the potential divorce for all family members, possibly informing CF's acting out and CM's withdrawal.

Gender, sex orientation, etc.: Although AF maintains many traditional Mexican views on family and even her role as a wife and mother, she also holds modern American views on women's rights in relationships, especially related to accepting her husband's affair.

Other social influences: CF is now hanging around with a "party" crowd, which is shifting how she defines herself and her family.

Identity Narratives that have developed around problem for AF, AM, and/or CM/F: AF feels extremely conflicted between her traditional cultural and religious values and her modern gender identity; AM reports some guilt but a stronger pull to do what is true in his heart—he appears to be trying to reclaim an emotional side of himself that he has not frequently acted upon; CF reports feeling a sense of power and freedom with her new party lifestyle that separates her from the chaos at home; CM is focusing all of his energy into his studies but slowly losing connection with friends and family.

Local or Preferred Discourses: Both parents report that they believe divorce is the best choice in this situation, but are afraid to move forward because of AF's family reaction.

Other Influential Discourses: AF's family views the divorce as sin and may choose to cut her off if she goes this route.

V. Genogram

Construct a family genogram and include all relevant information, including:

- ages, birth/death dates
- names
- relational patterns
- occupations
- medical history
- psychiatric disorders
- abuse history

Also include a couple of adjectives for persons frequently discussed in session (these should describe personal qualities and/or relational patterns, e.g., quiet, family caretaker, emotionally distant, perfectionist, helpless, etc.). Genogram should be attached to report.

VI. Client Perspectives

Areas of Agreement: Based on what the client(s) has(ve) said, what parts of the above assessment do they agree with or are likely to agree with? Role of AF family, family dynamics.

Areas of Disagreement: What parts do they disagree with or are likely to disagree with? Why?

Depiction of CM potentially having problems down the road because they view him as the "star" right now.

How do you plan to respectfully work with areas of disagreement?

Tentatively raise issues related to CM functioning, perhaps after CF has shown initial improvements.

©2007 Diane R. Gehart

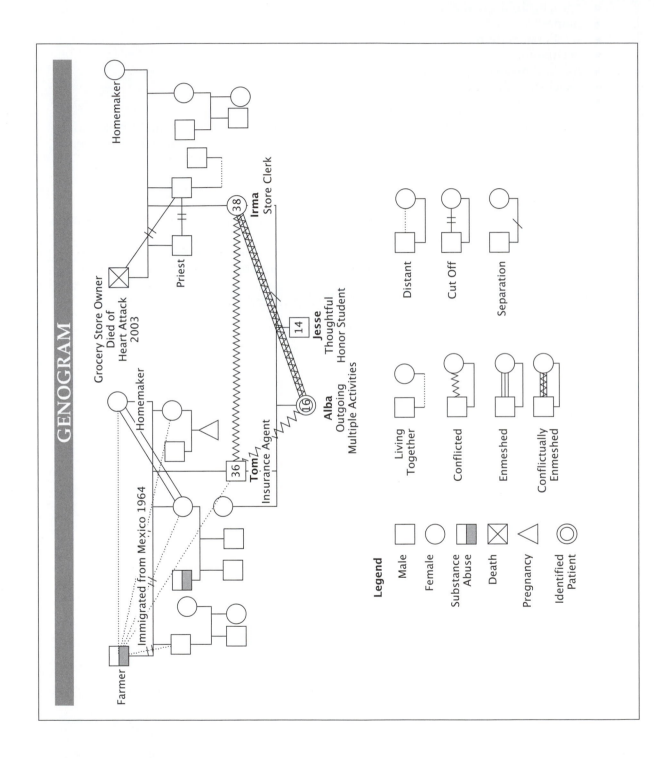

GENOGRAM

CLINICAL ASSESSMENT

Client ID # (do not use name): 8101	Ethnicities: Mexican-American	Primary Language: ☒ Eng ☒ Span ☐ Other: _____

List all participants/significant others: Put a [★] for Identified Patient(IP); [✔] for sig. others who **WILL** attend; [✕] for sig. others who will **NOT** attend.

Adult: Age: Profession/Employer	Child: Age: School/Grade
[✔] AM† 36: Insurance agent	[✔] CM 14: 8th grade; honor student
[✔] AF 38: Department store clerk	[★] CF 16: 10th grade; theater, sports
[ ] AF/M #2: _____	[ ] CF/M _____

Presenting Problems

☐ Depression/hopelessness
☐ Anxiety/worry
☒ Anger issues
☒ Loss/grief
☐ Suicidal thoughts/attempts
☐ Sexual abuse/rape
☒ Alcohol/drug use
☐ Eating problems/disorders
☐ Job problems/unemployed

☐ Couple concerns
☐ Parent/child conflict
☐ Partner violence/abuse
☒ Divorce adjustment
☐ Remarriage adjustment
☐ Sexuality/intimacy concerns
☒ Major life changes
☐ Legal issues/probation
☐ Other: _____

Complete for children
☒ School failure/decline performance
☐ Truancy/runaway
☐ Fighting w/peers
☐ Hyperactivity
☐ Wetting/soiling clothing
☐ Child abuse/neglect
☐ Isolation/withdrawal
☐ Other: _____

Mental Status for IP

Interpersonal issues	☐ NA	☒ Conflict ☒ Enmeshment ☐ Isolation/avoidance ☐ Emotional disengagement ☐ Poor social skills ☐ Couple problems ☐ Prob w/friends ☐ Prob at work ☐ Overly shy ☐ Egocentricity ☐ Diff establish/maintain relationship ☐ Other: _____
Mood	☐ NA	☐ Depressed/sad ☐ Hopeless ☐ Fearful ☐ Anxious ☒ Angry ☒ Irritable ☐ Manic ☐ Other: _____
Affect	☐ NA	☒ Constricted ☐ Blunt ☐ Flat ☐ Labile ☐ Dramatic ☐ Other: _____
Sleep	☐ NA	☐ Hypersomnia ☐ Insomnia ☒ Disrupted ☒ Nightmares ☐ Other: _____
Eating	☐ NA	☒ Increase ☐ Decrease ☐ Anorectic restriction ☐ Bingeing ☐ Purging ☐ Body image ☐ Other: _____
Anxiety symptoms	☒ NA	☐ Chronic worry ☐ Panic attacks ☐ Dissociation ☐ Phobias ☐ Obsessions ☐ Compulsions ☐ Other: _____

(continued)

† *Abbreviations:* AF: Adult Female; AM: Adult Male; CF#: Child Female with age, e.g., CF12; CM#: Child Male with age; Hx: History; Cl: Client.

Mental Status for IP *(continued)*

Trauma symptoms	☒ NA	☐ Acute ☐ Chronic ☐ Hypervigilance ☐ Dreams/nightmares ☐ Dissociation ☐ Emotional numbness ☐ Other: _____
Psychotic symptoms	☒ NA	☐ Hallucinations ☐ Delusions ☐ Paranoia ☐ Loose associations ☐ Other: _____
Motor activity/ speech	☐ NA	☐ Low energy ☐ Restless/hyperactive ☒ Agitated ☐ Inattentive ☐ Impulsive ☐ Pressured speech ☐ Slow speech ☐ Other: _____
Thought	☐ NA	☐ Poor concentration/attention ☒ Denial ☐ Self-blame ☒ Other-blame ☐ Ruminative ☐ Tangential ☐ Illogical ☐ Concrete ☐ Poor insight ☒ Impaired decision making ☐ Disoriented ☐ Slow processing ☐ Other: _____
Socio-Legal	☐ NA	☐ Disregards rules ☒ Defiant ☐ Stealing ☐ Lying ☐ Tantrums ☐ Arrest/incarceration ☐ Initiates fights ☐ Other: _____
Other symptoms	☒ NA	

Diagnosis for IP

Contextual Factors considered in making Dx: ☒ Age ☒ Gender ☒ Family dynamics ☒ Culture ☒ Language ☒ Religion ☐ Economic ☐ Immigration ☐ Sexual orientation ☐ Trauma ☐ Dual dx/comorbid ☒ Addiction ☐ Cognitive ability ☐ Other: _____

Describe impact of identified factors: Used teen-friendly language with CF using gender and ethnic similarity to connect; considered current family dynamics when assessing CF mood and behavior; although Spanish is spoken with extended family, CF identifies English as her primary language and prefers to speak in English in session; the family speaks English together at home. Family's religious beliefs and intergenerational history of addiction also considered as part of assessment.

Axis I
Primary: 309.28 Adjustment Disorder w Disturbance of Mood and Conduct, Acute

Secondary: R/O 305.00 Alcohol Abuse 305.20 Cannabis Abuse

Axis II: V71.09 no dx

Axis III: None reported

Axis IV:
☒ Problems with primary support group
☐ Problems related to social environment/school
☒ Educational problems
☐ Occupational problems
☐ Housing problems
☐ Economic problems
☐ Problems with accessing health care services

List DSM symptoms for Axis I Dx (include frequency and duration for each). Client meets 5 of 5 criteria for Axis I Primary Dx.

1. Stressor: parents separated; father moved out; father had affair
2. Began drinking and smoking pot on weekends with friends
3. No incidents of drinking/driving or severe intoxication
4. Grades have dropped from 3.5 GPA to 2.75 GPA
5. More arguing and defiance at home
6. Will continue to monitor substance use to rule out abuse

☐ Problems related to interactions with the legal system
☐ Other psychosocial problems

Axis V: GAF 65 GARF 60

Have medical causes been ruled out?
☐ Yes ☐ No ☒ In process
**Has patient been referred for psychiatric/
medical eval?** ☒ Yes ☐ No
Has patient agreed with referral?
☒ Yes ☐ No ☐ NA
List psychometric instruments or consults used
for assessment:
☐ None or MAST _____

**Medications (psychiatric & medical)
Dose /Start Date**
☒ None prescribed
1. _____ / ___ mg; _____
2. _____ / ___ mg; _____
3. _____ / ___ mg; _____

Client response to diagnosis:
☒ Agree ☐ Somewhat agree ☐ Disagree
☐ Not informed for following reason:
_____

Medical Necessity (*Check all that apply*): ☒ Significant impairment ☒ Probability of significant impairment
☒ Probable developmental arrest
Areas of impairment: ☒ Daily activities ☒ Social relationships ☒ Health ☒ Work/school
☒ Living arrangement ☐ Other: _____

Risk Assessment

Suicidality
☐ No indication
☒ Denies
☐ Active ideation
☐ Passive ideation
☐ Intent without plan
☐ Intent with means
☐ Ideation past yr
☐ Attempt past yr
☐ Family/peer hx of completed suicide

Homicidality
☐ No indication
☒ Denies
☐ Active ideation
☐ Passive ideation
☐ Intent w/o means
☐ Intent with means
☐ Ideation past yr
☐ Violence past yr
☐ Hx assault/temper
☐ Cruelty to animals

Hx Substance:
Alcohol abuse:
☐ No indication
☐ Denies
☐ Past
☒ Current
Freq/Amt: 2–3 beers/week

Drug:
☐ No indication
☐ Denies
☐ Past
☒ Current
Drugs: Marijuana
Freq/Amt: 1–2 times/week
☒ Family/sig. other abuses

Sexual & Physical Abuse and Other Risk Factors
☐ Current child w abuse hx:
  ☐ Sexual ☐ Physical ☐ Emotional ☐ Neglect
☐ Adult w childhood abuse:
  ☐ Sexual ☐ Physical ☐ Emotional ☐ Neglect
☐ Adult w abuse/assault in adulthood:
  ☐ Sexual ☐ Physical ☐ Current
☐ History of perpetrating abuse:
  ☐ Sexual ☐ Physical
☐ Elder/dependent adult abuse/neglect
☐ Anorexia/bulimia/other eating disorder
☒ Cutting or other self-harm:
  ☐ Current
  ☒ Past; Method: Cut 1–2 times 6 mo ago
  ☐ Criminal/legal hx: _____
  ☐ None reported

(continued)

Risk Assessment *(continued)*

Indicators of Safety: ☒ At least one outside person who provides strong support ☒ Able to cite specific reasons to live, not harm self/other ☐ Hopeful ☐ Has future goals ☒ Willing to dispose of dangerous items ☒ Willingness to reduce contact with people who make situation worse ☒ Willing to implement safety plan, safety interventions ☐ Developing set of alternatives to self/other harm ☒ Sustained period of safety: 6 mos. ☐ Other: _____

Safety Plan includes: ☒ Verbal no harm contract ☐ Written no harm contract ☒ Emergency contact card ☒ Emergency therapist/agency number ☐ Medication management ☒ Specific plan for contacting friends/support persons during crisis ☐ Specific plan of where to go during crisis ☒ Specific self-calming tasks to reduce risk before reach crisis level (e.g., journaling, exercising, etc.) ☐ Specific daily/weekly activities to reduce stressors ☐ Other: _____

Notes: Legal/Ethical Action Taken: ☐ NA _____

Case Management

Date 1st visit: 6/24/08 _____ Last visit: 7/2/08 _____ **Session Freq:** ☒ Once week ☐ Every other week ☐ Other: _____ **Expected Length of Treatment:** _____	**Modalities:** ☐ Individual adult ☒ Individual child ☒ Couple ☒ Family ☐ Group: _____ _____	**Is client involved in mental health or other medical treatment elsewhere?** ☐ No ☒ Yes: Divorce group at school **If Child/Adolescent:** Is family involved? ☒ Yes ☐ No

Patient Referrals and Professional Contacts

Has contact been made with social worker?
☐ Yes ☐ No: explain: _____ ☒ NA

Has client been referred for medical assessment?
☒ Yes ☐ No evidence for need

Has client been referred for psychiatric assessment?
☒ Yes; cl agree ☐ Yes, cl disagree ☐ Not nec.

Has contact been made with treating physicians or other professionals?
☒ Yes ☐ No ☐ NA

Has client been referred for social/legal services?
☐ Job/training ☐ Welfare/food/housing ☐ Victim services
☐ Legal aid ☐ Medical ☐ Other: _____ ☒ NA

Anticipated forensic/legal processes related to treatment:
☐ No ☒ Yes: Custody hearings _____

Has client been referred for group or other support services?
☒ Yes ☐ No ☐ None recommended

Client social support network includes:
☐ Supportive family ☐ Supportive partner ☒ Friends ☒ Religious/spiritual organization ☐ Supportive work/social group ☐ Other: _____

Anticipated effects treatment will have on others in support system; (Parents, children, siblings, sig. others, etc.):
Addressing CF issues may increase focus on CM and need for divorce.

Is there anything else client will need to be successful?
Parents may benefit from individual therapy.

Client Sense of Hope: Little 1----------X----------10 High

Expected Outcome and Prognosis

☒ Return to normal functioning

☐ Expect improvement, anticipate less than normal functioning

☐ Maintain current status/prevent deterioration

Evaluation of Assessment/Client Perspective

How was assessment method adapted to client needs?

Used client-friendly language and form for alcohol/substance use.

Age, culture, ability level, and other diversity issues adjusted for by:

Asked diagnostic questions in language client could understand without family present.

Systemic/family dynamics considered in following ways:

Family included for history but not for individual mental health assessment.

Describe actual or potential areas of client-therapist agreement/disagreement related to the above assessment:

CF sees her "partying" as normal; parents see it as abuse. As she is still functioning fairly well at school and keeping up with most major commitments and relationships, does not qualify for abuse at this point in time, but is likely to if trend continues.

_____ , _____ _____

Therapist signature   License/Intern status   Date

_____ , _____ _____

Supervisor signature   License   Date

TREATMENT PLAN

Therapist: Maria Sanchez, MFT Trainee   **Client ID #:** 8101

Theory: Systemic

Primary Configuration: ☐ Individual ☐ Couple ☒ Family ☐ Group: _____

Additional: ☒ Individual ☒ Couple ☐ Family ☐ Group: _____

Medication(s): ☒ NA ☐ _____

Contextual Factors considered in making plan: ☒ Age ☒ Gender ☒ Family dynamics
☒ Culture ☒ Language ☒ Religion ☐ Economic ☐ Immigration ☐ Sexual orientation
☐ Trauma ☐ Dual dx/comorbid ☒ Addiction ☐ Cognitive ability
☐ Other: _____

Describe how plan is adapted to contextual factors: Plan designed to engage teen by using techniques and language that are comfortable to her; the larger family dynamics that contribute to CF current symptoms will be directly addressed in session; culture, language, and religious beliefs will be considered when defining goals and interventions that are likely to be meaningful to family.

I. Initial Phase of Treatment (First 1–3 Sessions)

I.A. Initial Therapeutic Tasks

Therapeutic Relationship

> TT1: Develop therapeutic relationship with all members. Note: Particular attention to **multipartiality** given division between parents and CF and parents.

> I1: Intervention: Maintain **neutrality** and use **client language** to build relationship with all members.

Assessment

> TT2: Assess individual, systemic, and broader cultural dynamics. Note: What is the role of CF alcohol use in **maintaining family homeostasis** during separation?

> I1: Intervention: Assess **interaction cycle** to identify how CF "partying" helps family maintain homeostasis.

> I2: Intervention: **Circular questions** to assess family meaning system and roles of each.

Set Goals

> TT3: Define and obtain client agreement on treatment goals. Note: _____

> I1: Intervention: Define goal in behavioral terms that all family members can agree upon.

Note: **BOLDFACE** indicates Systemic Therapy assessment and techniques.

Referrals and Crisis

TT4: Identify needed referrals, crisis issues, and other client needs. Note: _____

I1: Intervention: Refer CF for medical/psychiatric evaluation due to alcohol/substance use.

I.B. Initial Client Goals (1–2 Goals): Manage crisis issues and/or reduce most distressing symptoms

Goal #1: ☒ Increase ☐ Decrease **direct communication** about divorce between family members (personal/relational dynamic) to reduce CF's need to drink and smoke to distract family from the issues they are avoiding (symptom).

Measure: Able to sustain responsible alcohol/substance use behavior for period of 2 ☐ wks ☒ mos with no more than 1 mild episode of intoxication.

I1: Intervention: Use **positive connotation** of CF drinking as her way of sacrificing self and grades in order to distract parents from their pain.

I2: Intervention: **Circular questions** to reframe CF's drinking: who does her drinking hurt the most in the present? Who will be hurt by it most in the long run? If she were to stop partying, who would be the most surprised? The least? What positive/negative effects would this have on the family?

II. Working Phase of Treatment (Sessions 2+)
II.A. Working Therapeutic Tasks
Monitor Progress

TT1: Monitor progress toward goals. Note: Emphasis on keeping CF safe.

I1: Intervention: Monitor effectiveness of weekly tasks; adjust **hypothesis** as necessary to improve outcome.

Monitor Relationship

TT2: Monitor quality of therapeutic alliance as therapy proceeds. Note: _____

I1: Intervention: Use **humor** and **irreverence** to connect with CF and family.

II.B. Working Client Goals (2–3 Goals): Target individual and relational dynamics in case conceptualization using theoretical language (e.g., reduce enmeshment, increase differentiation, increase agency in relational narrative, etc.).

Goal #1: ☒ Increase ☐ Decrease effectiveness of the **parental coalition** in relating to children (personal/relational dynamic) to reduce the need for CF to act out to get them on the same team (symptom).

(continued)

II. Working Phase of Treatment (Sessions 2+) *(continued)*

Measure: Able to sustain <u>effective parenting</u> for period of <u>2</u> ☐ wks ☒ mos with no more than <u>2</u> mild episodes of <u>defiance</u>.

    I1: Intervention: <u>Use variation of **invariant prescription** in which parents clearly communicate</u> <u>alliance by maintaining secrets from kids.</u>

    I2: Intervention: **Directives** <u>to AM that increase emotional connection, such as a ritual greeting</u> <u>or good-bye during visits and for AF to increase consistency, such as writing a "house citation"</u> <u>instead of verbally disciplining.</u>

Goal #2: ☐ Increase ☒ Decrease <u>CF's **systemic role of sacrificing herself to maintain family homeostasis** and increase her freedom to attend to the developmental task of increased independence</u> (personal/relational dynamic) to reduce <u>poor decision making and increase her motivation for success at school and in extracurricular activities</u> (symptom).

Measure: Able to sustain <u>motivation</u> for period of <u>2</u> ☐ wks ☒ mos with no more than <u>2</u> mild episodes of <u>poor choices</u>.

    I1: Intervention: **Circular questions** <u>that reveal how her acting out is helping everyone but her</u> <u>in the family.</u>

    I2: Intervention: **Paradoxical "go slow" injunctions** <u>for her not to stop all the bad behavior too</u> <u>soon—so that parents have a reason to keep delaying the divorce.</u>

III. Closing Phase of Treatment (Last 2+ Weeks)

III.A. Closing Therapeutic Tasks
Termination Plan

    TT1: Develop aftercare plan and maintain gains. Note: <u>Emphasis on keeping CF safe.</u>

    I1: Intervention: **Restraining** and **go slow techniques** <u>to reinforce family's commitment to</u> <u>change; circular questions to develop relapse prevention plan.</u>

III.B. Closing Client Goals: Determined by theory's definition of health

Goal #1: ☒ Increase ☐ Decrease **family's ability** <u>to emotionally and practically navigate</u> <u>separation and divorce</u> (personal/relational dynamic) to reduce <u>CF acting out</u> (symptom).

Measure: Able to sustain <u>low conflict and effective problem solving</u> for period of <u>3</u> ☐ wks ☒ mos with no more than <u>2</u> mild episodes of <u>conflict or CF acting out.</u>

    I1: Intervention: **Circular questions** <u>to safely communicate about feelings, plans, desires,</u> <u>related to separation and divorce and identify possibilities for proceeding.</u>

    I2: Intervention: **Rituals** <u>to facilitate reparation between AM and family members related</u> <u>to the affair.</u>

IV. Client Perspective

Has treatment plan been reviewed with client? ☒ Yes ☐ No; If no, explain: _____

_____

Describe areas of client agreement and concern: <u>Both parents state that they believe the other</u> <u>person is the "real" problem but are willing to come to conjoint family sessions for their daughter's sake.</u> <u>AF prefers harsher punishments for CF than AM.</u>

_____ , _____

Therapist signature   Intern status   Date

_____ , _____

Supervisor signature   License   Date

_____

Abbreviations: TT: Therapeutic Task; I: Intervention; AM: Adult Male; AF: Adult Female; CM: Child Male; CF: Child Female; Dx: Diagnosis; NA: Not Applicable.

PROGRESS NOTES

Progress Notes for Client # <u>8101</u>

Date: <u>7/25/08</u> **Time:** <u>6:00</u> am/<u>pm</u> **Session Length:** ☒ 50 min. or ☐ _____

Present: ☒ AM ☒ AF ☒ CM ☒ CF ☒ _____

Billing Code: ☐ 90801 (Assess) ☐ 90806 (Insight-50 min) ☒ 90847 (Family-50 min)

☐ Other _____

Symptom(s)	Dur/Freq Since Last Visit	Progress: Setback----Initial----------------Goal
1. CF drinking	Report 1 beer; no marijuana	-5----------1------------5-X----------10
2. Conflict w/AM	Kids went on weekly visit; "ok time"	-5----------1------------5------X------10
3. Triangulation	Kids report no incidents of triangulation	-5----------1------------5-------X-----10

Explanatory Notes: CF reports willing to honor parents' desire for her not to smoke; reports doing more HW this week. Kids report less tension about separation and that AF saying less about AM. They also report AM "trying harder," so they are willing to visit.

(continued)

PROGRESS NOTES *(continued)*

Interventions/HW: Followed up on last week's directives; used circular questions to make overt divorce tensions that are being played out on kids. Developed plan to alter CF ordeal of writing e-mail to parents before going out to include "responsibility (safety) plan" for night; altered AM directive for special greeting to include "secret handshake"; continued invariant prescription with a closed parent-only meeting at the end of the session.

Client Response/Feedback: Family excited about progress and actively help develop assignments for week. CF responds well to defiance-based, paradoxical messages.

Plan: ☒ Continue with treatment plan; plan for next session: Follow up on homework, circular questions to further discussion of plans for family future.

☐ Modify plan: _____

Next session: Date: 8/2/08 Time: 6:00 am/**pm**

Crisis Issues: ☒ Denies suicide/homicide/abuse/crisis ☐ Crisis assessed/addressed:

CF denies heavy alcohol or drug use; parents report there is no indication of this; deny cutting.

_____ , _____ _____
Therapist signature   License/Intern status   Date

◇◇◇

Case Consultation/Supervision Notes: Supervisor encouraged focusing on interrupting family dynamics and moving toward raising the issue of divorce and how things will work in future.

Collateral Contacts: Date: 7/25/08 Time: 2:00 pm Name: Betty Anderson, School Counselor

Notes: Counselor reports grades slightly up; no other reported problems.

_____

☒ Written release on file: ☒ Sent ☐ Received ☐ In court docs ☐ Other: _____

_____ , _____ _____
Therapist signature   License/Intern status   Date

_____ , _____ _____
Supervisor signature   License   Date

_____

Abbreviations: AM: Adult Male; AF: Adult Female; CM: Child Male; CF: Child Female; HW: Homework.

Structural Therapy

"Training in family therapy should therefore be a way of teaching techniques whose essence is to be mastered, then forgotten. After this book is read, it should be given away, or put in a forgotten corner. The therapist should be a healer: a human being concerned with engaging other human beings, therapeutically, around areas and issues that cause them pain, while always retaining great respect for their values, areas of strength, and esthetic preferences. The goal in other words is to transcend technique."—Minuchin & Fishman, 1981, p. 1

Lay of the Land

Structural therapy is primarily associated with the work of Salvador Minuchin, and the majority of this chapter focuses on his work. In addition, the chapter highlights two evidence-based treatments that draw heavily from traditional structural family therapy: brief strategic family therapy and ecosystemic structural family therapy.

In a Nutshell: The Least You Need to Know

As the name implies, structural therapists map family structure—boundaries, hierarchies, and subsystems—to help clients resolve individual mental health symptoms and relational problems (Minuchin & Fishman, 1981). After assessing family functioning, therapists aim to restructure the family, realigning boundaries and hierarchies to promote growth and resolve problems. They are active in sessions, staging enactments, realigning chairs, and questioning family assumptions. Structural family therapy focuses on strengths, never seeing families as dysfunctional but rather as people who need assistance in expanding their repertoire of interaction patterns to adjust to their ever-changing developmental and contextual demands.

The Juice: Significant Contributions to the Field

If you remember a thing or two from this chapter, they should be these:

Juice 1: Boundaries, or Rules for Relating

Boundaries are one of the few family therapy terms that have trickled into the vernacular, so often that your clients come in talking about them. At first glance, the term seems two-dimensional, and much like Goldilocks, you are tempted to sum things up by saying they are too rigid, too weak, or just right. However, as you begin to work with the idea of boundaries, you quickly learn that boundaries are far more complex than they initially appear. But let's start with the simple definition.

Boundaries are rules for managing physical and psychological distance between family members, for defining the regulation of closeness, distance, hierarchy, and family roles (Minuchin & Fishman, 1981). Although they may sound static, they are organic, living processes. Structural therapists identify three basic types of boundaries:

- **Clear Boundaries:** Clear boundaries are "normal" boundaries that allow for close emotional contact with others while simultaneously allowing each person to maintain a sense of identity and differentiation (Colapinto, 1991). Each culture has a unique style of balancing closeness and distance, with different appropriate outward expressions of this balance. For example, some cultures require more physical space for clear boundaries than do others.

- **Enmeshment and Diffuse Boundaries:** Diffuse or weak boundaries lead to relational enmeshment (for those who like to be technically correct, boundaries are diffuse and relationships enmeshed). Families with overly diffuse boundaries do not make a clear distinction between members, creating a strong sense of mutuality and connection at the expense of individual autonomy (Colapinto, 1991). When talking with an enmeshed family, therapists typically see family members doing the following:

  - Interrupting one another or speaking for one another
  - Mind-reading and making assumptions
  - Insisting on high levels of protectiveness and overconcern
  - Demanding loyalty at the expense of individual needs
  - Feeling threatened when there is disagreement or difference

  How can you tell the difference between clear and close versus diffuse boundaries? Simple. If boundaries are diffuse, the family will report symptoms and problems in one or more individuals and/or complaints about family interactions. Moreover, behaviors that constitute problematic boundaries in one cultural context may be clear in another cultural context (Minuchin & Fishman, 1981). Immigrant and other bicultural families present special problems because there is more than one cultural context at play. Thus, although identifying problem boundaries seems straightforward at first, it quickly becomes murky in actual practice, requiring therapists to proceed mindfully and respectfully and to attend to each family's unique situation.

- **Disengagement and Rigid Boundaries:** Rigid boundaries lead to relational disengagement. Autonomy and independence are emphasized at the expense of emotional connection, creating isolation that may be more emotional than physical (Colapinto, 1991). These families have excessive tolerance for deviation, often failing to mobilize support and protection for one another. Therapists working with disengaged families notice the following:

  - Lack of reaction and few repercussions, even to problems
  - Significant freedom for most members to do as they please

- Few demands for or expressions of loyalty and commitment
- Consistently using parallel interactions (e.g., doing different activities in the same room) as substitutes for reciprocal interactions and engagement

Again, rigid boundaries cannot be accurately assessed without taking cultural and developmental variables into consideration; unless members are experiencing symptoms or problems, there is little ground for identifying boundaries as overly rigid.

Juice 2: Enactments

Perhaps the most distinctive of structural interventions, enactments are techniques in which the therapist prompts the family to re-enact a conflict or other interaction (Colapinto, 1991; Minuchin, 1974; Minuchin & Fishman, 1981). Regardless of the therapy model you choose to use in the end, enactments are one of the most important techniques for therapists to master. Why? Because most couples and families are going to start arguing in your office whether you ask them to or not, so you better be prepared! Enactments are one of the best ways to handle this..

Minuchin preferred enactments to talking about interactions because often people describe themselves as one way but behave quite differently, not because they are malicious or hypocritical but because it is often difficult to see clearly how our behavior looks from the outside (Minuchin & Fishman, 1981). Enactments are used to both assess and alter the problematic interactional sequences, allowing the therapist to *map, track,* and *modify* the family structure. In the case study at the end of the chapter, the therapist uses enactments to first assess the boundaries between the parents and their sons, (the eldest referred for fighting at school), and later uses enactments to strengthen the parental hierarchy and boundaries.

As therapists become more experienced, they require only a few minutes of watching a family interact to know where and how to *restructure* the family. Restructuring may take the form of creating a clearer boundary in enmeshed relationships (e.g., stopping people from interrupting and speaking for one another), increasing engagement by encouraging the expression of empathy or direct eye contact, or improving parental effectiveness by helping the parent successfully manage a child's in-session behavior.

An enactment occurs in three phases, as a "dance in three movements" (Minuchin & Fishman, 1981, p. 81):

1. **Observation of Spontaneous Interactions: Tracking and Mapping:** When talking with the family, the therapist closely follows both content and process, listening for the rules and assumptions that coordinate the family's interactions, such as demands for overconnectedness, extreme disconnection, or hierarchical confusion, as well as strengths and resources. The therapist tracks *actual transactions* more closely than verbal accounts (Colapinto, 1991), while developing a hypothesis that *maps* the family's boundaries and hierarchy (Minuchin & Fishman, 1981). Once therapists identify an area for change, they are ready to invite the family into the active phase of enactment.

2. **The Invitation: Eliciting Transactions:** The invitation for an enactment is issued in two ways: either the therapist directly asks the family to engage in an enactment, or the family spontaneously starts an enactment of at-home behavior, usually in the form of an argument (Colapinto, 1981). Obviously, the therapist does not need to do much when the family spontaneously begins; if the family does not, the therapist must issue an explicit invitation to "show" the problem:

   "Can you re-enact what happened last night?" or
   "Please show me what happens at home when he is 'defiant'; can you act out an incident of defiance that happened last week so I have a good idea of what the problem really is?"

3. **Redirecting Alternative Transactions:** This is the most important part. It really is not therapeutic to ask a family to start enacting problem behaviors if the therapist does not jump in and help redirect the behavior to clarify boundaries and hierarchies. How therapists redirect the interaction depends on the particular interaction that needs to be changed. Redirection often involves the following:

   - Stopping family members from interrupting or speaking for one another
   - Directing two people to directly engage each other while asking a third member to allow the other two to communicate
   - Encouraging emotional understanding and connection between disengaged parties
   - Rearranging chairs physically to increase or decrease emotional closeness
   - Requesting parents to actively establish an effective hierarchical position with a child

Enactments are beneficial because they provide live practice with new interactions and family patterns, increasing the likelihood of transitioning in-session gains and insights into everyday family life. They also reduce the illusion that the problem belongs to a single person; when a family demonstrate the problem in front of the therapist, it becomes clear that the reported problem does not belong to a single person but to the larger family unit. Finally, enactments increase the family's sense of competence and strength by helping them to successfully engage in new preferred behaviors (Minuchin & Fishman, 1981).

Rumor Has It: The People and Their Stories

Salvador Minuchin

Trained as a pediatrician and child psychiatrist, Salvador Minuchin is considered the progenitor of structural family therapy (Colapinto, 1991; Minuchin, 1974). Minuchin lived and worked on three continents; he was born and raised in Argentina and then lived in Israel during two periods of his life before settling in the United States. In 1954, after returning from a two-year period of working with displaced children in Israel, he began his psychiatry training with Harry Stack Sullivan, whose psychoanalytic work emphasized interpersonal relationships. After his training, Minuchin accepted a position at the Wiltwyck School for delinquent boys and suggested to his colleagues—Dick Auerswald, Charlie King, Braulio Montalvo, and Clara Rabinowitz—that they see the entire family. With no formal models to follow, they used a one-way mirror to observe each other and developed a working model as they went along. In 1962, Minuchin visited the Mental Research Institute, where Haley, Watzlawick, Fisch, and others were at the forefront of developing family therapy approaches. There he befriended Jay Haley, who developed the strategic approach to family therapy (see Chapter 9); the mutual influence of this friendship is evident in the work of both men.

From 1965 to 1976, Minuchin served as the director of the Philadelphia Child Guidance Clinic, and in 1975 he founded the Family Therapy Training Center (later renamed the Philadelphia Child and Family Therapy Training Center). In 1967, Minuchin, Montalvo, Guerney, Rosman, and Schumer published *Families of the Slums,* considered the first book to describe structural therapy and a book that discussed diversity issues before the term *multiculturalism* was coined. Over the years, Minuchin and his colleagues have written numerous books that detail how they have developed and refined this model to address changing cultural contexts and specific diagnoses (Minuchin, Rosman, & Baker, 1978). Minuchin is still an active leader in the field, continuing to teach new generations of therapists (Minuchin, Nichols, & Lee, 2007). His influential students and colleagues include Harry Aponte, Jorge Colapinto, Charles Fishman, Jay Lappin, and Michael Nichols.

Harry Aponte

Harry Aponte (1994, 1996) attends to issues of spirituality, poverty, and race in the practice of structural family therapy.

Marion Lindblad-Goldberg

Marion Lindblad-Goldberg succeeded Minuchin as the director of the Philadelphia Child and Family Therapy Training Center in 1986 and still serves as its director. She and her colleagues (Lindbald-Goldberg, Dore, & Stern, 1998) developed the empirically supported treatment called "ecosystemic structural family therapy" (ESFT), which they emphasize in current training programs at the center.

Jose Szapocznik

Jose Szapocznik and his colleagues at the Center for Family Studies in Florida developed the empirically supported brief strategic family therapy (BSFT) to address drug abuse problems with Cuban youth in Miami (Szapocznik & Williams, 2000).

The Big Picture: Overview of Treatment

Minuchin (1974) identifies three main *phases* of structural therapy:

1. Join the family and accommodate to their style (build an alliance)
2. Map the family structure, boundaries, and hierarchy (evaluate and assess)
3. Intervene to transform the structure to diminish symptoms (address the problems they identified in the assessment)

Generally, therapists alternate between phases two and three many times, revising and refining the map and hypotheses about family functioning until the problems are addressed and resolved. I like to think of it as similar to the golden rule with shampoo: "lather, rinse, repeat" until you achieve the desired effect.

Who Attends Therapy?

To be able to assess the system, structural therapists prefer to begin therapy with the entire family, but they do not insist on it (Colapinto, 1991). However, once the family system has been assessed, the therapist often meets with specific subsystems and individuals to achieve structural goals. For example, often sessions with the couple alone are necessary to strengthen the boundaries between the couple and parental subsystems and to sever cross-generational coalitions.

Making Connection: The Therapeutic Relationship

Joining and Accommodating

Structural family therapists have a unique term for the therapeutic relationship: *joining* (Minuchin, 1974; Minuchin & Fishman, 1981; Minuchin & Nichols, 1993). They "join" the system in the sense that they *accommodate* to its style: how people talk, what words they use, how they walk, and so forth. *Mimesis*, a Greek term that means "copy" (as in *mimeograph*; if you're too young to remember that, consider yourself lucky), has also been used to refer to the process of accommodating the family's way of being. In the historical context of psychotherapy, this is a radical concept, because unlike in psychodynamic, cognitive-behavioral, and even experiential therapies, the therapist does not take a superior role.

Minuchin (1974) compared the process of joining a family to an anthropologist studying a new culture, which always begins by sitting back and observing patterns, habits, and behaviors before beginning to address one's own agenda, in this case to alleviate the family's distress. The process of joining can also be likened to falling in rhythm with the family. Do they talk fast or slow? Do they talk over one another or wait for clear pauses to speak? Do they use teasing and humor, or are their words gentle and soft? A successful structural therapist needs to have a wide repertoire of social skills to successfully join with families, especially when working with diverse populations. In the case study at the end of this chapter, the therapist uses humor and sincerity to balance connecting with the parents while simultaneously gaining the trust of their often defiant teenage son.

Joining as an Attitude

Colapinto (1991) emphasizes that joining is more of an attitude than a technique; it is the glue that holds the therapeutic system together through the often turbulent and challenging journey called therapy (Minuchin & Fishman, 1981). The attitude of joining requires (a) a strong, clear sense of connection and affiliation (e.g., curiosity, openness, sensitivity, acceptance) and (b) an equally clear sense of distance and differentiation (e.g., questioning, dissenting, promoting change).

Therapeutic Spontaneity

Structural therapists strive to cultivate therapeutic spontaneity, which does not refer to a do-as-you-please attitude but rather a relationally and contextually responsive expression of self: "the therapist's spontaneity is constrained by the context of therapy" (Minuchin & Fishman, 1981, p. 3). Therapeutic spontaneity refers to the ability to flow naturally and authentically in a variety of contexts and situations. Much in the way riding a bike becomes natural after a painful period of training wheels and falls, therapeutic spontaneity is cultivated and shaped through the training process, which increases therapists' repertoire for "being natural" in a wide range of clinical situations.

Therapist's Use of Self

According to Minuchin, therapists must use themselves to relate to the family, varying from being highly involved to professionally detached (Minuchin & Fishman, 1981). They may be clearly detached from family interactions so that they can clarify boundaries or prescribe a specific intervention, maintain a moderate level of connection to coach the family in new interactions, or assume a fully engaged position by taking sides with one family member to "unbalance" the system (an intervention discussed later in the chapter). The therapist is highly flexible, adapting to each family's needs and cultural norms.

"Making It Happen"

> "The primary injunction from the model to the therapist can be summarized in three words: 'Make it happen.'"—Colapinto, 1991, p. 435

The therapist's job is to find a way to help the family achieve desired change, and he/she must do whatever it takes to make this happen. Therefore, therapists' roles can vary widely: they can be the "producer" who ensures conditions that make therapy possible, the "stage director" who pushes the family toward more functional patterns, the "protagonist" who directly uses himself/herself to alter stuck family interactions, or the "narrator" or "coauthor" who collaboratively helps the family revise their script. Thus therapists need to be open to playing whichever role will be most beneficial for a particular family in a given session, rather than being wedded to their own favorite roles.

Recent Adaptation: A Softer Style

In his later work, Minuchin has described a change in approach: "I have moved from being an active challenger—confronting, directing, and controlling—to a softer style, in which I use humor, acceptance, support, suggestion, and seduction on behalf of the same goals" (Minuchin et al., 2007, p. 6). Despite this change, Minuchin has not abandoned the expert role or the goal of achieving change in the present.

The Viewing: Case Conceptualization and Assessment

Structural family therapists conceptualize and assess the following factors:

STRUCTURAL ASSESSMENT

- Role of symptom in the family
- Subsystems
- Cross-generational coalitions
- Boundaries
- Hierarchy
- Complementarity
- Family development
- Strengths

Role of the Symptom

Structural therapists identify three possible relationships between the symptom and the family system (Colapinto, 1991):

1. **Family as Ineffectual Challenger of Symptom:** The family is *passive.* In order to maintain a highly enmeshed or disengaged family structure, it fails to challenge the symptomatic member.

2. **Family as "Shaper" of Individual's Symptoms:** The family structure shapes the individual's experience and behaviors.

3. **Family as "Beneficiary" of the Symptom:** The symptom performs a regulatory function in maintaining the family structure.

As in virtually all forms of family therapy, the *symptom bearer* or *identified patient* (IP) is never seen as the sole source of the problem, and instead the family interaction patterns are targeted for intervention.

Subsystems

Minuchin (1974) conceptualized a family as a single system that also had multiple *subsystems.* Some subsystems can be found in almost every family: couple, parental, sibling, and each individual as a separate subsystem. In addition, in some families other influential subsystems develop along gender lines, hobbies, interests (sports, music), and even personalities (serious versus fun-loving). When assessing a family (see Chapter 2), generally the most important subsystem issues to consider are (a) whether there is a clear distinction between the parental and couple subsystems and (b) whether there is a clear boundary between the parental and child/sibling subsystems. Alternatively stated, is there an effective parental hierarchy?

Cross-Generational Coalitions: Problematic Subsystems

One type of subsystem is particularly damaging: *cross-generational coalitions* (Minuchin & Fishman, 1981; Minuchin & Nichols, 1993). A cross-generational coalition is a subsystem that forms between a parent and child *against* the other parent or other key caretaker. This is a common family dynamic; often a mother has grown closer to her children and has unresolved marital or parenting conflicts with her spouse. The inverse, a father in coalition with the children against the mother, is also frequent, as is a family that divides into "teams," with the father and mother heading their team in overt or covert opposition to the other. These coalitions are especially common in divorces, and in fact, both parents typically try to create these coalitions simultaneously against the other: thus the children become the rope in a tug of war. These coalitions are often *covert*, meaning they are not directly addressed or spoken about in the family but are evident by secrets between the parent and child ("don't tell your mom/dad about this") or comments that compliment the child and disparage the other spouse ("I am so glad you didn't inherit your father's/mother's gene for X"). These coalitions can also involve other caretakers, such as grandparents or parentified children.

Boundary Assessment (see Juice 1)
Hierarchy

When working with reported problems in child behavior, therapists must first assess the parental hierarchy so that they know how to intervene (Colapinto, 1991; Minuchin, 1974; Minuchin & Fishman, 1981). There are three basic forms of parental hierarchy:

- **Effective:** When the parental hierarchy is appropriate and effective, parents can set boundaries and limits while still maintaining emotional connection with their children.

- **Insufficient:** When the parental hierarchy is insufficient, parents are not able to effectively manage the child's behavior and often adapt a permissive parenting style. This style is easy to identify in the therapy office: the parents are not able to keep younger children from tearing up the waiting room and office, or their teens act as though they have the right to set their own curfews and rules. Often the parents hope that the therapist will "teach" their children to listen, but this often requires intervening more with the parents than the children. Generally, these parents have enmeshed boundaries with their children, but not always. As with boundaries, the outward expression of effective versus insufficient can only be determined by examining the cultural context, family life stage of development, and symptomatic behavior.

- **Excessive:** When there is excessive hierarchy, the rules are developmentally too strict and unrealistic and consequences are too severe to be effective. In this situation, there is almost always a rigid boundary between children and parents. These parents need assistance in developing age-appropriate rules and expectations and in developing a stronger emotional bond with their children.

Complementarity

Much like systemic therapists (Chapter 9), structural therapists assess for rigid complementary patterns between family members (Colapinto, 1991). Like a jigsaw puzzle, family members develop complementary roles: the over/underfunctioner, good/bad child, understanding/strict parent, logical/emotional partner, and so forth. Over time, these systemically generated roles become viewed as inherent personality characteristics that seem unchangeable. The more exaggerated and rigid these roles become, the less adaptable the individuals and family become. Structural therapists recognize the mutually reinforced patterns and target the ones that need to change for members to grow.

Family Development

Rather than a static entity, the family is viewed as continually growing and changing in response to predictable stages of development as well as unexpected life events such as death, a move, or divorce (Minuchin & Fishman, 1981). Minuchin and Fishman (1981) identify four major stages in family development:

1. Couple formation
2. Families with young children

3. Families with school-age or adolescent children
4. Families with grown children

At each stage the members need to renegotiate boundaries to define the levels of closeness and differentiation that will support individual members' growth needs. Families often get stuck transitioning from one stage to another if they fail to renegotiate boundaries and hierarchy as the family develops.

Strengths

Minuchin strongly feels that therapists should avoid labeling families as dysfunctional and instead recognize their strengths, particularly their cultural and idiosyncratic strengths (Minuchin & Fishman, 1981; Minuchin & Nichols, 1993). He powerfully argues against seeing the family as an enemy of its individual members, as is frequent in psychological literature, encouraging therapists to recognize how the family provides support, protection, and a foundation for its members. Family strengths, such as a strong connection to extended family or community, are identified and used to promote the goals of individual and family growth as well as to reduce symptoms.

Targeting Change: Goal Setting

"A well-functioning family is not defined by the absence of stress, conflict, and problems, but by how effectively it handles them in the course of fulfilling its function. This, in turn, depends on the structure and adaptability of the family."—Colapinto, 1991, p. 422

Structural therapists target similar goals for all families (Colapinto, 1991; Minuchin, 1974):

- *Clear boundaries* between all subsystems that allow for connectedness and differentiation congruent with the family's cultural contexts.
- Clear distinction between the *marital/couple subsystem* and the *parental subsystem*.
- *Effective parental hierarchy* and the severing of cross-generational coalitions.
- A family structure that promotes the *development and growth of individuals and the family*.

The Doing: Interventions

Enactments and Modifying Interactions (see Juice 2)
Systemic Reframing

As the family begin to describe their problems, therapists reflect on their understanding using *systemic reframing* (Colapinto, 1991; Minuchin, 1974; Minuchin & Fishman, 1981). A systemic reframe takes into account that all behavior has reciprocal antecedents: person A affects person B's response, which then affects person A's response, ad infinitum (A $\leftrightarrows$ B). Reframes often highlight complementary relationships in the family, such as the pursuer/distancer pattern. Reframing usually involves removing the blame from one person (the identified patient) and "spreading" blame equally by describing how each person's response contributes to the problem dynamic. Once this is done, blame becomes a moot point.

Systemic reframing involves piecing together each member's description of the problem and reframing it to reveal the broader systemic dynamic. Thus, if the wife complains that her husband never listens to her, and he complains that she is always nagging him about something, the therapist can systemically reframe their descriptions to highlight how the more she pushes him to listen and interact, the more he withdraws; and the more he withdraws, the more she feels compelled to pursue him for interaction.

HOW TO GENERATE SYSTEMIC REFRAMES

- Assess broader interactional patterns (complementary relationships, hierarchy, boundaries, etc.)
- Redescribe the problem (use interactional patterns to describe the problem in a larger context)

Boundary Making

Boundary making is a special form of enactment that targets over- or underinvolvement to help families soften rigid boundaries or strengthen diffuse boundaries (Colapinto, 1991; Minuchin, 1974). Structural therapists use this technique to direct who participates and how. By actively setting boundaries, therapists interrupt the habitual interaction patterns, allowing members to experience underutilized skills and abilities. Boundary making may involve several different directives:

- Asking family members to change seats
- Asking family members to move seats further or closer together or turn toward one another
- Having separate sessions with individuals or subsystems to strengthen subsystem boundaries
- Asking one or more members to remain silent during an interaction
- Asking questions that highlight a problem boundary area (e.g., "Do you always answer for your son when he is asked a question?")
- Blocking interruptions or encouraging pauses for less dominant persons to speak

Challenging the Family's Worldview

Challenging the family's worldview and unproductive assumptions typically involves verbally questioning operational assumptions in the family system, whether overtly spoken or covertly acted upon (Colapinto, 1991; Minuchin, 1974; Minuchin & Fishman, 1981). Common assumptions that create problems for individuals, couples, and families include the following:

- "Kids' needs come first."
- "It's better to keep the peace than start conflict."
- "It is easier to sacrifice my needs than ask for what I want."
- "If I give here, you should give there."
- "It's better for the kids for us to stay in this unhappy marriage."

Structural therapists often challenge these assumptions by overtly questioning whether they are actually having the effect family members anticipate. The challenge can be delivered softly or strongly, depending on what will be most effective in the particular family structure.

Intensity and Crisis Inductions

Intensity and crisis inductions are interventions that use affect to create structural shifts in hierarchy and boundaries, especially when the family is having trouble "hearing" the therapist with other interventions (Minuchin, 1974; Minuchin & Fishman, 1981; Minuchin & Nichols, 1993). Because families differ in the degree of loyalty they demand to their reality, they need different levels and styles of intensity, depending on the issue being discussed. Intensity involves turning up the emotional heat by using tone of voice, pacing, and word choice to break through rigid and stuck interactional patterns. For example, a therapist may say to a couple who claims to have no time for a weekly date because of their children's numerous after-school activities, "Do you think your children would prefer to be in soccer and have divorced parents or to have fewer activities and an intact family?"

Closely related to intensity, *crisis induction* in structural therapy is used with families who chronically avoid a conflict or problem (Colapinto, 1991). For example, in families with anorectic children, the therapist may bring the symptom into the room by staging a meal and having the family deal with it. Similarly, with alcohol or substance abuse issues, the therapist often induces a crisis so that the family will acknowledge and finally address the problem. The therapist can then help the family develop new interactions and patterns.

Unbalancing

Unbalancing is used for more extreme difficulties in hierarchy or when the identified patient is being scapegoated. This intervention is used to realign boundaries between subsystems (Minuchin, 1974; Minuchin & Fishman, 1981). Therapists use their expert position to temporarily "join sides" with individuals who are being scapegoated or with subsystems that need to develop stronger boundaries by arguing their cause or helping to explain their perspective to others. At first glance, this may seem to go against the general rule of neutrality that characterizes structural therapy specifically and psychotherapy more generally. However, unbalancing is done only briefly and with specific realignment goals in mind, generally only after more direct interventions, such as enactments and challenging assumptions, have failed.

Expanding Family Truths and Realities

Each family develops a unique worldview that defines its realities and truths. When working with a highly rigid family structure, structural therapists directly challenge these beliefs and realities (already discussed under Challenging the Family's Worldview; Minuchin & Fishman, 1981). However, whenever possible, structural therapists cite these beliefs to *expand* the family's functioning in new directions. For example, they might say, "Because you obviously have such deep concern for your child, you are parents who are likely to understand that the child needs space to grow in order to really flourish" or "Since you are willing to go to such lengths to be helpful, it seems you are probably able to be helpful in an even more challenging way: allowing him to make his own mistakes." Rather than introduce an entirely foreign concept, the structural therapist takes the family's fundamental premise that has been supporting the problem and redirects its logic to support an alternative set of behaviors and interactions, allowing the family to maintain its core beliefs but use them in new ways.

Making Compliments and Shaping Competence

Minuchin and Fishman (1981) strongly caution therapists that professional training creates a "search and destroy" (diagnose and treat) approach to psychopathology that often blinds therapists to family strengths and positive interaction patterns. Instead, therapists should augment and reinforce the family's natural positive patterns and strengths. *Compliments* are used to bolster behaviors that support families in moving toward their goals, and *shaping competence* involves noticing small successes along the way to reaching goals. For example, families usually improve after enactments and refrain from interrupting or speaking for each other in later sessions. Therapists can shape competence by noticing these changes in session or as they are reported from week to week.

Shaping competence also involves refusing to function for the family in session. For example, rather than taking responsibility for having children focus and behave during a session, the therapist asks the parents to do so. If a child is kicking the furniture or gets up to play with a toy during a family session, rather than correct the child, the therapist asks the parents to have the child stop. Similarly, if the therapist is trying to strengthen the parental hierarchy, the therapist asks the parents to answer questions first and recognizes their authority by directing children to ask parents for permission to do such things as go to the bathroom or get some water. In the case study at the end of this chapter, the therapist uses shaping competence with a teen to increase his motivation to pursue his life goals rather than relying entirely on increased parental hierarchy to reduce his fighting at school and improve his grades.

Snapshot: Research and the Evidence Base

Quick Summary: Structural therapy has good research support, especially for newer treatments. Although no manual has been created to make structural family therapy an empirically supported treatment, the components of structural therapy have been used in many empirically supported treatments, especially those targeting youth:

- **Brief Strategic Family Therapy** (and two related models: structural ecosystemic therapy and structural ecodevelopmental preventive interventions; Szapocznik & Williams, 2000)

- **Ecosystemic Structural Family Therapy** (Lindblad-Goldberg, Dore, & Stern, 1998)

- **Multisystemic Family Therapy** (Henggeler, Schoenwald, Borduin, Rowland, & Cunningham, 1998)

- **Multidimensional Family Therapy** (Liddle, 2002)

These empirically supported treatments generally target adolescents from diverse families and integrate structural therapy components to assess and restructure the family.

Clinical Spotlight: Brief Strategic Family Therapy

Drawing on structural and strategic therapies, Jose Szapocznik and his colleagues at the Center for Family Studies developed brief strategic family therapy (BSFT) to address drug abuse problems with Cuban youth in Miami (Szapocznik & Williams, 2000). Expanded and adopted to treat African-Americans and other Hispanic populations, this therapy is recognized as an evidence-based approach; a complete manual is available through the National Institute for Drug Abuse website (www.nida.nih.gov/TXManuals/bsft; Szapocznick, Hervis, & Schwartz, 2003). BSFT is based on three central concepts: *systems, structure* (patterns of interaction), and *strategy*.

Goals

Brief strategic family therapy has two goals:

- Reduce or eliminate child drug use
- Change family interactions that are supporting the problem behaviors (youth drug use)

Case Conceptualization

In comparison with other evidence-based approaches, BSFT focuses primarily *within* family dynamics using structural and strategic family therapy concepts (Stantisteban, Suarz-Morales, Robbins, & Szapocznik, 2006; Szapocznik et al., 2003):

- **Structure and Organization:** The therapist uses traditional structural concepts such as subsystems, hierarchy, leadership, and coalitions to assess the structure, organization, and flow of information in the family.

- **Resonance:** Using the structural therapy concepts of boundaries, the therapist assesses emotional resonance within the broader context of cultural norms: enmeshed (high resonance) and disengaged (low resonance).

- **Developmental Stage:** The therapist uses the family's ability to adapt its structure to support members in their current life stage of development (e.g., increasing autonomy as children grow).

- **Life Context:** The therapist assesses the effects of the family's broader social life, such as extended family, community, school, peers, and courts.

- **Identified Patienthood:** The more the family believes the identified patient is to blame for all its problems, the more difficult it is to treat the family.

- **Conflict Resolution:** The therapist assesses the family's style of conflict resolution:
    - **Denial:** Conflict is not allowed to emerge: "We have no problems."
    - **Avoidance:** When conflict arises, it is quickly stopped or covered up, such as by procrastinating, minimizing, or postponing difficult conversations.
    - **Diffusion:** When the problem is brought up, the subject is switched to another problem topic, often as a personal attack against the person who raised the issue.
    - **Conflict Emergence Without Resolution:** Conflict occurs but no resolution is reached.
    - **Conflict Emergence with Resolution:** The family is able to resolve the conflict.

Principles of Intervention

Interventions are deliberately chosen to target the aspects of family interactions that are most likely to achieve the desired outcome.

- **Joining:** The therapist uses structural family therapy, joining, to connect with the family system.

- **Enactments:** Structural enactments are used to assess family functioning and restructure family interactions.

- **Working in the Present:** Interventions target current interactions with minimal focus on the past.

- **Reframing Negativity:** Therapists reframe negative interpretations to promote caring and concern within the family.

- **Reversals:** Therapists may coach one or more family members to do or say the *opposite* of what is typically done or said.

- **Working with Boundaries and Alliances:** Standard structural techniques are used to either loosen or strengthen boundaries to better meet developmental needs.

- **Detriangulation:** The therapist may remove a third, less powerful person from a conflict between two others.

- **Opening Closed Systems:** Systems in which open conflict is not allowed must be "opened" to allow effective expression and resolution of differences.

Clinical Spotlight: Ecosystemic Structural Family Therapy

Ecosystemic structural family therapy (ESFT), an empirically supported adaptation of structural family therapy (Minuchin, 1974), was developed by Marion Lindblad-Goldberg and her colleagues at the Philadelphia Child and Family Training

Center (formerly the Philadelphia Child Guidance Clinic) to treat children and adolescents with severe emotional or behavioral problems and their families within the context of their communities (Lindblad-Goldberg, Dore, & Stern, 1998). ESFT has addressed a wide range of child and adolescent clinical problems across all levels of severity and in diverse treatment settings. In the in-home or community setting, ESFT targets youth who are either at risk of out-of-home placement or who have already spent time in inpatient or residential settings. The families of these youth tend to be compromised by trauma-induced parental substance abuse, conflictual relationships, emotional disturbance, and the absence of emotional or concrete support.

Case Conceptualization

ESFT is a bio/developmental/systemic trauma-informed clinical model that examines the biological and developmental influences of family members as well as current and historical familial, cultural, and ecological influences. It is based on the fundamental assumption that both child and parental functioning are inextricably linked to their relational environment.

ESFT therapists are guided by five interrelated constructs:

- Family structure
- Family emotion regulation,
- Individual differences (historical, biological, cultural, developmental)
- Affective proximity (emotional attachment between parent and child and between parents)
- Family development

Goals

The primary targets of therapeutic change are the following:

- Parental executive functioning
- Child coping skills
- Co-parent alliances
- Nonadaptive emotional attachment patterns
- Emotional regulation
- Extrafamilial supports to family members

Interventions

The necessary agents of change in ESFT are (a) the family members in partnership with the therapist and (b) the family-therapist entity in partnership with extrafamilial helpers. ESFT incorporates techniques from many different models of psychotherapy to create relational change. It is the relational objective that determines an intervention's appropriateness. Structural techniques that are used to reorganize or restructure the way family members relate to one another include boundary making and rebalancing power or clarifying hierarchy. Like the structural family therapy model, ESFT emphasizes building strong therapeutic alliances with all family members. The most common structural interventions used in ESFT are behavioral enactments and validation of family members' strengths. The most common ESFT intervention is *enactment* to help family members practice new ways of relating: adjust the necessary emotional proximity between family members, learn to regulate emotions, and learn to tolerate distress. Other commonly used techniques address thinking, beliefs, or knowledge in the family; these techniques include reframing, constructing adaptive narratives, psychoeducation, and the use of rituals.

Snapshot: Working with Diverse Populations

"Every family has elements in their own culture, which if understood and utilized, can become levers to actualize and expand the family members' behavioral repertory. Unfortunately, we therapists have not assimilated this axiom. Though we pay lip service to the strengths of the family, and talk about the matrix of development and healing, we are trained as psychological sleuths. Our instincts are to 'search and destroy': pinpoint the psychological disorder, label it, and eradicate it."—Minuchin & Fishman, 1981, pp. 262–263

Minuchin and his colleagues developed the structural family therapy model to work with poor, ethnically diverse, urban families because they did not find that traditional insight-oriented approaches were effective with this population (Colapinto, 1991; Minuchin et al., 1967). From its inception, structural family therapy has attended to the dynamics and needs of diverse families, especially those with children who are having difficulties. Because Minuchin and many of the proponents of structural family therapy were themselves from diverse and immigrant backgrounds, they were aware of the strengths of diverse families. Structural family therapy employs an active, engaged approach in which the therapist often takes an expert stance in relation to the family, an approach that often fits with the values of traditional cultures.

Various types of diversity have been studied. Research on gay and lesbian families indicates that their basic structure and dynamics are similar to (not statistically different from) those of heterosexual couples (Gottman, 2008), and therefore the same restructuring techniques may be appropriate. Harry Aponte (1994, 1996) has focused on issues of spirituality, race, and poverty related to structural family work. The case example that follows this chapter demonstrates how structural therapy can be used for working with an Irish-Italian immigrant family whose eldest son is fighting with peers and failing high school.

ONLINE RESOURCES

Philadelphia Child and Family Therapy Training Center

www.philafamily.com

Brief Strategic Family Therapy Manual

www.nida.nih.gov/TXManuals/bsft

Brief Strategic Family Therapy Training

www.brief-strategic-family-therapy.com

REFERENCES

*Asterisk indicates recommended introductory readings.

Aponte, H. J. (1994). *Bread and spirit: Therapy with the new poor: Diversity of race, culture, and values.* New York: Norton.

Aponte, H. J. (1996). Political bias, moral values, and spirituality in the training of psychotherapists. *Bulletin of the Menninger Clinic, 60*(4), 488–502.

*Colapinto, J. (1991). Structural family therapy. In A. S. Gurman & D. P. Kniskern (Eds.), *Handbook of family therapy* (Vol. 2, pp. 417–443). New York: Brunner/Mazel.

Gottman, J. M. (2008, April). *Marriage counseling: Keynote address.* Annual Conference of the American Counseling Association, Honolulu, HI.

Henggeler, S. W., Schoenwald, S. K., Borduin, C. M., Rowland, M. D., & Cunningham, P. B. (1998). *Multisystemic treatment of antisocial behavior in children and adolescents.* New York: Guilford.

Liddle, H. A. (2002). *Multidimensional family therapy treatment for adolescent cannibis users.* Rockville, MD: Substance Abuse and Mental Health Services Administration.

Lindblad-Goldberg, M., Dore, M., & Stern, L. (1998). *Creating competence from chaos.* New York: Norton.

Minuchin, S. (1974). *Families and family therapy.* Cambridge, MA: Harvard University Press.

*Minuchin, S., & Fishman, H. C. (1981). *Family therapy techniques.* Cambridge, MA: Harvard University Press.

Minuchin, S., Montalvo, B., Guerney, B. G., Rosman, B., & Schumer, F. (1967). *Families of the slums.* New York: Basic Books.

Minuchin, S., & Nichols, M. P. (1993). *Family healing: Tales of hope and renewal from family therapy.* New York: Free Press.

Minuchin, S., Nichols, M. P., & Lee, W. Y. (2007). *Assessing families and couples: From symptom to system.* New York: Allyn & Bacon.

Minuchin, S., Rosman, B., & Baker, L. (1978). *Psychosomatic families: Anorexia in context.* Cambridge, MA: Harvard University Press.

Stantisteban, D. A., Suarz-Morales, L., Robbins, M. S., & Szapocznik, J. (2006). Brief Strategic Family Therapy: Lessons learned in efficacy research and challenges to blending research and practice. *Family Process, 45,* 259–271.

Szapocznik, J., Hervis, O. E., & Schwartz, S. (2003). *Brief strategic family therapy for adolescent drug abuse* (NIH Publication No. 03-4751). NIDA Therapy Manuals for Drug Addiction. Rockville, MD: National Institute for Drug Abuse.

Szapocznik, J., & Williams, R. A. (2000). Brief Strategic Family Therapy: Twenty-five years of interplay among theory, research and practice in adolescent behavior problems and drug abuse. *Clinical Child and Family Psychology Review, 3*(2), 117–134.

STRUCTURAL CASE STUDY

Bill and Sally bring their son, Tom, in for therapy after he was suspended a second time for getting into a fight at school. Six months ago the family moved across town when Bill was transferred, just before Tom was about to start high school. An above-average student in middle school, Tom is now in danger of failing the ninth grade. Bill and Sally have been arguing more since the move, with Bill working longer hours at the new job, leaving Sally to handle the kids. John, Tom's younger brother, is reportedly doing well with the move and tries to stay out of the conflict.

After meeting with the family, a structural family therapist developed the following case conceptualization.

Shaded Sections Emphasized in Structural Planning and Intervention

CASE CONCEPTUALIZATION FORM

Therapist: Albert Luis, MFT Trainee   **Client/Case #:** 9002   **Date:** 4/28/08

I. Introduction to Client and Significant Others *(Include age, ethnicity, occupation, grade, relevant identifiers, etc.). Put an * next to persons in session and/or IP for identified patient.*

*AF†:   40, Irish-American, pediatric nurse

*AM: 44, Italian-American (second-generation), bank executive

*CM: 14 (IP) 9th grade, Alexander High School, track team

*CM: 12 7th grade, Barton Middle School, jazz band

II. Presenting Concern

Client's/Family's Descriptions of Problem(s):

AF: States that AM is too harsh on CM14 and that CM14 is just adjusting to HS.

AM: States that AF is too lenient on CM14 and that CM14 is not learning responsibility and is on the road to becoming a failure.

CF14:   States that he is adjusting to HS and move; trying make friends at a new school and learning how to study.

CM12:   States that his brother and father fight more recently; believes CM14 is rebelling like all teenagers do.

Broader System Problem Descriptions (description of problem from referring party, teachers, relatives, legal system, etc.):

School counselor: States that she believes CM14 is not living up to his potential; has "defiance" issues; difficulty fitting in at school.

III. Background Information

Recent Background (recent life changes, precipitating events, first symptoms, stressors, etc.):

After performing above average in middle school, CM14 began high school six months ago after family moved across town due to AM's job transfer. He was suspended two weeks ago due to fist fight with peer (second incident); he is currently in danger of failing two classes. CM14 reports being motivated to keep his grades up to stay on the track team. He reports experimenting with drinking and pot in the past year. AF and AM have been arguing more since the move, and CM14 has been having problems in school. CM12 is reported doing well. AM has been working longer hours with the new job, and AF reports he is not helping out like he did before.

---

† *Abbreviations:* AF: Adult Female; AM: Adult Male; CF#: Child Female with age, e.g., CF12: CM#: Child Male with age; Hx: History; Ex: Explanation or Example; NA: Not Applicable.

(continued)

III. Background Information *(continued)*

Related Historical Background (family history, related issues, past abuse, trauma, previous counseling, medical/mental health history, etc.):

Report "normal" family before now: summer vacations, sports and music activities; nightly dinners. AM says he went through a "rebellious" period when he was a teen but he never let his grades drop or get suspended. There is a history of alcohol abuse on both sides of the family. Deny history of child abuse or domestic violence. No reported health concerns.

IV. Systemic Assessment

Client/Relational Strengths

Personal/individual: CM14 is motivated to get his grades up to stay on track team; he and CM12 have made new friends in the neighborhood; AM doing well in promotion; both parents motivated to improve situation at home.

Relational/social: CM14 has supportive counselor and good relationship with two teachers; CM14 is close with one uncle, who serves as mentor; has made some friends at new school.

Spiritual: AM and AF are Catholic and use their spiritual tradition to keep them connected; semi-active in local church.

Family Structure and Interaction Patterns

Couple Subsystem (to be assessed): ☒ Personal current ☐ Personal past ☐ Parents'

Couple Boundaries: ☐ Clear ☒ Enmeshed ☐ Disengaged ☐ Other: _____

Rules for closeness/distance: AM and AF expect the other to share opinion and emotional reactions; feel rejected when the other person sees things differently.

Couple Problem Interaction Pattern (A ⇆ B):

Start of tension: CM14 has an incident at school or home (talks back, poor grade, etc.).

Conflict/symptom escalation: AM yells at CM: AF tries to calm down the situation; when AM continues, AF tells him to "lay off" CM; AM feels unsupported and gets angry with AF, yelling at her in front of CM; afterwards, AM generally leaves the room; they go to bed angry.

Return to "normal"/homeostasis: In the morning, they are "cool" but by afternoon "warm up" without ever talking about or resolving the problem most of the time.

Couple Complementary Patterns: ☐ Pursuer/distancer ☐ Over/under functioner

☐ Emotional/logical ☒ Good/bad parent ☐ Other: _____ .

Ex: AF tends to take the side of CM14 and AM is the disciplinarian. The pattern was evident but not

as extreme when the kids were younger.

Satir Communication Stances:

AF: ☐ Congruent ☒ Placator ☐ Blamer ☐ Superreasonable ☐ Irrelevant

AM: ☐ Congruent ☐ Placator ☒ Blamer ☐ Superreasonable ☐ Irrelevant

Describe dynamic: AF tries to be the peacemaker in the family, often neglecting her own needs. AM

more direct with asserting his needs.

Gottman's Divorce Indicators:

Criticism: ☒ AF ☒ AM. Ex: Both quick to criticize the other's parenting and decisions.

Defensiveness: ☒ AF ☒ AM. Ex: Both respond to the other's criticism defensively.

Contempt: ☐ AF ☐ AM. Ex: NA

Stonewalling: ☐ AF ☐ AM. Ex: NA

Failed repair attempts: ☐ AF ☒ AM. Ex: _____

Not accept influence: ☐ AF ☐ AM. Ex: NA

Harsh startup: ☒ AF ☒ AM. Ex: Both begin with harsh startup.

Parental Subsystem: ☒ Family of procreation ☐ Family of origin

Membership in Family Subsystems: Parental: ☒ AF ☒ AM. ☐ Other: _____

Is parental subsystem distinct from couple subsystem? ☐ Yes ☒ No ☐ NA (divorce)

Sibling subsystem: CM14 and CM12; get along well.

Special interest: AF and CM14 are both active athletes.

Family Life Cycle Stage:

☐ Single adult ☐ Marriage ☐ Family with young children

☒ Family with adolescent children ☐ Launching children ☐ Later life

Describe struggles with mastering developmental tasks in one of these stages: Family having

difficulty adjusting to CM14 adjusting to high school; difficulty helping CM14 take on more freedom

and responsibility.

Hierarchy Between Child/Parents:

AF: ☐ Effective ☒ Insufficient (permissive) ☐ Excessive (authoritarian) ☒ Inconsistent

AM: ☐ Effective ☐ Insufficient (permissive) ☒ Excessive (authoritarian) ☐ Inconsistent

Ex: AF inconsistent and lenient; AM too harsh in response.

IV. Systemic Assessment *(continued)*

Emotional Boundaries with Children:

AF: ☐ Clear/balanced ☒ Enmeshed (reactive) ☐ Disengaged (disinterested)

☐ Other: _____

AM: ☐ Clear/balanced ☒ Enmeshed (reactive) ☐ Disengaged (disinterested)

☐ Other: _____

Ex: Both parents have enmeshed boundaries with children, AM becoming overly angry when son does not live up to his expectations, and AF responding by wanting to shield and protect him for the consequences of his choices.

Problem Interaction Pattern (A ⇆ B):

Start of tension: CM14 refuses to do chore.

Conflict/symptom escalation: AM gets angry and lectures about responsibility; AF volunteers to "fix things"; AM sends CM14 to room; AF does chore for CM14; CM12 goes to room to play video game.

Return to "normal"/homeostasis: Once dad calms down, AF talks to him into letting CM14 out of room, usually without consequences.

Triangles/Coalitions:

☒ AF and CM14 against AM: Ex: AF takes CM's side in most arguments.

☐ AM and C _____ against AF: Ex: _____

☐ Other: Ex: _____

Communication Stances:

AF or _____ : ☐ Congruent ☒ Placator ☐ Blamer ☐ Superreasonable ☐ Irrelevant

AM or _____ : ☐ Congruent ☐ Placator ☒ Blamer ☐ Superreasonable ☐ Irrelevant

CM14 _____ : ☐ Congruent ☐ Placator ☒ Blamer ☐ Superreasonable ☐ Irrelevant

CM12 or _____ : ☐ Congruent ☒ Placator ☐ Blamer ☐ Superreasonable ☐ Irrelevant

Ex: _____

Hypothesis (Describe possible role or function of symptom in maintaining family homeostasis):

CM14's behavior gives his mother a child to parent and protect and provides a sense of closeness for her, filling the gap of the long hours her husband is at work. Additionally, AM and AF have not adjusted their parenting to CM14's developmental needs by increasing his responsibility and freedom based on his ability.

Intergenerational Patterns

Substance/alcohol abuse: ☐ NA ☒ Hx: Both sides of the family have hx of alcohol and or substance abuse. Report no current abuse in family.

Sexual/physical/emotional abuse: ☒ NA ☐ Hx:

Parent/child relations: ☐ NA ☐ Hx: AM rebellious toward his father; conflict between AM father and oldest brother who is in same sex relationship.

Physical/mental disorders: ☒ NA ☐ Hx:

Historical incidents of presenting problem: ☐ NA ☒ Hx: Repeating pattern in father's family and variation of pattern in mother's family.

Family strengths: Strong connection with both sides of the extended family.

Previous Solutions and Unique Outcomes

Solutions that DIDN'T work: AM using harsher punishments; AF "giving him another chance".

Solutions that DID work: CM14 began studying more after the school counselor told him he would not be allowed to continue on track team unless grades improved.

Narratives, Dominant Discourses, and Diversity
Dominant Discourses informing definition of problem:

Cultural, ethnic, SES, etc.: Italian and Irish immigrant traditions of strong, connected families; always there for each other when it really matters; AM has continued his father's tradition of being the "responsible" man and worries his son is not headed in the right direction.

Gender, sex orientation, etc.: Strong themes related to what it means to be a "man," esp for AM. CM14 generally agrees with dad's ideals but not how he expects these to be lived out by a teenager.

Other social influences: CM14 attending HS in wealthier neighborhood and feels a lot of pressure to be accepted by his peers.

Identity Narratives that have developed around problem for AF, AM, and/or CM/F: CM14 is beginning to develop a reputation as a "problem" kid, esp in the eyes of his father. CM12 is increasingly the "good" kid, distinctions the family never had before. AM is aware he is becoming the mean parent; he dislikes label but feels he has to make his son a real man.

Local or Preferred Discourses: When questioned, CM14 believes that he is just going through a "phase" and that he will get his grades up and stay out of trouble. He is worried about where he will fall in the school's social hierarchy, which has been influencing his decisions about substance use, fights, etc.

Other Influential Discourses: AF and AM are also struggling with how to balance their value of family with their desire to "get ahead" financially; CM14 experiencing parallel struggle trying to fit in with the "rich kids."

(continued)

V. Genogram *(continued)*

Construct a family genogram and include all relevant information, including:

- ages, birth/death dates
- names
- relational patterns
- occupations
- medical history
- psychiatric disorders
- abuse history

Also include a couple of adjectives for persons frequently discussed in session (these should describe personal qualities and/or relational patterns, e.g., quiet, family caretaker, emotionally distant, perfectionist, helpless, etc.). Genogram should be attached to report.

VI. Client Perspectives

Areas of Agreement: Based on what the client(s) has(ve) said, what parts of the above assessment do they agree with or are likely to agree with?

Family members agree with descriptions of "sides" that have been taken and each parent's role.

Areas of Disagreement: What parts do they disagree with or are likely to disagree with? Why?

AF and AM define the issues of lenient and strict very differently; both believe they are right on the issue. AM is less concerned about couple issues.

How do you plan to respectfully work with areas of disagreement?

Avoid taking sides or defining what "proper" parents would do and instead work with parents to identify what strategies work with CM14, working toward an effective system of clear limits and consequences that are equally enforced by both parents. Begin working on parenting before introducing couples as an area of treatment.

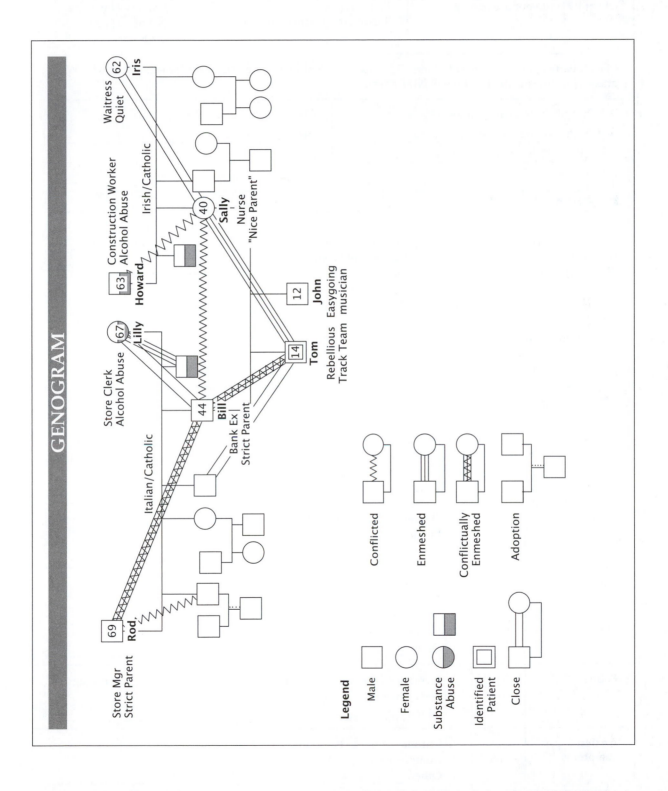

CLINICAL ASSESSMENT

Client ID #: (do not use name): 9002	Ethnicity(ies): Italian-American, Irish-American	Primary Language: ☒ Eng ☐ Span ☐ Other: _____

List all Participants/Significant others: Put a [★] for Identified Patient (IP); [✔] for sig. others who **WILL** attend; [✕] for sig. others who will *NOT* attend.

Adult: Age: Profession/Employer	Child: Age: School/Grade
[✔] AM†: 44 Italian-American; bank executive	[★] CM: 14 9th grade; track team
[✔] AF: 42 Irish-American; pediatric nurse	[ ] CF:
[ ] AF/M #2: _____	[✔] CM: 12 7th grade; jazz band

Presenting Problems

		Complete for children
☐ Depression/hopelessness	☐ Couple concern	☒ School failure/decline performance
☐ Anxiety/worry	☒ Parent/child conflict	
☒ Anger issues	☐ Partner violence/abuse	☐ Truancy/runaway
☐ Loss/grief	☐ Divorce adjustment	☒ Fighting w/peers
☐ Suicidal thoughts/attempts	☐ Remarriage adjustment	☐ Hyperactivity
☐ Sexual abuse/rape	☐ Sexuality/intimacy concerns	☐ Wetting/soiling clothing
☒ Alcohol/drug use	☒ Major life changes	☐ Child abuse/neglect
☐ Eating problems/disorders	☐ Legal issues/probation	☐ Isolation/withdrawal
☐ Job problems/unemployed	☐ Other: _____	☐ Other: _____

Mental Status for IP

Interpersonal issues	☐ NA	☒ Conflict ☒ Enmeshment ☐ Isolation/avoidance ☐ Emotional disengagement ☐ Poor social skills ☐ Couple problems ☐ Prob w/friends ☐ Prob at work ☐ Overly shy ☐ Egocentricity ☐ Diff establish/maintain relationship ☐ Other: _____
Mood	☐ NA	☐ Depressed/sad ☐ Hopeless ☐ Fearful ☐ Anxious ☒ Angry ☒ Irritable ☐ Manic ☐ Other: _____
Affect	☐ NA	☒ Constricted ☐ Blunt ☐ Flat ☐ Labile ☐ Dramatic ☐ Other: _____
Sleep	☐ NA	☐ Hypersomnia ☐ Insomnia ☒ Disrupted ☐ Nightmares ☐ Other: _____
Eating	☒ NA	☐ Increase ☐ Decrease ☐ Anorectic restriction ☐ Bingeing ☐ Purging ☐ Body image ☐ Other: _____
Anxiety symptoms	☒ NA	☐ Chronic worry ☐ Panic attacks ☐ Dissociation ☐ Phobias ☐ Obsessions ☐ Compulsions ☐ Other: _____

† *Abbreviations:* AF: Adult Female; AM: Adult Male; CF#: Child Female with age, e.g., CF12; CM#: Child Male with age; Hx: History; Cl: Client.

Trauma symptoms	☒ NA	☐ Acute ☐ Chronic ☐ Hypervigilance ☐ Dreams/nightmares ☐ Dissociation ☐ Emotional numbness ☐ Other: _____
Psychotic symptoms	☒ NA	☐ Hallucinations ☐ Delusions ☐ Paranoia ☐ Loose associations ☐ Other: _____
Motor activity/ speech	☐ NA	☐ Low energy ☒ Restless/Hyperactive ☐ Agitated ☐ Inattentive ☐ Impulsive ☐ Pressured speech ☐ Slow speech ☐ Other: _____
Thought	☐ NA	☒ Poor concentration/attention ☐ Denial ☐ Self-blame ☒ Other-blame ☐ Ruminative ☐ Tangential ☐ Illogical ☒ Concrete ☐ Poor insight ☒ Impaired decision making ☐ Disoriented ☐ Slow processing ☐ Other: _____
Socio-Legal	☐ NA	☐ Disregards rules ☒ Defiant ☐ Stealing ☐ Lying ☐ Tantrums ☐ Arrest/incarceration ☒ Initiates fights ☐ Other: _____
Other symptoms	☒ NA	

Diagnosis for IP

Contextual Factors considered in making Dx: ☒ Age ☒ Gender ☒ Family dynamics ☒ Culture ☐ Language ☐ Religion ☐ Economic ☐ Immigration ☐ Sexual orientation ☐ Trauma ☐ Dual dx/comorbid ☒ Addiction ☐ Cognitive ability ☐ Other: _____

Describe impact of identified factors: Father has specific expectations for sons based on his cultural background and gender roles; norms of teen behavior considered; substance use identified as potential problem and monitor.

Axis I
Primary: 309.3 Adjustment Disorder w Disturb of Conduct, Acute

Secondary: V61.20 Parent-Child relational problem; Rule Out Mood Disorder; Oppositional Disorder; Substance Abuse

Axis II: V71.09

Axis III: None Reported

Axis IV:

☒ Problems with primary support group: Parents
☒ Problems related to social environment/school: Move; new school
☒ Educational problems: New school
☐ Occupational problems
☐ Housing problems
☐ Economic problems
☐ Problems with accessing health care services
☐ Problems related to interactions with the legal system
☐ Other psychosocial problems

Axis V: GAF 62 GARF 60

List DSM symptoms for Axis I Dx (include frequency and duration for each). Client meets 5 of 5 criteria for Axis I Primary Dx.

1. Stressor: Move to new neighborhood/school; start HS

2. Significant drop in grades

3. Two physical fights at school

4. Increased defiance at home, esp with AM

5. Began experimenting with alcohol and pot use (1–2 times per week)

6. _____

(continued)

Diagnosis for IP *(continued)*

Have medical causes been ruled out?
☐ Yes ☐ No ☒ In process
**Has patient been referred for psychiatric/
medical eval?** ☐ Yes ☒ No
Has patient agreed with referral?
☐ Yes ☐ No ☒ NA
List psychometric instruments or consults used
for assessment:
☐ None or Youth Outcome Questionnaire

**Medications (psychiatric & medical)
Dose /Start Date**
☒ None prescribed
1. _____/_____ mg; _____
2. _____/_____ mg; _____
3. _____/_____ mg; _____

Client response to diagnosis:
☒ Agree; ☐ Somewhat agree ☐ Disagree;
☐ Not informed for following reason:
_____

Medical Necessity: *(Check all that apply):* ☒ Significant impairment ☐ Probability of significant impairment
☒ Probable developmental arrest
Areas of impairment: ☒ Daily activities ☒ Social relationships ☒ Health ☒ Work/school
☐ Living arrangement ☐ Other: _____

Risk Assessment

Suicidality:
☒ No indication
☐ Denies
☐ Active ideation
☐ Passive ideation
☐ Intent without plan
☐ Intent with means
☐ Ideation past yr
☐ Attempt past yr
☐ Family/peer hx of completed suicide

Homicidality:
☐ No indication
☒ Denies
☐ Active ideation
☐ Passive ideation
☐ Intent w/o means
☐ Intent with means
☐ Ideation past yr
☒ Violence past yr
☒ Hx assault/temper
☐ Cruelty to animals

Hx Substance:
Alc abuse:
☐ No indication
☐ Denies
☐ Past
☒ Current
Freq/Amt: drunk 1-2xs mo

Drug:
☐ No indication
☐ Denies
☐ Past
☒ Current
Drugs: Marijuana
Freq/Amt: 1-2x/mo
☒ Family/sig.other abuses

Sexual & Physical Abuse and Other Risk Factors:
☐ Current child w abuse hx:
   ☐ Sexual ☐ Physical ☐ Emotional ☐ Neglect
☐ Adult w childhood abuse:
   ☐ Sexual ☐ Physical ☐ Emotional ☐ Neglect
☐ Adult w abuse/assault in adulthood:
   ☐ Sexual ☐ Physical ☐ Current
☐ History of perpetrating abuse:
   ☐ Sexual ☐ Physical
☐ Elder/dependent adult abuse/neglect
☐ Anorexia/bulimia/other eating disorder
☐ Cutting or other self-harm:
   ☐ Current
   ☐ Past; Method: _____
   ☐ Criminal/legal hx: _____
☒ None reported

Indicators of Safety: ☒ At least one outside person who provides strong support ☒ Able to cite specific reasons to live, not harm self/other ☐ Hopeful ☒ Has future goals ☐ Willing to dispose of dangerous items ☐ Willingness to reduce contact with people who make situation worse ☐ Willing to implement safety plan, safety interventions ☒ Developing set of alternatives to self/other harm ☐ Sustained period of safety: _____ ☐ Other: _____

Safety Plan includes: ☒ Verbal no harm contract ☐ Written no harm contract ☒ Emergency contact card ☒ Emergency therapist/agency number ☐ Medication management ☒ Specific plan for contacting friends/support persons during crisis ☐ Specific plan of where to go during crisis ☐ Specific self-calming tasks to reduce risk before reach crisis level (e.g., journaling, exercising, etc.) ☐ Specific daily/weekly activities to reduce stressors ☐ Other: _____

Notes: Legal/Ethical Action Taken: ☒ NA _____

Case Management

Date
1st visit: 4/28/08 _____
Last visit: 5/15/08 _____
Session Freq:
☒ Once week ☐ Every other week ☐ Other: _____
Expected Length of Treatment:
_____

Modalities:
☐ Individual adult
☒ Individual child
☒ Couple
☒ Family
☒ Group:
Teen _____

Is client involved in mental health or other medical treatment elsewhere?
☒ No
☐ Yes: _____

If Child/Adolescent: Is family involved?
☒ Yes ☐ No

Patient Referrals and Professional Contacts
Has contact been made with social worker?
☒ Yes ☐ No: explain: school counselor _____ ☐ N/A

Has client been referred for medical assessment?
☒ Yes ☐ No evidence for need

Has client been referred for psychiatric assessment?
☐ Yes; cl agree ☐ Yes, cl disagree ☒ Not nec.

Has contact been made with treating physicians or other professionals?
☒ Yes ☐ No ☐ NA

Has client been referred for social services?
☐ Job/training ☐ Welfare/Food/Housing ☐ Victim services
☐ Legal aid ☐ Medical ☒ Other: teen group at school _____ ☐ N/A

Anticipated forensic/legal processes related to treatment:
☒ No ☐ Yes: _____

Has client been referred for group or other support services?
☒ Yes ☐ No ☐ None recommended

Client social support network includes:
☒ Supportive family ☐ Supportive partner ☐ Friends ☒ Religious/spiritual organization ☐ Supportive work/social group ☐ Other: _____

Anticipated effects treatment will have on others in support system: (parents, children, siblings, sig. others, etc.):
Parents involved in treatment; adjust parenting; CM12 also attend. _____

Is there anything else client will need to be successful?
Parents may need to address couple issues. _____

(continued)

Case Management *(continued)*

Client Sense of Hope: Little 1----------5X----------10 High

Expected Outcome and Prognosis:
☒ Return to normal functioning
☐ Expect improvement, anticipate less than normal functioning
☐ Maintain current status/prevent deterioration

Evaluation of Assessment/Client Perspective

How was assessment method adapted to client needs?

Used language CM14 and CM12 could understand; respectful of cultural, gender expectations.

Age, culture, ability level, and other diversity issues adjusted for by:

Using teen language; allowing family to discuss traditions and values.

Systemic/family dynamics considered in following ways:

Considered CM14 behavior in broader system, including parents' conflicting parenting styles and confused parental

hierarchy cross-generational coalition.

Describe actual or potential areas of client-therapist agreement/disagreement related to the above assessment:

CM14 does not view situation as "big" problem; AM sees as bigger problem than AF.

_____ , _____ _____
Therapist Signature   License/Intern status   Date

_____ , _____ _____
Supervisor Signature   License   Date

TREATMENT PLAN

Therapist: Albert Luis, MFT Trainee   **Client ID #:** 9002

Theory: Structural

Primary Configuration: ☐ Individual ☐ Couple ☒ Family ☐ Group: _____

Additional: ☒ Individual ☒ Couple ☐ Family ☒ Group: Teen

Medication(s): ☒ NA ☐ _____

Contextual Factors considered in making plan: ☒ Age ☒ Gender ☒ Family dynamics

☒ Culture ☐ Language ☒ Religion ☐ Economic ☒ Immigration ☐ Sexual orientation

☐ Trauma ☐ Dual dx/comorbid ☒ Addiction issues ☐ Cognitive ability

☐ Other: _____

Describe how plan adapted to contextual factors: Considered cultural, religious, immigration issues, esp as relating to gender roles; extra time to join with teen; family dynamics and family developmental stage considered in conceptualizing treatment.

I. Initial Phase of Treatment (First 1–3 Sessions)
I.A. Initial Therapeutic Tasks
Therapeutic Relationship

TT1: Develop therapeutic relationship with all members. Note: Particular attention to **joining** with rebellious teen

I1: Intervention: **Mimesis** to join, carefully gaining CM14's trust while ensuring AM feels respected using cultural/religious norms; using humor with CM14.

Assessment

TT2: Assess individual, systemic, and broader cultural dynamics. Note: Include school functioning; cultural and gender issues.

I1: Intervention: **Enactments** to **map structure** to identify potential **cross-generational coalitions,** effectiveness of **parental hierarchy,** quality of parent/couple relationships.

I2: Intervention: Assess **boundaries** at home, school, and with extended family system.

Set Goals

TT3: Define and obtain client agreement on treatment goals. Note: _____

I1: Intervention: Discuss observations of family **structure;** obtain client agreement on goals.

Note: **BOLDFACE** indicates Structural Therapy assessment and techniques.

(continued)

I. Initial Phase of Treatment (First 1–3 Sessions) *(continued)*

Referrals and Crisis

> TT4: Identify needed referrals, crisis issues, and other client needs. Note: <u>Focus on recent violence. Develop safety plan with limits for substance use.</u>
>
> > I1: Intervention: <u>Rule out medical causes, substance abuse, danger to others (potential gang involvement).</u>

I.B. Initial Client Goals (1–2 Goals): Manage crisis issues and/or reduce most distressing symptoms.

> **Goal #1:** ☒ Increase ☐ Decrease **clarity of parent-child boundaries** by defining **parental hierarchy** while simultaneously increasing CM14's **responsibility** for his choices and actions (personal/relational dynamic) to reduce <u>violence</u> (symptom).
>
> *Measure:* Able to sustain <u>pro-social interactions</u> for period of 2 ☐ wks ☒ mos with no more than <u>0</u> mild episodes of <u>violence.</u>
>
> > I1: Intervention: **Reframing** to increase CM14's internal motivation to choose pursuing meaningful life goals over violence.
> >
> > I2: Intervention: **Separate parenting** sessions to strengthen **parental coalition** by developing an agreed-upon approach to parenting CM14 in regards to violence at school.

II. Working Phase of Treatment (Sessions 2+)

II.A. Working Therapeutic Tasks

Monitor Progress

> TT1: Monitor progress toward goals. Note: <u>Assess CM14 individually and family's progress.</u>
>
> > I1: Intervention: <u>Monthly progress questionnaires; call school counselor every 1–2 months.</u>

Monitor Relationship

> TT2: Monitor quality of therapeutic alliance as therapy proceeds. Note: _____
>
> > I1: Intervention: <u>Monitor CM14's responses to interventions and humor to ensure he is "on board"; monitor parents' responses to ensure they feel respected.</u>

II.B. Working Client Goals (2–3 Goals): Target individual and relational dynamics in case conceptualization using theoretical language (e.g., reduce enmeshment, increase differentiation, increase agency in relational narrative, etc.)

Goal #1: ☒ Increase ☐ Decrease **clarity of boundaries** and mutually satisfying **interactions** b/n AM and CM14 (personal/relational dynamic) to reduce **enmeshment** and clarify parental **hierarchy** and reduce fights (symptom).

Measure: Able to sustain mutually satisfying exchanges for period of 2 ☐ wks ☒ mos with no more than 1 mild episodes of arguing in a 2-week period.

> I1: Intervention: **Enactments** that reduce aggressive communications, reinforce parental hierarchy, and reduce enmeshment (e.g., direct family to begin re-enacting argument from past week and redirect to improve communication and clarify boundaries).

> I2: Intervention: Separate parental sessions to create **parental coalition** and alliance.

Goal #2: ☒ Increase ☐ Decrease **and strengthen CM14's personal boundaries** by increasing his responsibility for conduct and life direction (personal/relational dynamic) to reduce **parent-child enmeshment** to improve grades and motivation (symptom).

Measure: Able to sustain responsibilities at home and school for period of 2 ☐ wks ☒ mos with no more than 1–2 mild episodes of poor grades, failure to do chores, etc.

> I1: Intervention: Shaping competency by complimenting CM14 and highlighting areas of mature decision making, drawing on motivation to stay on track team (e.g., "Once you made the decision to improve your grades to stay on the team, you knew exactly what to do without your parents telling you").

> I2: Intervention: Reframe CM14 "rebelling" against father as "wanting to be seen as an adult"; extend metaphor to identify more effective ways of showing father that he is an adult than using drugs and alcohol; draw on cultural, religious, and intergenerational definitions of being a "man."

Goal #3: ☒ Increase ☐ Decrease **parental coalition** (personal/relational dynamic) to reduce **good/bad parent dichotomy** (symptom).

Measure: Able to sustain effective coalition for period of 2 ☐ wks ☒ mos with no more than 1 mild episodes of failing to support the other.

> I1: Intervention: **Reframe** each partner's parenting style as a complement to the other and having a place in the successful parenting; draw on religious, intergenerational, and cultural models of good parenting.

(continued)

II. Working Phase of Treatment (Sessions 2+) *(continued)*

I2: Intervention: Clarify **parental subsystem boundaries** and **strengthen hierarchy** by creating agreed-upon roles and limits as well as enable both parents to have a strong emotional connection with children; develop plan for addressing alcohol and substance issue if CM14 continues to make poor decisions related to use.

III. Closing Phase of Treatment (Last 2+ Weeks)

III.A. Closing Therapeutic Tasks
Termination Plan

TT1: Develop aftercare plan and maintain gains. Note: target long-term substance use; parenting of CM12.

I1: Intervention: **Shape competencies** by having family take proactive role in identifying potential future problems and solutions.

III.B. Closing Client Goals: Determined by theory's definition of health

Goal #1: ☒ Increase ☐ Decrease **clear boundaries** by encouraging each person's responsibility for self (personal/relational dynamic) to reduce **enmeshment** and increase family **cohesion** (symptom).

Measure: Able to sustain clear boundaries for period of 2 ☐ wks ☒ mos with no more than 2 mild episodes of fighting, etc.

I1: Intervention: Couple sessions for parents to strengthen **marital subsystem** and emotional intimacy.

I2: Intervention: Individual child sessions with CM14 to **reinforce strengths and positive** decisions related to grades, friends, and substance use.

IV. Client Perspective

Has treatment plan been reviewed with client? ☒ Yes ☐ No; If no, explain: _____

_____

Describe areas of client agreement and concern: Family willing to meet as family to work on issues.

_____ , _____ _____
Therapist signature   License/intern status   Date

_____ , _____ _____
Supervisor signature   License   Date

_____

Abbreviations: TT: Therapeutic Task; I: Intervention; AM: Adult Male; AF: Adult Female; CM: Child Male; CF: Child Female; Dx: Diagnosis; NA: Not Applicable.

PROGRESS NOTES

Progress Notes for Client # 9002

Date: 5/30/08 **Time:** 6:30 am/**pm**   **Session Length:** ☒ 50 min. or ☐ _____

Present: ☒ AM ☒ AF ☒ CM ☐ CF ☒ CM12 _____

Billing Code: ☐ 90801 (Assess) ☐ 90806 (Insight-50 min) ☒ 90847 (Family-50 min)

☐ Other _____

Symptoms(s)	Dur/Freq Since Last Visit	Progress: Setback------Initial----------Goal
1. Conflict w AM	2 moderate arguments w AM/ past wk	-5----------1---------X---5------------10
2. Fights with peers	No new incidents this week	-5----------1------------X------------10
3. Grades drop	Report increase in completing HW/5 days	-5----------1------------5------------10

Explanatory Notes: Denies drinking this week; report less defiance/arguing with AM; AF reports being more supportive of AM; report family had "fun" movie night on Saturday. CM14 reports meeting a new group of friends who are less "trouble prone" than those he had met previously.

Interventions/HW: Enactments in session to encourage CM14 to take greater responsibility for choices, clarify boundaries between AF, AM, and CM14, and interrupt cross-generational coalition. Identified rules for going out and how greater freedom can be earned. Met with AM and AF alone briefly to discuss parental coalition issues: agreeing on rules and limits. HW: continue with one fun weekend activity.

Client Response/Feedback: CM14 receptive to viewing self as taking responsibility for his life direction. Family receptive to redirection in enactments and open to working with parents alone. Enthusiastic about HW.

Plan: ☒ Continue with treatment plan: plan for next session: Parents only to discuss parenting next week; CM14 only following.

☐ Modify plan: _____

Next session: Date: 6/7/08 Time: 6:30 am/**pm**

Crisis Issues: ☒ Denies suicide/homicide/abuse/crisis ☐ Crisis assessed/addressed:

CM14 denies current alcohol and substance use; no reported fighting or plans for fighting.

_____ , _____   _____

Therapist signature License/intern status Date

Abbreviations: AM: Adult Male; AF: Adult Female; CM: Child Male; CF: Child Female; HW: Homework.

(continued)

PROGRESS NOTES *(continued)*

◇◇

Case Consultation/Supervision Notes: Supervisor recommended individual session with parents to address parenting and one alone with CM14 to increase his motivation.

Collateral Contacts: Date: 5/30/08 Time: 2:00 pm Name: Janet Rodriguez

Notes: School counselor reports working on plan to make up work to ensure passes 9th grade; will have to take summer school; report CM14 participating well in teen group; report no new fights at school.

☒ Written release on file: ☒ Sent ☐ Received ☐ In court docs ☐ Other: _____

_____ , _____ _____
Therapist signature   License/Intern status   Date

_____ , _____ _____
Supervisor signature   License   Date

Experiential Family Therapies

"Life is not the way it's supposed to be. It's the way it is. The way you cope with it is what makes the difference."—Virginia Satir

Lay of the Land

Experiential family therapies include two traditional approaches, the Satir growth model and symbolic-experiential therapy, and a recently developed evidence-based approach to couples emotionally focused therapy.

- **The Satir Growth Model:** Focuses on family communication using warmth and support

- **Symbolic-Experiential Therapy:** Focuses on symbolic meanings and emotional exchanges within the family using a balance of warmth and confrontation to promote change

- **Emotionally Focused Therapy (EFT):** The leading evidence-based approach to couples therapy that uses experiential, systemic, and attachment theories

Common Assumptions and Practices

Targeting Emotional Transactions

Whereas systemic, strategic, structural, and cognitive-behavioral family therapists primarily track *behavioral* interaction sequences, experiential family therapists focus on the *emotional* layer of those same interactions—while still attending to behavior and cognition (Johnson, 2004; Satir, Banmen, Gerber, & Gomori, 1991; Whitaker & Bumberry, 1988). Assessment and intervention target the emotional exchanges between family members and significant others in relation to the presenting problem.

Warmth, Empathy, and the Therapist's Use of Self

More so than strategic, structural, and intergenerational family therapists, experiential family therapists use warmth and empathy in building relationships with clients (Johnson, 2004; Satir, 1988; Satir et al., 1991; Whitaker & Bumberry, 1988). Therapists use themselves—their personhood—to make this strong affective connection with clients. This approach creates a sense of safety that allows clients to explore areas of emotional vulnerability.

Individual and Family Focus

Experiential family therapies address individual and family concerns as distinct sets of problems (Johnson, 2004; Satir et al., 1991; Whitaker & Bumberry, 1988). In contrast, systemic, structural, and intergenerational therapies conceptualize individual systems as part of the family system, assuming that if the family system is treated the individual symptoms will be resolved. Experiential therapists may not entirely disagree with this perspective but are much more deliberate in treating problems at the individual level.

The Satir Growth Model
In a Nutshell: The Least You Need to Know

One of the first prominent women in the field, Virginia Satir began her career in family therapy at the Mental Research Institute (MRI; see Chapter 9) working alongside Jay Haley, Paul Watzlawick, Richard Fisch, and the other leading family therapists in Palo Alto (Satir, 1967, 1972). She eventually left the MRI to develop her own ideas, which can broadly be described as infusing humanistic values into a systemic approach. She brought a warmth and enthusiasm for human potential that is unparalleled in the field of family therapy. Her therapy focused on fostering individual growth as well as improving family interactions. She used experiential exercises (e.g., family sculpting; see later section on Sculpting), metaphors, coaching, and the self of the therapist to facilitate change (Satir et al., 1991; Satir & Baldwin, 1983). Her work is practiced extensively internationally, with Satir practitioners connecting through the Satir Global Network.

The Juice: Significant Contributions to the Field

If you remember one thing from this chapter, it should be:

Communication Stances

The communication stances in the Satir growth model offer a clinician of any theoretical orientation an efficient and effective means of conceptualizing how best to communicate and interact with a client (Satir, 1967/1983, 1988; Satir et al., 1991). As already described in Chapter 2, there are five communication stances: congruent, placator, blamer, superreasonable, and irrelevant. Each stance either acknowledges or minimizes three realities: self, other, and context. Four of the stances—placator, blamer, superreasonable, and irrelevant—are *survival stances* that were used to "survive" as a child during difficult times. Everyone uses one of these to some extent because all children are put in situations they are not ready to handle as they move from one life stage to another. Survival stances often fit together like puzzle pieces within a family, with people assuming complementary stances to create balance. In all cases, the goal is to move people toward more congruent communication, communication in which they respectfully balance the needs of *self* and *others* while responding appropriately within and acknowledging the *context*.

At first glance, these stances appear too simplistic to be of much clinical relevance. I believed this myself until I started teaching case conceptualization (see Chapter 2). Over time, however, I began to appreciate their remarkable sophistication and the insights they offer. Identifying a client's communication stance can help therapists design interventions more effectively and use almost every utterance to move clients toward their goals, whether working solely from a Satir approach or from an entirely

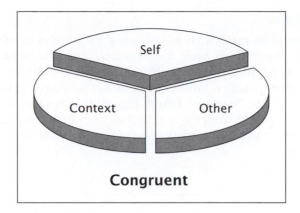

Congruent

different approach. Therapists can also communicate with a wide range of clients, adjusting their comments and interventions to accommodate the client and using consistent and focused language to reinforce therapeutic movement with every communication, from scheduling an appointment to wording interventions from any model.

Communication Strategies for Survival Stances

Unlike the congruent stance, each survival stance minimizes one or more essential parts of the total picture, as illustrated by the dark shading in the following diagrams.

Placator

Because placators have people-pleasing tendencies, therapists use less directive therapy methods, such as multiple-choice questions and open-ended reflections, to require them to voice their opinion and take a stand. Often this is quite painful and scary for placators. With clients who tend toward placating, therapists should carefully avoid giving opinions, making it seem that they have an opinion, or offering too much personal information. Clients will use this type of information to know what parts of themselves to hide and what parts to foreground to gain therapist approval. Never underestimate placators; they are skilled in the art of people pleasing. Research indicates that some clients make up things to give the impression that therapy is progressing (Gehart & Lyle, 2001). Not until the placator regularly and openly *disagrees* with the therapist has rapport been established.

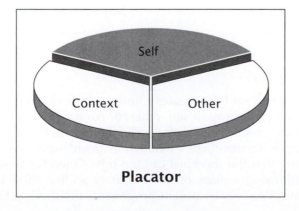

Placator

Blamer

Therapists must increase blamers' awareness of others' thoughts and feelings and help them learn how to communicate their personal perspectives in ways that are respectful of others. With these clients, direct confrontation often strengthens the therapeutic relationship (counter to what one might expect). Most blamers lose respect for "wimpy" (think placating) therapists who do not speak their minds honestly and directly, a skill that blamers have mastered. Blamers generally prefer more upfront and direct communication than is generally tolerated in polite society.

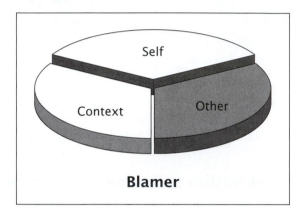

Superreasonable

When working with superreasonable clients, logic and rules reign supreme. Therapists must refer to context to gain validity in their world. The goal with this stance is to help clients value the internal, subjective realities of themselves and others.

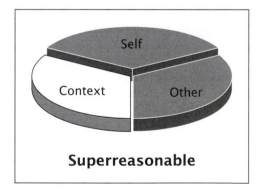

Irrelevant

The irrelevant type creates a unique challenge for therapists because there is no consistent grounding in self, other, or context for the therapist to use in understanding and communicating with the client. Instead, the therapist must spend time "floating" along with the client's distractions to identify the unique "anchors" of the client's reality that the therapist can tap into. Often the first step is to make the therapeutic relationship a place of utmost safety so that there is less need for distracting communication. As treatment progresses, the therapist works with irrelevant clients to

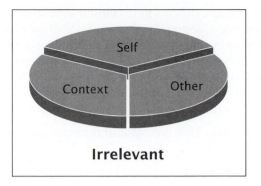

increase their ability to recognize the thoughts and feelings of self and others and to acknowledge the demands of context. Progress is typically slower with those who use this stance frequently.

Rumor Has It: The People and Their Stories

Virginia Satir

A true pioneer, Virginia Satir was one of the first therapists to work with entire families. She began her private practice in 1951, and by 1955 she was training therapists at the Illinois Psychiatric Institute to work with families. She then joined the newly established MRI in Palo Alto, California, to continue her research. A grant from the National Institute of Mental Health in 1962 provided funding to establish the first family therapy training program. In 1964, she published her first book, *Conjoint Family Therapy*, which outlines the key aspects of her model. She left the MRI to become the director of Esalen Institute in Big Sur, California, offering workshops facilitating personal growth. She also founded the AVANTA network (also called the Virginia Satir Global Network) to connect practitioners of the model.

John Banmen

Having trained and worked closely with Virginia Satir (et al., 1991), Banmen now teaches the Satir growth model internationally, particularly in China, Taiwan, and Hong Kong where Satir's work is highly influential, and continues to publish on current applications of her work (Banmen, 2002, 2003).

Maria Gomori

Having trained and studied with Satir (Satir et al., 1991), Maria Gomori (2002) now runs the Satir Professional Development Institute of Manitoba, which offers comprehensive training in the model.

Lynne Azpeitia

Having trained and worked closely with Satir, Lynne continues training the next generation of Satir practitioners and developing strength-oriented applications for working with nonclinical populations (Azpeitia, 1991, 1995).

The Big Picture: Overview of Treatment

Satir et al. (1991) use a six-stage model of change that is based on Satir's research at the MRI on cybernetic systems and that draws from humanistic principles, including the assumption that people naturally strive toward growth. Her six-stage model describes how the therapy process helps families move toward a *second-order change* in the family structure (see Chapter 8). The model also emphasizes that the therapist perturbs the system, shakes it up and respects its ability to naturally reorganize itself in a more useful way, rather than attempting to direct and control the system from the outside. Thus, even though Satir uses education and coaches clients on how to better communicate, the aim is not for clients to literally follow her instructions but rather to adapt and respond to the instructions in a way that works for their system. The six stages are as follows:

1. **Status Quo:** This is a state of homeostasis that includes at least one symptomatic member.

2. **Introduction of Foreign Element:** A foreign element, which may be a life crisis, tragedy, or therapeutic intervention, gets the system off balance.

3. **Chaos:** The new perspective creates a *positive feedback* loop that throws the system into a state of chaos; at this point the "natural" response is to feel uncomfortable, and in almost all cases the family tries to regain the status quo (stage 1), which may or may not be possible.

4. **Integration of New Possibilities:** Eventually the family system interprets the new information in a meaningful way; the therapist needs to be respectful of how the system uses the information and responds to therapist-client interactions, honoring and trusting the system's autonomy.

5. **Practice:** The system develops a new set of interaction patterns based on the new information. This may or may not look like what the therapist expects, but the therapist asks two key evaluative questions: (a) Are the symptoms improving?; (b) Is each person able to self-actualize and grow?

6. **New Status Quo:** This is a state of new homeostasis that does not include a symptomatic member and that allows all members to grow and flourish.

In most cases, therapy involves going through these six stages several times, with the discomfort and relative sense of chaos diminishing each time the client cycles through, becoming increasingly comfortable with change.

Making Connection: The Therapeutic Relationship

Humanistic and Systemic Foundations

Satir et al. (1991, pp. 14–15) state four primary assumptions about people and therapy; the first two reflect *humanistic* assumptions and the latter two a *systemic* view.

ASSUMPTIONS OF SATIR'S GROWTH MODEL

1. People naturally tend toward positive growth (humanistic principle).

2. All people possess the resources for positive growth (humanistic principle).

3. Every person and every thing or situation impacts and is impacted by everyone and everything else (systemic principle).

4. Therapy is a process that involves interaction between therapist and client; in this relationship, each person is responsible for him/herself (systemic and humanistic principle).

These assumptions clarify the therapist's role in the process (the therapist is "responsible for him/herself"), but also how the therapist believes the therapeutic process works: clients already possess the natural inclination toward growth and the resources for it, and it is the therapist's job to activate these tendencies. These assumptions inform the role of the therapist as a *guide* to the process of becoming more fully human.

Therapeutic Presence: Warmth and Humanity

Carl Rogers (1961, 1981), a leader in humanistic, experiential therapies, based his client-centered approach on three therapist qualities: (a) congruence or genuineness, (b) accurate empathy, and (c) unconditional positive regard. These conditions are the theoretical foundation of the warmth and humanity for which Satir is legendary (Satir et al., 1991). Her way of being in the world radiated an unshakable hope and deep-felt respect for her clients. Her presence in the room put people at ease and allowed them to feel secure enough to nondefensively relate to one another. She created a safe haven that made it easy for her clients to address the issues in their lives. How she did this is a much more difficult question to answer. This quality of being, or *therapeutic presence,* is difficult to define, and there are few methods for systematically developing it (Gehart & McCollum, 2008). The more *congruent* therapists are—that is, able to communicate authentically while responding to the needs of both self and others—the better they can create the therapeutic warmth and humanity that characterized the work of Satir.

Making Contact

Satir et al. (1991) describe establishing a therapeutic relation as "making contact," which refers to a series of connections both within the therapist and between the therapist and the other. Making contact begins with the therapist being in contact with himself/herself, including all resources of the self as defined in the *self mandala:* physical, intellectual, emotional, sensual, interactional, nutritional, contextual, and spiritual. In addition, the therapist prepares to meet another "miracle," a fellow human being. Then, the therapist works to make contact with each client in the room, engaging them on "all channels": mind, body, and spirit. Thus open-body positioning and congruent communication are critical. Once the therapist has made contact with each person, the therapist works to help family members make contact with each other and ultimately with others in their broader social system. The therapy process cannot move forward until the therapist has made contact with the client. When contact is made, clients feel valued for who they are, regardless of their problem, and they feel free to make mistakes in the therapist's presence. Making contact involves the following:

- Making direct eye contact with clients
- Touching clients (e.g., shaking hands)
- Sitting or standing at the same physical level so that eye contact is easy (i.e., leaning down to talk with children)
- Asking each person's name and how he or she prefers to be called (Satir et al., 1991)

Empathy

Satir practitioners convey their understanding of clients' subjective, inner realities by expressing *empathy*, an accurate understanding of another's emotional reality. Empathy does not mean that a therapist takes the client's side, avoids confronting inconsistencies, or ignores the client's responsibility. Don't get me wrong; clients *like* therapists who take their side, don't confront them, and ignore their responsibility in the problem situation. It feels good to be "validated" in this way, but this type of "validation" is detrimental to therapeutic progress. Similarly, comments that imply a client has a "right" to feel a certain way can also shut down the process of reflecting on the client's responsibility for his/her half of an interaction. On the other hand, expressing empathy emphasizes that it is not wrong or right, normal or abnormal, to feel a certain way—that this is simply how the client feels and this is his/her "truth," at least for the moment (e.g., "It sounds like you felt betrayed"). Honoring the client's unique experience without validating it as right or normal makes it much easier to move the client toward seeing that the other person has his/her unique experience that is also "true" for that person, creating a context from which to understand how these two (or more) realities may collide and create problematic interactions.

Conveying Hope

In joining with clients, therapists instill hope that they can change and that things can be better, even if they seem hopeless at the moment. Satir et al. (1991) emphasize that clients must have faith that change is possible before they can move forward with treatment.

Establishing Credibility

Clients also need to believe that therapy and their particular therapist can help them resolve their problems. Therapists establish credibility by making a personal connection (making contact) and by being confident and competent (modeling high self-esteem; Satir et al., 1991).

The Viewing: Case Conceptualization and Assessment

In the Satir growth model, both family functioning and individual functioning are assessed.

Assessment of Family Functioning

- Role of the symptom in the system
- Family dynamics
- Family roles
- Family life chronology
- Survival triad

Assessment of Individual Functioning

- Survival stances
- Six levels of experience: the iceberg
- Self-worth and self-esteem
- Mind-body connection

Role of the Symptom in the System

Much like other systemic therapists, Satir (1972) viewed the symptom as having a role in the family system. For example, a child's exaggerated acting out, such as with drug use or sexual activity, may serve to reduce tension in the marriage by getting the parents on the same page about the child's issue. Similarly, a person's depression may be a means of avoiding an unpleasant confrontation with a spouse or boss. Basically, symptoms always have an emotional function in the family system, even if they are consciously and logically unwanted. The question is, Why this particular symptom in this particular family (or relationship)? If the therapist can understand how the symptom makes emotional sense in the family dance, it will be easier to help the family find ways to interact successfully without the need for the symptom.

Family Dynamics

Along with assessing family roles, Satir et al. (1991) identify problematic family dynamics:

- **Power Struggles:** These can be within the family and couple or with extended family members.

- **Parental Conflicts:** These can involve parents disagreeing about how to parent and care for children.

- **Lack of Validation:** The family openly expresses little emotional support or validation.

- **Lack of Intimacy:** There is minimal sharing of significant personal information and one's emotional life.

Family Roles

Satir (1972, 1988) assessed each person's role in the family system to understand the function of the problem. Possible roles include the following:

- The martyr
- The victim or helpless one
- The rescuer
- The good child or parent
- The bad child or parent

Family Life Chronology

The family life chronology (Satir, 1967/1983; Satir et al., 1991) is a timeline that includes the major events in an individual's or family's life:

- Births and deaths
- Important family events: marriages, moves, tragedies, major illnesses, job loss
- Important historical events: wars, natural disasters, economic downturns

This chronology gives both the therapist and client a "big picture" view of the context for the potential problem and provides clues as to what old wounds may be fueling the current problems, as well as what potential strengths and resources might exist.

Survival Triad

Another area for assessment is the survival triad (Satir, 1988)—the child, mother, and father—and the quality of the relationship between all three. Satir asserted that it was in this primary triad that a child learns how to be human (Azpeitia, 1991). Is there an emotional bond between each parent and the child, or do the parents have significantly different levels of connection with the child? Because the survival triad should serve as a nurturing system for the child, when the child is experiencing difficulty, the therapist considers how the nurturing function of these relationships can be improved.

Survival Stances (see Juice)
Six Levels of Experience: The Iceberg

Satir practitioners use the *six levels of experience* to help clients *transform* their feelings about feelings to make lasting change (Satir et al., 1991). These levels are likened to an *iceberg*, with the behavior the only visible layer and the other five layers unseen beneath the surface. The six layers of the iceberg are as follows:

- **Behavior:** The behavior on the surface; the external manifestation of the person's inner world

- **Coping:** Defenses and survival stances: placating, blaming, superreasonable, and irrelevant; these come out in times of stress, and a person may use different stances in different relational contexts

- **Feelings:** Present feelings that are strongly past-based, using past events to interpret the present

- **Perceptions:** Beliefs, attitudes, and values that inform one's sense of self; most perceptions are formed when very young and are based on a limited view of reality

- **Expectations:** A strong belief about how life should go, how people should behave, and how one should perform; most expectations are formed while young and are often unrealistic and/or may not apply to a particular situation

- **Yearnings:** Universal longings to be loved, accepted, validated, and confirmed

In therapy Satir practitioners use the six levels of experience to assess the motivation behind problematic behaviors and interactions. By understanding the *yearnings* as well as *perceptions* and *expectations* that fuel problematic behavior, coping, and feelings, therapists are able to help clients transform their feelings about feelings to more effectively meet the underlying longing for love and acceptance.

Self-Worth and Self-Esteem

Satir was one of the first to recognize the importance of self-worth and self-esteem, and she always assessed a person's level of self-esteem (Satir, 1972). Clinically, it is generally unhelpful to assess self-esteem in an all-or-none fashion (i.e., high vs. low), as is frequently done by teachers, parents, and concerned others who believe they have identified the secret cause behind a child's poor behavior. Instead, it is more useful to consider the specific *aspects of the self* that a client *values* and the aspects of which he/she is ashamed. For example, a child may value and have confidence in her ability to make friends but have less confidence in her scholastic abilities.

More recent research on self-esteem indicates that *self-compassion,* or acceptance of one's strengths and weaknesses, is a better indicator of happiness than self-esteem, which can be artificially high (Neff, 2003). People who overestimate their abilities and worth often have high self-esteem but significant problems in their interpersonal and work or school relationships because they have unrealistic expectations of "what is due them." The best indicator of health, self-compassion is one's ability to accept strengths and weaknesses in oneself and others. People who are judgmental, impatient, or intolerant of others' weaknesses are almost always equally harsh on themselves; conversely, those who are hard on themselves are almost always equally harsh on others, even if it is not verbalized. As self-compassion and self-worth rise, people become more realistic and tolerant of their own and others' weaknesses while realistically assigning and assuming responsibility for their actions.

Mind-Body Connection

Satir et al. (1991) also consider the mind-body connection: how emotional issues may be manifesting in the body, either *symbolically* or *functionally*. For example, if a person is feeling burdened, this emotional feeling may manifest symbolically as stooped shoulders ("should-ers") or as a "burdened" posture. Similarly, if a person is feeling overwhelmed, this may manifest functionally in often being ill or exhausted. In addition, the role of nutrition and exercise is assessed. Finally, Satir maintained that the way the body is used indicates the person's communication stance:

- **Congruent Communication and Self-Esteem:** Open and relaxed body postures
- **Placating:** Timid and reserved postures
- **Blaming:** Pointing, angry, and stiff postures
- **Superreasonable:** Cold and distant postures
- **Irrelevant:** Hyper and distracted

Targeting Change: Goal Setting

At the most general level, the goal of Satir's growth model is transformation: to achieve optimal realization of a person's full potential (Azpeitia, 1991). This goal translates into two broad sets of practical goals for treatment planning:

1. Relational, family, or systemic goals
2. Individual goals

Satir therapists' attention to individual goals reflects their humanistic foundations and is unique among systemically based therapists; symbolic-experiential therapists, who share this humanistic foundation, also have systemic and individual goals (see discussion of symbolic-experiential therapy later in chapter).

Relationally Focused Goals: Congruent Communication

The heart of relational goals in Satir's approach is congruent communication: the ability to communicate authentically while responding to the needs of both self and others. Specifically, the goal is to help the family develop ways for all members to communicate so that the system's homeostasis no longer needs the initial symptoms (problems) to maintain balance. The following are examples of specific goals (Satir, 1967/1983; Satir et al., 1991).

EXAMPLES OF RELATIONALLY FOCUSED GOALS

- Increase congruent communication in relationships with spouse, parent, child, etc.
- Change family rules and "shoulds" to general guidelines

Individually Focused Goals: Self-Actualization

The overarching individual goal is consistent with other humanistic approaches: to promote the self-actualization of all members of the system. Self-actualization means fulfilling one's potential and living an authentic and meaningful life. The more a person self-actualizes, the greater his/her sense of self-worth and self-esteem. Examples of specific goals (Satir et al., 1991) are as follows.

EXAMPLES OF INDIVIDUALLY FOCUSED GOALS

- Increase a sense of self-worth and self-compassion
- Reduce defensiveness and the use of survival stances

In the case study at the end of this chapter, the goals focus on (a) helping a teen who has been sexually abused regain her sense of self-worth (especially after the abuse) and autonomy (developmental task), and (b) helping the couple and family develop congruent communication regarding the abuse as well as resolve couple concerns that were there prior to the abuse.

The Doing: Interventions

Therapist's Use of Self

Therapists' use of self—being authentically who they are—is one of the most essential interventions in Satir's approach (1988). By being authentic, therapists provide a role model for how to communicate congruently and also show the effects of increased self-actualization. Furthermore, the use of the therapist's self in therapy, which may include self-disclosure, creates a safe relationship in which clients can practice communicating congruently without negative consequences and learn to tap into more authentic modes of expression.

Ingredients of an Interaction

The foundation for all other interventions (Azpeitia, 1991), the *ingredients of an interaction* details the internal communication process and can be used to teach clients about internal and relational processes (Satir et al., 1991). The ingredient questions are used to help people better understand their interactions with others and can be used with individuals, couples, or families. When a client shares a troubling interaction with another, the therapist uses the following seven questions to walk the client through the "ingredients of an interaction" (Azpeitia, 1991; Satir et al., 1991):

1. **What do I HEAR AND SEE?** The therapist prompts clients to describe behaviorally what happened without adding interpretations; this is similar to "videotalk" in solution-based therapies (Chapter 14) (e.g., "My child did not take out the trash immediately upon my asking her to do so").

2. **What MEANINGS do I make of what I hear and see?** After obtaining a clear, behavioral description, the therapist facilitates a discussion of how the clients interpreted these behaviors; meanings often connect back to past experiences (e.g., "My child does not respect me; I would never have spoken to my parents that way").

3. **What FEELINGS do I have about the meanings I make?** Next, the therapist helps clients identify specific feelings about the meanings and interpretations (e.g., "This makes me angry and hurt"). Therapists use "facilitation of emotional expression" techniques, described in detail in next section.

4. **What FEELINGS do I have *ABOUT* THESE FEELINGS?** Then the therapist asks clients about whether they can accept and tolerate the feelings; the more congruent a person is, the more accepting he/she is of various feelings. If a person is not accepting, survival stances will be triggered (e.g., *congruent*: "I don't like these feelings, but I know that they are natural"; *incongruent*: "I don't like these feelings and need my child to do what I say so that I don't have such feelings anymore"). Subsequent interventions target this level of feeling, not the emotions attached to the interpretation.

5. **What DEFENSES do I use?** When people use incongruent communication, they respond in the interaction using defense mechanisms such as projection, denial, ignoring, or one of the communication stances (e.g., "I get angry and yell at my child for not following my request"; "I blame my spouse for spoiling the child").

6. **What RULES FOR COMMENTING do I use?** Each person's family of origin and early significant others impart rules for commenting on interpersonal interactions that may limit self-worth, restrict choices, and determine what actions are "allowed" and "appropriate"; most of these rules are unspoken and brought into future relationships without reflection on whether they are appropriate or useful (e.g., "It is not okay for a parent to be vulnerable with a child"; "Parents should always be in charge"). These rules are transformed using "softening" techniques (described in Softening Family Rules).

7. **What is my RESPONSE in the situation?** How does the client respond behaviorally and verbally (e.g., "I tell my child 'You don't respect me' in an angry, hostile tone and stay angry even after the child does the chore"; "I also get angry at my spouse for not being stricter with the children")? Incongruent and problematic responses are targeted for change.

Facilitating Emotional Expression

Satir therapists work with clients to help them express difficult-to-articulate emotions related to the presenting problem (Satir, 1991). If clients complain about family members or a difficult life situation, experiential therapists listen closely for the emotions, expressed or unexpressed, that are related to the problem circumstance. They listen not just for the surface emotions (e.g., "I am angry that my partner was late") but also for deeper levels of emotion (e.g., "My partner does not care about me") and use questions and empathetic reflections to focus clients on those deeper emotions.

Softening Family Rules

Satir et al. (1991) coached families in softening rigid family rules by changing them to *guidelines*. For example, rather than saying "I should not get angry," a client or family was encouraged to revise the limiting rule to "When I am angry, I will express this anger in a way that is respectful to the others and myself." In addition, Satir encouraged families to have as few rules as possible and to be flexible, adapting them for each context and as children's developmental needs change.

Communication Enhancement: Coaching, Role Play, and Enactment

A hallmark of Satir's approach, coaching clients in how to have authentic, congruent communication in session, involves the "ingredients of an interaction" (previously discussed) combined with specific communication coaching strategies (Satir, 1988; Satir et al., 1991). When coaching communication, Satir had clients turn their chairs toward one another and gave the clients prompts, such as "Tell your partner how you feel about what happened on Saturday night." If the client was able to congruently address his/her partner about this, she then prompted the partner to respond in kind, continuing this process until the problem was resolved. When a person had trouble communicating congruently and reverted to a survival stance, Satir interrupted the conversation and suggested how to rephrase the statement or how to make the client's nonverbal communications more congruent (e.g., "Now, can you say that starting the statement with 'I' instead of 'you'?" or "Can you show the emotion you say you are feeling when you speak to your wife?").

COMMON AREAS OF COMMUNICATION COACHING

- Asking clients to start statements using "I" rather than "You"
- Taking full responsibility for one's feelings rather than blaming others (e.g., "Instead of 'You made me feel...,' try 'When X happened, I felt...'")
- Encouraging clients to be direct and honest rather than expecting the other to read between the lines
- Identifying double binds (e.g., "You asked your husband to show more affection, but when he does, you are upset and say he only did so because you asked")

In addition, the "ingredients of an interaction" technique (see previous discussion) was used to help coach clients through what they heard and saw, how they interpreted and felt about it, and the feelings about feelings and family-of-origin rules for communicating about what happened. In the case study at the end of the chapter, the therapist plans to use role play to help a teen who has been sexually abused regain her sense of safety, ability to set boundaries, and confidence in her ability to say "no."

Sculpting or Spatial Metaphor

Satir's most distinctive intervention is family sculpting, which is done either with the family or in a group setting (Satir, 1988; Satir et al., 1991). Sculpting involves putting family members in physical positions that represent how the "sculptor" sees each person's role in the family. For example, if a child sees a parent as blaming or harshly punitive, he may sculpt that parent with a harsh look and angry pointing finger and perhaps himself as the child cowering or hiding. Typically, either the therapist or the client may direct the sculpting. If family members are directing the sculpting, each person in the family is given an opportunity to sculpt the family as he or she sees it. Sometimes the sculptor assigns each family member a line to say that represents how he or she might be feeling, thinking, or viewing the situation. Usually, however, the essence of this intervention is to give a nonverbal, symbolic depiction of the family process from each person's perspective.

In most cases sculpting is a highly effective nonverbal confrontation that bypasses cognitive defenses. Through the sculpting process, a person is able to literally *see* how he or she is contributing to the problematic family process far more quickly than when the same information is provided with words. For example, if a person places herself far away from the rest of the family because she feels scapegoated or ostracized, this often communicates the emotional reality of her situation far more effectively than if she were to use words, which would generally be responded to with a verbal rationalization. When all family members are sculpting, it is generally best to let each person sculpt how he/she sees the family before allowing the family members to discuss one another's sculpting. Therapists encourage family members to respect each person's subjective experience as illustrated in the sculpting and to use the experience to deepen their understanding of one another.

In the case study at the end of this chapter, the therapist uses sculpting with a teen who has been sexually abused at a time when her mother is significantly increasing her business travel; to assess the emotional impact of these changes, the therapist has the family sculpt what the family was like prior to the abuse and after.

Touch

Satir (1988) used touch in therapy to initially connect with clients and to encourage and reassure them when they were practicing new ways of communicating, thereby underscoring emotional content and providing palpable support. She also used touch with children to help teach alternatives to violent behavior and to model for parents how to manage difficult children. The fact that she was an extremely nurturing female figure contributed significantly to how clients experienced her touch. In today's practice environments, touching is generally discouraged because it can easily be misinterpreted as sexual harassment or may make a client feel uncomfortable. Thus therapists need to carefully consider the legal and ethical issues of using touch. That said, touch may be appropriate in certain practice and cultural contexts. At minimum, therapists can learn from Satir the importance of coaching clients in touching *each other*—their children and spouses—in more loving and helpful ways. For example, rather than using a demonstration, therapists can guide a parent on how to hold children who are having a tantrum.

Interventions for Special Populations

Family Reconstruction: Group Intervention

A form of group psychodrama, the family reconstruction is used to allow clients to safely explore unresolved family issues and life events in the safety of the group setting (Satir et al., 1991). The client, who is called the "star," first identifies key events in his/her life chronology and significant sources of influence. The star then picks people from the group to re-enact pivotal life experiences and relationships. The therapist facilitates the re-enactment with the following three goals in mind:

- Identify the roots of old learning and their role in the present
- Develop a more realistic picture of the client's parents
- Discover unique strengths and potentials

Parts Party

A group activity similar to the family reconstruction, the parts party involves the client identifying group members to represent aspects of the self (Satir et al., 1991). The person may have members enact generic characteristics (martyr, victim, savior) or use famous figures to represent different aspects of self. In this way, the therapist facilitates a process in which the client is better able to accept different aspects of self and to identify the contexts in which they have been and continue to be useful. The language of "parts" can also be used to facilitate similar discussions and insights in individual, couple, and family therapy.

Symbolic-Experiential Therapy
In a Nutshell: The Least You Need to Know

Symbolic-experiential therapy is an experiential family therapy model developed by Carl Whitaker. Whitaker referred to his work as "therapy of the absurd," highlighting the unconventional and playful wisdom he used to help transform families (Whitaker, 1975). Relying almost entirely on emotional logic rather than cognitive logic, his work is often misunderstood as nonsense, but it is more accurate to say that he worked with "heart sense." Rather than intervene on behavioral sequences like strategic-systemic therapists, Whitaker focused on the emotional process and family structure (Roberto, 1991). He intervened directly at the emotional level of the system, relying heavily on "symbolism" and real life experiences as well as humor, play, and affective confrontation.

For the astute observer, Whitaker's work embodied a deep and profound understanding of families' emotional lives; to the casual observer, he often seemed rude or inappropriate. When he was "inappropriate," it was always for the purpose of confronting or otherwise intervening on emotional dynamics that he wanted to expose, challenge, and transform. He was adamant about balancing strong emotional confrontation with warmth and support from the therapist (Napier & Whitaker, 1978). In many ways, he encouraged therapists to move beyond the rules of polite society and invite themselves and clients to be genuine and real enough to speak the whole truth.

The Juice: Significant Contributions to the Field

If you remember one thing from this chapter, it should be this:

The Battle for Structure and the Battle for Initiative

Whitaker referred to two "battles" in therapy: the battle for structure and the battle for initiative. Even if you are turned off by the war metaphor, every competent therapist should consider the principles he is describing. The battle for *structure* should be won by the *therapist*, who sets the boundaries and limits for therapy (Whitaker & Bumberry, 1988). Therapists need to win this battle because they are responsible for setting up a program for change and therefore need to ensure that the necessary structure for change is in place:

- That the necessary people attend therapy
- That therapy occurs frequently enough to produce progress
- That the session content and process will produce change

The "battle" occurs when the therapist must insist on these key pieces. Whitaker was quite clear that if clients were not able to meet the minimal structure requirements, he would not do therapy. He saw the therapist's personal integrity at the heart of this battle:

> The key point here is for the therapist to face the need to act with personal and professional integrity. You must act on what you believe. Betrayals help no one. The Battle for Structure is really you coming to grips with yourself and then presenting this to them. It's not a technique or power play. It's a setting of the minimum conditions you require before beginning. (Whitaker & Bumberry, 1988, p. 54)

Although it is unethical to do therapy if you do not believe that you can render successful treatment, frequently therapists "settle" for trying to do marital or family therapy without the key players attending sessions or do not direct the content or process to the areas they believe need to be addressed. Losing this battle results in stagnant therapy.

Conversely, the battle for *initiative* needs to be won by the *client*. It is the client who must have the most investment and initiative to pursue change. This insight is often summarized as: *therapists should never work harder than their clients*. This is a particularly challenging battle for new therapists, who can be overly helpful and often want to move faster than their clients are able. However, if the therapist wants change more than the client, this creates a problematic dynamic and, paradoxically, often stalls change. The therapist needs to wait and sometimes let the tension and crisis build until the client develops the incentive and motivation to make changes. If the therapist has more initiative toward change, clients feel they are being dragged or forced and then start to dig in their heels or find little ways to sabotage the therapist's efforts at change. Instead, when the client has the greater motivation for change, the process flows more smoothly. Thus therapists must be ready to follow clients' lead on how hard to work, following their flow of energy and enthusiasm.

The battle for initiative can be interpersonally uncomfortable, involving awkward silences, "I don't know" answers, or tension. Clients may feel frustrated that the therapist is not taking the lead in choosing topics of discussion and providing ready solutions. Whitaker and Bumberry (1988) explain the purpose of allowing this tension to build: "It's an issue of the family becoming somebody. They need to grapple with each other. It's an invitation to them to come alive and stop play-acting" (p. 66).

Rumor Has It: The People and Their Stories

Carl Whitaker

Along with his colleagues, Thomas Malone and John Warkentin, Whitaker began seeing families in the 1940s and so was one of the earliest pioneers in the field (Roberto, 1991). A psychoanalytically trained psychiatrist, he began to shift away from conceptualizing client problems as internal conflicts toward viewing problems as part of dysfunctional interactions. In his early work with psychosis and trauma, he focused on the emotional dynamics in session and within the family system. As his work evolved, he increasingly focused on affect and here-and-now experiences within family relationships. While Whitaker was chair of the Department of Psychiatry at Emory University, Whitaker and Malone began to use co-therapy, a hallmark of the approach. Whitaker's best-known colleagues include Augustus Napier, Whitaker's co-author on *The Family Crucible;* William Bumberry, Whitaker's co-author on Dancing with the Family; David Keith (Keith, Connell, & Connell, 2001); and Gary Connell (Connell, Mitten & Bumberry, 1999).

The Big Picture: Overview of Treatment

Therapy of the Absurd

Symbolic-experiential therapy is often referred to as the "therapy of the absurd" (Whitaker, 1975). However, absurdity in this case is not absurdity for absurdity's sake (whatever that might be); instead, symbolic-experiential therapists employ a specific form of absurdity for a specific purpose. Absurdity is used to *perturb* (shake or wake up) the system in a compassionate and caring way. Sometimes the "caring" takes the form of speaking a truth no one else has been willing to speak, but the therapist is always careful to convey the spirit of caring behind such brutally honest comments (Whitaker & Bumberry, 1988). Usually, however, therapy of the absurd involves humor, playfulness, and silliness. By being able to play with otherwise "serious matters," therapists invite themselves as well as their clients into a more resourceful position in relation to the problem. A new attitude of lightness and hope emerges from this playfulness. Therapy of the absurd also uses paradoxical techniques that take the symptom and exaggerate it 10% so that clients can see the folly of their fears and habits. Symbolic-experiential therapists almost always employ paradox in a playful way.

Making Connection: The Therapeutic Relationship

"Families do not fail, therapists do."—Whitaker & Ryan, 1989, p. 56

Therapist's Authentic Use of Self

Symbolic-experiential therapists strive to be authentic and genuine and, arguably, are the most authentic of family therapists in that they do not follow many of the pretenses that many would consider professional or appropriate boundaries; they are the first to point out that the emperor has no clothes (Connell et al., 1999; Napier & Whitaker, 1978; Whitaker & Bumberry, 1988). They are fully themselves and do not hide this from their clients. If they are bored, they show it; if they are annoyed, they express it. If they see an elephant in the middle of the room, they say something. This level of authenticity requires extensive supervision and training to ensure that therapists are able to maintain exceptionally clear boundaries between their personal issues and clients' issues. For this reason, therapists who do not work this way are often baffled when watching symbolic-experiential therapists in action because they use a different set of relational rules for being "professional." In the end, being authentic at this level is primarily for the benefit of the client: to model the type of authenticity the therapist wants the client to develop and to create an environment in which the client can do this. If the therapist is hiding behind professional boundaries and the "role," the client has little chance of fully developing this type of authenticity.

Personal Integrity

Whitaker insisted that the therapist maintain a clear and unwavering integrity as a person (Whitaker & Bumberry, 1988). This integrity requires a fierce adherence to personal beliefs and the willingness to stand up for them, even when they are unpopular and may make people upset. Integrity is required to push families to address the painful issues they have been avoiding.

Therapist's Responsibility

Symbolic-experiential therapists strive "to be responsive *to* the family without being responsible *for* them" (Whitaker & Bumberry, 1988, p. 44). They are careful not to take on responsibility for clients' lives, but instead are responsibile for pushing clients to accept full responsibility for their own lives. The therapist's greatest responsibility is to ensure that the therapeutic process promotes change: to win the battle for structure. The therapist is *active* but not directive.

Stimulating Mutual Growth

The therapeutic process in symbolic-experiential therapy stimulates mutual growth: both the therapist and client grow together through their authentic encounter with each other (Connell et al., 1999; Napier & Whitaker, 1978). Because therapists are fully authentic—the same people they are in other relationships—they learn about their own limitations, blind spots, and weaknesses and use the encounters with clients to also grow and become more fully authentic people themselves. The encounter touches each participant—client and therapist—at a deeply profound level, leaving both transformed.

Use of Co-Therapists

Whitaker encouraged the use of a co-therapist, recommending that one therapist be nurturing and the other more confrontational so that the family has a strong base of support as well as a process for having difficult issues raised and addressed (Napier & Whitaker, 1978). In providing a balance of support and challenge, the co-therapy team models a co-parenting relationship.

The Viewing: Case Conceptualization and Assessment

Authentic Encounters and the Affective System

Case conceptualization in symbolic-experiential therapy is one of the most difficult to fully capture in words. In one sense, the therapist relies primarily on the in-the-moment *authentic encounters* with the client to directly experience who the other is in a holistic way (Connell et al., 1999; Whitaker & Bumberry, 1988). To anyone new to the practice, that statement is a bit too vague to be helpful. It is much like riding a bike: beginners need each step broken down, whereas those who are experienced say, "it's easy; just pedal," forgetting how difficult it was to get started (and how long dad pushed from behind). The little steps that allow symbolic-experiential therapists to effortlessly "roll" along and "intuit" their case conceptualization are grounded in a systemic understanding of the family: boundaries, homeostasis, triangles, and other factors. However, symbolic-experiential therapists focus primarily on the family's *emotional system* rather than their behavioral interactions. When they get a sense of boundaries or triangles, they focus on the emotional exchange between parties rather than actions. Therapists "feel" their way through the system.

Trial of Labor

The assessment of the family is accomplished through a *trial of labor*, which refers to observing how the family responds to the therapist's interventions and interactions (Whitaker & Keith, 1981). During the trial of labor, the therapist tries to understand each person's preferred family roles, beliefs about life, values within relationships, developmental and family histories, and interactional patterns. More specifically, the therapist attends to two broad patterns: (a) the structural organization of the family and (b) the emotional processes and exchanges within the family (Roberto, 1991). In assessing structure, Whitaker used many of the same criteria as structural therapists.

Assessing Structural Organization

- **Permeable Boundaries Within the Family:** Interpersonal boundaries should be permeable, not overly rigid or diffuse.

- **Clear Boundaries with Extended Family and Larger Systems:** Boundaries with larger systems should allow for the autonomy of the nuclear family as well as connection with broader systems.

- **Role Flexibility:** Family roles, including the scapegoat or good/bad child, should rotate frequently.

- **Flexible Alliances and Coalitions:** Alliances and coalitions are inevitable but should be flexible, changing with each new situation or challenge rather than always involving the same people on the same team.

- **Generation Gap:** Generations should have clear boundaries, resulting in strong marital and sibling subsystems.

- **Gender-Role Flexibility:** Gender roles should be negotiable, resisting stereotyped gender norms in favor of the ability of each parent or partner to assume a wide range of roles as necessary.

- **Transgenerational Mandates:** Transgenerational behavioral expectations and values are assessed across three to four generations; in healthy families, these are open to renegotiation.

- **"Ghosts":** Therapy identifies deceased or living extended family members who are creating cross-generational stress.

Assessing Emotional Process

- **Differentiation and Individuation:** Each family member should be able to hold unique opinions and speak for himself or herself.

- **Tolerance of Conflict:** Healthy families are able to tolerate the overt and explicit expression of differences and conflict.

- **Conflict Resolution and Problem Solving:** Healthy families are able to engage in overt conflict and successfully resolve conflicts and solve problems, which may involve win-win scenarios, compromises, or acceptance of differences.

- **Sexuality:** In healthy families, couples share sexual intimacy, and sexuality is contained within generational lines.

- **Loyalty and Commitment:** Members experience a clear sense of loyalty and commitment while allowing for individual autonomy.

- **Parental Empathy:** Parents should demonstrate empathy for children's experience while still maintaining boundaries and structure; parents who were abused as children often fail to have sufficient empathy or are overly empathetic and do not set healthy boundaries.

- **Playfulness, Creativity, and Humor:** Fun and laughter are signs of healthy family functioning.

- **Cultural Adaptations:** Immigrant families are able to balance the needs of their culture of origin and their current cultural context.

- **Symbolic Process:** Each family has particular symbols and images that are "affectively loaded" and thus helpful in facilitating change.

Focus on Competency

When assessing families, symbolic-experiential therapists emphasize strengths, competencies, and resources for change (Roberto, 1991). Families are viewed as highly resilient and resourceful, and therapists focus on activating these resources (Whitaker & Bumberry, 1988).

Symptom Development

Symptoms develop when dysfunctional structures and processes persist over time (Roberto, 1991). Healthy families experience periods of dysfunction and difficulty, but these do not become chronic. The persistence of dysfunction can occur over generations, with offspring feeling obligated to adhere to family myths and legacies or to make up for prior losses.

Targeting Change: Goal Setting

Symbolic-experiential therapists have three primary long-term goals for all clients:

- **Increase Family Cohesion:** Create a sense of nurturance and confidence in problem solving (Roberto, 1991)

- **Promote Personal Growth:** Support the completion of developmental tasks for all family members (Roberto, 1991; Whitaker & Bumberry, 1988)

- **Expand the Family's Symbolic World** (Whitaker & Bumberry, 1988)

Increase Family Cohesion

The first goal involves increasing cohesion and the authenticity of family relationships, which means increasing the sense of love and meaningful connection between family members. Therapists focus on two key areas to achieve this goal:

- **Cohesion:** More than many other family therapists, symbolic-experiential therapists focus on increasing the sense of family cohesion, the emotional connection between family members. The outer expression of cohesion and connection varies across cultures and genders, but it is generally characterized by a strong sense of belonging, being loved, being wanted, and loyalty.

- **Interpersonal Boundaries:** Symbolic-experiential family therapists also use the term *boundaries* to refer to the relational rules that regulate closeness and distance. Boundaries should allow (a) each person to have enough freedom to be fully himself or herself (i.e., authentic), and (b) strong emotional connection and intimacy between family members.

- **Transgenerational Boundaries:** Transgenerational boundaries should allow for sufficient autonomy of the nuclear family while encouraging connection with extended families.

Promote Personal Growth

Symbolic-experiential family therapists aim to increase each person's level of personal growth by successfully navigating developmental tasks, a process also referred to as *self-actualization*. Because self-actualization is a lifelong process, how a therapist and client know when therapy is done can be a tricky question. At minimum, client self-actualization and growth should be promoted to the point where the client is no longer experiencing symptoms at the individual level, such as depression or anxiety, and can function in most areas of daily life, such as school or work. Beyond a base level of individual functioning, therapists aim to promote personal growth and a more authentic experience of self and self-expression. This is a more difficult quality to quantify, but it is generally easy for clients to articulate a sense of growth or being more of who they are. Therapists encourage clients to pursue specific self-growth goals that relate to their presenting problem. Examples include the following:

- Increase ability to express thoughts and feelings respectfully with others and decrease people-pleasing behaviors
- Increase ability to connect with others at a deeper emotional level and to express this connection verbally
- Increase ability to consciously respond to stress rather than react with anger or fear
- Increase proactive handling of problems and reduce procrastination and avoidance

Expand the Family's Symbolic World

Symbolic-experiential therapists believe that people filter their lives through relatively few constructs or beliefs about life; these constructs constitute a person's *symbolic world*.

All experiences are filtered through this system of symbolic meaning to interpret life events as good or bad, problematic or joyful. As a growth-oriented approach, experiential therapy aims to expand the meaning of experience and broaden the client's life horizons: "If we can aid in the expansion of the symbolic world of the families we see, they can live richer lives" (Whitaker & Bumberry, 1988, p. 75). For example, if a family identifies itself with hard work and success at the expense of personal relationships, the therapist explores the source of this identity and may try to expand the meaning of success to include relational, health, and other spheres of life in addition to work.

The Doing: Interventions

Creating Confusion and Disorganization

In the early phases of therapy, symbolic-experiential therapists create confusion and disorganization to break the family out of their rigid interaction patterns: "confusion is, by itself, one of the most potent ways to symbolically open up the infrastructure of the family" (Whitaker & Bumberry, 1988, p. 82). Confusion can be created with absurd comments (e.g., offering ridiculous solutions), role reversals (e.g., relabeling a child's correcting of the parent as the child trying to parent the parent), or appealing to universal principles that are at odds with the family's beliefs (e.g., that teen rebellion is normal or a rite of passage).

Here-and-Now Experiencing

Believing that people rarely grow emotionally by intellectual education, symbolic-experiential therapists use present-moment interactions and their own affect to promote change (Mitten & Connell, 2004; Whitaker & Bumberry, 1988). In fact, Whitaker and Bumberry (1988) go so far as to quip: "Nothing worth learning can be taught" (p. 85). Thus therapists use the immediacy of what is in the room—including their own negative emotional responses to clients—to highlight and redirect structural change and confront dysfunctional patterns and beliefs.

Redefining and Expanding Symptoms

Symbolic-experiential therapists often choose to redefine symptoms as ineffective efforts toward growth, thus pointing in the direction of needed change (Connell et al., 1999; Roberto, 1991). Although similar to positive connotation in the Milan approach, the symbolic-experiential approach uses the specific reframe of striving for *growth and authenticity*. For example, a child's refusal to do homework is redefined as fear of failing at a new level of challenge at school. In addition, therapists expand the symptom from an individual matter to a family matter, often extending this to an intergenerational problem (e.g., fear of failure kept grandfather from pursuing his dream of owning his own business; Mitten & Connell, 2004).

Spontaneity, Play, and "Craziness"

Experiential therapists use spontaneity and fun toward several ends (Mitten & Connell, 2004; Roberto, 1991; Whitaker & Bumberry, 1988). First, by being playful, therapists build a strong therapeutic relationship that allows them to directly and honestly confront clients without encountering resistance. When working alone, they position themselves to be the type of person whom the client trusts enough to listen to the raw truth; when working as co-therapists, one therapist tends to be nurturing and the other confrontational. Playfulness also helps to reframe problems that have been unrealistically magnified, as is often the case with parents or spouses who magnify a single flaw in the other and de-emphasize the balance of good qualities. As folk wisdom teaches, laughter is the best medicine, and symbolic-experiential therapists are skilled in using laughter to help their clients heal.

The use of humor and play often goes against common stereotypes about therapists and therapy, which are based primarily on psychodynamic therapies, but most clients find laughter helpful, or at least enjoyable.

Separating Interpersonal from Personal Distress

Symbolic-experiential therapists help clients learn how to separate personal issues from interpersonal issues (Roberto, 1991). Often people get into trouble because they do not know how to allow each person in a relationship to have personal autonomy while also being intimately connected with others. When clients are unreasonably demanding to their partners or children, the therapist helps them sort out where their spheres of influence should begin and end. For example, if a parent is demanding that a child play a certain instrument or sport that the child clearly does not enjoy, the therapist will confront the family about where the parenting ends and the child's autonomy begins. Similarly, with couples, if one partner insists that the other feel a certain way about an issue (e.g., be equally upset about a friend's comment), the therapist will invite the couple to separate out and honor each person's unique response to the situation as well as the underlying need for validation in wanting the partner to respond a certain way.

Affective Confrontation of Rigid Patterns and Roles

Symbolic-experiential family therapists use affective confrontation to interrupt rigid patterns. The goals may be (a) to raise clients' awareness when they do not know how they are contributing to the problem, (b) to raise a taboo subject that the client and others have been avoiding, or (c) to increase motivation to make changes when there is cognitive awareness but no change in action (Roberto, 1991). Whitaker explained:

> I am comfortable pushing the family because of my belief that they have unlimited potential. They have the capacity to expand and progress, if only they have the courage to try. My job is to struggle to mobilize that courage.... Not to push, under the assumption that I might make things worse, is to decide for the family that they're too sick to care and too inept to grow. (Whitaker & Bumberry, 1988, p. 37)

"When did you divorce your husband and marry your son?" and "You are aware that you have abandoned the family to advance your career" are examples of confrontations used to interrupt dysfunctional patterns. In addition, affective confrontation is useful for increasing motivation when the insight is there but no action has followed. For example, with parents who need to save their marriage but have no time for a date because the kids have too many after-school activities, a therapist can say, "What do you think would be more detrimental for your daughter: missing dance practice once a week for a few months or having her parents divorce? Do you want to ask your child what her preference is?"

Augmenting Despair and Amplifying Deviation

With clients who are unrealistically hopeless (pessimists), symbolic-experiential therapists use paradoxical techniques such as augmenting despair and amplifying deviation (Roberto, 1991). As with other paradoxical techniques, the therapist exaggerates the client's symptom, such as despair, slightly—perhaps 10–20%—just enough to get outside the client's comfort zone (or normal range of despair) so that the client can see how out of proportion the despair and negative assumptions are with the facts. This can be done in a playful way or in a more direct and literal way, depending on what would be most useful to the client and most congruent with his/her personality. For example, the therapist may jokingly suggest to a client who feels hopeless about meeting the man of her dreams at age 25 that she perhaps consider a career that will substitute for a marriage, perhaps even join a convent; if such a comment is well timed and delivered, the client is likely to see how unrealistic her despair is.

Absurd Fantasy Alternatives

Symbolic-experiential therapists enjoy inviting clients into absurd fantasy scenarios to shake them out of their patterns and to make realistic solutions more palatable (Mitten & Connell, 2004; Roberto, 1991). Designed to increase the family's flexibility and openness to new behaviors, fantasy alternatives get clients out of their habitual ways of looking at things by playfully perturbing or shaking up the system so that new symbolic meanings, ideas, and perspectives can emerge. Therapists may suggest, "If washing dishes is such a problem, why don't you invest in paper plates?" or "If you need that much space, why don't you build a private cell in the backyard where you can really be alone? I guess that would lead to a fight with your wife as to whether or not to install a heating system."

Reinforcing Parental Hierarchy

Symbolic-experiential therapists are careful to reinforce the parental hierarchy and clearly establish generational boundaries between parents and children (Whitaker & Bumberry, 1988). This involves supporting parents when they make a request of a child, instructing parents to manage a child's behavior in session (rather than having the therapist take over), beginning with parents, and greeting parents first.

Stories, Free Associations, and Metaphors

Symbolic-experiential therapists share stories, free-associate, and offer metaphors to provide powerful images and examples that will inspire clients to change (Mitten & Connel, 2004). Clients can often receive a message more easily through a fictional story or metaphor because it is about somebody else—not them—and so there is less resistance or debate about details.

Emotionally Focused Therapy
In a Nutshell: The Least You Need to Know

Emotionally focused therapy (EFT) is one of the most thoroughly researched approaches in the field and is an empirically validated treatment for treating couples (Johnson, 2004); thus it qualifies as an "evidence-based therapy." Sue Johnson and Les Greenberg (1985, 1994) developed the model using a combination of (a) attachment theory, (b) experiential theory (specifically, Carl Rogers's person-centered therapy), and (c) systems theory (specifically, systemic-structural therapies; see Chapters 9 and 10; Johnson, 2004). Emotionally focused therapists focus on the emotional system of the couple and use heightened affect to help couples restructure their interactional patterns, increase emotional intimacy, and address their attachment needs.

The Juice: Significant Contributions to the Field

If you remember one thing from this chapter, it should be this:

Softening Emotions

A hallmark EFT technique, softening of emotions is used to create emotional bonding, change interactional positions, and redefine the relationship as safe and connected. A softening occurs when a previously blaming, critical partner asks, from a position of emotional vulnerability, a newly accessible partner to meet his/her attachment needs and longings (Johnson, 2004). The more critical partner softens his/her stance and words, allowing the more vulnerable or anxious partner to reduce emotional reactivity and defensiveness. Therapists can facilitate softening by encouraging partners to express their underlying attachment-based fears, including hurt and disappointment, when discussing conflict areas. Typically, this is done by underscoring the attachment issues, such as fear of rejection, in a particular area of tension. For example, if the wife is complaining that the husband does not spend enough time with her and the children, emotionally focused therapists help her to articulate the fear of abandonment and/or feelings of rejection that underlie the complaint, thus revealing the wife's vulnerability and fears rather than her anger and frustration. When she expresses these softer emotions of vulnerability and asks her husband directly for comfort and connection, generally a more productive and healing conversation occurs that creates new bonding events.

Rumor Has It: The People and Their Stories

Susan Johnson

With Les Greenberg, Sue Johnson began developing emotionally focused therapy in the 1980s. They developed this approach by refining their methods based on the outcomes of their research on what worked and what did not work. Sue Johnson has continued research on the model, particularly as it applies to couples and families, and also teaches internationally. She has applied emotionally focused therapy to the treatment of a host of issues, including couples therapy with trauma survivors (Johnson, 2002), depression, and couples with chronically ill children (Johnson, 2004). She has also created, with her colleagues, a detailed workbook for people learning EFT (Johnson, Bradley, Furrow, Lee, Palmer, Tilley, & Woolley, 2005).

Les Greenberg

With Sue Johnson, Les Greenberg co-developed EFT while serving as a professor at York University in Toronto and the director of the York University Psychotherapy Research Clinic. He teaches internationally and continues to research and refine a version of the model he calls emotion-focused therapy. Although he has focused primarily on its application to individuals, he has recently written a book called *Emotion-Focused Couple Therapy: The Dynamics of Emotion, Love, and Power* (Greenberg & Goldman, 2008).

The Big Picture: Overview of Treatment

Johnson (2004) identifies three primary therapeutic tasks:

Task 1: Creating and maintaining alliance
Task 2: Assessing and formulating emotion
Task 3: Restructuring interactions

She also identifies *three stages with nine steps* that describe the progression of therapy (Johnson, 2004):

Stage 1: De-escalation of Negative Cycles

Step 1: Create an alliance and delineate conflict in the attachment struggle
Step 2: Identify the negative interaction cycle
Step 3: Access unacknowledged emotions and underlying interactional positions
Step 4: Reframe problem in terms of negative cycle and attachment needs, with the cycle being the common enemy

Stage 2: Change Interactional Patterns

Step 5: Promote identification of disowned attachment needs and aspects of self, integrating these into relational interactions

Step 6: Promote acceptance of the partner's experience along with new interaction sequences

Step 7: Encourage expression of needs and wants while increasing emotional engagement and bonding to redefine the couple's attachment

Stage 3: Consolidation and Integration

Step 8: Facilitate new solutions to old problems

Step 9: Consolidate new positions and new cycles of attachment

Making Connection: The Therapeutic Relationship

Empathetic Attunement

The therapist attunes to each partner's emotions with the intent to make contact with each of their emotional worlds (Johnson, 2004). Empathetic attunement requires listening to clients, connecting what they say with the therapist's personal experience, and then staying within the client's subjective perspective. Such attunement typically happens more at the nonverbal level, both in perceiving the client's emotional state and in reflecting it back through nonverbal communication (e.g., by softening the voice, nodding the head).

Acceptance

Therapists maintain a nonjudgmental stance that is grounded in a positive view of human nature and acceptance of human struggles. Acceptance involves honoring and prizing clients *as they are* and acknowledging the fullness of their humanity.

Genuineness

Genuineness requires that the therapist be real and emotionally present with clients without being impulsive or constantly disclosing personal information. Therapists are humble and able to admit mistakes and misunderstandings. As a result, clients experience the relationship between them and the therapist as an authentic human encounter.

Continuous Monitoring of the Alliance

The therapist continually monitors the therapeutic alliance with each partner to ensure that a strong affective connection and sense of safety continue through all stages of therapy. When expressing empathy in couples therapy, it is particularly easy for the alliance with one partner to weaken as the therapist expresses an understanding of the other partner, because for a moment the therapist may appear to be taking sides in an attempt to understand. Thus therapists need to constantly balance their focus between the two partners.

Joining the System

The therapist must build an alliance not only with each individual but also with the relationship as a system, accepting it as it is, just as each individual is accepted. Joining the system involves not only identifying relational patterns (e.g., nag/withdraw, pursue/distance, criticize/defend) but also reflecting these back to the couple so that they can better understand their relationship.

The Therapist's Role

According to Johnson (2004), the therapist is the following:

- A process consultant who helps the couple reprocess their emotional experiences
- A choreographer who helps the couple restructure their relationship dance
- A collaborator who follows and leads the therapeutic alliance

The therapist is *not* the following:

- A coach teaching communication skills
- A "wise creator of insight" into the past and/or future
- A strategist employing paradox or problem prescription

Expression of Empathy: RISSSC

Johnson (2004) uses the following techniques (RISSSC) to express understanding of the client's affective reality:

- **Repeat:** Repeat key words and phrases the client says
- **Images:** Use images to capture emotion in a way that abstract words cannot
- **Simple:** Use simple words and phrases
- **Slow:** Maintain a slow pace that enables emotional experience to unfold
- **Soft:** Use a voice to soothe and encourage deeper experiencing and risk taking
- **Clients' Words:** Adopt clients' words and phrases in a validating way

The Viewing: Case Conceptualization and Assessment

Intrapsychic and Interpersonal Issues

Much like other experiential family therapists, the EFT therapist attends to both intrapsychic and interpersonal issues.

- **Intrapsychic:** How individuals process their experiences, particularly their key attachment-oriented emotional responses
- **Interpersonal:** How partners organize their interactions into patterns and cycles

Attachment and Adult Love

Using Bowlby's (1988) theory of attachment to conceptualize adult love, Johnson (2004) identifies 10 tenets of this theory (pp. 25–32).

1. **Attachment Is an Innate Motivating Force:** The desire to be connected to others is intrinsic.

2. **Secure Dependence Complements Dependency:** Neither complete independence nor overdependence is possible, only effective or ineffective dependency.

3. **Attachment Offers an Essential Safe Haven:** Secure attachment provides a buffer against stress and uncertainty.

4. **Attachment Offers a Secure Base:** A secure base allows for exploration, innovation, and openness.

5. **Emotional Accessibility and Responsiveness Build Bonds:** Secure attachment is established by being emotionally accessible and responsive.

6. **Fear and Uncertainty Activate Attachment Needs:** When threatened, a person experiences a strong emotional need for comfort and connection.

7. **The Process of Separation Distress Is Predictable:** If attachment needs are not met, the person experiences predictable responses of anger, clinging, depression, and despair.

8. **There Are a Finite Number of Insecure Attachment Styles:**
   - **Anxious and Hyperactivated:** When needs are not met, the person becomes anxiously clingy, relentlessly pursues connection, and may become aggressive, blaming, and critical.

- **Avoidance:** When needs are not met, the person suppresses attachment needs and instead focuses on tasks or other distractions.
    - **Combination Anxious and Avoidant:** In this style, the person pursues closeness and then avoids it once offered.

9. **Attachment Involves Working Models of Self and Other:** People use the quality of attachments to define themselves and others as lovable, worthy, and competent.

10. **Isolation and Loss Are Inherently Traumatizing:** Isolation and loss of connection are inherently traumatic experiences.

Primary and Secondary Emotions

How does an emotionally focused therapist know which emotions to focus on? Is any emotion a client expresses worthy of focus? The answers to these questions are multilayered. First, emotionally focused therapists distinguish between primary emotions and secondary emotions:

- **Primary Emotions:** Stem from attachment fears and needs (usually softer, more vulnerable emotions, such as helplessness)
- **Secondary Emotions:** Such as anger, frustration, and withdrawal

In the early phases of therapy, the therapist focuses on the salient secondary emotions, encouraging partners to express their own emotions rather than blame the other. As therapy progresses, the therapist begins to raise each partner's awareness of the primary emotion underlying the secondary emotion, such as the hurt that is beneath the anger of having one's partner no longer expressing sexual interest.

Negative Interaction Cycle

One of the therapist's first tasks is to identify negative interaction cycles, such as nag/withdraw, pursuer/distancer, or criticize/defend interactions. Therapists focus on the *command* aspect of communication (see Chapter 8), which is the relationship-defining aspect of any communication. By understanding this command aspect, the therapist can quickly identify often-unexpressed emotions that are related to unmet attachment needs.

Targeting Change: Goal Setting

The goals of EFT include the following:

- Creating secure attachment for both partners
- Developing new interaction patterns that nurture and support each partner
- Increasing direct expression of emotions, especially those related to attachment needs

The Doing: Interventions

Reflection of Emotion

The EFT therapist attends to poignant emotions and *reflects* back to the client a deep understanding and acceptance of these emotions (Johnson, 2004). The goal of reflection is to help clients more fully experience their emotions, both primary (attachment-based) and secondary. As therapy progresses, reflections should highlight unmet attachment needs: "What I hear you saying is not only that you get angry when he does not call but that you begin to fear he does not love you anymore."

Validation

Rather than imply approval, validation communicates to clients that their emotional experiences are understandable and understood by the therapist. Therapists use validation to convey that each partner is entitled to his or her experience and emotional responses, helping to articulate the underlying logic and emotions of each person's behaviors: "At first you feel very sad that he does not seem to want to spend time with you, but after a while you become angry and then try to force him to spend time with you."

Evocative Responding: Reflections and Questions

Whether phrased as reflections or questions, therapists use evocative responses to bypass superficial issues and identify unexpressed emotions and needs (Johnson, 2004). Because evocative responses are based on conjecture, the therapist offers these *tentatively*, allowing the client to correct or rephrase: "I think that part of the reason you may be pulling away is that you want closeness and connection so badly; if you were to be rejected, you would be devastated."

Heightening

The therapist heightens key emotions and interactions that play a crucial role in maintaining the couple's negative cycle (Johnson, 2004). The therapist can heighten by repeating a high-impact phrase (e.g., "feeling betrayed"), using nonverbal gestures like leaning forward or lowering the voice, using images and metaphors, or directing clients to enact responses. The therapist may also ask the client to repeat poignant moments: "Can you say that again—that you need her? Can you look at her and say that again?"

Empathetic Conjecture and Interpretation

At times the EFT therapist will offer an empathetic conjecture or interpretation, typically addressing defensive strategies, attachment longings, and attachment fears (Johnson, 2004). In the later phases of therapy, conjecture is used to *seed attachment* by highlighting the desire for attachment that is blocked by fear or anger.

Tracking and Reflecting Interaction Patterns

Therapists track patterns and cycles of interactions and then reflect on these patterns to help couples better understand the nature of their relationship (Johnson, 2004). For example, they look for common pursue/withdrawal and blame/defend patterns and attend to the unique sequences of each couple's interactions.

Reframing Problems Contextually

Consistent with Johnson's systemic perspective, problems are reframed in the broader context of the relationship to emphasize the underlying vulnerabilities and attachment processes (Johnson, 2004). For example, anger may be reframed as attachment protest or withdrawal as fear of rejection. To increase solidarity, the negative interaction cycle is always framed as the couple's common enemy.

Enactments, Restructuring, and Choreography

As in structural therapy, couples are asked to enact their present positions so that the therapist can help them more fully experience their underlying emotions (Johnson, 2004). The therapist then redirects or "choreographs" the couple's interaction to be less constricting and more accepting, perhaps by asking a partner to share a new affective insight directly with the other or by physically repositioning the couple to increase emotional intensity. In the later stages of therapy, the therapist usually uses enactments to choreograph partners' requests of each other and to create new positive responses that will lead to new bonding experiences that redefine the relationship as safe and secure.

Turning the New Emotional Experience into a New Response

After helping one partner explore an emotional experience, the therapist uses this experience to allow the other partner to respond in new ways, creating a positive interaction cycle in which each partner is better able to understand himself/herself and the other: "What is happening for you when you hear him say that his avoidance is not motivated by disinterest but by fear of rejection?" (Johnson, 2004).

Self-Disclosure

Used infrequently, self-disclosure can build rapport or intensify validation of client responses (Johnson, 2004). However, the therapist keeps self-disclosure to a minimum to maintain a focus on the emotional process of the couple.

Snapshot: Research and the Evidence Base

Quick Summary: *There is excellent research support for EFT, few systematic outcome studies on other experiential approaches, and strong support for the experiential approach to forming therapeutic relationships.*

Research on Humanistic Principles

With the notable exception of emotionally focused couples therapy (Johnson, 2004), an empirically supported treatment (see Chapter 7), there is minimal outcome research on the effectiveness of experiential family therapies. However, what has received attention is the therapeutic relationship as defined by experiential and humanistic therapies. The common factors model (Sprenkle, Davis, & Lebow, 2009; see Chapter 7) purports that 30% of therapeutic outcome in any form of therapy can be attributed to the therapeutic relationship as defined in the humanistic tradition: nonjudgmental, empathetic, and engaged (Miller, Duncan, & Hubble, 1997). Therefore, although the specific interventions and overall outcome have not received significant research support, the principles behind the humanistic approach to therapeutic relationships have strong, consistent support.

Research on EFT Effectiveness

Researched for over 25 years, EFT is currently the only empirically validated couples therapy. EFT has a 70–73% recovery rate in 10 to 12 sessions, with 90% of all couples showing significant improvement (Johnson, Hunsley, Greenberg, & Schindler, 1999), compared with a 35% recovery rate in behavioral couples therapy (Jacobson, Follette, & Pagel, 1986). Relapse is rarely a problem in EFT, whereas in behavioral couples therapy gains are rarely maintained at a two-year follow-up (Jacobson & Addis, 1993). Research has demonstrated EFT's effectiveness with two difficult-to-treat couples: trauma survivors and parents of chronically ill children (Clotheir, Manion, Gordon-Walker, & Johnson, 2002; Johnson, 2005).

Snapshot: Working with Diverse Populations

Quick Summary: *Experiential approaches are used internationally, especially EFT and Satir's growth model; however, these approaches should be carefully adapted for patterns of and attitudes toward emotional expression in a specific subpopulation.*

Used with a wide range of clients, experiential approaches value clear, congruent emotional expression and the willingness to be vulnerable. Therefore, when working with populations that have different attitudes toward emotional expression and/or are in a treatment context where such vulnerability feels unsafe, therapists need to proceed thoughtfully. For example, the emotional expression often promoted in Satir's communication approach may not be comfortable for some men or East Asian-Americans, populations that generally value less dramatic and more indirect emotional expression. Similarly, an experiential approach may be too threatening for mandated clients, who often feel that they might be in a worse position with the courts or social agencies that mandated their treatment if they express too much or certain emotions. Given the fact that a report will be sent to an outside party, these clients are less trusting of the therapeutic relationship.

Additionally, therapists need to monitor their expectations for women's level and style of emotional expression; nontraditional female clients report feeling that their therapists expect that they express their emotions in a certain way and report feeling judged and misunderstood because they do not subscribe to stereotyped modes of female emotional expression (Gehart & Lyle, 2001). Therapists working with such clients must be very careful to (a) avoid inaccurate assessment due to different cultural and gender standards and values concerning emotional expression, (b) adjust the level of intimacy in the therapeutic alliance to fit with the client's level of comfort, and (c) choose interventions that actively engage clients at their comfortable level. The case study that follows this chapter details how an experiential therapy would design treatment for a Greek-Armenian family whose teenage daughter has been sexually molested.

ONLINE RESOURCES

Emotionally Focused Therapy: Sue Johnson, Canada
www.eft.ca

Emotionally Focused Therapy: San Diego, California
www.sdeft.us

Emotionally Focused Therapy: Los Angeles and Houston
www.theeftzone.com

Emotion-Focused Therapy: Les Greenberg, Canada
www.emotionfocusedtherapy.org

Satir Global Network (formerly AVANTA): Includes links to training institutes in Asia, Europe, South America
www.avanta.net

Satir Institute of the Pacific: John Banmen
http://www.satirpacific.org/

Satir Institute of the Rockies
http://www.satirtraining.org

Satir Institute of the Southeast
http://www.satirinstitute.org/

Satir Training Centre Ottawa
http://www.satirottawa.ca/main/

Science and Behavior Books: Publishing books on the Satir Model
www.sbbks.com

REFERENCES

*Asterisk indicates recommended introductory readings.

Azpeitia, L. M. (1991). The Satir model in action [course reader]. Encino, CA: California Family Study Center.

Azpeitia, L. M. (1995). Blossoms in Satir's garden: Lynne Azpeitia's work with gifted adults. *Advanced Development, Special Edition,* 127–146.

Banmen, J. (Guest Ed.). (2002). The Satir model: Yesterday and today (Special issue). *Contemporary Family Therapy, 24.*

Banmen, J. (2003). *Meditations of Virginia Satir.* Palo Alto, CA: Science and Behavioral Books.

Bowlby, J. (1988). *A secure base: parent-child attachment and healthy human development.* London: Routledge.

Clotheir, P., Manion, I., Gordon-Walker, J., & Johnson, S. M. (2002). Emotionally focused interventions for couples with chronically ill children: A two year follow-up. *Journal of Marital and Family Therapy, 28,* 391–399.

Connell, G., Mitten, T., & Bumberry, W. (1999). *Reshaping family relationships: The symbolic-experiential therapy of Carl Whitaker.* Philadelphia: Brunner/Mazel.

Gehart, D. R., & Lyle, R. R. (2001). Client experience of gender in therapeutic relationships: An interpretive ethnography. *Family Process, 40,* 443–458.

Gehart, D., & McCollum, E. (2008). Teaching therapeutic presence: A mindfulness-based approach. In S. Hicks (Ed.), *Mindfulness and the healing relationship.* New York: Guilford.

Gomori, Maria. (2002). *Passion for freedom.* Palo Alto, CA: Science and Behavior Books.

Greenberg, L. S., & Goldman, R. N. (2008). *Emotion-focused couple therapy: The dynamics of emotion, love, and power.* Washington, DC: American Psychological Association.

Jacobson, N. S., & Addis, M. E. (1993). Research on couples and couples therapy: What do we know? Where are we going? *Journal of Consulting and Clinical Psychology, 57,* 5–10.

Jacobson, N. S., Follette, W. C., & Pagel, M. (1986). Predicting who will benefit from behavioral marital therapy. *Journal of Counsulting and Clinical Psychology, 54,* 518–522.

*Johnson, S. M. (2004). *The practice of emotionally focused marital therapy: Creating connection* (2nd ed.). New York: Brunner/Routledge.

Johnson, S. M. (2005). *Emotionally focused couple therapy with trauma survivors: Strengthening attachment bonds.* New York: Guilford.

Johnson, S. M., Bradley, B., Furrow, J., Lee, A., Palmer, G., Tilley, D., & Woolley, S. (2005). *Becoming an emotionally focused couples therapist: A workbook.* New York: Brunner/Routledge.

Johnson, S. M., & Greenberg, L. S. (1985). The differential effects of experiential and problem solving interventions in resolving marital conflicts. *Journal of Consulting and Clinical Psychology, 53,* 175–184.

Johnson, S. M., & Greenberg, L. S. (Eds.). (1994). *The heart of the matter: Perspectives on emotion in marital therapy.* New York: Brunner/Mazel.

Johnson, S. M., Hunsley, J., Greenberg, L. S., & Schindler, D. (1999). Emotionally focused couples therapy: Status and challenges. *Clinical Psychology: Science and Practice, 6,* 67–79.

Keith, D., Connell, G., & Connell, L. (2001). *Defiance in the family: Finding hope in therapy.* New York: Routledge.

Miller, S. D., Duncan, B. L., & Hubble, M. (1997). *Escape from Babel: Toward a unifying language for psychotherapy practice.* New York: Norton.

Mitten, T. J., & Connel, G. M. (2004). The core variables of symbolic-experiential therapy: A qualitative study. *Journal of Marital and Family Therapy, 30,* 467–478.

*Napier, A. Y., & Whitaker, C. (1978). *The family crucible: The intense experience of family therapy.* New York: Harper.

Neff, K. (2003). Self-compassion: An alternative conceptualization of a healthy attitude toward oneself. *Self and Identity, 2,* 85–101.

*Roberto, L. G. (1991). Symbolic-experiential family therapy. In A. S. Gurman & D. P. Kniskern (Eds.), *Handbook of family therapy* (Vol. 2, pp. 444–476). New York: Brunner/Mazel.

Rogers, Carl. (1961). *On becoming a person: A therapist's view of psychotherapy.* London: Constable.

Rogers, C. (1981). *Way of being.* Boston: Houghton Mifflin.

Satir, V. (1967/1983). *Conjoint family therapy* (3rd revised ed.). Palo Alto, CA: Science and Behavior Books.

Satir, V. (1972). *Peoplemaking.* Palo Alto, CA: Science and Behavior Books.

Satir, V. (1988). *The new peoplemaking.* Palo Alto, CA: Science and Behavior Books.

Satir, V., & Baldwin, M. (1983). *Satir step by step: A guide to creating change in families.* Palo Alto, CA: Science and Behavior Books.

*Satir, V., Banmen, J., Gerber, J., & Gomori, M. (1991). *The Satir model: Family therapy and beyond.* Palo Alto, CA: Science and Behavior Books.

Sprenkle, D. H., Davis, S. D., & Lebow, J. (2009). *Beyond our sacred models: Common factors in couple, family, and relational psychotherapy.* New York: Guilford.

Whitaker, C. A. (1975). Psychotherapy of the absurd: With a special emphasis on the psychotherapy of aggression. *Family Process, 14,* 1–15.

*Whitaker, C. A., & Bumberry, W. M. (1988). *Dancing with the family.* New York: Brunner/Mazel.

*Whitaker, C. A., & Keith, D. V. (1981). Symbolic-experiential family therapy. In A. S. Gurman & D. P. Kniskern (Eds.), *Handbook of family therapy* (pp. 187–224). New York: Brunner/Mazel.

Whitaker, C. A., & Ryan, M. C. (1989). *Midnight musings of a family therapist.* New York: Norton.

EXPERIENTIAL CASE STUDY

Brad and Sophie have sought counseling because they just discovered that recently a female babysitter had sexually abused their daughter, Briana. A report was made to child protective services, and the baby sitter, who was 16, is currently being charged with the abuse. Briana has become socially withdrawn and reports intrusive thoughts about the abuse. Both practicing lawyers, the couple report increased arguing over the past year since Sophie has had to travel more for work and Brad has had to pick up more of the childcare duties. Sophie feels guilty about the abuse because her travel schedule necessitated the increased use of babysitters.

After an initial consultation, an experiential family therapist developed the following case conceptualization.

Shaded Sections Emphasized in Experiential Planning and Intervention

CASE CONCEPTUALIZATION FORM

Therapist: Sharee Lee   **Client/Case #:** 1020   **Date:** 9/04/09

I. Introduction to Client and Significant Others *(Include age, ethnicity, occupation, grade, relevant identifiers, etc.). Put an * next to persons in session and/or IP for identified patient.*

*AF†:   36, lawyer, Greek-American, bipolar diagnosis

*AM: 44, lawyer, Armenian-American

CF: 12 (IP) 7th grade, honor student

CM or _____ : _____

II. Presenting Concern

Client's/Family's Descriptions of Problem(s):

AF: Blames self for abuse and feels guilty about pursuing her career.

AM: Although he does not blame AF for the abuse, he is concerned about the weakening of AF's relationship with CF over the past year or two due to her increased focus at work.

CF12:   Feels supported by parents and is happy that her parents believed her; reports feeling increasingly uncomfortable around her peers; having nightmares and intrusive thoughts.

CM or: _____ : _____

Broader System Problem Descriptions (description of problem from referring party, teachers, relatives, legal system, etc.):

Child Protective Services Social Worker: Believes CF's report and has referred her for therapy to address trauma issues.

_____ : _____

III. Background Information

Recent Background (recent life changes, precipitating events, first symptoms, stressors, etc.):

Sophie began traveling more for work a year ago, which necessitated hiring more babysitters for Briana after school and on weekends. Six months ago a female babysitter began molesting Briana, which continued for almost two months before it escalated to a point where Briana told her parents. Her parents promptly made a report and swift action was taken by CPS. Sophie and Brad have been arguing more since she has been traveling, and her relationship with Briana has reportedly weakened during this period also.

---

† *Abbreviations:* AF: Adult Female; AM: Adult Male; CF#: Child Female with age, e.g., CF12; CM#: Child Male with age; IP: Identified patient; Hx: History; Ex: Explanation or Example; NA: Not Applicable.

(continued)

III. Background Information *(continued)*

Related Historical Background (family history, related issues, past abuse, trauma, previous counseling, medical/mental health history, etc.):

Sophie was diagnosed with bipolar, as was her mother and sister, and has had prior therapy related to the mood disorder. She is currently taking medications and reports being stable. There have been several divorces by Brad and Sophie's siblings, which alarms them both.

IV. Systemic Assessment
Client/Relational Strengths

Personal/individual: All three are highly intelligent and well educated. Parents accomplished professionals. AF has learned to manage her bipolar. AM is a highly involved father. CF is talented and well liked at school.

Relational/social: Parents immediately believed CF and did not make her feel guilty for waiting to tell. Both families of origin have frequent family gatherings and stay connected.

Spiritual: AF and AM share the Orthodox tradition and attend church fairly regularly. The couple use church to help them work through their marital difficulties.

Family Structure and Interaction Patterns
Couple Subsystem (to be assessed): ☐ Personal current ☐ Personal past ☒ Parents'

Couple Boundaries: ☐ Clear ☒ Enmeshed ☐ Disengaged ☒ Other: _____

Rules for closeness/distance: Frequently argue over how the other is not making choices he/she approves of. Both put pressure on the other to conduct self according to other's values/wishes.

Couple Problem Interaction Pattern (A ⇄ B):

Start of tension: AF informs AM that she has accepted another case that will require significant travel out of state.

Conflict/symptom escalation: AM gets angry, saying that it is unfair to him and to CF; AF retorts that she had to give up the last 10 years to take care of CF while he moved ahead in his career; the couple continue defending personal positions.

Return to "normal"/homeostasis: Ends by AM saying that he cannot stop her and AF withdrawing to reading, television, or other room.

Couple Complementary Patterns: ☒ Pursuer/distancer ☐ Over/under functioner ☐ Emotional/logical ☐ Good/bad parent ☒ Other: Engaged/disengaged parent; Ex: AM pursues AF for engagement at home; AF withdrawing from family life to fulfill her career aspirations that she feels she is entitled to due to the years lost to raising CF when young.

Satir Communication Stances:

AF: ☐ Congruent ☐ Placator ☒ Blamer ☐ Superreasonable ☐ Irrelevant
AM: ☐ Congruent ☐ Placator ☐ Blamer ☒ Superreasonable ☐ Irrelevant

Describe dynamic: AF focuses on her needs to the exclusion of what others need or what is contextually appropriate; AM is focused on "what needs to get done" with less attention to emotional needs of self or other. This has enabled him to pick up parenting duties as AF works longer hours.

Gottman's Divorce Indicators:

Criticism: ☐ AF ☒ AM. Ex: AM critical of AF's choices to prioritize work.

Defensiveness: ☒ AF ☐ AM. Ex: AF very defensive about choices; easily triggered.

Contempt: ☐ AF ☐ AM. Ex: NA

Stonewalling: ☒ AF ☒ AM. Ex: Both tend to stonewall other to manage conflict.

Failed repair attempts: ☐ AF ☐ AM. Ex: Neither frequently extends repair attempt.

Not accept influence: ☒ AF ☐ AM. Ex: AF refusing to accept influence of AM at this point in relationship due to her sense of entitlement to "catch up" in work life.

Harsh startup: ☐ AF ☒ AM. Ex: AM increasingly harsh in raising issues.

Parental Subsystem: ☒ Family of procreation ☐ Family of origin

Membership in Family Subsystems: Parental: ☒ AF ☒ AM ☐ Other: _____
Is parental subsystem distinct from couple subsystem? ☒ Yes ☐ No ☐ NA (divorce) Couple do have distinct marital subsystem, with their shared profession a significant binding force.

Sibling subsystem: NA.

Special interest: AF and AM have professional connection: lawyers. CF "joins" this system by maintaining high grades and showing interest in history and politics.

Family Life Cycle Stage:
☐ Single adult ☐ Marriage ☐ Family with young children
☒ Family with adolescent children ☐ Launching children ☐ Later life
Describe struggles with mastering developmental tasks in one of these stages:

AF conformed to stereotypical mother role through young childhood, but as CF is approaching teenage years, AF feels more entitled to pursue her career aspirations. She is feeling her job is "mostly done" because CF is already so high functioning.

Hierarchy Between Child/Parents:
AF: ☐ Effective ☐ Insufficient (permissive) ☐ Excessive (authoritarian) ☒ Inconsistent
AM: ☒ Effective ☐ Insufficient (permissive) ☐ Excessive (authoritarian) ☐ Inconsistent
Ex: AM has established a consistent, effective hierarchy with CF. AF had a more effective hierarchy before she began to turn over her parenting duties and authority to AM. CF wants to connect with AF: thus she has some influence; but CF is also angry about AF's choice to travel.

(*continued*)

IV. Systemic Assessment *(continued)*

Emotional Boundaries with Children:

AF: ☐ Clear/balanced ☐ Enmeshed (reactive) ☒ Disengaged (disinterested)

   ☐ Other: _____

AM: ☒ Clear/balanced ☐ Enmeshed (reactive) ☐ Disengaged (disinterested)

   ☒ Other: Limited emotional connection.

Ex: AF was much more emotionally engaged prior to the past year; AM maintains a fairly clear emotional boundary with CF but it is limited in its emotional depth; their connection is through joint activities and intellectual discussion.

Problem Interaction Pattern (A $\rightleftarrows$ B):

Start of tension: CF crying and upset related to memories of abuse.

Conflict/symptom escalation: AM tries to calm her with logical discussion. CF knows he is trying but does not get her emotional needs met. AM calls AF and tells her to talk with CF on phone, but CF does not want to talk.

Return to "normal"/homeostasis: CF eventually calms down, generally going to bed and waking up in a better mood.

Triangles/Coalitions:

☐ AF and CM _____ against AM: Ex: _____.

☒ AM and CF against AF: Ex: In past year, AM and CF have become much closer, each angry at AF's life decision.

☐ Other: Ex: _____

Communication Stances:

AF or _____ : ☐ Congruent ☐ Placator ☒ Blamer ☐ Superreasonable ☐ Irrelevant

AM or _____ : ☐ Congruent ☐ Placator ☐ Blamer ☒ Superreasonable ☐ Irrelevant

CF or _____ : ☐ Congruent ☒ Placator ☐ Blamer ☐ Superreasonable ☐ Irrelevant

CM or _____ : ☐ Congruent ☐ Placator ☐ Blamer ☐ Superreasonable ☐ Irrelevant

Ex: CF is the peacemaker in the family and the most emotionally attuned to others. AF is more focused on her needs. AM tends to be very logical and have difficulty connecting emotionally, which is what CF needs most right now.

Hypothesis (Describe possible role or function of symptom in maintaining family homeostasis):

CF's emotional needs as she recovers from the abuse have forced the family to address dynamics that were only mildly problematic in the past: AF's travel, AM's lack of emotional availability, and the couple's unresolved issues related to AF's career dilemma.

Intergenerational Patterns

Substance/alcohol abuse: ☒ NA ☐ Hx: _____

Sexual/physical/emotional abuse: ☐ NA ☒ Hx: AF's parents had emotionally abusive relationship.

Parent/child relations: ☐ NA ☒ Hx: Mothers on both sides have close relationships to one child that fulfill unmet needs from marriage.

Physical/mental disorders: ☐ NA ☒ Hx: AF, her mother, and younger sister all diagnosed with bipolar or believed to have it (mother).

Historical incidents of presenting problem: ☐ NA ☒ Hx: AF and sister were both sexually abused as children by cousin; both parents come from professional families in which mother able to pursue careers; all married siblings on both sides have had conflictual marriages.

Family strengths: Religious faith; strong immigrant work ethics; professionals.

Previous Solutions and Unique Outcomes

Solutions that DIDN'T work: The couple arguing about AF's work priority has not helped; parents have not been particularly helpful in supporting CF with the abuse.

Solutions that DID work: Parents believed CF and took *actions* that made CF feel supported and protected; when AF is home long enough to relax, she can connect better with CF. AM's choice to take up more of the parenting duties demonstrates to CF that he really cares.

Narratives, Dominant Discourses, and Diversity
Dominant Discourses informing definition of problem:

Cultural, ethnic, SES, etc.: Their Greek/Armenian immigrant and Orthodox heritage informs multiple values: the drive for success, hard working, dedicated to family (for AF this was true with CF until she became more independent), dedicated to marriage, acceptance of open conflict, and open emotional expression. The parents feel significant shame and guilt in not protecting daughter better.

Gender, sex orientation, etc.: AF in particular is struggling with traditional definition of her role in the family as a woman and modern standards of women's success professionally. Up to this point, she has found these two roles incompatible, able to do one or the other at a time. Furthermore, AF is angry at herself for letting her daughter be abused the way she and her sister were. By taking up the primary parenting role, AM has stepped out of strong cultural gender stereotypes.

Other social influences: As lawyers, AF and AM have intense fights and can use very sharp words with each other. Their cultural background, professions, and favored survival stances (blamer and superreasonable) enable them to have more intense conflict with less emotional damage than is typical.

Identity Narratives that have developed around problem for AF, AM, and/or CM/F: AF feels extremely guilty about her travel creating the conditions that led to abuse and yet she feels powerless

IV. Systemic Assessment (*continued*)

to stop her current career path with significant damage to her clients and feeling like a failure. AM has surprised himself in how much he has enjoyed taking on as primary caregiver, although a dark cloud hangs over it because it feels like he is losing his wife in the process. CF feels "damaged" from the abuse and "unwanted" due to her mother's perceived abandonment.

Local or Preferred Discourses: AF wants to find a way to balance her role as mother and wife with her role as a high-powered professional. AM wants to have AF more engaged in the family while maintaining his more involved role as father.

Other Influential Discourses: AF and AM are both afraid of the divorce patterns their siblings have and want to avoid this for themselves. AF and her sister want to ensure that CF overcomes the abuse and gets more help than they did when they were young.

V. Genogram

Construct a family genogram and include all relevant information, including:

- ages, birth/death dates
- names
- relational patterns
- occupations
- medical history
- psychiatric disorders
- abuse history

Also include a couple of adjectives for persons frequently discussed in session (these should describe personal qualities and/or relational patterns, e.g., quiet, family caretaker, emotionally distant, perfectionist, helpless, etc.). Genogram should be attached to report.

VI. Client Perspectives

Areas of Agreement: Based on what the client(s) has(ve) said, what parts of the above assessment do they agree with or are likely to agree with?

Family would agree with description of basic tension due to AF's work priorities and impact of abuse on CF.

Areas of Disagreement: What parts do they disagree with or are likely to disagree with? Why? AF does not see herself as disengaged the way CF and AM describe her and has a difficult time understanding why they are so unable to understand her need to excel at work.

How do you plan to respectfully work with areas of disagreement? Approach issue of how CF and AM perceive AF's choices gently and without judgment and try to increase each person's understanding of the other's needs and perceptions.

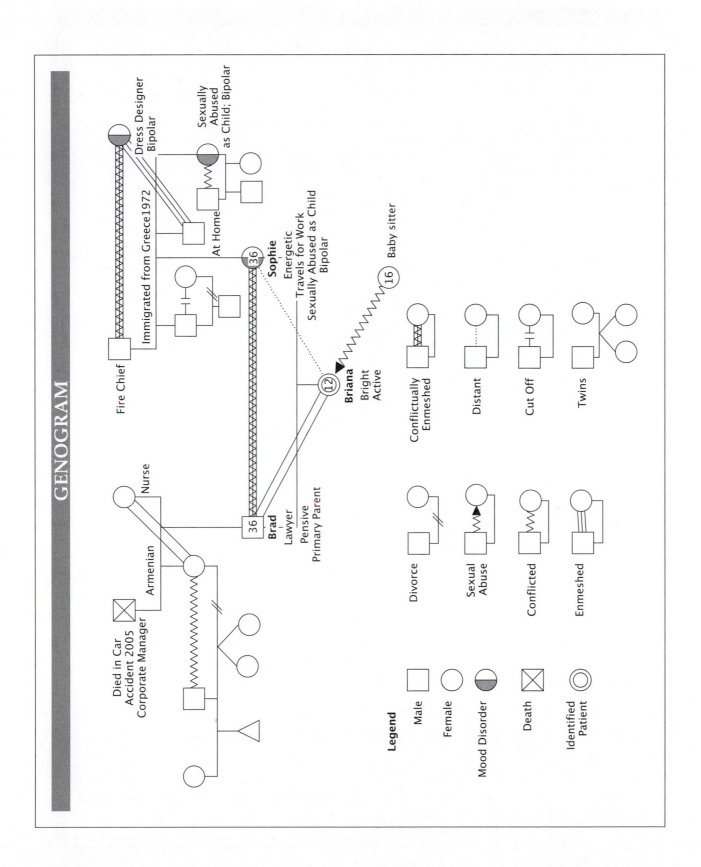

CLINICAL ASSESSMENT

Client ID # (do not use name): 1020	Ethnicities: Armenian-American/ Greek-American	Primary Language: ☒ Eng ☐ Span ☒ Other: 2nd Lang Greek

List all participants/significant others: Put a [★] for Identified Patient [IP]; [✔] for Sig. others who **WILL** attend; [×] for Sig. others who will *NOT* attend.

Adult: Age: Profession/Employer	Child: Age: School/Grade
[✔] AM† 44: Lawyer; Armenian-American	[ ] CM _____
[✔] AF 36: Lawyer; Greek-American	[★] CF 12: 7th Grade _____
[ ] AF/M #2 _____	[ ] CF/M #2 _____

Presenting Problem

		Complete for children
☒ Depression/hopelessness	☒ Couple concerns	☒ School failure/decline performance
☐ Anxiety/worry	☐ Parent/child conflict	
☐ Anger issues	☐ Partner violence/abuse	☐ Truancy/runaway
☒ Loss/grief	☐ Divorce adjustment	☐ Fighting w/peers
☐ Suicidal thoughts/attempts	☐ Remarriage adjustment	☐ Hyperactivity
☒ Sexual abuse/rape	☐ Sexuality/intimacy concerns	☐ Wetting/soiling clothing
☐ Alcohol/drug use	☒ Major life changes	☒ Child abuse/neglect
☐ Eating problems/disorders	☐ Legal issues/probation	☒ Isolation/withdrawal
☐ Job problems/unemployed	☒ Other: Nightmares; trauma	☐ Other: _____

Mental Status for IP

Interpersonal issues	☐ NA	☐ Conflict ☐ Enmeshment ☒ Isolation/avoidance ☒ Emotional disengagement ☐ Poor social skills ☐ Couple problems ☐ Prob w/friends ☐ Prob at work ☐ Overly shy ☐ Egocentricity ☐ Diff establish/maintain relationship ☐ Other: _____
Mood	☐ NA	☐ Depressed/sad ☐ Hopeless ☒ Fearful ☒ Anxious ☐ Angry ☒ Irritable ☐ Manic ☐ Other: _____
Affect	☐ NA	☒ Constricted ☐ Blunt ☐ Flat ☐ Labile ☐ Dramatic ☐ Other: _____
Sleep	☐ NA	☐ Hypersomnia ☐ Insomnia ☒ Disrupted ☒ Nightmares ☐ Other: _____
Eating	☒ NA	☐ Increase ☐ Decrease ☐ Anorectic restriction ☐ Bingeing ☐ Purging ☐ Body image ☐ Other: _____
Anxiety symptoms	☐ NA	☐ Chronic worry ☐ Panic attacks ☐ Dissociation ☐ Phobias ☐ Obsessions ☐ Compulsions ☒ Other: Intrusive thoughts

† *Abbreviations*: AF: Adult Female; AM: Adult Male; CF#: Child Female with age, e.g. CF12; CM# Child Male with age; Hx: History; Cl: Client.

Trauma symptoms	☐ NA	☒ Acute ☐ Chronic ☒ Hypervigilance ☒ Dreams/nightmares ☐ Dissociation ☒ Emotional numbness ☐ Other: _____
Psychotic symptoms	☒ NA	☐ Hallucinations ☐ Delusions ☐ Paranoia ☐ Loose associations ☐ Other: _____
Motor activity/ speech	☐ NA	☒ Low energy ☐ Restless/hyperactive ☐ Agitated ☐ Inattentive ☐ Impulsive ☐ Pressured speech ☐ Slow speech ☐ Other: _____
Thought	☐ NA	☐ Poor concentration/attention ☐ Denial ☐ Self-blame ☐ Other-blame ☒ Ruminative ☐ Tangential ☐ Illogical ☐ Concrete ☐ Poor insight ☐ Impaired decision making ☐ Disoriented ☐ Slow processing ☐ Other: _____
Socio-Legal	☒ NA	☐ Disregards rules ☐ Defiant ☐ Stealing ☐ Lying ☐ Tantrums ☐ Arrest/ incarceration ☐ Initiates fights ☐ Other: _____
Other symptoms	☒ NA	

Diagnosis for IP

Contextual Factors considered in making Dx: ☒ Age ☒ Gender ☒ Family dynamics ☒ Culture ☒ Language ☒ Religion ☒ Economic ☒ Immigration ☐ Sexual orientation ☐ Trauma ☐ Dual dx/comorbid ☐ Addiction ☐ Cognitive ability ☐ Other: _____

Describe impact of identified factors: Sexual abuse trauma; change in family dynamic also had significant emotional impact. Age, culture, religion norms considered when assessing emotional expression (parents from emotionally expressive cultures). English primary language.

Axis I
Primary: 309.81 Post Traumatic Stress Disorder, Acute

Secondary: V61.20 Parent-Child Relational Problem

Axis II: V71.09 None

Axis III: None reported

Axis IV:
☒ Problems with primary support group
☐ Problems related to social environment/school
☒ Educational problems
☐ Occupational problems
☐ Housing problems
☐ Economic problems
☐ Problems with accessing health care services
☐ Problems related to interactions with the legal system
☒ Other psychosocial problems

Axis V: GAF 60 GARF 60

List DSM symptoms for Axis I Dx (include frequency and duration for each). Client meets 6 of 6 criteria for Axis I Primary Dx.

1. Life-threatening trauma: Sexually molested for 3 months

2. Intrusive thoughts and nightmares most days

3. Detachment from others; social withdrawal

4. Restricted affect

5. Exaggerated startle response; difficulty falling and staying asleep

6. Symptoms for more than 1 month

(continued)

Diagnosis for IP *(continued)*

Have medical causes been ruled out?
☒ Yes ☐ No ☐ In process
**Has patient been referred for psychiatric/
medical eval?** ☒ Yes ☐ No
Has patient agreed with referral?
☒ Yes ☐ No ☐ NA
List psychometric instruments or consults used
for assessment:
☒ None or _____

**Medications (psychiatric & medical)
Dose /Start Date**
☒ None prescribed
1. _____ / _____ mg; _____
2. _____ / _____ mg; _____
3. _____ / _____ mg; _____

Client response to diagnosis:
☒ Agree ☐ Somewhat agree ☐ Disagree
☐ Not informed for following reason:

Medical Necessity *(Check all that apply):* ☒ Significant impairment ☐ Probability of significant impairment
☒ Probably developmental arrest
Areas of impairment: ☒ Daily activities ☒ Social relationships ☐ Health ☒ Work/school
☐ Living arrangement ☐ Other: _____

Risk Assessment

Suicidality
☒ No indication
☒ Denies
☐ Active ideation
☐ Passive ideation
☐ Intent without plan
☐ Intent with means
☐ Ideation past yr
☐ Attempt past yr
☐ Family/peer hx of completed suicide

Homicidality
☒ No indication
☒ Denies
☐ Active ideation
☐ Passive ideation
☐ Intent w/o means
☐ Intent with means
☐ Ideation past yr
☐ Violence past yr
☐ Hx assault/temper
☐ Cruelty to animals

Hx Substance
Alc abuse:
☒ No indication
☒ Denies
☐ Past
☐ Current
Freq/Amt: _____
Drug:
☒ No indication
☒ Denies
☐ Past
☐ Current
Drugs: _____
Freq/Amt: _____
☐ Family/sig.other abuses

Sexual & Physical Abuse and Other Risk Factors
☒ Current child w abuse hx:
    ☒ Sexual ☐ Physical ☐ Emotional ☐ Neglect
☐ Adult w childhood abuse:
    ☐ Sexual ☐ Physical ☐ Emotional ☐ Neglect
☐ Adult w abuse/assault in adulthood:
    ☐ Sexual ☐ Physical ☐ Current

☐ History of perpetrating abuse:
    ☐ Sexual ☐ Physical
☐ Elder/dependent adult abuse/neglect
☐ Anorexia/bulimia/other eating disorder
☐ Cutting or other self-harm:
    ☐ Current
    ☐ Past; Method: _____
    ☐ Criminal/legal hx: _____
    ☐ None reported

Indicators of Safety: ☒ At least one outside person who provides strong support ☐ Able to cite specific reasons to live, not harm self/other ☐ Hopeful ☒ Has future goals ☐ Willing to dispose of dangerous items ☒ Willingness to reduce contact with people who make situation worse ☒ Willing to implement safety plan, safety interventions ☐ Developing set of alternatives to self/other harm ☐ Sustained period of safety: ____
☐ Other: _____

Safety Plan includes: ☐ Verbal no harm contract ☐ Written no harm contract ☒ Emergency contact card ☒ Emergency therapist/agency number ☐ Medication management ☐ Specific plan for contacting friends/ support persons during crisis ☐ Specific plan of where to go during crisis ☒ Specific self-calming tasks to reduce risk before reach crisis level (e.g., journaling, exercising, etc.) ☐ Specific dailfy/weekly activities to reduce stressors ☐ Other: _____

Notes: Legal/Ethical Action Taken: ☐ NA Report to Child Protective Services; report taken by Susan Roth 7:30 pm 9/4/09.

Case Management

Date
1st visit: 9/4/09 _____

Last visit: 9/11/08 _____

Session Freq:
☒ Once week ☐ Every other week ☐ Other: _____

Expected Length of Treatment:
_____

Modalities:
☐ Individual adult
☒ Individual child
☒ Couple
☒ Family
☒ Group:
Teen survivor group

Is client involved in mental health or other medical treatment elsewhere?
☒ No
☐ Yes:

_____

If Child/Adolescent: Is family involved?
☒ Yes ☐ No

Patient Referrals and Professional Contacts

Has contact been made with social worker?
☒ Yes ☐ No: explain: _____ ☐ NA

Has client been referred for medical assessment?
☒ Yes ☐ No evidence for need

Has client been referred for psychiatric assessment?
☒ Yes; cl agree ☐ Yes, cl disagree ☐ Not nec.

Has contact been made with treating physicians or other professionals?
☒ Yes ☐ No ☐ NA

Has client been referred for social services?
☐ Job/training ☐ Welfare/food/housing ☒ Victim services
☐ Legal aid ☐ Medical ☐ Other: _____ ☐ NA

Anticipated forensic/legal processes related to treatment:
☐ No ☒ Yes: CPS Case _____

Has client been referred for group or other support services?
☒ Yes ☐ No ☐ None recommended

Client social support network includes:
☒ Supportive family ☐ Supportive partner ☐ Friends ☒ Religious/spiritual organization ☐ Supportive work/social group ☐ Other: _____

Anticipated effects treatment will have on others in support system (parents, children, siblings, significant others, etc.):
Parents will be part of treatment.

Is there anything else client will need to be successful?
Address family dynamics

(continued)

Case Management (*continued*)

Client Sense of Hope: Little 1-------------5X----------10 High

Expected Outcome and Prognosis
☒ Return to normal functioning
☐ Expect improvement, anticipate less than normal functioning
☐ Maintain current status/prevent deterioration

Evaluation of Assessment/Client Perspective
How was assessment method adapted to client needs?
Created safe space for CF to talk; used age-appropriate language.

Age, culture, ability level, and other diversity issues adjusted for by:

Asked about language preference; cultural norms for emotional expression and family boundaries considered when

making diagnosis and evaluating family. Involved family, honoring cultural norms for involvement.

Systemic/family dynamics considered in following ways:
Family dynamics and change in mother's role at home considered in assessment.

Describe actual or potential areas of client-therapist agreement/disagreement related to the above assessment:
Family agrees with PTSD diagnosis and agrees that "something" needs to change in family dynamics to get "back on track."

_____ , _____   _____
Therapist Signature   License/Intern status   Date

_____ , _____   _____
Supervisor Signature   License   Date

TREATMENT PLAN

Therapist: Sharee Lee   **Client ID #:** 1020

Theory: Satir Growth Model

Primary Configuration: ☒ Individual ☐ Couple ☒ Family ☐ Group _____

Additional: ☐ Individual ☒ Couple ☐ Family ☐ Group: _____

Medication(s): ☒ NA ☐ _____

Contextual Factors considered in making plan: ☒ Age ☒ Gender ☒ Family dynamics

☒ Culture ☒ Language ☒ Religion ☒ Economic ☒ Immigration ☐ Sexual orientation

☒ Trauma ☐ Dual dx/comorbid ☐ Addiction ☐ Cognitive ability

☐ Other: _____

Describe how plan adapted to contextual factors: Per family preference and cultural norms, the family is included in all phases of treatment, although CF will also have some individual sessions. As a pre-teen, play will be offered as an option if CF prefers, although she is quite verbal for her age (only child and highly educated parents). Religious faith and community will be considered as possible resources for healing. English is preferred language for therapy.

I. Initial Phase of Treatment (First 1–3 Sessions)

I.A. Initial Therapeutic Tasks
Therapeutic Relationship

     TT1: Develop therapeutic relationship with all members. Note: Focus on culture, age differences, education level.

     I1: Intervention: **Make contact** using **warmth** and **empathy**. Clearly establish **hope** that CF will have a normal life and that therapy will help with that process.

Assessment

     TT2: Assess individual, system, and broader cultural dynamics. Note: Family and culture.

     I1: Intervention: **"Before and after" sculpting** of each person's perspective of how the family changed both relative to AF increasing travel and the abuse incidents.

     I2: Intervention: Assess each member's **survival communication stance** and how affecting individuals and family since abuse.

Note: **BOLDFACE** indicates Satir Growth Model assessment and techniques.

(continued)

I. Initial Phase of Treatment (*continued*)

Set Goals

> **TT3:** Define and obtain client agreement on treatment goals. Note: Attend to CF and family's desire for family vs. individual sessions.

> > **I1:** Intervention: Identify goals for (a) **individual growth** of each and (b) **improved communication** and **emotional connection** between family members.

Referrals and Crisis

> **TT4:** Identify needed referrals, crisis issues, and other client needs. Note: Stabilize abuse.

> > **I1:** Intervention: Connect CF with available resources for abuse victims, including Victim of Crime, and work with CPS and other authorities on reporting and investigation.

I.B. Initial Client Goals (1–2 Goals): Manage crisis issues and/or reduce most distressing symptoms

> **Goal #1:** ☐ Increase ☐ Decrease CF sense of **physical and emotional safety** and sense of normalcy (personal/relational dynamic) to reduce nightmares and intrusive thoughts (symptom).
>
> *Measure:* Able to sustain sense of safety for period of 2 ☒ wks ☐ mos with no more than 1 mild episodes of nightmares or intrusive thoughts.
>
> > **I1:** Intervention: Allow CF to tell her story, **share her fears,** and **validate** her sense of safety and ability to protect self; discuss her present fears and fears of what the abuse may mean for her future.
>
> > **I2:** Intervention: **Role play** and **sculpting** to reinforce sense of being able to protect self.

II. Working Phase of Treatment (Sessions 2+)

II.A. Working Therapeutic Tasks

Monitor Progress

> **TT1:** Monitor progress toward goals. Note: Check in individually and as family.

> > **I1:** Intervention: Every 3–4 sessions ask if family is satisfied with progress and is seeing changes.

Monitor Relationship

> **TT2:** Monitor quality of therapeutic alliance as therapy proceeds. Note: Check in individually and as family.

> > **I1:** Intervention: Each week establish **"emotional contact"** with each client; monitor throughout session.

II.B. Working Client Goals (2–3 Goals): Target individual and relational dynamics in case conceptualization using theoretical language (e.g., reduce enmeshment, increase differentiation, increase agency in relational narrative, etc.).

Goal #1: ☒ Increase ☐ Decrease CF **sense of safety and esteem** in peer relationships (personal/relational dynamic) to reduce social withdrawal (symptom).

Measure: Able to sustain engagement in pre-abuse social activities for period of 1 ☐ wks ☒ mos with no more than 2 mild episodes of withdrawal.

    I1: Intervention: **Give voice** to fears and anxieties that fuel withdrawal.

    I2: Intervention: **Coaching** and **role play** on how to interact with others and maintain safety and boundaries.

Goal #2: ☒ Increase ☐ Decrease **emotional connection** between CF and AF (personal/relational dynamic) to reduce disengagement and increase CF's sense of **personal support** (symptom).

Measure: Able to sustain emotional connection for period of 2 ☐ wks ☒ mos with no more than 1 mild episodes of disconnection

    I1: Intervention: **Sculpting** to increase AF awareness of loss that CF is experiencing.

    I2: Intervention: **Coaching on congruent communication** to help AF and CF more readily connect.

Goal #3: ☒ Increase ☐ Decrease **congruent communication** between all family members (personal/relational dynamic) to reduce **triangulation** and **parental conflict** (symptom).

Measure: Able to sustain direct, congruent communication for period of 2 ☐ wks ☒ mos with no more than 2 mild episodes of conflict and riangulation.

    I1: Intervention: **Coaching family to communicate congruently** in session.

    I2: Intervention: **Coaching family to detriangulate** in session, increasing CF and AM's direct communication to AF.

III. Closing Phase of Treatment (Last 2+ Weeks)

III.A. Closing Therapeutic Tasks
Termination Plan

    TT1: Develop aftercare plan and maintain gains. Note: Coordinate with social worker

    I1: Intervention: Identify family and community resources, such as church, to continue to provide support and safety.

(continued)

III. Closing Phase of Treatment (*continued*)

III.B. Closing Client Goals: Determined by theory's definition of health

Goal #1: ☒ Increase ☐ Decrease CF sense of **autonomy** and **self-definition** as she enters adolescence (personal/relational dynamic) to reduce **low self-esteem** (symptom).

Measure: Able to sustain sense of agency and worth for period of 2 ☐ wks ☒ mos with no more than 2 mild episodes of **placating** and feeling like "damaged goods."

  I1: Intervention: Individual sessions with CF to increase **valuing of self** and reduce victim and **placating** stance.

  I2: Intervention: **Art therapy collages** to develop vision of who she is becoming and increasing ownership of self-identity as enters adolescence.

IV. Client Perspective

Has treatment plan been reviewed with client? ☒ Yes ☐ No; If no, explain: _____

_____

Describe areas of client agreement and concern: Clients are particularly enthusiastic about wanting family sessions, especially early in therapy. _____

_____ , _____ _____
Therapist signature   Intern status   Date

_____ , _____ _____
Supervisor signature   License   Date

Abbreviation: TT: Therapeutic Task; I: Intervention; AM: Adult Male; AF: Adult Female; CM: Child Male; CF: Child Female; Dx: Diagnosis; NA: Not Applicable.

PROGRESS NOTES

Progress Notes for Client # 1020

Date: 9/30/09 **Time:** 3:00 am/**pm**   **Session Length:** ☒ 50 min or ☐ _____

Present: ☒ AM ☒ AF ☐ CM ☒ CF ☐ _____
Billing Code: ☐ 90801 (Assess) ☐ 90806 (Insight-50 min) ☒ 90847 (Family-50 min)

☐ Other _____

Symptoms(s)	Dur/Freq Since Last Visit	Progress: Setback----------Initial----------Goal
1. Nightmares/intrusive thoughts	1 nightmare this week; intrusive thoughts last for less than 1 minute—2–3 times/day	-5----------1-------------5----X--------10
2. Disengagement	AF spent Sat afternoon with CF	-5----------1------------X--------------10
3. Social withdrawal	CF spent lunch with friends all days this wk	-5----------1-------------5-X-----------10

Explanatory Notes: Report CF feeling "safer" and engaging more socially; CF reporting that she feels more like AF cares; AF still traveling for work but more open to finding ways to minimize the effect it has on CF and AM. Continued arguing between AM and AF but less severe than prior.

Interventions/HW: Facilitated sharing of each person's emotional response to reported progress and changes, especially related to AF spending more quality time with CF. Coached family members on congruent communication, helping each to reduce use of survival stance and defenses.

Client Response/Feedback: Clients responded well to sharing of positive affect related to progress; AF's eyes watered when CF shared her appreciation for AF spending time with her. Family responsive to communication coaching and report trying to use what learned in session at home.

Plan: ☐ Continue with treatment plan; plan for next session: _____

☒ Modify plan: Couple session next week to discuss balancing AF work and home; following week CF alone.

Next session: Date: 10/7/08 Time: 5:00 am/**pm**
Crisis Issues: ☒ Denies suicide/homicide/abuse/crisis ☐ Crisis assessed/addressed:

_____

_____ , _____ _____
Therapist signature   License/Intern status   Date

◇◇◇

(continued)

PROGRESS NOTES *(continued)*

Case Consultation/Supervision Notes: Now that CF is stabilized, supervisor encouraged separate couple and child sessions to reinforce generational boundaries and allow CF to discuss more personal issues related to the abuse in private.

Collateral Contacts: Date: 9/29/09 Time: 10:00 Name: Dora James, CPS Social Worker

Notes: Returned social worker's call; requested update on progress.

☒ Written release on file: ☒ Sent ☐ Received ☒ In court docs ☐ Other: _____

_____ , _____ _____
Therapist signature   License/Intern status   Date

_____ , _____ _____
Supervisor signature   License   Date

_____

Abbreviations: AM: Adult Male; AF: Adult Female; CM: Child Male; CF: Child Female; HW: Homework.

Intergenerational and Psychoanalytic Family Therapies

"Bowen theory is really not about families per se, but about life."—Friedman, 1991, p. 134

Lay of the Land

Although distinct from each other, Bowenian intergenerational therapy and psychoanalytic family therapy share the common roots of (a) psychoanalytic theory and (b) systemic theory. A psychoanalytically trained psychiatrist, Bowen (1985) developed a highly influential and unique approach to therapy that is called Bowen intergenerational therapy. Drawing heavily from object relations theory, psychoanalytic or psychodynamic family therapies have developed several unique approaches, including *object relations family therapy* (Scharff & Scharff, 1987), *family-of-origin therapy* (Framo, 1992), and *contextual therapy* (Boszormenyi-Nagy & Krasner, 1986). These therapies share several key concepts and practices:

- Examining a client's early relationships to understand present functioning
- Tracing transgenerational and extended family dynamics to understand a client's complaints
- Promoting insight into extended family dynamics to facilitate change
- Identifying and altering destructive beliefs and patterns of behavior that were learned early in life in one's family of origin

Bowen Intergenerational Therapy
In a Nutshell: The Least You Need to Know

Bowen intergenerational theory is more about the nature of being human than it is about families or family therapy (Friedman, 1991). The Bowen approach requires therapists to work from a broad perspective that considers the evolution of the human species and the characteristics of all living systems. Therapists use this broad perspective to conceptualize client problems and then rely primarily on the therapist's use of self to effect change. As part of this broad perspective, therapists routinely consider the *three-generational emotional process* to better understand the current presenting symptoms. The process of therapy involves increasing clients' awareness of how their current behavior is connected to multigenerational processes and the resulting family dynamics. The therapist's primary tool for promoting client change is the therapist's personal level of *differentiation*, the ability to distinguish self from other and manage interpersonal anxiety.

The Juice: Significant Contributions to the Field

If you remember a couple of things from this chapter, they should be:

Differentiation

Differentiation is one of the most useful concepts for understanding interpersonal relationships, although it can be difficult to grasp at first (Friedman, 1991). An *emotional or affective* concept, differentiation refers to a person's ability to separate intrapersonal and interpersonal distress:

- **Intrapersonal:** Separate thoughts from feelings in order to *respond* rather than *react*
- **Interpersonal:** Know where oneself ends and another begins without loss of self

Bowen (1985) also described differentiation as the ability to balance two life forces: the need for *togetherness* and the need for *autonomy*. Differentiation is conceptualized on a *continuum* (Bowen, 1985): a person is more or less differentiated rather than differentiated or not differentiated. Becoming more differentiated is a lifelong journey that is colloquially referred to as "maturity" in the broadest sense.

A person who is more differentiated is better able to handle the ups and downs of life and, more importantly, the vicissitudes of intimate relationships. The ability to clearly separate thoughts from feelings and self from others allows one to more successfully negotiate the tension and challenges that come with increasing levels of intimacy. For example, when one's partner expresses disapproval or disinterest, this does not cause a differentiated person's world to collapse or inspire hostility. Of course, feelings may be hurt, and the person experiences that pain. However, he/she doesn't immediately *act on* or *act out* that pain. Differentiated people are able to reflect on the pain: clearly separate out what is their part and what is their partner's part and identify a respectful way to move forward. In contrast, less differentiated people feel compelled to immediately react and express their feelings before thinking or reflecting on what belongs to whom in the situation. Partners with greater levels of differentiation are able to tolerate difference between themselves and others, allowing for greater freedom and acceptance in all relationships.

Because differentiated people do not immediately react in emotional situations, a common misunderstanding is that differentiation implies lack of emotion or emotional expression (Friedman, 1991). In reality, highly differentiated peeople are actually able to engage *more* difficult and intense emotions because they do not overreact and instead can thoughtfully reflect on and tolerate the ambiguity of their emotional lives.

It can be difficult to assess a client's level of differentiation because it is expressed differently depending on the person's culture, gender, age, and personality (Bowen, 1985). For example, to the untrained eye, emotionally expressive cultures and genders may look more undifferentiated, and emotionally restricted people and cultures may appear more differentiated. However, emotional coolness often is a result of *emotional cut-off* (see later section on Emotional Cut-Off), which is how a less differentiated person manages intense emotions. Therapists need to assess the actual functioning intrapersonally (ability to separate thought from feeling) and interpersonally (ability to separate self from other) to sift through the diverse expressions of differentiation.

Genograms

Introduced in Chapter 2, the genogram has become one of the most commonly used family assessment instruments (McGoldrick, Gerson, & Petry, 2008). At its most basic level, a genogram is a type of family tree or genealogy that specifically maps key multigenerational processes that illuminate for both therapist and client the emotional dynamics that contribute to the reported symptoms.

New therapists are often reluctant to do genograms. When I ask students to do their own, most are enthusiastic. However, when I ask them to do one with a client, most are reluctant. They may say, "I don't have time" or "I don't think these clients are the type who would want to do a genogram." Yet after completing their first genogram with a client, they almost always come out saying, "That was more helpful than I thought it was going to be." Especially for newer therapists—and even for seasoned clinicians—genograms are always helpful in some way. Although originally developed for the intergenerational work in Bowen's approach, the genogram is so universally helpful that many therapists from other schools adapt it for their approach, creating solution-focused genograms (Kuehl, 1995) or culturally focused genograms (Hardy & Laszloffy, 1995; Rubalcava & Waldman, 2004).

The genogram is simultaneously (a) an assessment instrument and (b) an intervention, especially in the hands of an intergenerational therapist. As an assessment instrument, the genogram helps the therapist identify intergenerational patterns that surround the problem, such as patterns of parenting, managing conflict, and balancing autonomy with togetherness. As an intervention, genograms can help clients see their patterns more clearly and how they may be living out family patterns, rules, and legacies without conscious awareness. As a trainee, I worked with one client who had never spoken to her parents about how her grandfather had sexually abused her and had no intention of doing so because she believed it would tear the family apart. This changed the day we constructed her genogram. I had her color in each person she knew he had also abused. When she was done, the three-generation genogram had over 12 victims colored in red; she went home and spoke to her mother that night and began a multigenerational process of healing for her family.

Rumor Has It: The People and Their Stories

Murray Bowen

A psychoanalytically trained psychiatrist, Bowen (1966, 1972, 1976, 1985) began working with people diagnosed with schizophrenia at the Menninger Clinic in the 1940s and continued his research in the 1950s at the National Institute for Mental Health (NIMH), where he hospitalized entire families with schizophrenic members to study their emotional processes. He then spent the next 30 years at Georgetown University developing one of the most influential theories of family and natural systems, which has influenced generations of family therapists.

Georgetown Family Center: Michael Kerr

A longtime student of Bowen, Michael Kerr has also been one of his most influential students and has served as director of the Georgetown Family Center where Bowen refined his clinical approach.

The Center for Family Learning: Philip Guerin and Thomas Fogarty

Guerin and Fogarty co-founded the Center for Family Learning in New York, one of the premier training centers for family therapy. Both Guerin and Fogarty have written extensively on the clinical applications of Bowen's model.

Monica McGoldrick and Betty Carter

Betty Carter and Monica McGoldrick (1999) used Bowen's theory to develop their highly influential model of the *family life cycle,* which uses the Bowenian concept of balancing the need for togetherness and independence to understand how families develop. McGoldrick's work with genograms is the definitive work on this tool subject (McGoldrick, Gerson, and Petry, 2008).

David Schnarch

Grounded in Bowen's intergenerational approach, Schnarch developed a unique approach to working with couples, the Sexual Crucible Model, which is designed to increase a couple's capacity for intimacy by increasing their level of differentiation. One of the hallmarks of this approach is harnessing the intensity in the couple's sexual relationship to promote the differentiation process.

The Big Picture: Overview of Treatment

Much like other approaches that have psychodynamic roots, intergenerational therapy is a *process*-oriented therapy that relies heavily on the *self-of-the-therapist,* most specifically the therapist's level of differentiation, to promote client change (Kerr & Bowen, 1988). This therapy does not emphasize techniques and interventions. Instead, therapists use genograms and assessment to promote insight and then intervene as differentiated persons. For example, when one partner tries to get the therapist to take his/her side in an argument, the therapist responds by simultaneously modeling differentiation and gently promoting it in the couple. By refusing to take sides and also helping the couple tolerate their resulting anxiety (their problem is still not fixed, and neither partner has been "validated" by the therapist), the therapist creates a situation in which the couple can increase their level of differentiation: they can use self-validation to soothe their feelings and learn how to tolerate the tension of difference between them. Change is achieved through alternately using insight and the therapeutic relationship to increase clients' levels of differentiation and tolerance for anxiety and ambiguity.

Making Connection: The Therapeutic Relationship

Differentiation and the Emotional Being of the Therapist

More than in any other family therapy approach, in intergenerational therapy the therapist's level of differentiation (Bowen, 1985; Kerr & Bowen, 1988) and emotional being (Friedman, 1991) are central to the change process. Intergenerational therapists focus on developing a therapeutic relationship that encourages all parties to further their differentiation process: *"the differentiation of the therapist is technique"* (Friedman, 1991, p. 138; italics in original). Intergenerational therapists believe that clients can only differentiate as much as their therapists have differentiated (Bowen, 1985). For this reason, the therapist's level of differentiation is often the focus of supervision early in training, and therapists are expected to continually monitor and develop themselves so that they can be of maximum assistance to their clients. Bowen therapists assert that the theory cannot be learned through books (such as this one) but can only be learned through a relationship with a supervisor or teacher who uses these ideas to interact with the student (Friedman, 1991).

A Nonanxious Presence

The greater a therapist's level of differentiation, the more the therapist can maintain a nonanxious presence with clients (Kerr & Bowen, 1988). This is not a cold, detached stance but rather an emotionally engaged stance that is *nonreactive,* meaning that the therapist does not react to attacks, "bad" news, and so forth without careful reflection. The therapist does not rush in to rescue clients from anxiety every time they feel overwhelmed by anger, sadness, or another strong emotion; instead, the therapist calmly wades right into the muck the client is trying to avoid and guides the client through the process of separating self from other and thought from feelings (Friedman, 1991). The therapist's calm center is used to help clients move through the differentiation process in a safe, contained environment in which differentiation is modeled. When clients are upset, the "easiest" thing to do is to soothe and calm their anxieties, fears, and strong emotions; this makes everyone calmer sooner, but nothing is learned. The intergenerational therapist instead shepherds a more difficult process of slowly coaching clients through that which they fear or detest in order to facilitate growth.

The Viewing: Case Conceptualization and Assessment

Viewing is the primary "intervention" in intergenerational therapy because the approach's effectiveness relies on the therapist's ability to accurately assess the family dynamics and thereby guide the healing process (Bowen, 1985). Although this is true with all therapies, it is truer with intergenerational therapies because the therapist's level of differentiation is critical to the ability to accurately "see" what is going on.

Emotional Systems

Bowen viewed families, organizations, and clubs as emotional systems that have the same processes as those found in all natural systems: "Bowen has constantly emphasized over the years that we have more in common with other forms of protoplasm (i.e., life) than we differ from them" (Friedman, 1991, p. 135). He viewed humans as part of an *evolutionary emotional process* that goes back to the first cell that had a nucleus and was able to differentiate its functions from other cells (i.e., human life begins with one cell that divides to create new cells, which then differentiate to create the different systems and structures of the body: blood, muscle, neurons, etc.). This process of differentiating yet remaining part of a single living organism (system) is a primary organizing concept in Bowen's work, and the family's emotional processes are viewed as an extension (not just a metaphor) of the differentiation process of cells. Thus Bowen's theory of natural systems focuses on the relationship between the human species and all life past and present.

Of particular interest in family therapy are natural systems that have developed emotional interdependence (e.g., flocks of birds, herds of cattle, and human families; Friedman, 1991). The resulting system or emotional field profoundly influences all of its members, defining what is valued and what is not. When a family lacks sufficient differentiation, it may become emotionally fused, an undifferentiated family "ego mass." Intergenerational therapists focus squarely on a family's unique emotional system rather than on environmental or general cultural factors, and they seek to identify the rules that structure the particular system.

This approach is similar to other systemic conceptualizations of the family as a single organism or system; however, Bowen emphasizes that it is fundamentally an *emotional* system. Because this system has significant impact on a person's behavior, emotions, and symptoms, one must always assess this context to understand a person's problems. For example, in the case study at the end of this chapter, the therapist explores how Wei-Wei's panic attacks fit within the broader fabric of the family system, her immigration history, and her professional life, rather than focusing solely on the medical and psychological aspects of the attacks.

Chronic Anxiety

Bowen viewed chronic anxiety as a biological phenomenon that is present in all natural systems. Chronic anxiety involves automatic physical and emotional reactions that are not mediated through conscious, logical processes (Friedman, 1991). Families exhibit chronic anxiety in their responses to crises, loss, conflict, and difficulties. The process of differentiation creates a clearheadedness that allows individuals and families to reduce the reactivity and anxiety associated with survival in natural systems and instead make conscious choices about how to respond. For example, chronic anxiety in a family may result from a mother feeling guilty about a child's lack of success, in which case it is the therapist's job to help the mother increase her level of differentiation so that she can respond to the child's situation from a clear, reasoned position rather than with a blind emotional reactivity that rarely helps the situation. In the case study at the end of the chapter, the therapist works with the mother to reduce her anxiety and panic as her son finishes medical school and begins his independent life as an adult.

The Multigenerational Transmission Process

The multigenerational transmission process is based on the premise that emotional processes from prior generations are present and "alive" in the current family emotional system (Friedman, 1991). In this process, children may emerge with higher, equal, or lower levels of differentiation than their parents (Bowen, 1985). Families with severe emotional problems result from a multigenerational process in which the level of differentiation has become lower and lower with each generation. Bowen's approach is designed to help an individual create enough distance from these processes to comprehend the more universal processes that shape human relationships and individual identities (Friedman, 1991). Thus, in the case study at the end of this chapter, the therapist will assess the emotional content of the parents' prior life in China, which is viewed as an ongoing aspect of the family's current reality.

Multigenerational Patterns

Intergenerational therapists assess multigenerational patterns, specifically those related to the presenting problem. Using a genogram or oral interview, the therapist identifies patterns of depression, substance use, anger, conflict, the parent-child relationship, the couples relationship, or whatever issues are most salient for the client. The therapist then identifies how the current situation fits with these patterns. Is the client replicating or rebelling against the pattern? How has the pattern evolved with this generation? The therapist thereby gains greater clarity into the dynamics that are feeding the problem. In cases of immigration, such as that at the end of this chapter, the historic family patterns may change because of different cultural contexts (e.g., the family attempts or is forced to blend and adapt), may be rigidly the same (e.g., the family wants to adhere to traditions), or may be radically different (e.g., the family wants to "break" from the past).

Level of Differentiation (see Juice)

When differentiation is used as part of case conceptualization, the therapist assesses the client's level of differentiation along a continuum, which Bowen developed into a differentiation scale that ranges from 1 to 100, with lower levels of differentiation represented by lower numbers (Bowen, 1985). Bowen maintained that people rarely reach higher than 70 on this scale.

Although there are pen-and-paper measures such as the Chabot Emotional Differentiation Scale (Licht & Chabot, 2006), most therapists simply note patterns of where and how a person is able or unable to separate self from other and thought from emotion. What is most useful for treatment is not some overall score or general assessment of differentiation, but the specific places where clients need to increase their level of differentiation to resolve the presenting problem. For example, a couple may need to increase their ability to differentiate self from other in the area of sex so that they can create a better sexual relationship that allows each person to have preferences, discuss them, and find ways to honor these preferences without becoming emotionally overwhelmed.

Emotional Triangles

Bowen identified triangles as one of the most important dynamics to assess because they are the basic building block of families (Bowen, 1985; Friedman, 1991; Kerr & Bowen, 1988). A triangle is a process in which a dyad draws in a third person (or some thing, topic, or activity) to stabilize the primary dyad, especially when there is tension in the dyad. Because triangles use a third person or topic to alleviate tension, the more you try to change the relationship with the third entity, the more you ironically reinforce the aspects you want to change. Thus, therapists assess triangles to identify the primary relationship that needs to be targeted for change.

Bowen maintained that triangulation is a fundamental process in natural systems (Bowen, 1985). Everyone triangulates to some degree: going down the hall to complain about your boss or coworker is triangulation. However, when this becomes the primary means for dealing with dyadic tension and the members of the dyad never actually resolve the tension themselves, then pathological patterns emerge. The more rigid the triangle, the greater the problems.

The classic family example of a triangle is a mother who becomes overinvolved with her children to reduce unresolved tension in the marriage. This overinvolvement can take the form of positive interactions (overinvolvement in school and social activities, emotional intimacy, constant errands or time devoted to the child) or negative interactions (nagging and worrying about the child; the therapist suspects that this is what is going on in the case study at the end of the chapter). Another common form of triangulation is seen in divorced families, in which both parents often triangulate the child, trying to convince the child to take their side against the other parent. Triangulation can also involve using alcohol or drugs to create dyadic stability, complaining or siding with friends or family of origin against one's spouse, or two siblings siding against a third.

The Family Projection Process

The family projection process describes how parents "project" their immaturity onto one or more children (Bowen, 1985), causing decreased differentiation in subsequent generations. The most common pattern is for a mother to project her anxiety onto one child, focusing all her attention on this child to soothe her anxiety, perhaps becoming overly invested in the child's academic or sporting activities. The child or children who are the focus of the parent's anxiety will be less differentiated than the siblings who are not involved in this projection process.

Emotional Cut-Off

A particularly important process to assess is emotional cut-off, which refers to situations in which a person no longer emotionally engages with another in order to manage anxiety; this usually occurs between children and parents. Emotional cut-off can take the form of no longer seeing or speaking to the other or, alternatively, being willing to be at the same family event with virtually no interaction. Often people who display cut-off from their family believe that doing so is a sign of mental health (e.g., "I have set good boundaries") or even a sign of superiority (e.g., "It makes no sense for me to spend time with *that type* of person"). They may even report that this solution helps them manage their emotional reactivity. However, cut-off is almost always a sign of lower levels of differentiation (Bowen, 1985). Essentially, the person is so emotionally fused with the other that he/she must physically separate to be comfortable. The higher a person's level of differentiation, the less need there is for emotional cut-off. This does not mean that a highly differentiated person does not establish boundaries. However, when differentiated people set boundaries and limit contact with family, they do so in a way that is respectful and preserves emotional connection, and not out of emotional reactivity (e.g., after an argument).

Emotional cut-off requires a little more attention in assessment because it can "throw off" an overall assessment of differentiation and family dynamics. People who emotionally cut themselves off as a means of coping often appear more differentiated than they are; it may also be harder to detect certain family patterns because in some cases the client "forgets" or honestly does not know the family history. However, at some times and in certain families, more cut-off is necessary because of extreme patterns of verbal, emotional, or childhood abuse. In such cases, where contact is not appropriate or possible, the therapist still needs to assess the *emotional* part of the cut-off. The more people can stay emotionally engaged (e.g., have empathy and cognitive understanding of the relational dynamics) without harboring anger, resentment, or fear, the healthier they will be, and this should be a therapeutic goal.

Sibling Position

Intergenerational therapists also look at sibling position as an indicator of the family's level of differentiation; all things being equal, the more the family members exhibit the expected characteristics of their sibling position, the higher the level of differentiation (Bowen, 1985; Kerr & Bowen, 1988). The more intense the family projection process is on a child, the more that child will exhibit characteristics of an infantile younger child. The roles associated with sibling positions are informed by a person's cultural background, with immigrants generally adhering to more traditional standards than later generations. Most often, older children identify with responsibility and authority, and later-born children respond to this domination by identifying with underdogs and questioning the status quo. The youngest child is generally the most likely to avoid responsibility in favor of freedom.

Societal Regression

When a society experiences sustained chronic anxiety because of war, natural disaster, economic pressures, and other traumas, it responds with emotionally based reactive decisions rather than rational decisions (Bowen, 1985) and regresses to lower levels of functioning, just like families. These Band-Aid solutions to social problems generate a vicious cycle of increased problems and symptoms. Societies can go through cycles in which their level of differentiation rises and falls.

Targeting Change: Goal Setting

Two Basic Goals

Like any theory with a definition of health, intergenerational therapy has clearly defined long-term therapeutic goals that can be used with all clients:

1. To increase each person's level of differentiation (in specific contexts)
2. To decrease emotional reactivity to chronic anxiety in the system

Increasing Differentiation

Increasing differentiation is a general goal that should be operationally defined for each client. For example, "increase AF's and AM's level of differentiation in the marital relationship by increasing the tolerance of difference while increasing intimacy" is a better goal than "increase differentiation."

Decreasing Emotional Reactivity to Chronic Anxiety

Decreasing anxiety and emotional reactivity is closely correlated with the increasing differentiation. *As differentiation increases, anxiety decreases.* Nonetheless, it can be helpful to include these as separate goals to break the process down into smaller steps. Decreasing anxiety generally precedes increasing differentiation and therefore may be included in the working rather than the termination phase of therapy. As with the general goal of increasing differentiation, it is clinically helpful to tailor this to an individual client. Rather than stating the general goal of "decrease anxiety," which can easily be confused with treating an anxiety disorder (as may or may not be the case), a more useful clinical goal would address a client's specific dynamic: "decrease emotional reactivity to child's defiance" or "decrease emotional reactivity to partner in conversations about division of chores and parenting."

The Doing: Interventions

Theory Versus Technique

The primary "technique" in Bowen intergenerational theory is the therapist's ability to embody the theory. The premise is that if therapists understand Bowen's theory of natural systems and work on their personal level of differentiation, they will naturally interact with clients in a way that promotes the clients' level of differentiation (Friedman, 1991). Thus understanding—"living" the theory—is the primary technique for facilitating client change.

Process Questions

Intergenerational therapists' embodiment of the theory most frequently expresses itself through *process questions*, questions that help clients see the systemic process or the dynamics that they are enacting. For example, a therapist can use process questions to help clients see how the conflict they are experiencing with their spouse is related to patterns they observed in the parents' relationship: "How do the struggles you are experiencing with your spouse now compare with those of each of your parents? Similar or different? Is the role you are playing now similar to that of one of your parents in their marriage? Is it similar to the type of conflict you had with your parents when you were younger? Who are you most like? Least like?" These questions are generated naturally from the therapist's use of the theory to conceptualize the client's situation.

Encouraging Differentiation of Self

According to Bowenian theory, families naturally tend toward togetherness and relationship as part of survival. Thus therapeutic interventions generally target the counterbalancing force of differentiation (Friedman, 1991) by encouraging clients to use *"I" positions* to maintain individual opinions and mood states while in relationships with others. For example, if spouses are overreactive to the moods of the other, every time one person is in an angry or unhappy mood, the other feels there is no other choice but to also be in that mood state. Therapists promote differentiation by coaching the second spouse to maintain his/her emotional state without undue influence from the other. In this chapter's case study, the therapist will work with Wei-Wei, who is having panic attacks, to increase her sense of differentiation, particularly in relationship to her son but also in relationship to her husband, from whom she has become distant.

Genograms

The genogram is used both as an assessment tool and an intervention (McGoldrick, Gerson, & Petry, 2008). As an intervention, the genogram identifies not only problematic intergeneration patterns but also alternative ways for relating and handling problems. For example, if a person comes from a family in which one or more children in each generation have strongly rebelled against their parents, the genogram can be used to identify this pattern, note exceptions in the larger family, and identify ways to prevent or intervene on this dynamic. The genogram's visual depiction of the pattern across generations often inspires a greater sense of urgency and commitment to change than when the dynamics are only discussed in session. Constructing the genogram often generates a much greater sense of urgency and willingness to take action compared to relying strictly on process questions and a discussion of the dynamics. Chapter 2 includes a description of how to construct a genogram and use it in session.

Detriangulation

Detriangulation involves the therapist maintaining therapeutic neutrality (differentiation) in order to interrupt a client's attempt to involve the therapist or someone else in a triangle (Friedman, 1991). Whether working with an individual, couple, or family, most therapists at some point will be "invited" by clients to triangulate with them against a third party who may or may not be present in the room. When this occurs, the therapist "detriangulates" by refusing to take a side, whether literally or more subtly. For example, if a client says, "Don't you think it is inappropriate for a child to talk back?" or "Isn't it inappropriate for a husband to go to lunch with a single woman who is attracted to him?," the quickest way to relieve the client's anxiety is to agree: this makes the relationship between the client and therapist comfortable, allowing the client to immediately feel "better," "understood," and "empathized with." However, by validating the client's position and taking the client's side against another, the therapist undermines the long-term goal of promoting differentiation. Thus, if therapy becomes "stuck," therapists must first examine their role in a potential triangle (Friedman, 1991).

Rather than take a side, the therapist invites clients to validate *themselves*, examine their own part in the problem dynamic, and take responsibility for their needs and wants. There is often significant confusion in the therapeutic community about "validating" a client's feelings. *Validation* implies approval; however, approval from the therapist undermines a client's sense of autonomy. Intergenerational therapists emphasize that when therapists "validate" by saying "It is normal to feel this way," "It sounds like he really hurt you," or in some way imply "You are entitled to feel this way," they close down the opportunity for differentiation. Instead, clients are coached to approve or disapprove of their own thoughts and feelings and then take responsibility and action as needed.

Relational Experiments

Relational experiments are behavioral homework assignments that are designed to reveal and change unproductive relational processes in families (Guerin, Fogarty, Fay, & Kautto, 1996). These experiments interrupt triangulation processes by increasing direct communication between a dyad or by reversing pursuer/distancer dynamics that are fueled by lack of differentiation.

Going Home Again

Most adults are familiar with this paradox: you seem to be a balanced person who can manage a demanding career, an educational program, and a complex household; yet, when you go home to visit family for the holidays, you find yourself suddenly acting like a teenager—or worse. Intergenerational therapists see this difference in functioning as the result of unresolved issues with the family of origin that can be improved by increasing differentiation. Even if you cannot change a parent's critical comments or a sibling's arrogance, you can be in the presence of these "old irritants" and not regress to past behaviors but instead keep a clear sense of self. As clients' level of differentiation grows, they are able to maintain a stronger and clearer sense of self in the family nuclear system. The technique of "going home" refers to when therapists encourage clients to interact with family members while maintaining a clearer boundary between self and other and to practice and/or experience the reduced emotional reactivity that characterizes increases in differentiation (Friedman, 1991).

Interventions for Special Populations

The Sexual Crucible Model

One of the most influential applications of Bowen intergenerational theory is the Sexual Crucible Model developed by David Schnarch (1991). The model proposes that marriage functions as a "crucible," a vessel that physically contains a volatile transformational process. In the case of marriage, the therapist achieves transformation by helping both partners differentiate (or more simply, forcing them to "grow up"). As with all crucibles, the contents of marriage must be contained because they are unstable and explosive.

Schnarch views sexual and emotional intimacy as inherently intertwined in the process of differentiation. He directs partners to take responsibility for their individual needs rather than demand that the other change to accommodate their needs, wants, and desires. To remain calm, each person learns to self-soothe rather than demand that the other change. Schnarch also includes exercises like "hugging to relax" in which he helps couples develop a greater sense of physical intimacy and increased comfort with being "seen" by the other. He has developed this model for therapists to use with clients and has also made it accessible to general audiences (Schnarch, 1998).

Schnarch has developed a comprehensive and detailed model for helping couples create the type of relationship most couples today expect: a harmonious balance of emotional, sexual, intellectual, professional, financial, parenting, household, health, and social partnerships. However, Schnarch points out that this multifaceted intimacy has never been the norm in human relationships. His model is most appropriate for psychologically minded clients who are motivated to increase intimacy.

Psychoanalytic Family Therapies
In a Nutshell: The Least You Need to Know

Many of the founders of family therapy were psychoanalytically trained, including Don Jackson, Carl Whitaker, Salvador Minuchin, Nathan Ackerman, and Boszormenyi-Nagy. Although some disowned their academic roots as they developed methods for working with families, others, such as Nathan Ackerman and Boszormenyi-Nagy, did not. In the 1980s, renewed interest in object relations therapies led to the development of *object relations family therapy* (Scharff & Scharff, 1987).

These therapies use traditional psychoanalytic and psychodynamic principles that describe inner conflicts and extend these principles to external relationships. In contrast to individual psychoanalysts, psychoanalytic family therapists focus on the family as a nexus of relationships that either support or impede the development and functioning of its members. As in traditional psychoanalytic approaches, the process of therapy involves analyzing intrapsychic and interpersonal dynamics, promoting client insight, and working through these insights to develop new ways of relating to self and others. Some of the more influential approaches are *contextual therapy* (Boszormenyi-Nagy & Krasner, 1986), *family-of-origin therapy* (Framo, 1992), and *object relations family therapy* (Scharff & Scharff, 1987).

The Juice: Significant Contributions to the Field

If you remember one thing from this chapter, it should be this:

Ethical Systems and Relational Ethics

Boszormenyi-Nagy (1986; Boszormenyi-Nagy & Krasner, 1986) introduced the idea of an *ethical system* at the heart of families that, like a *ledger,* keeps track of *entitlement* and *indebtedness.* Families use this system to maintain trustworthiness, fairness, and loyalty between family members; its breakdown results in individual and/or relational symptoms. Thus the goal of therapy is to re-establish an ethical system in which family members are able to trust one another and to treat one another with fairness.

Clients often present in therapy with a semiconscious awareness of this ethical accounting system. Their presenting complaint may be that things are no longer fair in the relationship; parents are not sharing their duties equitably or one child is being treated differently than another. In these cases, an explicit dialogue about the family's ethical accounting system—what they are counting as their entitlement and what they believe is owed them—can be helpful in increasing empathy and understanding among family members.

Rumor Has It: The People and Their Stories

Nathan Ackerman and the Ackerman Institute

A child psychiatrist, Nathan Ackerman (1958, 1966) was one of the earliest pioneers in working with entire families, which he posited were split into factions, much the way an individual's psyche is divided into conflicting aspects of self. After developing his family approach at the Menninger Clinic in the 1930s and at Jewish Family Services in New York in the 1950s, he opened his own clinic in 1960, now known as the Ackerman Institute, which has remained one of the most influential family therapy institutes in the country. With Don Jackson, he co-founded the field's first journal, *Family Process*.

Ivan Boszormenyi-Nagy

With one of the most difficult names to pronounce in the field (Bo-zor-ma-nee Naj), Boszormenyi-Nagy was an early pioneer in psychoanalytic family therapy. His most unique contribution was his idea that families had an ethical system, which he conceptualized as a *ledger of entitlement and indebtedness* (Boszormenyi-Nagy & Krasner, 1986).

James Framo

A student of Boszormenyi-Nagy, James Framo is best known for developing *family-of-origin therapy*; as part of treatment with individuals, couples, and families, he invited a client's entire family of origin in for extended sessions (Boszormenyi-Nagy & Framo, 1965/1985; Framo, 1992). Framo located the primary problem not only in the family unit but also in the larger extended family system.

David and Jill Scharff

A husband-and-wife team, David and Jill Scharff (1987) developed a comprehensive model for object relations family therapy. Rather than focusing on individuals, they apply principles from traditional object relations therapy to the family as a unit.

The Women's Project

Bowenian trained social workers Marianne Walters, Betty Carter, Peggy Papp, and Olga Silverstein (1988) reformulated many foundational family therapy concepts through a feminist lens. Their work challenged the field to examine gender stereotypes that were being reinforced in family therapy theory and practice, within and beyond the practice of Bowen family therapy.

The Big Picture: Overview of Treatment

The psychodynamic tradition includes a number of different schools that share the same therapeutic process. The first task is to create a caring therapeutic relationship, or *holding environment* (Scharff & Scharff, 1987), between the therapist and client. Then the therapist analyzes the intrapsychic and interpersonal dynamics—both conscious and unconscious, current and transgenerational—that are the source of symptoms (Boszormenyi-Nagy & Krasner, 1986; Scharff & Scharff, 1987). The therapist's next task is to promote client insight into these dynamics, which requires getting through client defenses. Once clients have achieved insights into the intrapsychic and interpersonal dynamics that fuel the problem, the therapist facilitates *working through* these insights to translate them into action in clients' daily lives.

Making Connection: The Therapeutic Relationship

Transference and Countertransference

A classic psychoanalytic concept, *transference* refers to when a client projects onto the therapist attributes that stem from unresolved issues with primary caregivers; therapists use the immediacy of these interactions to promote client insight (Scharff & Scharff, 1987). *Countertransference* refers to when therapists project back onto clients, losing their therapeutic neutrality and having strong emotional reactions to the client; these moments are used to help the therapist and client better understand the reactions the client brings out in others. In therapy with couples and families, the processes of transference and countertransference vacillate more than in individual therapy because of the complex web of multiple relationships.

Contextual and Centered Holding

In contrast to traditional psychoanalysts, who are viewed as neutral "blank screens," object relations family therapists are more relationally focused, creating a nurturing relationship they call a *holding environment*. They distinguish between two aspects of holding in family therapy: contextual and centered (Scharff & Scharff, 1987). *Contextual holding* refers to the therapist's handling of therapy arrangements: conducting sessions competently, expressing concern for the family, and being willing to see the entire family. *Centered holding* refers to connecting with the family at a deeper level by expressing empathetic understanding to create a safe emotional space.

Multidirected Partiality

The guiding principle for relating to clients in contextual family therapy is *multidirectional partiality*, that is, being "partial" with all members of the family (Boszormenyi-Nagy & Krasner, 1986). Therapists must be accountable to everyone who is potentially affected by the interventions, including those not immediately present in the room, such as extended family members. This principle of inclusiveness means that the therapist must bring out the humanity of each member of the family, even the "monster member" (Boszormenyi-Nagy & Krasner, 1986). In practice, multidirectional partiality generally involves *sequential siding* with each member by empathizing with each person's position in turn.

The Viewing: Case Conceptualization and Assessment

Interlocking Pathologies

Expanding the classic psychodynamic view of symptomology, Ackerman (1956) held that the constant exchange of unconscious processes within families creates interlocking or interdependent pathologies and that any individual's pathology reflects those family distortions and dynamics, a position similar to that of systemic therapies. Thus, when working with a family, the therapist seeks to identify *how* the identified patient's symptoms relate to the less overt pathologies within the family.

Self-Object Relations Patterns

Object relations therapists emphasize the basic human need for relationship and attachment to others. Thus they assess *self-object relations*: how people relate to others based on expectations developed by early experiences with primary attachment objects, particularly mothers (Scharff & Scharff, 1987). As a result of these experiences, external objects are experienced as ideal, rejecting, or exciting:

- **Ideal Object:** An internal mental representation of the primary caretaker that is desexualized and deaggressivized and maintained as distinct from its rejecting and exciting elements

- **Rejecting Object:** An internal mental representation of the caregiver when the child's needs for attachment were rejected, leading to anger

- **Exciting Object:** An internal mental representation of the caretaker formed when the child's needs for attachment were overstimulated, leading to longing for an unattainable but tempting object

Splitting

The more intense the anxiety resulting from frustration related to the primary caregiver, the greater the person's need to spilt these objects, separating good from bad objects by repressing the rejecting and/or exciting objects, thus leaving less of the *ego*, or conscious self, to relate freely. To the degree that splitting is not resolved, there is an "all good" or "all bad" quality to evaluating relationships. In couples, splitting often results in seeing the partner as "perfect" (all good) in the early phases of the relationship, but when the partner no longer conforms to expectations, the partner becomes the enemy (all bad). In families, splitting can also take the form of the perfect versus the problem child.

Projective Identification

In couples and other intimate relationships, clients defend against anxiety by projecting certain split-off or unwanted parts of themselves onto the other person, who is then manipulated to act according to these projections (Scharff & Scharff, 1987). For example, a husband may project his interest in other women onto his wife in the form of jealousy and accusations of infidelity; the wife then decides to hide innocent information that may feed the husband's fear, but the more she tries to calm his fears by hiding information, the more suspicious and jealous he becomes.

Repression

Object relations therapists maintain that children must *repress* anxiety when they experience separation with their primary caregiver (attachment object), which results in less of the ego being available for contact with the outside world. Until this repressed material is made conscious, the adult unconsciously replicates these repressed object relationships. One of the primary aims of psychoanalytic therapy is to bring repressed material to the surface.

Parental Interjects

Framo (1976) believes that the most significant dynamic affecting individual and family functioning is parental introjects, the internalized negative aspects of parents. People internalize these attributes and unconsciously strive to make all future intimate relationships conform to them, such as when they hear a parent's critical comments in the neutral comments of a partner. Therapists help clients become conscious of these introjects to increase their autonomy in intimate relationships.

Transference Between Family Members

Similar to the way they assess transference from client to therapist, object relations therapists assess for transference from one family member onto another (Scharff & Scharff, 1987). Transference between family members involves one person projecting onto other members introjects and repressed material. The therapist's job is to help the family disentangle their transference, using interpretation to promote insight into intrapsychic and interpersonal dynamics. It is often easier to promote insight into transference patterns in family therapy than in individual therapy because these patterns happen "live" in the room with the therapist, thus reducing the potential for a client to rationalize or minimize.

Ledger of Entitlement and Indebtedness

Boszormenyi-Nagy (1986; Boszormenyi-Nagy & Krasner, 1986) conceptualized the moral and ethical system within the family as a *ledger of entitlements and indebtedness,* or more simply a *ledger of merits,* an internal accounting of what one believes is due and what one owes others. Of course, because in families each person has his/her own internal accounting system that has a different bottom line, tensions arise over who is entitled to what, especially if there is no consensus on what is fair and how give-and-take should be balanced in the family.

- **Justice and Fairness:** The pursuit of justice and fairness is viewed as one of the foundational premises of intimate relationships. Monitoring fairness is an ongoing process that keeps the relationship *trustworthy.* A "just" relationship is an ideal, and all relationships strive to achieve this never fully attainable goal.

- **Entitlements:** Entitlements are "ethical guarantees" to merits that are earned in the context of relationships, such as the freedom that parents are entitled to because of the care they extend to children. The person's sense of entitlement may only be evident in a crisis or extreme situation, such as a parent becoming suddenly ill. *Destructive entitlements* result when children do not receive the nurturing to which they are entitled and later project this loss onto the world, which they see as their "debtors."

- **Invisible Loyalties:** Family ledgers extend across generations, fostering invisible loyalties. For example, new couples may have unconscious commitments to their family of origin when starting their partnership. Invisible loyalties may manifest as indifferences, avoidance, or indecisiveness in relation to the object of loyalty, blocking commitment in a current relationship.

- **Revolving Slate:** This is a destructive relational process in which one person takes revenge (or insists on entitlements) in one relationship based on the relational transactions in another relationship. Instead of reconciling the "slate" or account in the relationship in which the debt was accrued, the person treats an innocent person as if he or she was the original debtor.

- **Split Loyalties:** This term refers to when a child feels forced to choose one parent (or significant caregiver) over another because of mistrust between the caregivers. Common in divorces, this highly destructive dynamic results in pathology in the child.

- **Legacy:** Each person inherits a legacy, a transgenerational mandate that links the endowments of the current generation to its obligations to future generations. "Legacy is the present generation's ethical imperative to sort out what in life is beneficial for posterity's quality of survival" (Boszormenyi-Nagy & Krasner, 1986, p. 418). Legacy is a positive force in the chain of survival.

Mature Love: Dialogue Versus Fusion

Boszormenyi-Nagy (1986) describes mature love as a form of dialogue between two people who are conscious of the family dynamics that have shaped their lives. This type of love is quite different from fusion, experienced as an amorphous "we" similar to an infant and its caregiver. Thus clients are encouraged to make invisible loyalties overt so that they can be critically examined, allowing for conscious choice and action rather than the fear and anxiety that characterize fused relationships.

Targeting Change: Goal Setting

Goals in psychoanalytic therapies include several long-term changes in both individual and relational functioning (Boszormenyi-Nagy & Krasner, 1986; Scharff & Scharff, 1987). General goals include the following:

- Increase autonomy and ego-directed action by making unconscious processes conscious
- Decrease interactions based on projections or a revolving slate of entitlements
- Increase capacity for intimacy without loss of self (fusion with object)
- Develop reciprocal commitments that include a fair balance of entitlements and indebtedness

The Doing: Interventions

Listening, Interpreting, and Working Through

In general, psychoanalytic therapies use three generic interventions:

- **Listening and Empathy:** The primary tool of psychoanalytic therapists is listening objectively to the client's story without offering advice, reassurance, validation, or confrontation. Empathy may be used to help the family to nondefensively hear the therapist's interpretation of their unconscious dynamics.

- **Interpretation and Promoting Insight:** Like other psychoanalytic therapists, family psychoanalytic therapists encourage insights into interpersonal dynamics by offering interpretations to the client, such as by analyzing self-object relations or analyzing ledgers of entitlement and indebtedness.

- **Working Through:** Working through is the process of translating insight into new action in family and other relationships. Changing one's behavior on the basis of new insight is often the most difficult part of therapy. Understanding that you are projecting onto your partner feelings and expectations that really belong in your relationship with your mother is not too difficult; changing how you respond to your partner when you feel rejected and uncared for is more challenging.

Eliciting

In contextual therapy, *eliciting* uses clients' spontaneous motives to move the family in a direction that is mutually beneficial and dialogical (Boszormenyi-Nagy & Krasner, 1986). The therapist facilitates this process by integrating the facts of the situation, each person's individual psychology, and interactive transitions to help the family rework the balances of entitlement and indebtedness, helping each member to reinterpret past interactions and identify new ways to move forward.

Detriangulating

Like other systemic therapists, psychoanalytic therapists identify situations in which the parents have triangulated a symptomatic child into the relationship to deflect attention from their couple distress (Framo, 1992). Once the child's role is made clear, the therapist dismisses the symptomatic child from therapy and proceeds to work with the couple to address the issues that created the need for the child's symptoms.

Family-of-Origin Therapy

Framo (1992) developed a three-stage model for working with couples that involved couples therapy, couples group therapy, and family-of-origin therapy. Therapists begin working with the couple alone to increase insight into their personal and relational dynamics. Next, the couple join a couples group, where they receive feedback from other couples and also view their dynamics; for many couples, insight comes more quickly when they see their problem dynamic acted out in another couple. Finally, each individual member of the couple is invited to have a four-hour-long session with his/her family of origin without the other partner present. These extended family-of-origin sessions are used to clarify and work through past and present issues, thereby freeing individuals to respond to their partners and children without the "ghosts" of these past attachments.

Interventions for Special Populations

Women's Project

Trained as social workers, Betty Carter, Olga Silverstein, Peggy Papp, and Marianne Walters (Walters et al., 1988) joined together to promote a greater awareness of women's issues in the field of family therapy. They raised the issue of gender power dynamics within traditional families and identified how family therapists were reinforcing stereotypes that were detrimental to women. In particular, they explicated how the misuse of power and control in abusive and violent relationships made it impossible for women to end or escape their victimization, a perspective that is now accepted by most therapists and the public at large. They also asserted that therapists should be *agents of social change*, challenging sexist attitudes and beliefs in families.

Walters et al. (1988) made several suggestions for how family therapists can reduce sexism in their work with couples and families:

- Openly discuss the *gender role expectations* of each partner and parent and point out areas where the couple or family hold beliefs that are unfair or unrealistic.
- Encourage women to take *private time* for themselves to avoid losing their individual identity to the roles of wife and mother.
- Use the self-of-the-therapist to model an *attitude of gender equality*.
- Push men to take on equal responsibility both in family relationships and in the household, as well as for scheduling therapy, attending therapy with children, and/or arranging for babysitting for couples sessions.

Snapshot: Research and the Evidence Base

Quick Summary: Research has focused more on theoretical constructs than on therapeutic outcome.

The focus of research on Bowenian and psychoanalytic therapies has not been on outcome, as is required to be labeled as empirically validated studies (Chapter 7), but rather on the validity of the concepts. Miller, Anderson, and Keala (2004) provide an overview of the research on the validity of the theoretical constructs. They found that research supports the relation between differentiation and (a) chronic anxiety, (b) marital satisfaction, and (c) psychological distress. However, there was little support for Bowen's assumption that people marry a person with a similar level of differentiation or his theories on sibling position; his concept of triangulation received partial empirical support.

Of particular interest to researchers is Bowen's concept of differentiation of self, which has been the focus of scores of research studies on topics such as client perceptions of the therapeutic alliance (Lambert, 2008), adolescent risk-taking behaviors (Knauth, Skowron, & Escobar, 2006), parenting outcomes in low-income urban families (Skowron, 2005), and adult well-being (Skowron, Holmes, & Sabatelli, 2003). Lawson and Brossart (2003) conducted a study that predicted therapeutic alliance and therapeutic outcome from the therapist's relationship with his or her parents, providing support for the Bowenian emphasis on the self-of-the-therapist. In regards to psychoanalytic family therapies, significant research has been conducted on the nature of attachment in problem formation (Wood, 2002). The concept of attachment is also central to two empirically supported family therapies: emotionally focused therapy (Chapter 11; Johnson, 2004) and multidimensional therapy (Chapter 9; Liddle, Dakof, Parker, Diamond, Barrett, & Tejeda, 2001). Research is needed on the outcomes and effectiveness of Bowen and psychoanalytic family therapies so that these models can be refined and further developed.

Snapshot: Working with Diverse Populations

Quick Summary: When working with diverse populations, therapists should use these insight-oriented approaches carefully, attending to the client's attitude toward introspection, rationality, and psychological analysis.

Apart from the work of the Women's Project (Walters et al., 1988), the application of Bowen intergenerational and psychoanalytic therapies to diverse populations has not been widely explored or studied. In general, these therapies are aimed at "thinking" or psychologically minded clients (Friedman, 1991). Thus minority groups who prefer action and concrete suggestions from therapists may have difficulty with these approaches. However, the therapist's stance as an expert fits with the expectations of many immigrant and marginalized populations. The work of Bowen, Framo, and Boszormenyi-Nagy that emphasizes the role of extended family members and intergenerational patterns may be particularly useful with diverse clients whose cultural norms dictate the primacy of extended family over the nuclear family system. In these families, it is expected that the nuclear family subordinate their will to that of the larger family system. In addition, research on the concept of differentiation of self provides initial support for its cross-cultural validity (Skowron, 2004).

In general, the greatest danger in using Bowenian or psychoanalytic therapies with diverse clients is that the therapist will use inappropriate cultural norms to analyze family dynamics, thereby imposing a set of values and beliefs that are at odds with the clients' culture. For example, if a therapist, without reflection, proceeds on the Bowenian premise that the nuclear family should be autonomous and develops therapeutic goals to move an immigrant family in that direction, the therapist could put the client in the difficult situation of being caught between the therapist's goals and the extended family's expectations. Similarly, if the therapist assumes that attachment in all cultures looks the same, the client may be inaccurately and unfairly evaluated, resulting in a therapy that is ineffective at best and destructive at worst. Because these theories have highly developed systems of assessing "normal" behavior, therapists must be mindful when working with clients who do not conform to common cultural norms. The case study that concludes this chapter applies intergenerational therapy to a Chinese immigrant couple in which the wife has had a recent onset of panic attacks.

ONLINE RESOURCES

Ackerman Institute: Psychoanalytic Therapy and Family Therapy Training
www.ackerman.org

The Bowen Center
thebowencenter.org

Center for Family Learning: Bowen Intergenerational Therapy
jrlobdellwebdesign.com/centerforfamilylearning/index.html

Georgetown Family Center: Bowen Center for the Study of the Family
www.thebowencenter.org/

Family Process: Journal
www.familyprocess.org

Sexual Crucible Model
www.passionatemarriage.com

REFERENCES

*Asterisk indicates recommended introductory readings.

Ackerman, N. W. (1956). Interlocking pathology in family relationships. In S. Rado & B. G. Daniels (Eds.), *Changing conceptions of psychoanalytic medicine* (pp. 135–150). New York: Grune & Stratton.

Ackerman, N. W. (1958). *The psychodynamics of family life.* New York: Basic Books.

Ackerman, N. W. (1966). *Treating the troubled family.* New York: Basic Books.

Boszormenyi-Nagy, I., & Framo, J. L. (1965/1985). *Intensive family therapy: Theoretical and practical aspects.* New York: Brunner/Mazel.

*Boszormenyi-Nagy, I., & Krasner, B. R. (1986). *Between give and take: A clinical guide to contextual therapy.* New York: Brunner/Mazel.

Bowen, M. (1966). The use of family theory in clinical practice. *Comprehensive Psychiatry* 7, 345–374.

Bowen, M. (1972). Being and becoming a family therapist. In A. Ferber, M. Mendelsohn, & A. Napier (Eds.), *The book of family therapy.* New York: Science House.

Bowen, M. (1976). Theory in practice of psychotherapy. In P. J. Guerin (Ed.), *Family therapy: Theory and practice.* New York: Gardner Press.

*Bowen, M. (1985). *Family therapy in clinical practice.* New York: Jason Aronson.

*Carter, B., & McGoldrick, M. (1999). *The expanded family life cycle: Individual, family, and social perspectives* (3rd ed.). Boston: Allyn & Bacon.

Framo, J. L. (1976). Family of origin as a therapeutic resource for adults in marital and family therapy: You can and should go home again. *Family Process 15*(2), 193–210.

*Framo, J. L. (1992). *Family-of-origin therapy: An intergenerational approach.* New York: Brunner/Mazel.

Friedman, E. H. (1991). Bowen theory and therapy. In A. S. Gurman and D. P. Kniskern (Eds.), *Handbook of family therapy* (Vol. 2, pp. 134–170). Philadelphia: Brunner/Mazel.

Guerin, P. J., Fogarty, T. F., Fay, L. F., & Kautto, J. G. (1996). *Working with relationship triangles: The one-two-three of psychotherapy.* New York: Guilford.

Hardy, K. V., & Laszloffy, T. A. (1995). The cultural genogram: Key to training culturally competent family therapists. *Journal of Marital and Family Therapy, 21,* 227–237.

Johnson, S. M. (2004). *The practice of emotionally focused marital therapy: Creating connection* (2nd ed.). New York: Brunner/Routledge.

*Kerr, M., & Bowen, M. (1988). *Family evaluation.* New York: Norton.

Knauth, D. G., Skowron, E. A., & Escobar, M. (2006). Effect of differentiation of self on adolescent risk behavior. *Nursing Research, 55,* 336–345.

Kuehl, B. P. (1995). The solution-oriented genogram: A collaborative approach. *Journal of Marital and Family Therapy, 21,* 239–250.

Lambert, J. (2008). Relationship of differentiation of self to adult clients' perceptions of the alliance in brief family therapy. *Psychotherapy Research, 18,* 160–166.

Lawson, D. M., & Brossart, D. F. (2003). Link among therapist and parent relationship, working alliance, and therapy outcome. *Psychothrapy Research, 13,* 383–394.

Licht, C., & Chabot, D. (2006). The Chabot Emotional Differentiation Scale: A theoretically and psychometrically sound instrument for measuring Bowen's intrapsychic aspect of differentiation. *Journal of Marital and Family Therapy, 32*(2), 167–180.

Liddle, H. A., Dakof, G. A., Parker, K., Diamond, G. S., Barrett, K., & Tejeda, M. (2001). Multidimensional family therapy for adolescent drug abuse: Results of a randomized clinical trial. *American Journal of Drug and Alcohol Abuse, 27,* 651–688.

*McGoldrick, M., Gerson, R., & Petry, S. (2008). *Genograms: Assessment and intervention* (3rd ed.). New York: Norton.

Miller, R. B., Anderson, S., & Keala, D. K. (2004). Is Bowen theory valid? A review of basic research. *Journal of Marital and Family Therapy, 30,* 453–466.

Rubalcava, L. A., & Waldman, K. M. (2004). Working with intercultural couples: An intersubjective-constructivist perspective. *Progress in Self Psychology, 20,* 127–149.

*Scharff, D., & Scharff, J. (1987). *Object relations family therapy.* New York: Aronson.

Schnarch, D. M. (1991). *Constructing the sexual crucible: An integration of sexual and marital therapy.* New York: Norton.

Schnarch, D. M. (1998). *Passionate marriage: Keeping love and intimacy alive in committed relationships.* New York: Holt.

Skowron, E. A. (2004). Differentiation of self, personal adjustment, problem solving, and ethnic group belonging among persons of color. *Journal of Counseling and Development, 82,* 447–456.

Skowron, E. A. (2005). Parental differentiation of self and child competence in low-income urban families. *Journal of Counseling Psychology, 52,* 337–346.

Skowron, E. A., Holmes, S. E., & Sabatelli, R. M. (2003). Deconstructing differentiation: Self regulation, interdependent relating, and well-being in adulthood. *Contemporary Family Therapy, 25,* 111–129.

*Walters, M., Carter, B., Papp, P., & Silverstein, O. (1988). *The invisible web: Gender patterns in family relationships.* New York: Guilford.

*Wood, B. L. (2002). Attachment and family systems (Special issue). *Family Process, 41.*

INTERGENERATIONAL CASE STUDY

Wei-Wei is seeking therapy because she recently started having panic attacks. She lives with her husband who is a surgeon and reports that life has been going well: she was recently promoted to rank of full professor at a prestigious university and her only son recently finished medical school. She reports no particular stress at the moment and is unsure why she is having these attacks. Her only prior history of mental disorders was anorexia as a teen as a way with coping with being sexually abused by an uncle while growing up in China.

After an initial consultation, an intergenerational family therapist developed the following case conceptualization.

Shaded Sections Emphasized in Intergenerational Treatment Planning and Intervention

CASE CONCEPTUALIZATION FORM

Therapist: Mei Zhou   **Client/Case #:** 1121   **Date:** 2/3/09

I. Introduction to Client and Significant Others *(Include age, ethnicity, occupation, grade, relevant identifiers, etc.). Put an * next to persons in session and/or IP for identified patient.*

AF†:   *53 (IP), professor of dance, immigrated from China to seek graduate education

AM: *55, surgeon, immigrated from China to seek education, met AF in school.

CF or _____ :

CM: 26, recently graduated from medical school, starting residency in Oregon, girlfriend moved with him

II. Presenting Concern

Client's/Family's Descriptions of Problem(s):

AF: Reports not knowing why she is having panic attacks; reports that life is otherwise "fine."

AM: Believes that panic is related to AF's perfectionism and loss of CM at home.

CF or _____ :

CM: Describes AF as "high strung" and always wanting things to look perfect.

Broader System Problem Descriptions (description of problem from referring party, teachers, relatives, legal system, etc.):

AF's friend: Believes AF is having a midlife crisis with CM leaving home and having finally reached her

last major personal goal: tenure.

III. Background Information

Recent Background (recent life changes, precipitating events, first symptoms, stressors, etc.):

After a period of positive life transitions—she was promoted at a prestigious university last year and

her son finished his residency six months prior—AF had her first panic attack 4 months ago while at the

opera with her husband. She reports feeling suddenly overwhelmed and had to leave in the middle of

the performance. Since then she has had an attack every 2–4 weeks with no identifiable trigger.

Related Historical Background (family history, related issues, past abuse, trauma, previous counseling, medical/mental health history, etc.):

AF reports being sexually abused by her uncle as a child growing up in Beijing, China. Her parents

were active in the Communist Party and were very concerned about how they were viewed in the com-

munity; when she told them about the abuse, they did not believe her. The abuse continued until

---

† *Abbreviations:* AF: Adult Female; AM: Adult Male; CF#: Child Female with age, e.g., CF12; CM#: Child Male with age; Hx: History; Ex: Explanation or Example; NA: Not Applicable.

(continued)

III. Background Information *(continued)*

she was old enough to fight him off, at around 16. During this time she reports eating very little to gain a sense of control over her life. She made it a goal to get a visa to study in the United States, which she did at 22. Lee is also an immigrant from China, coming to the U.S. to study. The couple met in college through the Chinese student association. The couple see their families every 4–5 years, AF rarely communicating with hers any longer.

IV. Systemic Assessment

Client/Relational Strengths

Personal/individual: AF and AM are both highly intelligent with a "survivor" attitude. Both are hardworking, accomplished professionals and dedicated to raising their son.

Relational/social: AF and AM have created a strong social network in the local Chinese community; they have two couples with whom they spend time on weekends.

Spiritual: Although neither was raised in a religious tradition, AF turns to Daoist and Buddhist writings for inspiration in learning how to create balance in her life.

Family Structure and Interaction Patterns

Couple Subsystem (to be assessed): ☒ Personal current ☐ Personal past ☐ Parents'

Couple Boundaries: ☐ Clear ☐ Enmeshed ☒ Disengaged ☐ Other: _____

Rules for closeness/distance: Both AF and AM are highly involved in their careers, which demand long hours. Although they have little conflict, they also have minimal emotional engagement, less so than what may be expected culturally although typical in a couple in which one partner has never been treated for sexual abuse.

Couple Problem Interaction Pattern (A ⇆ B):

Start of tension: AF has panic attack "out of the blue."

Conflict/symptom escalation: AM initially tries to calm her down: first gently reassuring but later becoming more agitated with her illogical response that typically demands that he drop what he is doing to take her home.

Return to "normal"/homeostasis: AM eventually takes her home and she calms down; they stay distant for the rest of the day but then return to normal by the next day.

Couple Complementary Patterns: ☐ Pursuer/distancer ☐ Over/under functioner

☐ Emotional/logical ☐ Good/bad parent ☒ Other: Symmetrical pattern of intellectual achievement; Ex: AF and AM compete intellectually and with their professional achievements.

Satir Communication Stances:

AF: ☐ Congruent ☐ Placator ☐ Blamer ☒ Superreasonable ☐ Irrelevant

AM: ☐ Congruent ☐ Placator ☐ Blamer ☒ Superreasonable ☐ Irrelevant

Describe dynamic: <u>Both partners are highly logical, focusing on what is contextually "appropriate"</u>

<u>and logical rather than what either is feeling.</u>

Gottman's Divorce Indicators:

Criticism: ☐ AF ☐ AM. Ex: <u>NA</u>

Defensiveness: ☐ AF ☐ AM. Ex: <u>NA</u>

Contempt: ☐ AF ☐ AM. Ex: <u>NA</u>

Stonewalling: ☒ AF ☒ AM. Ex: <u>If there is conflict or tension, it is handled with stonewalling or con-</u>

<u>flict avoidance.</u>

Failed repair attempts: ☐ AF ☐ AM. Ex: <u>NA</u>

Not accept influence: ☐ AF ☐ AM. Ex: <u>NA</u>

Harsh startup: ☐ AF ☐ AM. Ex: <u>NA</u>

Parental Subsystem: ☒ Family of procreation; ☐ Family of origin

Membership in Family Subsystems: Parental: ☒ AF ☒ AM. ☐ Other: _____

Is parental subsystem distinct from couple subsystem? ☒ Yes ☐ No ☐ NA (divorce)

Sibling subsystem: <u>NA</u>

Special interest: <u>AM and CM are both medical doctors</u>

Family Life Cycle Stage:

☐ Single adult ☐ Marriage ☐ Family with young children

☐ Family with adolescent children ☒ Launching children ☐ Later life

Describe struggles with mastering developmental tasks in one of these stages:

<u>CM has just left home and AF is having unexplained symptoms; it is possible that the panic attacks</u>

<u>are related to her adjusting to the launching of her only child.</u>

Hierarchy Between Child/Parents:

AF: ☒ Effective ☐ Insufficient (permissive) ☐ Excessive (authoritarian) ☐ Inconsistent

AM: ☒ Effective ☐ Insufficient (permissive) ☐ Excessive (authoritarian) ☐ Inconsistent

Ex: _____

Emotional Boundaries with Children:

AF: ☐ Clear/balanced ☒ Enmeshed (reactive) ☐ Disengaged (disinterested)

☐ Other: _____

(continued)

IV. Systemic Assessment (*continued*)

AM: ☒ Clear/balanced ☐ Enmeshed (reactive) ☐ Disengaged (disinterested)

   ☐ Other: _____

Ex: _____

Problem Interaction Pattern (A ⇆ B):

Start of tension: CM needs to complete applications for residency.

Conflict/symptom escalation: AF frequently inquires as to his progress with his applications; CM begins to feel smothered and avoids her; she pursues more; he gets angry but then rushes to do it all at once.

Return to "normal"/homeostasis: Once CM does what AF has asked, she lavishly compliments him and cheers on his efforts toward success.

Triangles/Coalitions:

☐ AF and C _____ against AM: Ex: _____

☐ AM and C _____ against AF: Ex: _____

☒ Other: Ex: AF and AM focus on CM rather than each other; CM has been the "glue" that keeps them together.

Communication Stances

AF or _____ : ☐ Congruent ☐ Placator ☐ Blamer ☒ Superreasonable ☐ Irrelevant

AM or _____ : ☐ Congruent ☐ Placator ☐ Blamer ☒ Superreasonable ☐ Irrelevant

CF or _____ : ☐ Congruent ☒ Placator ☐ Blamer ☐ Superreasonable ☐ Irrelevant

CM or _____ : ☐ Congruent ☐ Placator ☐ Blamer ☐ Superreasonable ☐ Irrelevant

Ex: CM uses placating to deal with his mother's anxiety and attention.

Hypothesis (Describe possible role or function of symptom in maintaining family homeostasis):

When CM left for his residency, AF had lost the emotional focal point of her life, as did the couple lose the focal point of their relationship. AF had recently also achieved her last major professional goal; thus her future focus is unclear, resulting in anxiety that has taken the form of panic attacks.

Intergenerational Patterns

Substance/alcohol abuse: ☒ NA ☐ Hx: _____

Sexual/physical/emotional abuse: ☐ NA ☒ Hx: CF abused for over 6 years by uncle.

Parent/child relations: ☐ NA ☒ Hx: AM and AF both have distant relationships with their parents.

Physical/mental disorders: ☐ NA ☒ Hx: AF's family has hx of heart disease; AM cancer.

Historical incidents of presenting problem: ☒ NA ☐ Hx: _____

Family strengths: History of professionals on both sides; continued in the U.S.

Previous Solutions and Unique Outcomes

Solutions that DIDN'T work: Removing AF from situations when she has panic disorder works in the short term but has not prevented future attacks.

Solutions that DID work: AF reports not having an attack while at work.

Narratives, Dominant Discourses, and Diversity

Dominant Discourses informing definition of problem:

Cultural, ethnic, SES, etc.: AF immigrated from China, the daughter of mid-level Chinese communist leaders who privileged family reputation over AF's report of sexual abuse. They valued hiding emotional problems at all costs; AF dealt with the abuse by controlling her eating. This pattern may relate to her current panic attacks as possible symptoms related to the launching of CM.

Gender, sex orientation, etc.: As a child, AF learned that women should be equal to men and should not burden others with their emotional pain.

Other social influences: In the eyes of the local Chinese community, AF and AM have been very successful, especially in raising their son, who has become an MD. This leads AF to feel the pressure to "be perfect" on the outside even if she feels otherwise on the inside.

Identity Narratives that have developed around problem for AF, AM, and/or CM/F:

AF reports that "life is great" and is thus puzzled by the emergence of panic attacks, which make her feel weak and victimized again. AM is frustrated because his wife who has been so competent historically is now acting on unexplained, childlike fears; thus, he also is feeling powerless.

Local or Preferred Discourses: AF is now questioning "what is success?" and "what comes after achieving her life goals?"

Other Influential Discourses: As MDs, both AM and CM feel a certain pressure to help AF fix this problem.

V. Genogram

Construct a family genogram and include all relevant information, including:

- ages, birth/death dates
- names
- relational patterns
- occupations
- medical history
- psychiatric disorders
- abuse history

V. Genogram *(continued)*

Also include a couple of adjectives for persons frequently discussed in session (these should describe personal qualities and/or relational patterns, e.g., quiet, family caretaker, emotionally distant, perfectionist, helpless, etc.). Genogram should be attached to report.

VI. Client Perspectives

Areas of Agreement: Based on what the client(s) has(ve) said, what parts of the above assessment do they agree with or are likely to agree with?

AM is more convinced than AF that her symptoms are related to CM moving away.

Areas of Disagreement: What parts do they disagree with or are likely to disagree with? Why?

AF is hesitant to link her symptoms to her son's moving away; she is also hesitant to see the relevancy of

her childhood abuse on her symptoms today.

How do you plan to respectfully work with areas of disagreement?

Tentatively make associations between past and present and between AF's symptoms and other recent

life changes, openly acknowledging that there may be other explanations or causes.

GENOGRAM

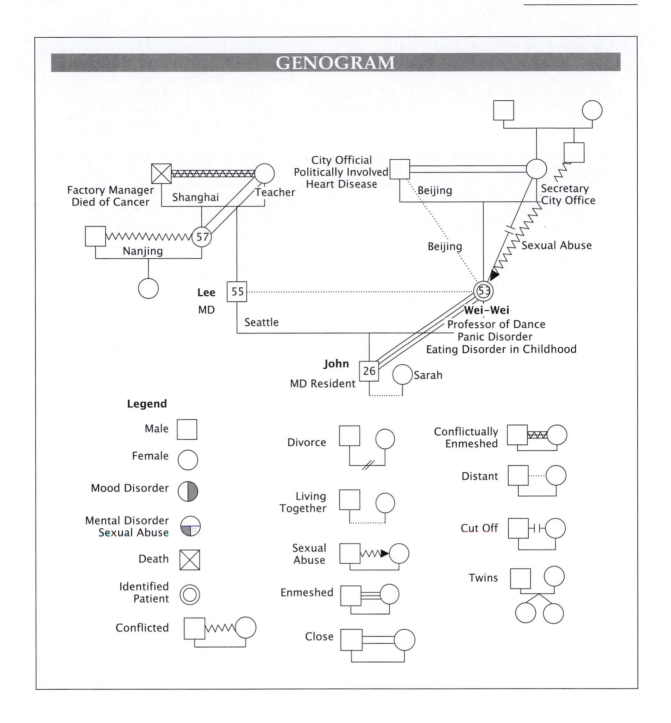

Factory Manager
Died of Cancer

Shanghai

Teacher

City Official
Politically Involved
Heart Disease

Beijing

Secretary
City Office

Nanjing

57

Beijing

Sexual Abuse

Lee | 55

MD

53

Wei–Wei
Professor of Dance
Panic Disorder
Eating Disorder in Childhood

Seattle

John | 26

MD Resident

Sarah

Legend

Male	☐
Female	○
Mood Disorder	◑
Mental Disorder Sexual Abuse	⊙
Death	☒
Identified Patient	◎
Conflicted	☐〜〜○

Divorce

Living Together

Sexual Abuse

Enmeshed

Close

Conflictually Enmeshed

Distant

Cut Off

Twins

CLINICAL ASSESSMENT

Client ID # (do not use name): 1121	Ethnicity(ies): Chinese Immigrants	Primary Language: ☐ Eng ☐ Span ☒ Other: Mandarin

List all participants/significant others: Put a [★] for Identified Patient (IP); [✔] for sig. others who **WILL** attend; [✕] for sig. others who will **NOT** attend

Adult: Age: Profession/Employer	Child: Age: School/Grade
[✔] AM 55: Immigrant from Shang-hai; surgeon	[✕] CM 26: MD in residency; lives with girlfriend
[★] AF 53: Immigrant from Beijing; professor of dance	[ ] CF _____
[ ] AF/M #2: _____	[ ] CF/M _____

Presenting Problems

☐ Depression/hopelessness
☒ Anxiety/worry
☐ Anger issues
☒ Loss/grief
☐ Suicidal thoughts/attempts
☒ Sexual abuse/rape
☐ Alcohol/drug use
☐ Eating problems/disorders
☐ Job problems/unemployed

☐ Couple concerns
☐ Parent/child conflict
☐ Partner violence/abuse
☐ Divorce adjustment
☐ Remarriage adjustment
☐ Sexuality/intimacy concerns
☒ Major life changes
☐ Legal issues/probation
☐ Other: _____

Complete for children
☐ School failure/decline performance
☐ Truancy/runaway
☐ Fighting w/peers
☐ Hyperactivity
☐ Wetting/soiling clothing
☐ Child abuse/neglect
☐ Isolation/withdrawal
☐ Other: _____

Mental Status for IP

Interpersonal issues	☐ NA	☐ Conflict ☒ Enmeshment ☐ Isolation/avoidance ☒ Emotional disengagement ☐ Poor social skills ☐ Couple problems ☐ Prob w/friends ☐ Prob at work ☐ Overly shy ☐ Egocentricity ☐ Diff establish/maintain relationship ☐ Other: _____
Mood	☐ NA	☐ Depressed/sad ☐ Hopeless ☐ Fearful ☒ Anxious ☐ Angry ☐ Irritable ☐ Manic ☐ Other: _____
Affect	☐ NA	☒ Constricted ☐ Blunt ☐ Flat ☐ Labile ☐ Dramatic ☐ Other: _____
Sleep	☐ NA	☐ Hypersomnia ☐ Insomnia ☒ Disrupted ☐ Nightmares ☐ Other: _____
Eating	☐ NA	☐ Increase ☐ Decrease ☐ Anorectic restriction ☐ Bingeing ☐ Purging ☐ Body image ☒ Other: Hx of anorexia
Anxiety symptoms	☐ NA	☐ Chronic worry ☒ Panic attacks ☐ Dissociation ☐ Phobias ☐ Obsessions ☐ Compulsions ☐ Other: _____

† *Abbreviations:* AF: Adult Female; AM: Adult Male; CF#: Child Female with age, e.g., CF12; CM#: Child Male with age; Hx: History; CI: Client.

Trauma symptoms	☐ NA	☐ Acute ☐ Chronic ☐ Hypervigilance ☐ Dreams/Nightmares ☐ Dissociation ☒ Emotional numbness ☒ Other: Untreated childhood sexual abuse.
Psychotic symptoms	☒ NA	☐ Hallucinations ☐ Delusions ☐ Paranoia ☐ Loose associations ☐ Other:
Motor activity/ speech	☐ NA	☒ Low energy ☐ Restless/hyperactive ☐ Agitated ☐ Inattentive ☐ Impulsive ☐ Pressured speech ☐ Slow speech ☐ Other:
Thought	☐ NA	☐ Poor concentration/attention ☒ Denial ☒ Self-blame ☐ Other-blame ☐ Ruminative ☐ Tangential ☐ Illogical ☐ Concrete ☒ Poor insight ☐ Impaired decision making ☐ Disoriented ☐ Slow processing ☐ Other:
Socio-Legal	☒ NA	☐ Disregards rules ☐ Defiant ☐ Stealing ☐ Lying ☐ Tantrums ☐ Arrest/ incarceration ☐ Initiates fights ☐ Other:
Other symptoms	☒ NA	

Diagnosis for IP

Contextual Factors considered in making Dx: ☐ Age ☒ Gender ☒ Family dynamics ☒ Culture ☒ Language ☒ Religion ☐ Economic ☒ Immigration ☐ Sexual orientation ☒ Trauma ☐ Dual dx/comorbid ☐ Addiction ☐ Cognitive ability ☐ Other:

Describe impact of identified factors: Services provided in Mandarin Chinese; Chinese norms for emotional expression and interpersonal connection considered when assessing family; untreated childhood trauma considered in assessing current symptoms.

Axis I

Primary: 300.01 Panic Disorder Without Agoraphobia

Secondary: _____

Axis II: V71.09

Axis III: Client reports hypertension

Axis IV:
☐ Problems with primary support group
☐ Problems related to social environment/school
☐ Educational problems
☐ Occupational problems
☐ Housing problems
☐ Economic problems
☐ Problems with accessing health care services
☐ Problems related to interactions with the legal system
☒ Other psychosocial problems

Axis V: GAF 58 GARF 65

List DSM Symptoms for Axis I Dx (include frequency and duration for each). Client meets 9 **of** 13 **criteria for Axis I Primary Dx.**

1. Panic attacks: palpitations, sweating, trembling, shortness of breath, feeling of choking, chest pain, dizziness, derealization, fear of losing control

2. Worry about implications of attacks; fear of another attack

3. Absence of agoraphobia

4. _____

5. _____

(continued)

Diagnosis for IP *(continued)*

Have medical causes been ruled out?
☒ Yes ☐ No ☐ In process
Has patient been referred for psychiatric/ medical eval? ☒ Yes ☐ No
Has patient agreed with referral?
☒ Yes ☐ No ☐ NA
List psychometric instruments or consults used for assessment:
☒ None or _____

Medications (psychiatric & medical)
Dose /Start Date
☐ None prescribed
1. Xanax _____ / .5 ___ mg; 2/15/09
2. _____ / _____ mg; _____
3. _____ / _____ mg; _____

Client response to diagnosis:
☒ Agree ☐ Somewhat agree ☐ Disagree
☐ Not informed for following reason:
_____

Medical Necessity *(Check all that apply):* ☒ Significant impairment ☐ Probability of significant impairment
☐ Probable developmental arrest
Areas of impairment: ☒ Daily activities ☒ Social relationships ☐ Health ☒ Work/school
☐ Living arrangement ☐ Other: _____

Risk Assessment

Suicidality:
☒ No indication
☒ Denies
☐ Active ideation
☐ Passive ideation
☐ Intent without plan
☐ Intent with means
☐ Ideation past yr
☐ Attempt past yr
☐ Family/peer hx of completed suicide

Homicidality:
☒ No indication
☒ Denies
☐ Active ideation
☐ Passive ideation
☐ Intent without means
☐ Intent w/o means
☐ Ideation past yr
☐ Violence past yr
☐ Hx assault/temper
☐ Cruelty to animals

Hx Substance:
Alc abuse:
☒ No indication
☒ Denies
☐ Past
☐ Current
Freq/Amt: _____
Drug:
☒ No indication
☒ Denies
☐ Past
☐ Current
Drugs: _____
Freq/Amt: _____
☐ Family/sig. other abuses

Sexual & Physical Abuse and Other Risk Factors:
☐ Current child w abuse hx:
    ☐ Sexual ☐ Physical ☐ Emotional ☐ Neglect
☒ Adult w childhood abuse:
    ☒ Sexual ☐ Physical ☒ Emotional ☐ Neglect
☐ Adult w abuse/assault in adulthood:
    ☐ Sexual ☐ Physical ☐ Current
☐ History of perpetrating abuse:
    ☐ Sexual ☐ Physical
☐ Elder/dependent adult abuse/neglect
☒ Anorexia/bulimia/other eating disorder; Past
☐ Cutting or other self-harm:
    ☐ Current
    ☐ Past; Method: _____
    ☐ Criminal/legal hx: _____
    ☐ None reported

Indicators of Safety: ☒ At least one outside person who provides strong support ☒ Able to cite specific reasons to live, not harm self/other ☐ Hopeful ☐ Has future goals ☐ Willing to dispose of dangerous items ☐ Willingness to reduce contact with people who make situation worse ☒ Willing to implement safety plan, safety interventions ☐ Developing set of alternatives to self/other harm ☐ Sustained period of safety: _____ ☐ Other: _____

Safety Plan includes: ☐ Verbal no harm contract ☐ Written no harm contract ☒ Emergency contact card ☒ Emergency therapist/agency number ☒ Medication management ☐ Specific plan for contacting friends/support persons during crisis ☒ Specific plan of where to go during crisis ☒ Specific self-calming tasks to reduce risk before reach crisis level (e.g., journaling, exercising, etc.) ☐ Specific daily/weekly activities to reduce stressors ☐ Other: _____

Notes: Legal/Ethical Action Taken: ☐ NA Called legal consultant about abuse reporting in foreign country; advised that since in past and no potential identified victims, no action needs to be taken.

Case Management

Date
1st visit: 2/3/09 _____

Last visit: 2/10/09 _____

Session Freq:
☒ Once week ☐ Every other week ☐ Other: _____

Expected Length of Treatment:

_____

Modalities:
☒ Individual Adult
☐ Individual Child
☒ Couple
☐ Family
☐ Group:

_____

Is client involved in mental health or other medical treatment elsewhere?
☒ No
☐ Yes:

_____

If Child/Adolescent: Is family involved?
☐ Yes ☐ No

Patient Referrals and Professional Contacts

Has contact been made with social worker?
☐ Yes ☐ No: explain: _____ ☒ NA

Has client been referred for medical assessment?
☒ Yes ☐ No evidence for need

Has client been referred for psychiatric assessment?
☒ Yes; cl agree ☐ Yes, cl disagree ☐ Not nec.

Has contact been made with treating physicians or other professionals?
☒ Yes ☐ No ☐ NA

Has client been referred for social services?
☐ Job/training ☐ Welfare/Food/Housing ☐ Victim services
☐ Legal aid ☐ Medical ☐ Other: _____ ☒ NA

Anticipated forensic/legal processes related to treatment:
☒ No ☐ Yes: _____

Has client been referred for group or other support services?
☐ Yes ☐ No ☒ None recommended

Client social support network includes:
☐ Supportive family ☒ Supportive partner ☐ Friends ☐ Religious/spiritual organization ☒ Supportive work/social group ☐ Other: _____

Anticipated effects treatment will have on others in support system?: (Parents, children, siblings, sig. others, etc.): Husband will attend sessions; likely to have positive effect on rp with son.

Is there anything else client will need to be successful? NA

Client Sense of Hope: Little 1----------5----X----10 High

Expected Outcome and Prognosis:
☒ Return to normal functioning
☐ Expect improvement, anticipate less than normal functioning
☐ Maintain current status/prevent deterioration

(continued)

Case Management *(continued)*

Evaluation of Assessment/Client Perspective

How was assessment method adapted to client needs?

Services provided in Mandarin.

Age, culture, ability level, and other diversity issues adjusted for by:

Used professional vocabulary and medical language; considered cultural norms for emotional expression and relationships.

Systemic/family dynamics considered in following ways:

Assess current changes in family system; include AM in assessment.

Describe actual or potential areas of client-therapist agreement/disagreement related to the above assessment:

Client is in full agreement with assessment; therapist has consulted with psychiatrist on diagnosis; client reports medications compliance.

_____ , _____ _____
Therapist signature   License/Intern status   Date

_____ , _____ _____
Supervisor signature   License   Date

TREATMENT PLAN

Therapist: Mei Zhou   **Client ID #:** 1121

Theory: Bowen Intergenerational Therapy

Primary Configuration: ☐ Individual ☒ Couple ☐ Family ☐ Group

Additional: ☒ Individual ☐ Couple ☐ Family ☐ Group: _____

Medication(s): ☐ NA ☒ Xanax

Contextual Factors considered in making plan: ☒ Age ☒ Gender ☒ Family dynamics

☒ Culture ☒ Language ☒ Religion ☒ Economic ☒ Immigration ☐ Sexual orientation

☒ Trauma ☐ Dual dx/comorbid ☐ Addiction ☐ Cognitive ability

☐ Other: _____

Describe how plan adapted to contextual factors: Services provided in Mandarin; included AM in session per request; mindful of cultural and family norms of saving face when discussing concerns.

I. Initial Phase of Treatment (First 1–3 Sessions)

I.A. Initial Therapeutic Tasks

Therapeutic Relationship

TT1: Develop therapeutic relationship with all members. Note: Bilingual, bicultural therapist.

I1: Intervention: Use **nonanxious presence;** attend to culture and education level.

Assessment

TT2: Assess individual, system, and broader cultural dynamics. Note: _____

I1: Intervention: Begin creating **genogram** to identify **intergenerational patterns.**

I2: Intervention: Identify how family system manages **chronic anxiety.**

Set Goals

TT3: Define and obtain client agreement on treatment goals. Note: _____

I1: Intervention: Frame goals in terms of how AF and family manage **anxiety.**

Referrals and Crisis

TT4: Identify needed referrals, crisis issues, and other client needs. Note: _____

I1: Intervention: Encourage AF to work with psychiatrist in managing medications and keeping open communication with psychiatrist about progress and side effects.

Note: **BOLDFACE** indicates Intergenerational Therapy assessment and techniques.

(continued)

I. Initial Phase of Treatment *(continued)*

I.B. Initial Client Goals (1–2 Goals): Manage crisis issues and/or reduce most distressing symptoms.

Goal #1: ☐ Increase ☒ Decrease daily stress and **chronic anxiety** (personal/relational dynamic) to reduce potential for panic attacks (symptom).

Measure: Able to sustain low stress levels for period of 2 ☐ wks ☒ mos with no more than 2 mild episodes of panic.

> I1: Intervention: Identify most obvious sources of stress and identify ways to increase AF's responsibility for her own thoughts and feelings, thereby increasing her level of **differentiation**.

> I2: Intervention: Develop plan with AF and AM for how to identify panic warning signs and how best to manage, encouraging them to increase their **emotional connection** while maintaining **clear boundaries.**

II. Working Phase of Treatment (Sessions 2+)
II.A. Working Therapeutic Tasks
Monitor Progress

> TT1: Monitor progress toward goals. Note: _____

>> I1: Intervention: Check in weekly on panic episodes; track progress in **differentiation**.

Monitor Relationship

> TT2: Monitor quality of therapeutic alliance as therapy proceeds. Note: _____

>> I1: Intervention: Ask client about alliance as well as check for nonverbal indicators that relationship may be off track given cultural norm for not revealing disapproval of professional.

II.B. Working Client Goals (2–3 Goals): Target individual and relational dynamics in case conceptualization using theoretical language (e.g., reduce enmeshment, increase differentiation, increase agency in relational narrative, etc.)

Goal #1: ☒ Increase ☐ Decrease AF's awareness of impact of launching CM (personal/relational dynamic) to reduce **enmeshment** with CM and the related **anxiety** (symptom).

Measure: Able to sustain greater acceptance of change for period of 2 ☐ wks ☒ mos with no more than _____ mild episodes of diffuse boundaries and relational anxiety.

> I1: Intervention: **Process questions** to help AF identify impact of CM leaving home; compare with her leaving her parents and never returning.

> I2: Intervention: Encourage **relational experiments** to reduce enmeshment and take action on insight.

Goal #2: ☒ Increase ☐ Decrease couple's **emotional intimacy** and connection (personal/relational dynamic) to reduce disengagement and anxiety (symptom).

Measure: Able to sustain emotional connection for period of 2 ☐ wks ☒ mos with no more than 2 mild episodes of disengagement.

> I1: Intervention: **Detriangulate** CM and work from marital relationship by increasing conversations about each other's emotional and personal lives.

> I2: Intervention: **Process questions** to help couple identify how their lack of conflict is symptomatic of disconnection and how immigration and abuse history have contributed to fear of intimacy.

III. Closing Phase of Treatment (Last 2+ Weeks)

III.A. Closing Therapeutic Tasks

Termination Plan

> TT1: Develop aftercare plan and maintain gains. Note: _____

> > I1: Intervention: Identify how couple will continue to increase **differentiation** and effective management of anxiety.

III.B. Closing Client Goals: Determined by theory's definition of health

Goal #1: ☒ Increase ☐ Decrease AF's ability to maintain **emotional center in anxious moments** (personal/relational dynamic) to reduce anxiety and panic (symptom).

Measure: Able to sustain increased differentiation for period of 3 ☐ wks ☒ mos with no more than mild episodes of anxiety (no panic attacks).

> I1: Intervention: **Process questions** to help AF identify her emotional responses and how to effectively manage so that panic attacks are not triggered.

> I2: Intervention: Promote **differentiation** by helping AF and AM envision a hopeful future after launching CM and rediscovering each other as marital partners.

IV. Client Perspective

Has treatment plan been reviewed with client? ☒ Yes ☐ No; If no, explain: _____

_____

(continued)

IV. Client Perspective *(continued)*

Describe areas of client agreement and concern: <u>AF is willing to explore potential of CM's launching</u> <u>as having an effect on her panic as it is one of the only recent changes, although she is not 100% con-</u> <u>vinced it is the cause; couple willing to discuss how they will redefine relationship without CM at home.</u>

_____ , _____   _____
Therapist Signature   Intern status   Date

_____ , _____   _____
Supervisor Signature   License   Date

_____

Abbreviations: TT: Therapeutic Task; I: Intervention; AM: Adult Male; AF: Adult Female; CM: Child Male; CF: Child Female; Dx: Diagnosis; NA: Not Applicable.

PROGRESS NOTES

Progress Notes for Client # 1121

Date: 3/10/09 **Time:** 2:00 am/pm **Session Length:** ☒ 50 min or ☐ _____

Present: ☒ AM ☒ AF ☐ CM ☐ CF ☐ _____
Billing Code: ☐ 90801 (Assess) ☐ 90806 (Insight-50 min) ☒ 90847 (Family-50 min)

☐ Other _____

Symptoms(s)	Dur/Freq Since Last Visit	Progress: Setback---------Initial---------Goal
1. Panic attack	None this week; second week in a row	-5----------1---------X---5-------------10
2. Worry/general stress	AF rate 5 on 10-pt scale	-5----------1------------X-------------10
3. Emotional connection	Report had good date night	-5----------1------------5-------------10

Explanatory Notes: AF reports no panic attack this week even during active weekend. Report she has been successful in eliminating several small daily stressors. Couple report had good date night without discussing CM.

Interventions/HW: Process questions to explore dynamics between AF and CM and AF and AM; triangulation process. Therapist used self and nonanxious presence to detriangulate from couple and to avoid overreacting to AF wanting therapist to side with her on issues related to CM. Design relational experiment for next call with CM this weekend.

Client Response/Feedback: Clients respond well to insight-oriented discussion about dynamics, although are more resistant to taking action on insights. Still some hesitancy from AF on reducing focus on CM both personally and within marriage.

Plan: ☒ Continue with treatment plan: plan for next session: Follow up on relational experiment.

☐ Modify plan: _____

Next session: Date: 3/17/09 Time: 2:00 am/pm
Crisis Issues: ☒ Denies suicide/homicide/abuse/crisis ☐ Crisis assessed/addressed:

_____

_____

_____ , _____ _____
Therapist signature   License/Intern status   Date

◇◇

(continued)

PROGRESS NOTES *(continued)*

Case Consultation/Supervision Notes: Supervisor reviewed genogram; continued focus on helping AF clarify boundaries with AM and CM.

Collateral Contacts: Date: _____ Time: _____ Name: _____

Notes: Faxed clinical update to psychiatrist

☒ Written release on file: ☒ Sent ☐ Received ☐ In court docs ☐ Other: _____

_____ , _____ _____
Therapist signature   License/Intern status   Date

_____ , _____ _____
Supervisor signature   License   Date

_____

Abbreviations: AM: Adult Male; AF: Adult Female; CM: Child Male; CF: Child Female; HW: Homework.

©2007. Diane R. Gehart

Behavioral and Cognitive-Behavioral Couple and Family Therapies

"The key thread that binds these diverse perspectives [behavioral therapies] *is a demand for continual empirical challenge.* Every strategy, and every case, is subjected to empirical scrutiny that aims to define the specific therapeutic ingredients that facilitate the achievement of the specific benefits desired by the family. In other words, every family presents a new experiment with the potential to advance therapeutic frontiers."—Falloon, 1991, p. 65, italics in original

Lay of the Land

Behavioral and cognitive-behavioral couple and family therapies (in this book called cognitive-behavioral family therapy, or CBFT—to save trees) are a group of related therapies based on the behavioral and cognitive-behavioral approaches originally developed for working with individuals. The most influential of these therapies are the following:

- **Behavioral Family Therapy:** This therapy focuses on parent training (Patterson & Forgatch, 1987).

- **Cognitive-Behavioral Family Therapy:** This therapy was developed by several therapists to integrate cognitive elements into therapy with couples and families (Dattilio, 2005; Epstein & Baucom, 2005).

- **Integrative Behavioral Couples Therapy:** This is an enhanced version of *behavioral couples therapy,* which was demonstrated to be effective in the short term but not in the long term; a humanistic component emphasizing *acceptance* of one's partner was added in an attempt to improve long-term outcomes (Jacobson & Christensen, 1996).

- **Gottman Method Couples Therapy:** This is a scientifically based approach to couples therapy based on Gottman's 30 years of research on the key differences between happy and unhappy marriages (Gottman, 1999). Although Gottman's approach is not an empirically supported treatment, its treatment goals are well supported by research data.

- **Functional Family Therapy:** This is an empirically supported treatment for working with troubled teens and their families.

Behavioral and Cognitive-Behavioral Family Therapies
In a Nutshell: The Least You Need to Know

In the general mental health field, cognitive-behavioral therapies (CBTs) are some of the most commonly used therapeutic approaches. They have their roots in behaviorism—Pavlov's research on stimulus-response pairings with dogs and Skinner's research on rewards and punishments with cats—the premises of which are still widely used with phobias, anxiety, and parenting. Until the 1980s, most of the cognitive-behavioral family therapies were primarily behavioral: behavioral family therapy (Falloon, 1991) and behavioral couples therapy (Holtzworth-Munroe & Jacobson, 1991). In recent years, approaches that more directly incorporate cognitive components have developed: cognitive-behavioral family therapy (Epstein & Baucom, 2000; Dattilio, 2005) and Gottman method couples therapy approach (1999).

Cognitive-behavioral family therapies integrate systemic concepts into standard cognitive-behavioral techniques by examining how family members—or any two people in a relationship—*reinforce* one another's behaviors to maintain symptoms and relational patterns. Therapists generally assume a directive, "teaching," or "coaching" relationship with clients, which is quite different from other approaches of "joining" or "empathizing" with clients to form a relationship. Because this approach is rooted in experimental psychology, research is central to its practice and evolution, resulting in a substantial evidence base.

The Juice: Significant Contributions to the Field

If you remember one thing from this chapter, it should be this:

Parent Training

Arguably, CBFTs greatest influence has been in the area of parenting (Patterson & Forgatch, 1987). Most therapists who work with families with young children, regardless of their primary orientation, use classic behavioral concepts of reinforcement and consistency to help improve parental efficiency (Dattilio, 2005; Patterson & Forgatch, 1987). The basic behavioral principle of *reinforcement*—that the positive or negative responses from the environment shape future behavior—is hard-wired into reptilian and mammalian nervous systems, and to a large extent all living creatures. Therefore, if a dog is given a treat each time it sits on command, it learns the command by pairing compliance with the positive reinforcer, the treat. *Consistency*—reinforcing every time—is the key, especially in the beginning. Kids, employees, graduate students, and to a certain extent spouses work essentially on the same principle.

Patterson and Forgatch (1987) developed one of the most prominent approaches to parent training. Their approach is based on the following key concepts and techniques:

- **Teaching Compliance and Socialization:** Therapists aim to teach children to comply with parental requests with the broader goal of socializing children to function in society.

- **Improving Parental Requests:** Parental requests should be (a) few in number, (b) polite, (c) statements rather than questions, (d) made only once before enforcing a consequence, (e) specific, and (f) well timed.

- **Monitoring and Tracking:** Parents must monitor their children's behavior away from home by always asking four basic questions: Who? Where? What? When?

- **Creating a Contingent Environment:** Parents are encouraged to develop positive contingencies (rewards) to encourage desired behavior in children using *point charts*.

- **Five-Minute Work Chore:** Parents are taught to assign a lesser punishment, such as the five-minute work chore, with initial infractions before removing privileges or using harsher punishments.

Being consistent and reinforcing behaviors are not the only skills parents need to master, but they are essential and therefore used widely when child behavior is a presenting concern. In the case study at the end of the chapter, the therapist includes parent training to treat ADHD in their seven-year-old son.

Rumor Has It: The People and Their Stories

Gerald Patterson and Marion Forgatch

Researchers at the Oregon Social Learning Center, Patterson and Forgatch (1987) have developed one of the most influential behavioral parent training programs.

Neil Jacobson and Andrew Christensen

In the early 1970s, Neil Jacobson developed behavioral couples therapy, which was later recognized as an empirically validated treatment (Jacobson & Addis, 1993; Jacobson & Christensen, 1996). Although effective in improving couple functioning in the short term, therapeutic gains were generally lost at the two-year follow-up. Therefore, Jacobson decided to add a more affective, humanistic focus that emphasizes *acceptance* of one's partner, calling this new model "integrative behavioral couples therapy." Christensen has carried on the development of this approach since Jacobson's death in 1999.

Norman Epstein

A professor at the University of Maryland, Norman Epstein has been a leader in developing cognitive and cognitive-behavioral approaches for working with couples (Epstein, 1982; Epstein & Baucom, 2002) and families (Epstein, Schlesinger, & Dryden, 1988; Freeman, Epstein, & Simon, 1987).

John Gottman

For over 30 years, John Gottman (1999) has studied key factors in couples communication, divorce, and marital satisfaction. On the basis of this research, he has developed a scientifically based couples therapy, originally called the marriage clinic approach, that reduces behaviors that predict divorce, and increases those that predict long-term marital satisfaction. He has written several books for the general public, including *The Seven Principles for Making Marriages Work* (Gottman, 2002) and *And Baby Makes Three* (Gottman & Gottman, 2008).

Frank Dattilio

In recent years, Frank Dattilio (2005) developed *cognitive-behavioral family therapy*, adopting traditional cognitive therapy. Specifically, work adapts Aaron Beck's (1976, 1988) concept of schemas—underlying core beliefs—for working with families.

James Alexander, Bruce Parsons, and Thomas Sexton

James Alexander and colleagues (Alexander & Parsons, 1982; Alexander & Sexton, 2002) developed functional family therapy, an empirically validated approach to working with defiant and conduct-disordered youth.

The Big Picture: Overview of Treatment

The therapy process for most CBFTs includes the following steps:

- **Step 1. Assessment:** Obtain a detailed behavioral and/or cognitive assessment of *baseline functioning,* including the frequency, duration, and context of problem behaviors and thoughts.

- **Step 2. Target Behaviors and Thoughts for Change:** Cognitive-behavioral therapists identify *specific* behaviors and thoughts for intervention (e.g., rather than using the general goal of "improve communication," the therapist targets tantrum frequency, name calling, curfew compliance, and other problem behaviors).

- **Step 3. Educate:** Therapists educate clients on their irrational thoughts and dysfunctional patterns.

- **Step 4. Replace and Retrain:** Interventions are designed to replace dysfunctional behaviors and thoughts with more productive ones.

Making Connection: The Therapeutic Relationship

Directive Educator and Expert

Although the affective quality of connection exhibited by CBFT therapists varies greatly (i.e., from cool and detached to warm and friendly), the primary role of the therapist is the same: to serve as an expert who *directs* and *educates* the client and family on how to better manage their problems (Falloon, 1991). Following the classic medical model, traditional CBFT therapists maintained a distance from clients, much like medical doctors today, simply diagnosing and prescribing interventions without achieving much emotional connection. Influenced by recent research such as the common factors model, which indicates that the affective quality of the therapeutic relationship is a strong predictor of positive outcomes (see Chapter 7), many CBFT therapists are increasing their use of empathy and warmth to create connection with their clients.

However, the following distinction is crucial: *the reason a CBFT therapist uses empathy is quite different from the reason an experiential therapist uses empathy.* This is frequently misunderstood, so I am going to say it again in case your mind was wandering: *CBFT therapists use empathy for entirely different reasons than experiential therapists.* CBFT therapists use it to create rapport, which then allows them to get to the "real" interventions that will change clients' behaviors, thoughts, and emotions. In dramatic contrast, for an experiential therapist, empathy *is* the intervention: they maintain that empathy is curative in and of itself (Rogers, 1961). The CBFT therapist who uses empathy should not be seen as manipulative because usually the idea is to make clients feel more comfortable with the process, not to trick them. They should also not be seen as integrating experiential concepts, because they are not using an experiential concept in the way an experiential therapist would use it. Instead, they are *adapting* it to work within their philosophical assumptions about therapy and the change process.

Written Contracts

CBFT therapists are perhaps the most businesslike of all therapists in their relationship with clients (Holtzworth-Munroe & Jacobson, 1991), at least in their written descriptions—and more than other therapists, they put this relationship on paper. CBFT therapists frequently use *written contracts* spelling out goals and expectations to help structure the relationship and to increase clients' motivation and dedication. Putting goals and agreements in writing and having clients sign that they agree can be a very motivating experience that creates commitment to the process.

The Viewing: Case Conceptualization and Assessment

Problem Analysis

From a CBFT therapist's perspective, most families do not come in with usefully defined problems. When a CBFT therapist hears, "We don't communicate anymore" or "My son is defiant," the therapist still has not heard a problem description. Problem analysis is the process of taking these vague descriptions and developing them into a clear description of behavioral interactions and their emotional consequences.

Problem analysis focuses on *present-day* behaviors, emotions, and cognitions. When clients tell their story about relationship distress or personal disappointments, CBFT therapists listen for (a) the behaviors, (b) emotions, and (c) thoughts that make the situation a problem. For example, if a client says that she is feeling depressed that her husband has left her, the therapist focuses on specific problematic *behaviors* (e.g., she no longer wants to see her friends), *feelings* (e.g., feeling worthless and hopeless), and *thoughts* (e.g., I will never find anyone again). These concrete, definable symptoms are the "problem," not that she is divorced. The focus of treatment is on reducing these undesirable thoughts, feelings, and behaviors and increasing more desirable ones. For example, in the case study at the end of the chapter, the child is diagnosed with ADHD; however, the therapist does not rely on this generic description of the problem but instead works with the family to define clear, specific behaviors that can be targeted for change, such as "not able to do more than 15 minutes of homework," or "gets up out of seat in class during reading periods."

Assessment of Baseline Functioning: Monitoring and Tracking

At the beginning of treatment, sometimes even before the first session, CBFT therapists conduct a baseline assessment of functioning, which provides a starting point for measuring change. They ask clients to log the (a) frequency, (b) duration, and (c) severity of specific behavioral symptoms, such as tantrums, anger, social withdrawal, or conflict. Therapists may also identify antecedent events that may have triggered the symptoms. Patterson and Forgatch (1987) use monitoring and tracking charts to help parents obtain a baseline description of their child's behavior. Although clients' verbal recall of their symptoms may seem sufficient, usually a baseline assessment provides more detailed and accurate information than recall alone, especially when remembering a child's behavior. A baseline log may look like this:

SAMPLE BASELINE LOG

PROBLEM BEHAVIOR	WHEN?	HOW LONG?	HOW SEVERE?	EVENTS BEFORE?	EVENTS AFTER?
Tantrum when did not get candy at grocery store; cried, said, "I hate you" to mother; refused to follow instructions	Before lunch and after doing several other errands	5 minutes of crying; 1 hour pouting afterwards	Moderate; stopped crying when left store	Very hot day; slept poorly night before; fight with brother earlier; mother did not give in to his first two requests	Another fight with brother in afternoon; mother yelled at him once got in car; refused to go to bed on time

Functional Analysis and Mutual Reinforcement

Originating in systemic theory, functional analysis identifies the precise contexts, antecedents, and consequences of the problem behavior (Falloon, 1991). However, family interactions are rarely as simple as the basic formula that works with laboratory rats: antecedent → behavior → consequence. Thus, Falloon (1991, p. 76) recommends the following questions to facilitate functional analysis in families:

FUNCTIONAL ANALYSIS QUESTIONS FOR FAMILIES

- How does this specific problem handicap this person (and/or the family) in everyday life?
- What would happen if the problem were reduced in frequency?
- What would this person (and his or her family) gain if the problem were resolved?
- Who (or what) reinforces the problem with attention, sympathy, and support?
- Under what circumstances is the specific problem reduced in intensity?
- Under what circumstances is the specific problem increased in intensity?
- What do family members currently do to cope with the problem?
- What are the assets and deficits of the family as a problem-solving unit?

When assessing couples, Holtzworth-Munroe and Jacobson (1991) recommend the following:

FUNCTIONAL ANALYSIS QUESTIONS FOR COUPLES

1. *Strengths and Skills of the Relationship*
   - What are the major strengths of the relationship?
   - What is each spouse's capacity to reinforce the other?
   - What behaviors are highly valued by the other?
   - What activities and interests do the couple currently share?
   - What relational competencies does each possess?

2. *Presenting Problems*
   - What are the primary complaints (defined behaviorally)?
   - What behaviors occur too frequently? Under what circumstances and with what reinforcements do they occur?
   - What behaviors occur too infrequently? Under what circumstances and with what reinforcements do they occur?
   - How did these problems develop over time?
   - Is there consensus about what needs to change?

3. *Sex and Affection*
   - Is either unsatisfied with the frequency or quality of their sex life? What behaviors are associated with the dissatisfaction?
   - Is either unsatisfied with the frequency or quality of nonsexual physical affection? What behaviors are associated with the dissatisfaction?
   - Is either in an extramarital affair? Is there a history of affairs?

4. *Future Prospects*
- Are both seeking to improve the relationship, or is one or both contemplating separation?
- Have steps been taken toward separation or divorce?

5. *Social Environment*
- What are the alternatives to this relationship, and how attractive are they?
- Is their social network supportive of separation?
- If there are children, what are the current effects, and what might be the effects of divorce?

6. *Individual Functioning*
- Does either have a significant mental or physical health disorder?
- What is the relationship history of each, and how does it affect the present relationship?

Adapted from Holtzworth-Munroe & Jacobson, 1991, pp. 106–107

When conducting a functional analysis, the therapist also looks for mutually reinforcing behaviors between parties and examines how these patterns are maintaining the symptom. This concept is similar to the systemic therapy concept of seeing the family's interactional patterns as interlocking steps in a dance. For example, if a parent inconsistently reinforces a child's problematic behavior (e.g., sometimes sets a consequence for talking back and sometimes does not), the behavior is likely to continue (e.g., because of an intermittent schedule of reinforcement); in the case study at the end of the chapter, the therapist is equally interested in assessing *how* the parents respond to their son's hyperactivity as she is in assessing the child's behaviors because the parents' responses reinforce—for better or worse—the son's behavior. Similarly, if a wife's depression results in less conflict in the marriage, this creates a positive reinforcement for the depression.

A-B-C Theory

Originally developed by Albert Ellis (1962) to analyze irrational thinking with individuals, the A-B-C theory has also been applied to working with families (Ellis, 1978, 1994). In this model, **A** is the "activating event," **B** is the "belief" about the meaning of that event, and **C** is the emotional or behavioral "consequence" based on the belief.

ELLIS'S A-B-C THEORY

A = Activating event → **B** = Belief about A → **C** = Emotional and behavioral consequence

Most clients come in able to see only the connection between A and C, and thus report that A *causes* C: "I am depressed *because* my husband does not help out with the kids" or "I am *angry* because my son doesn't listen to me." The therapist's job is to help the client identify the "B" belief that the client does not put into the equation, such as "If he does not help with the children in the ways I want him to, he really does not care about me" or "Good kids follow through on parental requests without questioning the parent." These irrational beliefs are identified in assessment and targeted for change in the intervention phase.

Family Schemas and Core Beliefs

The cognitive therapy of Aaron Beck (1976) focused on identifying and changing the schemas or core beliefs that were fueling the problems in an individual's life, such as the belief that one must be perfect or that life should be fair. More recently, Dattilio (2005) has developed a system for assessing family schemas, of which we all have two sets: (a) beliefs about our family of origin, and (b) beliefs about families in general. Drawing on Beck's work, he identifies eight types of common cognitive distortions about families:

1. **Arbitrary Inference:** A belief based on little evidence (e.g., assuming your child is trying to hide something because he did not answer the cell phone immediately)

2. **Selective Abstraction:** Focusing on one detail while ignoring the context and other obvious details (e.g., believing you've failed as a parent because your child is doing poorly in school)

3. **Overgeneralization:** Just like it sounds, generalizing one or two incidents to make a broad sweeping judgment about another's essential character (e.g., believing that because your son listens to acid rock he is not going to college and will end up on drugs)

4. **Magnification and Minimization:** Going to either extreme of overemphasizing or underemphasizing based on the facts (e.g., ignoring two semesters of your child's poor grades is minimizing; hiring a tutor for one low test score is magnification)

5. **Personalization:** A particular form of arbitrary influence in which external events are attributed to oneself; especially common in intimate relationships (e.g., my spouse has lost interest in me because she did not want to have sex tonight)

6. **Dichotomous Thinking:** All-or-nothing thinking: always/never, success/failure, or good/bad (e.g., if my husband isn't "madly in love" with me, he really doesn't love me at all)

7. **Mislabeling:** Assigning a personality trait to someone based on a handful of incidents, often ignoring exceptions (e.g., saying one's husband is lazy because he does not help immediately upon being asked)

8. **Mind-Reading:** A favorite in family and couple relationships: believing you know what the other is thinking or will do based on assumptions and generalizations; becomes a significant barrier to communication, especially when related to disagreements and hot topics such as sex, religion, money, and housework (e.g., before your spouse says a word, you are defending yourself)

Couple Cognition Types

Epstein and colleagues (Baucom, Epstein, Sayers, & Sher, 1989; Epstein, Chen, & Beyder-Kamjou, 2005) have identified five major types of cognitions that influence how couples emotionally and behaviorally respond to one another:

- **Selective Perceptions:** Focusing on certain events or information to the exclusion of others

- **Attributions:** Inferences about the causes of positive and negative aspects of the relationship

- **Expectancies:** Predictions about the likelihood of certain events in the relationship

- **Assumptions:** Basic beliefs or assumptions about the characteristics of the partner and/or the relationship

- **Standards:** Beliefs about the characteristics that the relationship and each partner "should" have

Targeting Change: Goal Setting

Specific treatment goals are identified through the previously discussed assessment procedures. Goals are stated in behavioral and measurable terms, such as "reduce arguments to no more than one per month." When working with couples and families, therapists use their authoritative role to identify goals that are agreeable to all (Holtzworth-Munroe & Jacobson, 1991). Immediately after clear goals are agreed upon, therapists also obtain a commitment from the couple or family to follow instructions and complete out-of-therapy assignments, often with a written contract. Getting clients to promise to complete assignments greatly increases the likelihood that clients will follow through.

Examples of Middle-Phase CBFT Goals

- Reduce CM tantrums by replacing positive and inconsistent reinforcements of tantrums with effective schedule of consistent consequences designed to extinguish the behaviors
- Replace perfectionist beliefs about child school performance with more realistic expectations
- Reduce generalizations and mind-reading between mother and father in their parenting discussions

Examples of Late-Phase CBFT Goals

- Develop positive mutual reinforcement cycle to reduce negativity and labeling
- Redefine family schemas to increase tolerance of difference between members
- Redefine couple schemas to reduce pressure for perfection and increase tolerance of weaknesses in other

The Doing: Interventions

Classical Conditioning: Pavlov's Dogs

Used primarily to treat anxiety disorders, classical conditioning was developed by Ivan Pavlov (1932) in his famous experiments with salivating dogs. Pavlov was able to train dogs to salivate at the sound of a bell by pairing the dog's natural response to salivate at the sight of food with a bell. When the bell was rung each time food was presented, the dog learned that the bell signaled that food was coming and began salivating. After enough repetition, the dog began to salivate with just the sound of the bell (as anyone who has owned more than one dog knows, the speed at which the dog learns this is highly breed specific). This procedure is technically described as *conditioned and unconditioned stimuli and responses.*

HOW CLASSICAL CONDITIONING WORKS

1. The Natural State of Affairs

Food (unconditioned stimulus; UCS) →
Salivation (unconditioned response; UCR)

2. Process of Pairing Conditional Stimulus with Response

Food (UCS) + *Bell* (conditioned stimulus; CS) →
Salivation (conditioned response: CR)

3. Resulting Pairing

Bell (conditioned stimulus; CS) → *Salivation* (conditioned response: CR)

Operant Conditioning and Reinforcement Techniques: Skinner's Cats

The bread and butter of CBFT interventions—especially parent training—is *operant conditioning*. Interventions based on operant conditioning use the principles identified by B. F. Skinner (1953) to modify human behavior, whether one's own or another's. The essential principle is to reward behavior in the direction of the desired behavior using small, incremental steps, a process called *shaping behavior*. Once a certain set of skills has been mastered, the bar is raised for which behavior will be reinforced (positively and/or negatively), with ever closer approximations to the desired behavior. Thus, if parents are trying to teach a child how to complete homework independently, they may begin by overseeing when, where, and how the child completes homework and reinforce success and failure under these conditions. Once the child regularly succeeds with full oversight, the child is given an area of responsibility to master—perhaps when the homework is done—and reinforced for success in this area. Next, the child may be rewarded for managing the list of homework assignments without oversight. This process continues until the child completes homework independently, much to the parents' delight. This type of reinforcement plan was used in the case study at the end of this chapter.

Forms of Reinforcement and Punishment

In operant conditioning, desired behaviors can be positively or negatively reinforced or punished, depending on the behavior. The following four options are used alone or in combination to shape desired behavior.

FOUR OPTIONS FOR SHAPING BEHAVIOR

- **Positive Reinforcement or Reward:** Rewards desired behaviors by *adding* something desirable (e.g., a treat)
- **Negative Reinforcement:** Rewards desired behaviors by *removing* something *un*desirable (e.g., relaxing curfew)
- **Positive Punishment:** Reduces undesirable behavior by *adding* something *un*desirable (e.g., assigning extra chores)
- **Negative Punishment:** Reduces undesirable behavior by *removing* something desirable (e.g., grounding)

SUMMARY OF OPERANT CONDITIONING

	INCREASE DESIRED BEHAVIOR	DECREASE UNDESIRABLE BEHAVIOR
Add Something	Positive reinforcement; reward	Positive punishment
Remove Something	Negative reinforcement	Negative punishment

Frequency of Reinforcement and Punishment

The frequency of reinforcement and punishment is key to increasing or decreasing behavior.

- **Immediacy:** The more immediate the reinforcement or punishment, the quicker the learning, especially with young children.

- **Consistency:** The more consistent the reinforcement or punishment, the quicker the learning. Consistency involves rewarding or punishing a behavior every time it occurs or on a consistent schedule (e.g., every other time) to create predictability.

- **Intermittent Reinforcement:** Random and unpredictable reinforcement increases the likelihood of a behavior, but not always the behavior you want. Inconsistent reinforcement of desired behaviors often *increases undesired behaviors*; thus, if a parent inconsistently reinforces curfew, the child is more likely to break it. However, random positive reinforcement of well-established desired behaviors helps sustain them (e.g., randomly reinforcing positive grades with periodic privileges).

The principles of positive and negative reinforcement and reward are incorporated into the following interventions.

Encouragement and Compliments

Patterson and Forgatch (1987) strongly encourage *positive reinforcement* to increase desired behavior with children. When working with distressed relationships, they coach families to increase compliments and expressions of appreciation to increase positive reinforcement.

Contingency Contracting

Contingency contracting can be used to promote new behaviors by creating a contingency that must be met to receive a desired reward. Parents can use contingency contracting with children that detail how privileges will be earned and lost (Falloon, 1988, 1991; Patterson & Forgatch, 1987). For example, if a child's grade point average (GPA) is above 3.0, the parents agree to an 11:00 P.M. curfew on Friday and Saturday.

Point Charts and Token Economies

Generally used with younger children, point charts (Patterson & Forgatch, 1987) or token economies (Falloon, 1991) are used to shape and reward positive behaviors by allowing children to build up points that they can apply to privileges, treats, or purchases. Because the rewards must be motivating for each particular child, siblings may have different rewards. In addition, the rewards should be appropriate and readily approved by the parent. For example, if parents offer a reward that is too expensive or takes too much time from their schedule, they will have difficulty keeping up their half of the bargain. In most cases, punishment is added to a token economy by having the child lose points for poor behavior. In the case study at the end of the chapter, the therapist implements such a system to help a family whose son has been diagnosed with ADHD.

Behavior Exchange and Quid Pro Quo

When working with couples, mutual behavior exchanges—called *quid pro quo* ("this for that") arrangements—can be useful to help the partners negotiate relational rules (e.g., "If you make dinner, I will do the dishes"; Holtzworth-Munroe & Patterson, 1991). However, research indicates that couples who rely primarily on quid pro quo arrangements tend to have lower levels of marital satisfaction (Gottman, 1999). Does that mean that using this technique is harmful when working with couples? Although a well-designed research study would best answer this question, it is wise to use behavior exchange judiciously with couples, balancing it with more affective techniques to increase understanding and acceptance and to avoid framing marriage as a business deal. To this end, Holtzworth-Munroe and Jacobson (1991) recommend having each partner select a behavior to "give" rather than have each "ask" for what he/she wants.

Communication and Problem-Solving Training

To help couples and families solve their problems, CBFT therapists also provide training in communication using the following guidelines (Falloon, 1991; Holtzworth & Jacobson, 1991):

- **Begin with the Positive:** When introducing a problem, each is instructed to begin with a statement of appreciation or a compliment.

- **Single Subject:** The communication training begins by identifying only one problem for the problem-solving session.

- **Specific, Behavioral Problems:** Problems are defined in specific behavioral terms rather than in global statements of feelings, characteristics, or attitudes (e.g., "he doesn't care" or "she's a nag").

- **Describe Impact:** When describing a complaint, the partner is encouraged to share the emotional impact of the behavior.

- **Take Responsibility:** Partners are encouraged to take responsibility for their half of the problem interaction.

- **Paraphrase:** After one person has spoken, the other summarizes what was heard so that misunderstandings can be immediately clarified.

- **Avoid Mind-Reading:** Clients are to avoid making inferences about the other's motivations, attitudes, or feelings.

- **Disallow Verbal Abuse:** Insults, threats, and other forms of verbal abuse are not allowed; the therapist redirects the couple in appropriate directions.

Psychoeducation

A hallmark of CBFT therapy, psychoeducation involves teaching clients psychological and relational principles about their problems and how best to handle them (Falloon, 1988, 1991; Patterson & Forgatch, 1987). Psychoeducation can be done in individual or group sessions. The content typically falls into three categories:

- **Problem-Oriented:** Information about the patient's diagnosis or situation, such as ADHD, divorced, alcohol dependence, or depression. Therapists use this type of education to motivate clients to take new action.

- **Change-Oriented:** Information about how to reduce problem symptoms, such as by improving communication, reducing anger, or decreasing depression. Therapists use this type of education to help clients actively solve their problems. For such education to be successful, clients need to be highly motivated, and therapists need to introduce the new behavior in small, practical steps using everyday language.

- **Bibliotherapy:** *Bibliotherapy* is a fancy term for assigning clients readings that will be (a) motivating and (b) instructional for dealing with their presenting problem. Typically, therapists assign a self-help or popular psychology book, but they may also assign fiction or professional literature.

- **Cinema Therapy:** Similar to bibliotherapy, cinema therapy involves assigning clients to watch a movie that will speak to the problem issues (Berg-Cross, Jennings, & Baruch, 1990).

Challenging Irrational Beliefs

Challenging irrational beliefs involves confronting unhelpful beliefs that are creating or sustaining the problem (Ellis, 1994). This can be done in session by the therapist or out of session with a thought record (see next section). A therapist challenges a client's irrational belief in two ways:

- **Direct Confrontation:** The client is explicitly told that the belief is irrational.

- **Indirect Confrontation:** The therapist uses a series of questions to help the client see how the belief or idea is irrational and/or contributing to the creation of the problem.

The decision to use a direct or indirect approach depends on the therapeutic relationship, the therapist's style, and the client's receptiveness to a particular approach; client and therapist cultural and gender issues also significantly affect this dynamic. The direct approach generally requires that the therapist use and the client accept a more hierarchical, expert stance, whereas the indirect approach typically is more appropriate when the therapeutic relationship is less hierarchical and the client has a greater need for autonomy.

Thought Records

Using Ellis's A-B-C Theory, therapists often ask clients to confront their own irrational thinking and problem behaviors by assigning "thought records" (Datillio, 2005). A type of structured journaling, thought records provide a means for clients to analyze their own cognitions and behaviors and develop more adaptive responses. Before assigning these as homework, therapists usually practice in session on a whiteboard to demonstrate the process. Thought records generally include the following information:

- **Trigger Situation** (e.g., argument with spouse)

- **"Automatic" or Negative Thoughts** (e.g., "he/she will never change"; "he is so selfish")

- **Emotional Response:** How automatic thoughts made person feel (e.g., hurt, rejected, betrayed)

- **Evidence For:** Evidence that supports the automatic or negative thoughts and interpretations (e.g., "he has done this before"; "he has not changed and does not seem to be trying")

- **Evidence Against:** Evidence that counters the automatic thoughts (e.g., "he did seem genuinely sorry"; "he has been really trying in other areas")

- **Cognitive Distortions:** Depending on the evidence, different types of cognitive distortions (e.g., arbitrary inference, selective abstraction, overgeneralization, magnification, minimization, personalization, dichotomous thinking, mislabeling, mind-reading)

- **Alternative Thought:** A more balanced perspective that incorporates both forms of "evidence" and corrects the cognitive distortion (e.g., "this is an area where we really seem to have differences; but we really do get along in so many other ways that are important to me; we are both trying to make this better")

SAMPLE THOUGHT RECORD

TRIGGER SITUATION	AUTOMATIC THOUGHT	EMOTIONAL RESPONSE	EVIDENCE FOR	EVIDENCE AGAINST	COGNITIVE DISTORTIONS	REALISTIC ALTERNATIVE
Argument over household chores	He'll never change; he's selfish and lazy	Hurt, anger, betrayal	Has done this before; not changing	Genuinely sorry; made progress in other areas; problem less frequent	Magnification; overgeneralization; selective abstraction	We have differences in this area; we are both trying to adjust to the other's need; he will probably never be exactly what I want in this area

With *relational issues* it is helpful to add the following:

- What did I do to contribute to this problem interaction? (e.g., I came on strong and blaming in the beginning; would not accept apology)
- What can I do differently next time? (e.g., be gentler when presenting my concern; listen with an open mind)

With *behavioral issues* the following can be added:

- Problem behaviors (e.g., yelling)
- Alternative behaviors (e.g., take time out, count to 10, take a deep breath)

Homework Tasks

CBFT therapists often assign homework tasks that are designed to solve the client's problem (Datillio, 2005; Falloon, 1991; Holtzworth-Munroe & Jacobson, 1991). For example, to reduce a couple's conflict, therapists may assign communication tasks, such as using a timer to take turns listening to and summarizing what the other is saying. They may also develop tasks for reducing depression, such as journaling positive thoughts or increasing recreational and social activities. In CBFT, the tasks are logical solutions to reported problems.

Homework Compared with Strategic Directives

CBFT tasks are linear and literal. In contrast, strategic and other systemic therapists assign tasks designed to (a) metaphorically make the covert overt (metaphorical task), (b) interrupt the problem interaction or behavioral pattern enough to allow the system to develop a new pattern (directive), or (c) make the uncontrollable controllable (paradox).

Homework Compared with Solution-Focused Tasks

In contrast to CBFT tasks, solution-focused tasks are designed to enact the *solution* rather than reduce the problem (see Chapter 14). In addition, solution-focused tasks are (a) broken into small steps, (b) developed from clients' ideas and past successes, and (c) designed to increase motivation and hope as much as to solve the problem.

Mindfulness Training

Mindfulness is a practice most commonly associated with Buddhist meditation, although most cultures and religious traditions have some form of mindfulness practice; in the Christian tradition this is referred to as contemplative or centering prayer (Keating, 2006). Although it has religious roots, mindfulness entered mental health as a nonreligious form of breathing or meditation exercise.

The most common form of mindfulness involves observing the breath (or focusing on a repeated word, a *mantra*) while quieting the mind of inner chatter and thoughts (Kabat-Zinn, 1990). By maintaining a focus on the breath, the practitioner remains grounded in the present moment without judging the experience as good or bad, preferred or not preferred. Usually within seconds, the mind loses focus and wanders off—thinking about the exercise, a fight that morning, to-do lists, past memories, future plans; feeling an emotion or itch; or hearing a noise in the room. At some point, the practitioner realizes that the mind has wandered off and then returns to the object of focus without berating the self for "failing" but rather with compassion, understanding that the loss of focus is part of the process—refraining from beating oneself up is usually the most difficult part. This process of focusing—losing focus—regaining focus—losing focus—regaining focus continues for an established period of time, usually 10 to 20 minutes.

A newer yet well-researched technique, mindfulness shows great promise as an effective treatment for a wide range of physical and mental health disorders, including chronic pain, fibromyalgia, psoriasis, depression, anxiety, ADHD, eating disorders, substance abuse, compulsive behaviors, and personality disorders (Baer, 2003). Mindfulness has been integrated in several forms of cognitive-behavioral therapies, including *dialectic behavioral therapy* (Linehan, 1993), *mindfulness-based stress reduction* (Kabat-Zinn, 1990), *mindfulness-based cognitive therapy* (Teasdale, Segal, and Williams, 1995), and *acceptance and commitment therapy* (Hayes, Strosahl, & Wilson, 1999).

Mindfulness-Based Group Programs

Jon Kabat-Zinn's (1990) *Mindfulness-Based Stress Reduction* (MBSR) program at the University of Massachusetts has been highly influential in making mindfulness a mainstream practice in behavioral medicine. The MBSR program is an eight-week group curriculum that teaches participants how to practice mindful breathing, mindful yoga postures, and mindful daily activities. Participants are required to practice daily at home for 20 to 45 minutes. Teasdale, Segal, and Williams (1995) have adapted this group curriculum for depression in their program called *Mindfulness-Based Cognitive Therapy* (MBCT), in which they use mindfulness to reduce the high depression relapse rate (50% of cases within a year). The findings on this approach are promising.

Mindfulness in Couple and Family Therapy

Family therapists are just beginning to explore the potential of mindfulness in couple and family therapy. Gehart and McCollum (2007) discuss the use of mindfulness in family therapy to inform a new attitude toward suffering; they encourage therapists to help clients meaningfully to engage certain forms of suffering rather than frantically to try to eliminate them as fast as possible. Gehart and McCollum (2008) also use mindfulness to teach therapeutic presence with family therapy trainees. Several studies suggest that mindfulness may be particularly helpful in treating couples. In a study by Wachs and Cordova (2008), mindfulness is positively correlated with marital adjustment. Similarly, Barnes, Brown, Krusemark, Campbell, and Rogge (2008) found that the personality trait of mindfulness predicted greater marital satisfaction, lower emotional stress after conflict, and better communication. Block-Lerner, Adair, Plumb, Rhatigan, and Orsillo (2008) found that mindfulness training increased empathetic responding in couples, and Carson, Carson, Gil, and Baucom (2008) found that couples in a mindfulness-based relationship enhancement group demonstrated greater relationship satisfaction and less relational distress. Given the promising results, therapists are likely to increase the use of mindfulness with couples.

Gottman Method Couples Therapy Approach
In a Nutshell: The Least You Need to Know

Gottman (1999) developed his scientifically based marital therapy from observational and longitudinal research on communication differences between couples who stayed together and ones who divorced. In the therapy based on these findings, the therapist coaches couples to develop the interaction patterns that distinguish successful marriages from marriages that end in breakup. Gottman's model is one of the few therapy approaches that are grounded entirely in research results rather than theory. However, a "scientifically based" therapy differs from an empirically supported treatment (see Chapter 7) in that the former uses research to set therapeutic goals whereas the latter requires research on treatment outcomes.

Debunking Marital Myths
Myth 1: Communication Training Helps

Gottman's (1999) research debunks several myths, including the myth that improving communication helps couples stay together. His research indicates that better communication produces short-term gains but that training couples to talk using "I" statements and "nonblaming" statements does not significantly affect whether or not they stay together. Instead, he found that both happily and unhappily married couples engage in defensiveness, criticism, and stonewalling (three of the Four Horsemen; contempt, the fourth, is seen mostly in marriages heading for divorce;

see following discussion of Four Horsemen). However, those who stay together maintain a ratio of 5:1 positive-to-negative interactions during conflict (20:1 during nonconflict conversations). Thus, simply improving communication is not as important as increasing the ratio of positive to negative interactions during conflict.

Myth 2: Anger Is a Dangerous Emotion

Contrary to what many therapists and the public may assume, Gottman (1999) found that expressing anger did not predict divorce; however, contempt (feeling superior to one's partner) and defensiveness do. Furthermore, although anger was associated with lower marital satisfaction in the short term, it was associated with increased marital satisfaction over the long term.

Myth 3: Quid Pro Quo Error

Gottman (1999) also found that *quid pro quo* ("this for that"; see previous discussion) actually characterizes *unhappy* marriages. Thus, he argued that contingency contracting is *not* appropriate when treating couples.

The Big Picture: Overview of Treatment

Gottman (1999) uses a highly detailed assessment system with numerous written and oral assessment tools to assess couples and target areas of change. The intervention process involves extensive psychoeducation about what works and what does not, as well as structured exercises that sometimes include videotaping couple conversations, replaying them for analysis, and identifying where and how improvements can be made. Gottman also believes that couples therapy should be characterized as the following:

- **A Positive Affect Experience:** Therapy should primarily be a positive affect experience; it should be enjoyable for clients, and therapists should avoid criticizing or implying blame.

- **Primarily Dyadic:** Therapy should primarily be a dyadic experience between the couple rather than triadic with the therapist moderating all interactions.

- **Emotional Learning:** Learning is "state"-dependent, meaning that, in order to change an emotional state, couples must be in that emotional state and then work through it; thus couples have difficult conversations in session to learn how to handle them differently.

- **Easy:** Interventions should seem easy and nonthreatening.

- **Nonidealistic:** Therapists should not be idealistic about the potential for marital bliss and instead aim for realistic goals, such as reducing conflict.

Making Connection: The Therapeutic Relationship

Therapist as Coach

The therapist serves as a relationship coach, empowering couples to take ownership of their relationship (Gottman, 1999). The therapist does not soothe the couple during difficult conversations but rather coaches them on how to soothe themselves and each other.

The Viewing: Case Conceptualization and Assessment

Assessing Divorce Potential

After studying couples for over 30 years, Gottman (1999) can predict a couple's potential for divorce in the next 5 years with 97.5% accuracy with only five variables, an impressive achievement. Furthermore, his careful research has identified several key predictors of divorce, the most notorious of which are the Four Horsemen of the Apocalypse.

The Four Horsemen of the Apocalypse

In Gottman's studies, the presence of the following four behaviors during a couple's argument predicted divorce with 85% accuracy.

1. **Criticism:** A statement that implies something is globally wrong with the partner (e.g., "always," "never," or a statement about personality). Women tend to criticize more than men.

2. **Defensiveness:** Used to ward off attack, defensiveness claims, "I'm innocent."

3. **Contempt:** The *single best predictor of divorce*, contempt is seeing oneself as superior to one's partner (e.g., "you are incapable of an intelligent thought"). Happy marriages had zero incidents of contempt.

4. **Stonewalling:** Stonewalling is when the listener withdraws from interaction, either physically or mentally. Men are more likely to stonewall than women.

5:1 Ratio

Most couples criticize, defend, and stonewall to a certain extent. The difference between those who stay together and those who do not lies in the ratio of positive to negative interactions during conflict conversations. Stable couples have five times as many positive interactions as negative interactions during conflict; distressed couples may have a 1:1 ratio. Many couples find this research result very helpful in learning how to improve their marriage.

Negative Affect Reciprocity

Negative affect reciprocity is the increased probability that one partner's emotions will be negative *immediately following* negativity in the other. Otherwise stated, "My negativity is *more predictable* after my partner has been negative than it ordinarily would be" (Gottman, 1999, p. 37). Negative affect reciprocity is the most consistent correlate of marital satisfaction and dissatisfaction, regardless of the culture studied, and is a far superior measure than the total amount of negative affect in the relationship.

Repair Attempts

Repair attempts refer to when one partner tries to "make nice" and end the conflict, soothe the other, or soften the complaint. Because happy couples are more responsive to repair attempts, they need fewer of them. Distressed couples frequently reject repair attempts, resulting in a higher number of total attempts. When failed repair attempts are combined with the Four Horsemen, Gottman (1999) can predict with 97.5% accuracy whether a couple will divorce in the next five years.

Accepting Influence

Marriages in which men are unwilling to accept influence from their wives (e.g., suggestions, requests) are 80% more likely to end in divorce.

Harsh Startup

Harsh startup is raising an issue using negative affect in the first minute of a conversation. For 96% of couples, only the first minute of data is necessary to predict divorce or stability (Gottman, 1999). Relationships in which the woman uses harsh startup are more likely to end in divorce.

Distance and Isolation Cascade

What if there are no horsemen in sight? Does that mean a couple is doing well? Not necessarily. If problems go unresolved, often couples become emotionally disengaged, starting the distance and isolation cascade (Gottman, 1999). These couples often say, "Everything is okay," but there is underlying tension and sadness. These couples are characterized by an absence of emotional expression, lack of friendship, unacknowledged tension, high levels of physiological arousal in conflict, and few efforts to soothe the other.

Typologies of Happy Marriages

Gottman (1999) has identified three different types of stable, happy marriages, which means that there is more than one way to get marriage right. All maintain the 5:1 ratio of positive-to-negative interactions but do so at different rates.

Volatile Couples: Volatile couples are more emotionally expressive, expressing more positive and negative emotions. Passionate fighting and passionate loving characterize their relationships.

Validating Couples: Validating couples have moderate emotional expression and strong marital friendships.

Conflict-Avoiding Couples: Conflict-avoiding couples have the least emotional expression, minimize problems, prefer to talk about the strengths of their marriage, and end conversations on a note of solidarity.

THE SOUND RELATIONSHIP HOUSE

Gottman (1999) maintains that marriages that work have two elements:

- An overall sense of positive affect
- An ability to reduce negative affect during conflict

He has designed a marriage therapy to increase these two qualities in ailing marriages in a model he terms *The Sound Marital House*, which has seven key aspects:

1. **Love Maps:** A cognitive understanding of who your partner is and what makes him/her happy is a basic component of *marital friendship*.

2. **Fondness and Admiration System:** This refers to the amount of respect and affection partners feel for each other and are willing to express.

3. **Turning Toward Versus Turning Away: The Emotional Bank Account:** This is a habitual turning toward and opening to each other emotionally in nonconflict interactions (e.g., wanting to share stories, spend time together).

4. **Positive Sentiment Override:** This refers to giving your partner "the benefit of the doubt," compared to negative sentiment override, in which even neutral comments are interpreted negatively.

5. **Problem Solving:** Another myth that Gottman's research has caused therapists to reconsider is that couples need to improve their problem-solving skills. That is only half the story, or more precisely 31%. Gottman's research indicates that both successful and unsuccessful couples argue about the same topics 69% of the time; he calls these the *perpetual problems*, which are due to inherent personality differences.

   - **Solving the Solvable:** Stable couples are able to successfully resolve solvable problems.

> ■ **Dialogue with Perpetual Problems:** Happy couples avoid gridlock and instead find a way to continue talking about their perpetual problems and core personality differences. Because it is impossible not to have perpetual problems, selecting a partner is really about choosing a particular set of perpetual problems.
>
> ■ **Physiological Soothing:** In successful marriages, partners are able to soothe themselves and their partner, enabling everyone to "calm down."
>
> 6. **Making Dreams Come True:** Couples avoid gridlock, especially around perpetual problems, by working together to make each partner's dreams come true.
>
> 7. **Creating Shared Meaning:** Happy couples develop a marital "culture" with rituals of connection and shared meanings, roles, and goals.

The Doing: Interventions

Session Format

Therapy begins with a highly structured assessment process. In the intervention phase, the typical session follows this format:

- **Catchup:** The couple check in on marital events, homework, and major issues; they are directed to talk to one another, not report to the therapist.

- **Pre-Intervention Marital Interaction: The Boxing Round:** The couple interact 6 to 10 minutes, usually by discussing a difficult topic.

- **Give an Intervention:** After the interaction, the therapist asks the couple for an intervention before suggesting one, based on the premise that people tend to accept their own ideas better.

- **The Spouses Make the Intervention Their Own:** The couple discuss their thoughts on how to improve their interactions, with the therapist facilitating and educating as necessary to help them master the process.

- **Got Resistance?** If there is resistance, the therapist needs to address the source of these concerns.

- **No Resistance?** Once the couple have a viable plan for altering their interaction, the therapist instructs them to engage in another 6-minute interaction to practice the suggested changes.

- **Homework:** Tasks are assigned based on the interactions in session.

Specific Interventions

Gottman uses highly detailed interventions that are outlined in *The Marriage Clinic* (Gottman, 1999). Some of the more notable interventions are as follows.

Love Maps

Couples are encouraged to develop their knowledge of each other by answering the following questions:

- Who are your partner's friends?
- Who are your partner's potential friends?
- Who are the rivals, competitors, "enemies" in your partner's world?
- What are the recent important events (in your partner's life)?
- What are some important upcoming events?

- What are some current stresses in your partner's life?
- What are your partner's current worries?
- What are some of your partner's hopes and aspirations for self and others? (Gottman, 1999, p. 205)

Soften Startup

Gottman teaches couples to use the following rules to help soften startup.

- **Be Concise:** Keep the initial statement brief and to the point.

- **Complain but Don't Blame:** Complain about a specific incident rather than blame or label.

- **Start with Something Positive:** Pose problems by starting with something positive.

- **Use "I" Instead of "You" Statements:** Start statements with "I" rather than "you" to avoid blaming and to increase personal responsibility.

- **Describe What Is Happening Rather than Judge:** Keep statements behavioral rather than global.

- **Ask for What You Need:** Clearly describe the behavioral changes you desire.

- **Be Polite and Appreciative:** Express appreciation for what your partner does do, and be respectful.

- **Express Vulnerable Emotions:** When possible, describe more vulnerable than blaming emotions.

Dreams Within Conflict

When working with the gridlock created by perpetual problems, the therapist asks each partner about the deeper meanings and dreams that are beneath his/her rigid stance in the gridlock. In session, partners are directed to ask each other the following questions in relation to a perpetual problem or gridlock issue:

- What do you believe about this issue?
- What do you feel about it? Tell me all of your feelings about it.
- What do you want to happen?
- What does this *mean* to you?
- How do you think your goals can be accomplished?
- What dreams or symbolic meanings (e.g., freedom, hope, caring) are behind your position on this issue? (Gottman, 1999, p. 248)

Negotiating Marital Power

Gottman facilitates couple discussion of gender roles using an extensive checklist (Gottman, 1999, pp. 298–300). He does not advocate a particular division of labor but instead helps the couple arrive at their own definition of "fair and equitable." The purpose of this exercise is to increase respect for the roles and duties of each partner.

Clinical Spotlight: Functional Family Therapy

An empirically validated treatment for working with conduct disorder and delinquency, functional family therapy (FFT) has been studied for over 30 years (Alexander & Parsons, 1982; Alexander & Sexton, 2002; Sexton & Alexander, 2000). The approach integrates cognitive theory, systems theory, and learning theory using a combination of strategic, cognitive, and behavioral interventions. FFT is a *family* therapy approach for working with delinquent youth that has three phases.

Early Phase: Engagement and Motivation

In the first phase, the therapist aims (a) to develop a connection with all members of the family and (b) to assess the *function* of the problem behaviors. During this phase the therapist works to reduce anger, blame, and hopelessness. Therapists create a context conducive to change by using cognitive techniques to reduce parents' tendencies to blame the problem on negative child characteristics (e.g., laziness or irresponsibility) and to replace these characterizations with descriptions that do not impute negative motives (e.g., experimenting with freedom, exploring identity).

All behavior is viewed as *adaptive* to serve a particular *function* in the system. Behaviors are viewed as attempts to achieve one of three functions:

- Contact or closeness (merging)
- Distance or independence (separating)
- A combination of the two (midpointing)

The therapist's primary task is to identify the function of the problem behaviors. Later interventions aim to achieve the desired goal or function without the negative consequences that brought the family to therapy.

Middle Phase: Behavioral Change

In the middle phase, the therapist aims to modify cognitive sets, attitudes, expectations, labels, and beliefs so that family members see how their actions are interrelated. Therapists specifically target parenting skills, negativity, and blaming and intervene by making comments about the impact of a behavior on others; describing the interrelation of feelings, thoughts, and behavior; offering interpretations; stopping negative interactions; relabeling behaviors in nonblaming terms; discussing the implications of symptom removal; changing the context of a symptom; and shifting the focus from one person or problem to another.

Once the therapist has changed the family's cognitive set, the therapist focuses on building interpersonal and problem-solving skills, using two general categories of interventions: *parent training* and *communication skills training.* Parent training is emphasized with younger children and follows traditional behavioral parenting interventions using operant conditioning principles. Communication skills training is based on traditional behavioral techniques that encourage brevity, directness, and active listening.

Late Phase: Generalization

The focus during this phase is to generalize change to the larger social systems in which the family interacts. The therapist now works more as a caseworker to encourage families to develop positive relations with community systems, such as mental health and juvenile justice authorities, and to develop a strong social network.

Snapshot: Research and the Evidence Base

Quick Summary: There is an excellent research foundation for CBFT approaches.

Because CBFT's conceptual home is in experimental psychology, research is part of its culture; therefore, CBFT therapies are some of the best-researched approaches in family therapy. Over the years, CBFT theorists have modified their approach based on research outcomes—sometimes dramatically—to incorporate more affective and relational components. Behavioral couples therapy is the premier example of this trend. Because of good short-term but poor long-term outcomes, Neil Jacobson reformulated his couples therapy to include more affective aspects; his new approach is called *integrative behavioral couples therapy* (Jacobson & Christensen, 1996). Similarly, because research indicates that a nonjudgmental therapeutic alliance is crucial, CBFT therapists have become increasingly attentive to this aspect of therapy.

Although CBFT has an extensive research history, therapists should not assume that it is therefore superior to other approaches. As discussed in Chapter 7, when confounding factors such as researcher allegiance are controlled for, no therapy is consistently found to be superior to any other (Sprenkle & Blow, 2004).

Snapshot: Working with Diverse Populations

Quick Summary: Although CBFT is used with a diverse range of clients, therapists must thoughtfully adapt their level of directiveness and their emphases on behavior, thought, and emotion when working with diverse populations.

Because CBFT defines behavioral norms, therapists must carefully apply this approach with diverse populations to avoid clashes in values and relational styles. CBFT's emphasis on the expert stance in relation to clients has strengths and weaknesses when working with diverse populations. Men and certain culture groups, such as Latinos, Asians, and Native Americans, often prefer active, directive therapy (Gehart & Lyle, 2001; Pedersen, Draguns, Lonner, & Trimble, 2002). However, hierarchical difference may cause a rebellious reaction in some clients (e.g., highly educated adults or teens) or an overly compliant and withholding response in others (e.g., women who have a habit of people pleasing; Gehart & Lyle, 2001).

By design, cognitive-behavioral goals conform to dominant cultural values. Therefore, therapists need to carefully evaluate treatment goals prior to intervention to ensure that they do not clash with religious, cultural, racial, socioeconomic, or other values and realities. In some cases, such as the Gottman (1999) method couples therapy approach, research has been conducted with major subpopulations (e.g., gay and lesbian couples) to determine if the theory-defined treatment goals are appropriate. Gottman found that same-sex couples exhibit similar interaction patterns as heterosexual couples, with few significant differences other than the obvious stressor of social stigmatization. The case study that concludes this chapter applies CBFT to an African-American family whose youngest son is diagnosed with ADHD.

ONLINE RESOURCES

Frank Dattilio

www.dattilio.com

Functional Family Therapy

www.fftinc.com

Gottman Method Couples theropy

www.gottman.com

Juvenile Justice Bulletin: Functional Family Therapy

www.ncjrs.org/pdffiles1/ojjdp/184743.pdf

Mindfulness Awareness Research Center: UCLA

www.marc.ucla.edu

Mindfulness Based Stress Reduction Clinic: Jon Kabit-Zinn

www.umassmed.edu/cfm/mbsr/

Oregon Social Learning Center: Patterson and Forgatch Parenting Program

www.oslc.org

REFERENCES

*Asterisk indicates recommended introductory readings.

*Alexander, J., & Parsons, B. V. (1982). *Functional family therapy.* Belmont, CA: Brooks/Cole.

Alexander, J., & Sexton, T. L. (2002). Functional Family Therapy (FFT) as an integrative, mature clinical model for treating high risk, acting out youth. In J. Lebow (Ed.), *Comprehensive handbook of psychotherapy, Vol IV: Integrative/Eclectic* (pp. 111–132). New York: Wiley.

Baer, R. A. (2003). Mindfulness training as a clinical intervention: A conceptual and empirical review. *Clinical Psychology: Science and Practice, 10*(2), 125–143.

Barnes, S., Brown, K. W., Krusemark, E., Campbell, W. K., & Rogge, R. D. (2008). The role of mindfulness in romantic relationship satisfaction and responses to relationship stress. *Journal of Marital and Family Thearpy, 33,* 482–500.

Baucom, D., Epstein, N., Sayers, S., & Sher, T. (1989). The role of cognitions in marital relationships: Definitional methodological, and conceptual issues. *Journal of Family Psychology, 10,* 72–88.

Beck, A. T. (1976). *Cognitive therapy and the emotional disorders.* New York: International Universities Press.

*Beck, A. T. (1988). *Love is never enough.* New York: Harper & Row.

Berg-Cross, L., Jennings, P., & Baruch, R. (1990). Cinematherapy: Theory and application. *Psychotherapy in Private Practice, 8,* 135–157.

Block-Lerner, J., Adair, C., Plumb, J. C., Rhatigan, D. L., & Orsillo, S. M. (2008). The case for mindfulness-based approaches in the cultivation of empathy: Does nonjudgmental, present-moment awareness increase capacity for perspective-taking and empathic concern? *Journal of Marital and Family Thearpy, 33,* 501–516.

Carson, J. W., Carson, K. M., Gil, K. M., & Baucom, D. H. (2008). Self expansion as a mediator of relationship improvements in a mindfulness intervention. *Journal of Marital and Family Therapy, 33,* 517–526.

*Dattilio, F. M. (2005). Restructuring family schemas: A cognitive-behavioral perspective. *Journal of Marital and Family Therapy, 31,* 15–30.

Ellis, A. (1962). *Reason and emotion in psychotherapy.* New York: Lyle Stuart.

Ellis, A. (1978). Family therapy: A phenomenological and active-directive approach. *Journal of Marriage and Family Counseling, 4,* 43–50.

Ellis, A. (1994). Rational-emotive behavior marriage and family therapy. In A. M. Horne (Ed.), *Family counseling and therapy* (pp. 489–514). San Francisco: Peacock.

Epstein, N. (1982). Cognitive therapy with couples. *American Journal of Family Therapy, 10,* 5–16.

Epstein, N., & Baucom, D. (2002). *Enhanced cognitive-behavioral therapy for couples: A contextual approach.* Washington, DC: American Psychological Association.

Epstein, N., Chen, F., & Beyder-Kamjou, I. (2005). Relationship standards and marital satisfaction in Chinese and American couples. *Journal of Marital and Family Therapy, 31,* 59–74.

Epstein, N., Schlesinger, S., & Dryden, W. (1988). *Cognitive-behavioral therapy with families.* New York: Brunner/Mazel.

*Falloon, I. R. H. (Ed.). (1988). *Handbook of behavioral family therapy.* New York: Guilford.

Falloon, I. R. H. (1991). Behavioral family therapy. In A. S. Gurman and D. P. Kniskern (Eds.), *Handbook of family therapy* (Vol. 2, pp. 65–95). Philadelphia: Brunner/Mazel.

Freeman, A., Epstein, N., & Simon, K. (1987). *Depression in the family.* New York: Routledge.

Gehart, D. R., & Lyle, R. R. (2001). Client experience of gender in therapeutic relationships: An interpretive ethnography. *Family Process, 40,* 443–458.

*Gehart, D., & McCollum, E. (2007). Engaging suffering: Towards a mindful revisioning of marriage and family therapy practice. *Journal of Marital and Family Therapy, 33,* 214–226.

Gehart, D., & McCollum, E. (2008). Teaching therapeutic presence: A mindfulness-based approach. In S. Hicks (Ed.), *Mindfulness and the healing relationship.* New York: Guilford.

*Gottman, J. M. (1999). *The marriage clinic: A scientifically based marital therapy.* New York: Norton.

Gottman, J. M. (2002). *The seven principles for making marriage work.* New York: Three Rivers Press.

Gottman, J. M., & Gottman, J. S. (2008). *And baby makes three.* New York: Three Rivers Press.

*Hayes, S. C., Strosahl, K. D., & Wilson, K. G. (1999). *Acceptance and commitment therapy: An experiential approach to behavior change.* New York: Guilford.

Holtzworth-Munroe, A., & Jacobson, N. S. (1991). Behavioral marital therapy. In A. S. Gurman and D. P. Kniskern (Eds.), *Handbook of family therapy* (Vol. 2, pp. 96–133). Philadelphia: Brunner/Mazel.

Jacobson, N. S., & Addis, M. E. (1993). Research on couples and couples therapy: What do we know? Where are we going? *Journal of Consulting and Clinical Psychology, 57,* 5–10.

*Jacobson, N. S., & Christensen, A. (1996). *Integrative couple therapy.* New York: Norton.

Kabat-Zinn, J. (1990). *Full catastrophe living: Using the wisdom of your body and mind to face stress, pain, and illness.* New York: Delta.

Keating, T. (2006). *Open mind open heart: The contemplative dimension of the gospel.* New York: Continuum International Publishing Group.

*Linehan, M. M. (1993). *Cognitive-behavioral treatment of borderline personality disorder.* New York: Guilford.

Patterson, G., & Forgatch, M. (1987). *Parents and adolescents: Living together: Part 1: The Basics.* Eugene, OR: Castalia.

Pavlov, I. P. (1932). Neuroses in man and animals. *Journal of the American Medical Association, 99,* 1012–1013.

Pedersen, P. B., Draguns, J. G., Lonner, W. J., & Trimble, J. E. (Eds.). (2002). *Counseling across cultures* (5th ed.) Thousand Oaks, CA: Sage.

Rogers, Carl. (1961). *On becoming a person: A therapist's view of psychotherapy.* London: Constable.

Sexton, T. L., & Alexander, J. F. (2000, December). Functional family therapy. *Juvenile Justice Bulletin,* U.S. Department of Justice, NCJ 184743.

Skinner, B. F. (1953). *Science and human behavior.* New York: MacMillian.

Sprenkle, D. H., & Blow, A. J. (2004). Common factors and our sacred models. *Journal of Marital and Family Therapy, 30,* 113–129.

Teasdale, J. D., Segal, Z. V., & Williams, J. M. C. (1995). How does cognitive therapy prevent depressive relapse and why should attentional control (mindfulness) help? *Behaviour Research and Therapy, 33,* 25–39.

Wachs, K., & Cordova, J. V. (2008). Mindful relating: Exploring mindfulness and emotional repertoires in intimate relationships. *Journal of Marital and Family Therapy, 33,* 464–481.

COGNITIVE-BEHAVIORAL CASE STUDY

Diamond and Tom are seeking counseling for their 7-year-old son Albert, who was just diagnosed with ADHD. They have been married for six years, each having children from a prior marriage. Diamond has two daughters from her prior marriage, Sharie (14) and Debbie (10), and Tom has a son from a former relationship, Desmond (10). The couple report reluctantly agreeing to put Albert on medications at the doctor's recommendation, but that they would like to find a better solution. They report that he is hyper at home and does not follow directions and that he has similar problems at school that have led to lower grades than they expect. They report the household as "hectic," with Diamond and Tom both working long, odd hours and Albert's siblings in and out of the house to visit with their other parents.

After meeting with the family, a cognitive-behavioral family therapist developed the following case conceptualization.

Shaded Sections Emphasized in Cognitive-Behavioral Planning and Intervention

---

CASE CONCEPTUALIZATION FORM

Therapist: Sally Wright   **Client/Case :** 1208   **Date:** 4/02/09

I. Introduction to Client and Significant Others *(Include age, ethnicity, occupation, grade, relevant identifiers, etc.). Put an * next to persons in session and/or IP for identified patient.*

*AF[†]:   34; hairstylist, African-American

*AM: 40; owns remodeling business, African-American/Native-American

*CF: 14 9th grade, track, honor student, visits biological dad on weekends

*CF: 10 5th grade, dance/cheer, visits biological dad on weekends

*CM: 10 5th grade, lives with mom 60% of time

CM: 7(IP) 2nd grade

II. Presenting Concern

Client's/Family's Descriptions of Problem(s):

AF: Concerned about CM7's ADHD diagnosis; blames self partially for not being around more. Believes she and AM need to get on the "same page" about the kids.

AM: Does not believe in ADHD; not concerned about CM7; believes "he's just a boy" and will grow out of it.

CF: 14 Helps by watching CM7 when parents are at work; believes his problem is that parents are too easy on him but also feels somewhat guilty because she has been watching him.

CF: 10 Believes the problem is that her mom spoils CM7; believes he is the "favorite" because he is their only child together.

CM: 10 Thinks something must be wrong with CM7 because he was not that hyper at his age.

CM: 7 He thinks the problem is that there is just too much going on in the house and that if Desmond were around to play with more, things would be better.

Broader System Problem Descriptions (description of problem from referring party, teachers, relatives, legal system, etc.):

Diamond's sister and mom: Think she is too easy on CM7 and should be home more with the kids.

CM7's teacher: Believes the parents are spread too thin to focus on CM7.

---

† *Abbreviations:* AF: Adult Female; AM: Adult Male; CF#: Child Female with age, e.g., CF12; CM#: Child Male with age; IP: Identified Patient; Hx: History; Ex: Explanation or Example; NA: Not Applicable.

(continued)

CASE CONCEPTUALIZATION FORM *(continued)*

III. Background Information

Recent Background (recent life changes, precipitating events, first symptoms, stressors, etc.):

AF and AM report that CM7 was always an active, energetic child that was difficult to parent. Since starting first grade, things have been difficult: frequent notes and calls from the teacher about his disruptive behavior and his grades have been inconsistent. His teacher requested they take him to the doctor to be evaluated for ADHD because he was in danger of not passing the second grade. CF14 is in charge of helping him with his homework and typically watches him in the afternoons.

Related Historical Background (family history, related issues, past abuse, trauma, previous counseling, medical/mental health history, etc.):

AF and AM married in 2003, after she got pregnant with CM7. AF had two children from a prior marriage, ages 14 and 10, and she has a conflictual relationship with their father, whom she tries to speak with rarely; they visit him every other weekend. AM has a 10-year-old son from a prior relationship and has physical custody 40% of the time.

IV. Systemic Assessment
Client/Relational Strengths

Personal/individual: CM7 is a buoyant, upbeat child who likes to have fun and keep people entertained. AF comes from a line of "strong woman" and is not afraid to do whatever needs to be done for her children. AM is a committed father. CM14 is very helpful taking care of CM7.

Relational/social: The family know how to have fun and especially enjoy going to the beach together. Generally, everyone tries to help out. Both AM and AF have close relationships with members of their families of origin.

Spiritual: AF has a deep Christian faith that has gotten her through the difficult times in her life, including sexual abuse by her older brother, a relationship she has since healed. CM14 also seems to have a similar budding faith. AM supports AF in her faith, going to church with her and using church to help him be a better father and husband.

Family Structure and Interaction Patterns
Couple Subsystem (to be assessed): ☐ Personal current ☐ Personal past ☒ Parents'

Couple Boundaries: ☐ Clear ☐ Enmeshed ☐ Disengaged ☒ Other: Close but conflictual

Rules for closeness/distance: The couple is emotionally close, sharing and supporting one another, but there is a lot of fighting, especially around parenting issues.

Couple Problem Interaction Pattern (A ⇆ B):

Start of tension: Teacher calls about CM7's problem behavior.

Conflict/symptom escalation: AF raises issue with AM, who minimizes the problem by saying: "boys will be boys." AF argues for him to take it seriously and help her discipline him. Return to "normal"/homeostasis: AM half-heartedly agrees with her plan but does not back her up; AF is so busy with work and tired of fighting she eventually gives up dealing with the issue too.

Couple Complementary Patterns: ☐ Pursuer/distancer ☐ Over/under functioner
☐ Emotional/logical ☒ Good/bad parent ☐ Other: _____.
Ex: AF almost always argues for discipline with the kids; AM is typically against it. _____

Satir Communication Stances:
AF: ☐ Congruent ☐ Placator ☒ Blamer ☐ Superreasonable ☐ Irrelevant
AM: ☐ Congruent ☒ Placator ☐ Blamer ☐ Superreasonable ☐ Irrelevant

Describe dynamic: _____

Gottman's Divorce Indicators:

Criticism: ☒ AF ☒ AM. Ex: Both criticize other's parenting style and choices. _____

Defensiveness: ☒ AF ☒ AM. Ex: Both defend against other's claims. _____

Contempt: ☐ AF ☐ AM. Ex: NA _____

Stonewalling: ☐ AF ☐ AM. Ex: NA _____

Failed repair attempts: ☐ AF ☐ AM. Ex: NA _____

Not accept influence: ☐ AF ☒ AM. Ex: AM placates but never honestly accepts AF's concerns. ____

Harsh startup: ☒ AF ☐ AM. Ex: AF typically brings up issues in harsh manner because it is "same old thing."

Parental Subsystem: ☒ Family of procreation ☐ Family of origin

Membership in Family Subsystems: Parental: ☒ AF ☒ AM. ☒ Other: CF14
Is parental subsystem distinct from couple subsystem? ☒ Yes ☐ No ☐ NA (divorce)

Sibling subsystem: CF14 and CF10 have strong subsystem. _____

Special interest: CM10 and CM7 connect in gender-typical play. _____

Family Life Cycle Stage:
☐ Single adult ☐ Marriage ☒ Family with young children
☒ Family with adolescent children ☐ Launching children ☐ Later life
Describe struggles with mastering developmental tasks in one of these stages:
The family are transitioning from having young children to having adolescents as well as struggling
to define their roles within the blended family. The couple have still not found a way to parent effectively
together and need to clarify these roles.

(continued)

IV. Systemic Assessment *(continued)*

Hierarchy Between Child/Parents:

AF: ☐ Effective ☐ Insufficient (permissive) ☒ Excessive (authoritarian) ☒ Inconsistent

AM: ☐ Effective ☒ Insufficient (permissive) ☐ Excessive (authoritarian) ☒ Inconsistent

Ex: Both parents are inconsistent, with AF tending to be the disciplinarian and AM tending to be the permissive parent.

Emotional Boundaries with Children:

AF: ☐ Clear/balanced ☒ Enmeshed (reactive) ☐ Disengaged (disinterested)

☐ Other: _____

AM: ☐ Clear/balanced ☐ Enmeshed (reactive) ☐ Disengaged (disinterested)

☒ Other: Varies by child _____

Ex: AF has become very reactive in relation to CM7; she is very close with CM14, treating her more as a peer at times. AM tends to have closer relationships with his sons and is more distant with his step-daughters, still not quite sure what role he should play.

Problem Interaction Pattern (A ⇆ B):

Start of tension: CM7 and CM10 start fighting over video game.

Conflict/symptom escalation: AF tells them to stop arguing; they ignore her; she then puts them on a time out; they sneak away before it should be over and go to the garage to help dad on project. When AF finds them there, she gives AM "the look" and tells him that they were supposed to be on time out; AM takes kids side by saying that they are doing fine now and getting along.

Return to "normal"/homeostasis: AF backs down because the boys do seem to be behaving and AM has them doing something productive.

Triangles/Coalitions:

☒ AF and C14 against AM: Ex: AF complains to CF14 how AM doesn't support her with CM7.

☒ AM and CM10/CM7 against AF: Ex: AM takes boys' side when AF sets limits.

☐ Other: Ex: _____

Communication Stances:

AF or _____ : ☐ Congruent ☐ Placator ☒ Blamer ☐ Superreasonable ☐ Irrelevant

AM or _____ : ☐ Congruent ☒ Placator ☐ Blamer ☐ Superreasonable ☐ Irrelevant

CF ___14___ : ☐ Congruent ☒ Placator ☐ Blamer ☐ Superreasonable ☐ Irrelevant

CF ___10___ : ☐ Congruent ☐ Placator ☒ Blamer ☐ Superreasonable ☐ Irrelevant

CM _____10_____: ☐ Congruent ☒ Placator ☐ Blamer ☐ Superreasonable ☐ Irrelevant

CM _____7_____: ☐ Congruent ☐ Placator ☐ Blamer ☐ Superreasonable ☒ Irrelevant

Ex: CM7 uses irrelevant behavior to cope with family stress. CF14 establishes her role in the family as a people pleaser, while CF10 is more like her mother. AM and CM10 both try to create peace whenever possible.

Hypothesis (Describe possible role or function of symptom in maintaining family homeostasis):

CM7's hyperactivity and distractibility serve to help focus and organize this hectic household and have become the symbol of both the blended family's unity and its lack of cohesiveness; CM7 has the simultaneous roles of "favorite" child and "problem" child.

Intergenerational Patterns

Substance/alcohol abuse: ☒ NA ☐ Hx: _____

Sexual/physical/emotional abuse: ☐ NA ☒ Hx: AF molested by older brother; stopped by parents.

Parent/child relations: ☐ NA ☒ Hx: Mothers on both sides have strong relationships with children; fathers are less emotionally engaged.

Physical/mental disorders: ☐ NA ☒ Hx: Diabetes on AM side.

Historical incidents of presenting problem: ☐ NA ☒ Hx: Both AM and AF have siblings that are also struggling with blended family issues.

Family strengths: Both families of origin are generally close and supportive.

Previous Solutions and Unique Outcomes

Solutions that DIDN'T work: AF setting harsh consequences and AM being lenient has not improved the situation. CF14 trying to set limits with CM7 has also not worked.

Solutions that DID work: CM7 does homework well in quiet area with someone helping him through each step; he is more cooperative when CM10 is around; he had fewer problems in first grade with a highly organized teacher; he does better with fewer choices and a less hectic environment/schedule.

Narratives, Dominant Discourses, and Diversity
Dominant Discourses informing definition of problem:

Cultural, ethnic, SES, etc.: AF identifies herself with a family tradition of strong, self-reliant African-American women, a tradition CF14 closely identifies with also. Both she and AM are proud of the comfortable standard of living they have achieved for their family.

Gender, sex orientation, etc.: AM is conscious of the negative stereotypes of African-American men as unavailable fathers and works hard to "be there" for his children. He did not marry the mother of CM10 because he was not ready and was afraid to fail. He feels very strongly that he wants his marriage with AF to work.

(continued)

IV. Systemic Assessment *(continued)*

Other social influences: Although they live in a minority-majority town, there is a relative minority of African-Americans, with the community being predominantly Hispanic. They are very active in their church, which is their primary community and very supportive.

Identity Narratives that have developed around problem for AF, AM, and/or CM/F:

AF fears that CM7's problems are an indicator that she and AM should not have had a child and that they have made things too complex for their kids. AM feels that his son is being picked on as one of only two black kids in the class. CM7 is beginning to see himself as the problem child at school.

Local or Preferred Discourses: AM sees CM7 as going through a developmental stage and also as having to deal with racism, which he sees as something his son is going to have to learn to cope with.

Other Influential Discourses: AF's friends from church encourage her to put her trust in the Lord and to use this experience to strengthen her family. Her sister and mother are saying this is a sign that she needs to put more energy into her parenting and her family.

V. Genogram

Construct a family genogram and include all relevant information, including:

- ages, birth/death dates
- names
- relational patterns
- occupations
- medical history
- psychiatric disorders
- abuse history

Also include a couple of adjectives for persons frequently discussed in session (these should describe personal qualities and/or relational patterns, e.g., quiet, family caretaker, emotionally distant, perfectionist, helpless, etc.). Genogram should be attached to report.

VI. Client Perspectives

Areas of Agreement: Based on what the client(s) has(ve) said, what parts of the above assessment do they agree with or are likely to agree with?

They are likely to agree with all of the above.

Areas of Disagreement: What parts do they disagree with or are likely to disagree with? Why?

The areas of disagreement are between AF's and AM's views of the problem.

How do you plan to respectfully work with areas of disagreement?

Questions and treatment planning will focus on reducing the symptoms rather than identifying the causes or assigning blame. A more science-based, educational approach will be used to reduce emphasis on who was right.

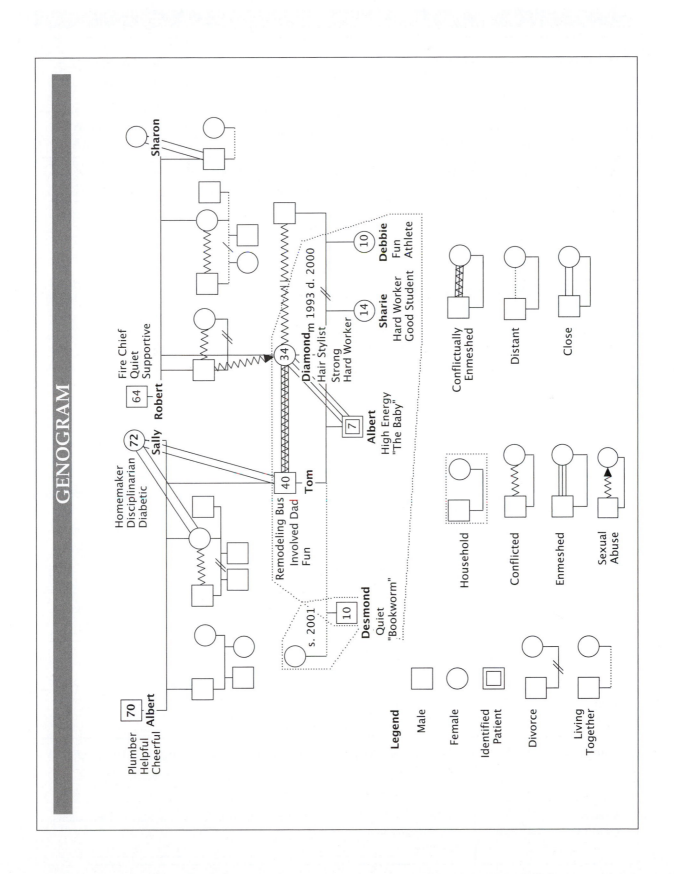

GENOGRAM

Albert
70
Plumber
Helpful
Cheerful

Sally
72
Homemaker
Disciplinarian
Diabetic

Robert
64
Fire Chief
Quiet
Supportive

Sharon

Tom
40
Remodeling Bus
Involved Dad
Fun

Diamond m 1993 d. 2000
Hair Stylist
Strong
Hard Worker

Desmond
10
Quiet
"Bookworm"

s. 2001

Albert
7
High Energy
"The Baby"

Sharie
14
Hard Worker
Good Student

Debbie
10
Fun
Athlete

Legend

Male ☐

Female ○

Identified Patient ☐

Divorce

Living Together

Household

Conflicted

Enmeshed

Sexual Abuse

Conflictually Enmeshed

Distant

Close

CLINICAL ASSESSMENT

Client ID # (do not use name): 1208	Ethnicity(ies): African American; AM part Native American	Primary Language: ☒ Eng ☐ Span ☐ Other: _____

List all Participants/Significant Others: Put a [★] for Identified Patient (IP); [✔] for sig. others who **WILL** attend; [✕] for Sig. others who will **NOT** attend.

Adult: Age: Profession/Employer	Child: Age: School/Grade
[✔] AM† 40: Owns remodeling business; African-American/Native-American	[✔] CM 10: 5ᵗʰ grade: dance/cheer: visits bio dad on weekends
[✔] AF 34: Hairstylist; African-American	[✔] CM 10: 5ᵗʰ grade: lives with mom 60% of time
[✔] CF 14: 9th grade; track; honor student; visits biological dad on weekends	[★] CM 7: 2ⁿᵈ grade

Presenting Problem

		Complete for children
☐ Depression/hopelessness	☐ Couple concerns	☒ School failure/decline performance
☐ Anxiety/worry	☒ Parent/child conflict	
☐ Anger issues	☐ Partner violence/abuse	☐ Truancy/runaway
☐ Loss/grief	☐ Divorce adjustment	☒ Fighting w/peers
☐ Suicidal thoughts/attempts	☒ Remarriage adjustment	☒ Hyperactivity
☐ Sexual abuse/rape	☐ Sexuality/intimacy concerns	☐ Wetting/soiling clothing
☐ Alcohol/drug use	☐ Major life changes	☐ Child abuse/neglect
☐ Eating problems/disorders	☐ Legal issues/probation	☐ Isolation/withdrawal
☐ Job problems/unemployed	☒ Other: Sibling conflict	☐ Other: _____

Mental Status for IP

Interpersonal issues	☐ NA	☒ Conflict ☐ Enmeshment ☐ Isolation/avoidance ☐ Emotional disengagement ☒ Poor social skills ☐ Couple problems ☐ Prob w/friends ☐ Prob at work ☐ Overly shy ☐ Egocentricity ☒ Diff establish/maintain relationship ☐ Other: _____
Mood	☐ NA	☐ Depressed/sad ☐ Hopeless ☐ Fearful ☐ Anxious ☐ Angry ☒ Irritable ☐ Manic ☐ Other: _____
Affect	☐ NA	☐ Constricted ☐ Blunt ☐ Flat ☒ Labile ☐ Dramatic ☐ Other: _____
Sleep	☒ NA	☐ Hypersomnia ☐ Insomnia ☐ Disrupted ☐ Nightmares ☐ Other: _____
Eating	☒ NA	☐ Increase ☐ Decrease ☐ Anorectic restriction ☐ Bingeing ☐ Purging ☐ Body image ☐ Other: _____
Anxiety symptoms	☒ NA	☐ Chronic worry ☐ Panic attacks ☐ Dissociation ☐ Phobias ☐ Obsessions ☐ Compulsions ☐ Other: _____

† *Abbreviations:* AF: Adult Female; AM: Adult Male; CF#: Child Female with age, e.g., CF12; CM#: Child Male with age; IP: Identified Patient; Hx: History; CI: Client NA: Not Applicable.

Trauma symptoms	☒ NA	☐ Acute ☐ Chronic ☐ Hypervigilance ☐ Dreams/Nightmares ☐ Dissociation ☐ Emotional numbness ☐ Other: _____
Psychotic symptoms	☒ NA	☐ Hallucinations ☐ Delusions ☐ Paranoia ☐ Loose associations ☐ Other: _____
Motor activity/ speech	☐ NA	☐ Low energy ☒ Restless/Hyperactive ☐ Agitated ☒ Inattentive ☒ Impulsive ☐ Pressured speech ☐ Slow speech ☐ Other: _____
Thought	☐ NA	☒ Poor concentration/attention ☐ Denial ☐ Self-blame ☐ Other-blame ☐ Ruminative ☒ Tangential ☐ Illogical ☐ Concrete ☐ Poor insight ☒ Impaired decision making ☐ Disoriented ☐ Slow processing ☐ Other: _____
Socio-Legal	☐ NA	☐ Disregards rules ☐ Defiant ☐ Stealing ☐ Lying ☒ Tantrums ☐ Arrest/incarceration ☒ Initiates fights ☐ Other: _____
Other symptoms	☒ NA	

Diagnosis for IP

Contextual Factors considered in making Dx: ☒ Age ☒ Gender ☒ Family dynamics ☒ Culture ☐ Language ☒ Religion ☐ Economic ☐ Immigration ☐ Sexual Orientation ☐ Trauma ☐ Dual dx/comorbid ☐ Addiction ☒ Cognitive ability ☒ Other: DX by MD

Describe impact of identified factors: Medical doctor's dx used in making dx; considered cultural, SES norms for CM7's behaviors; also considered blended family dynamics; religious resources considered as strength that can be used in treatment.

Axis I
Primary: 314.01 Attention-Deficit/Hyper-Activity Disorder, Combined Type

Secondary: V61.20 Parent-Child Relational Problem

Axis II: V71.09 No diagnosis

Axis III: None reported

Axis IV:
☒ Problems with primary support group
☒ Problems related to social environment/school
☒ Educational problems
☐ Occupational problems
☐ Housing problems
☐ Economic problems
☐ Problems with accessing health care services
☐ Problems related to interactions with the legal system
☐ Other psychosocial problems

Axis V: GAF 60 GARF 60

List DSM symptoms for Axis I Dx (include frequency and duration for each). Client meets 4 of 4 criteria for Axis I Primary Dx.

1. Inattention: carelessness, difficulty with sustained attention, does not listen, does not follow instructions, loses things, forgetful, distractable

2. Hyperactivity: fidgets, leaves seat, runs in classroom, talks excessively, blurts out answers, interrupts others

3. Symptoms at school, home, and Sunday school

4. Symptoms before age 7

(continued)

Diagnosis for IP *(continued)*

Have medical causes been ruled out?
☒ Yes ☐ No ☐ In process
**Has patient been referred for psychiatric/
medical eval?** ☒ Yes ☐ No
Has patient agreed with referral?
☒ Yes ☐ No ☐ NA
List psychometric instruments or consults used
for assessment:
☐ None or _Initial assessment conducted by MD; Youth_
Outcome Questionnaire

**Medications (psychiatric & medical)
Dose /Start Date**
☐ None prescribed
1. _Adderall 5 mg (school days)_ ; _4/02/09_
2. _____/_____ mg; _____
3. _____/_____ mg; _____

Client response to diagnosis:
☐ Agree ☒ Somewhat agree ☐ Disagree
☐ Not informed for following reason:
_____

Medical Necessity *(Check all that apply):* ☒ Significant impairment ☐ Probability of significant impairment
☒ Probable developmental arrest
Areas of impairment: ☒ Daily activities ☒ Social relationships ☐ Health ☒ Work/school
☐ Living arrangement ☐ Other: _____

Risk Assessment

Suicidality
☒ No indication
☒ Denies
☐ Active ideation
☐ Passive ideation
☐ Intent without plan
☐ Intent with means
☐ Ideation past yr
☐ Attempt past yr
☐ Family/peer hx of completed suicide

Homicidality
☒ No indication
☒ Denies
☐ Active ideation
☐ Passive ideation
☐ Intent without means
☐ Intent with means
☐ Ideation past yr
☐ Violence past yr
☐ Hx assault/temper
☐ Cruelty to animals

Hx Substance:
Alc abuse:
☒ No indication
☐ Denies
☐ Past
☐ Current
Freq/Amt: _____

Drug:
☒ No indication
☒ Denies
☐ Past
☐ Current
Drugs: _____
Freq/Amt: _____
☐ Family/sig.other abuses

**Sexual & Physical Abuse and Other Risk
Factors:**
☐ Current child w abuse hx:
    ☐ Sexual ☐ Physical ☐ Emotional ☐ Neglect
☐ Adult w childhood abuse:
    ☐ Sexual ☐ Physical ☐ Emotional ☐ Neglect
☐ Adult w abuse/assault in adulthood:
    ☐ Sexual ☐ Physical ☐ Current
☐ History of perpetrating abuse:
    ☐ Sexual ☐ Physical
☐ Elder/Dependent Adult Abuse/Neglect
☐ Anorexia/Bulimia/Other eating disorder
☐ Cutting or other self-harm:
    ☐ Current
    ☐ Past Method: _____
    ☐ Criminal/legal hx: _____
☒ None reported

Indicators of Safety: ☒ At least one outside person who provides strong support ☐ Able to cite specific reasons to live, not harm self/other ☒ Hopeful ☐ Has future goals ☐ Willing to dispose of dangerous items ☐ Willing to reduce contact with people who make situation worse ☐ Willing to implement safety plan, safety interventions ☐ Developing set of alternatives to self/other harm ☐ Sustained period of safety: ☐ Other: _____

Safety Plan includes: ☐ Verbal no harm contract ☐ Written no harm contract ☒ Emergency contact card ☒ Emergency therapist/agency number ☒ Medication management ☐ Specific plan for contacting friends/ support persons during crisis ☐ Specific plan of where to go during crisis ☒ Specific self-calming tasks to reduce risk before reach crisis level (e.g., journaling, exercising, etc.) ☐ Specific daily/weekly activities to reduce stressors ☐ Other: _____

Notes: Legal/Ethical Action Taken: ☒ NA Explain: _____

Case Management

Date

1st visit: 4/2/09 _____

Last visit: 4/9/09 _____

Session Freq:

☒ Once week ☐ Every other week ☐ Other: _____

Expected Length of Treatment:

_____

Modalities:
☐ Individual adult
☐ Individual child
☐ Couple
☒ Family
☐ Group: _____

Is client involved in mental health or other medical treatment elsewhere?

☐ No

☒ Yes:

Dr. Hamdad _____

If Child/Adolescent: Is family involved?

☒ Yes ☐ No

Patient Referrals and Professional Contacts

Has contact been made with social worker?

☐ Yes ☐ No: explain: _____ ☒ NA

Has client been referred for medical assessment?

☒ Yes ☐ No evidence for need

Has client been referred for psychiatric assessment?

☒ Yes; cl agree ☐ Yes, cl disagree ☐ Not nec.

Has contact been made with treating physicians or other professionals?

☒ Yes ☐ No ☐ NA

Has client been referred for social services?

☐ Job/training ☐ Welfare/Food/Housing ☐ Victim services

☐ Legal aid ☐ Medical ☐ Other: _____ ☒ NA

Anticipated forensic/legal processes related to treatment:

☒ No ☐ Yes _____

Has client been referred for group or other support services?

☒ Yes ☐ No ☐ None recommended <u>Parenting</u>

Client social support network includes:

☒ Supportive family ☐ Supportive partner ☐ Friends ☒ Religious/spiritual organization ☐ Supportive work/social group ☐ Other: _____

Anticipated effects treatment will have on others in support system (Parents, children, siblings, sig. others, etc.):

May raise issues in marriage

Is there anything else client will need to be successful?

Coordination with teacher

(continued)

Case Management *(continued)*

Client Sense of Hope: Little 1----------5X-----10 High

Expected Outcome and Prognosis
☒ Return to normal functioning
☐ Expect improvement, anticipate less than normal functioning
☐ Maintain current status/prevent deterioration

Evaluation of Assessment/Client Perspective
How was assessment method adapted to client needs?
Contacted MD and schoolteacher; did assessment with entire family present.

Age, culture, ability level, and other diversity issues adjusted for by:
Used child-friendly language; encourage sharing about religion; discussion of racism.

Systemic/family dynamics considered in following ways:
Considered blended family issues as significant contributors to reported problems.

Describe actual or potential areas of client-therapist agreement/disagreement related to the above assessment:
AF has made decision to use medication;

AM is against medications; parents willing to work on parenting and family issues to reduce or eliminate need for medication.

_____ , _____ _____
Therapist Signature   License/Intern status   Date

_____ , _____ _____
Supervisor Signature   License   Date

TREATMENT PLAN

Therapist: Sally Wright _____ **Client ID #:** 1208 _____

Theory: Cognitive-behavioral family therapy _____

Primary Configuration: ☐ Individual ☐ Couple ☒ Family ☐ Group

Additional: ☐ Individual ☒ Couple ☐ Family ☐ Group: _____

Medication(s): ☐ NA ☒ Adderall _____

Contextual Factors considered in making plan: ☒ Age ☒ Gender ☒ Family dynamics

☒ Culture ☐ Language ☒ Religion ☐ Economic ☐ Immigration ☐ Sexual orientation

☐ Trauma ☐ Dual dx/comorbid ☐ Addiction ☒ Cognitive ability

☐ Other: _____

Describe how plan is adapted to contextual factors: Include play activities (for boys); use child-friendly language; minimize distractions in room; include family; include discussion of race and religion; address blended family dynamics.

I. Initial Phase of Treatment (First 1–3 Sessions)

I.A. Initial Therapeutic Tasks

Therapeutic Relationship

> TT1: Develop therapeutic relationship with all members. Note: Include child-friendly, teen-friendly, and parent-appropriate language and activities.

> I1: Intervention: **Gain confidence** in family that therapist will be able to help.

Assessment

> TT2: Assess individual, system, and broader cultural dynamics. Note: _____

> I1: Intervention: Conduct **functional analysis** of CM7 symptoms; identify role in system.

> I2: Intervention: Assess **family schemas** related to blended family, parenting, sibling relationships, and CM7's behavior.

Set Goals

> TT3: Define and obtain client agreement on treatment goals. Note: _____

> I1: Intervention: Identify **measurable, behavioral goals** for CM7 and blended family issues.

Note: **BOLDFACE** indicates CBFT Therapy assessment and techniques.

(continued)

I. Initial Phase of Treatment *(continued)*

Referrals and Crisis

TT4: Identify needed referrals, crisis issues, and other client needs. Note: _____

 I1: Intervention: <u>Contact prescribing physician and teacher to discuss **baseline functioning** and</u>

  <u>related treatments.</u>

I.B. Initial Client Goals (1–2 Goals): Manage crisis issues and/or reduce most distressing symptoms.

> **Goal #1:** ☒ Increase ☐ Decrease **cooperation** <u>at school</u> (personal/relational dynamic) to reduce <u>academic problems and acting out at school</u> (symptom).
>
> *Measure:* Able to sustain <u>pro-social behavior</u> for period of <u>2</u> ☐ wks ☒ mos with no more than <u>2</u> mild episodes of <u>losing points for behavior or failure to turn in work.</u>
>
> I1: Intervention: <u>In session **role play** to practice ways to manage impulses and distractibility.</u>
>
> I2: Intervention: <u>Develop **reward system** for turning in homework, studying, and grades.</u>

II. Working Phase of Treatment (Sessions 2+)

II.A. Working Therapeutic Tasks

Monitor Progress

TT1: Monitor progress toward goals. Note: _____

 I1: Intervention: <u>Re-administer Youth Outcome Questionnaire every 2 months.</u>

Monitor Relationship

TT2: Monitor quality of therapeutic alliance as therapy proceeds. Note: _____

 I1: Intervention: <u>Verbally check in with family every month to inquire about their perspective on</u>

  <u>treatment.</u>

II.B. Working Client Goals (2–3 Goals): Target individual and relational dynamics in case conceptualization using theoretical language (e.g., reduce enmeshment, increase differentiation, increase agency in relational narrative, etc.).

> **Goal #1:** ☒ Increase ☐ Decrease <u>parental effectiveness in working together and</u> **reinforcing behavior** (personal/relational dynamic) to reduce <u>disruptive behaviors at home and at school</u> (symptom).
>
> *Measure:* Able to sustain **consistent reinforcement system** for period of <u>2</u> ☐ wks ☒ mos with no more than <u>3</u> mild episodes of <u>failing to support the other or failing to follow through on stated consequence.</u>
>
> I1: Intervention: <u>Parent-only sessions to conduct **parent training** on setting consistent consequences.</u>

I2: Intervention: Couple **problem solving and communication training** around parenting issues and family schemas related to parenting.

Goal #2: ☒ Increase ☐ Decrease **positive** and satisfying sibling **interactions** (personal/relational dynamic) to reduce conflict between siblings (symptom).

Measure: Able to sustain pro-social sibling interactions for period of 4 ☒ wks ☐ mos with no more than 2 mild episodes of fights that require parents to set consequences.

I1: Intervention: Family discussion of beliefs related to blended family to identify **unrealistic expectations** of others and family as a whole.

I2: Intervention: Puppet play to practice and play with new ways to **realign boundaries** and **redefine roles**.

Goal #3: ☒ Increase ☐ Decrease CM7 independence with schoolwork (personal/relational dynamic) to reduce academic failure (symptom).

Measure: Able to sustain doing homework with **monitoring** only at beginning and end of homework session for period of 4 ☒ wks ☐ mos with no more than 4 mild episodes of failing to complete assignments.

I1: Intervention: Use **operant conditioning** to begin increasing CM7's independence with homework.

I2: Intervention: Increase AM involvement in homework and decrease CF14's involvement.

III. Closing Phase of Treatment (Last 2+ Weeks)

III.A. Closing Therapeutic Tasks
Termination Plan

TT1: Develop aftercare plan and maintain gains. Note: Consult with psychiatrist and teacher about gains and follow-up care.

I1: Intervention: Encourage family to identify family and social resources to help maintain gains.

III.B. Closing Client Goals: Determined by theory's definition of health

Goal #1: ☒ Increase ☐ Decrease **family cohesion** (personal/relational dynamic) to reduce conflict (symptom).

Measure: Able to sustain effective family problem solving for period of 2 ☐ wks ☒ mos with no more than 2 mild episodes of conflict that last for no more than a day.

(continued)

TREATMENT PLAN *(continued)*

I1: Intervention: Art therapy to envision family as a supportive and nurturing place for all.

I2: Intervention: Create a written list of positive **family beliefs** and plans for how to enact.

IV. Client Perspective

Has treatment plan been reviewed with client? ☒ Yes ☐ No; If no, explain: _____

Describe areas of client agreement and concern: Clients asked if CM7 will be able to get off medication; informed clients that medication decisions need to be made by the psychiatrist; the current plan is designed to reduce the symptoms being treated by medication. They will need to consult with psychiatrist about need for medication as therapy progresses.

_____ , _____   _____
Therapist signature   Intern status   Date

_____ , _____   _____
Supervisor signature   License   Date

_____

Abbreviations: TT: Therapeutic Task; I: Intervention; AM: Adult Male; AF: Adult Female: CM: Child Male; CF: Child Female; Dx: Diagnosis; NA: Not Applicable.

©2007. Diane R. Gehart

PROGRESS NOTES

Progress Notes for Client # 1208

Date: 5/12/09   **Time:** 4:00 am/**pm**   **Session Length:** ☒ 50 min or ☐ _____

Present: ☒ AM ☒ AF ☒ CM7 ☒ CF 14 ☒ CF 10 ☒ CM 7
Billing Code: ☐ 90801 (Assess) ☐ 90806 (Insight-50 min) ☒ 90847 (Family-50 min)

☐ Other _____

Symptoms(s)	Dur/Freq Since Last Visit	Progress: Setback---------Initial---------Goal
1. Hyperactivity	No "red marks" in class this week	-5----------1-----------5---X----------10
2. Inattention/grades	Turned in all but one class assign; most HW	-5----------1---------X-----------------10
3. Family conflict	CM10 and CM7 one fight on Sat	-5----------1---------X-5-------------10

Explanatory Notes: Report role plays have helped with in-class behavior problems; AF and AM report supporting each other with reinforcing behaviors at school and doing homework and that they have had fewer conflicts since parent training session. Continued conflict between CM10 and CM7, but able to resolve more quickly.

Interventions/HW: Reviewed reward system and answered parents' questions related to it. Psycho-education on blended family issues; used art to have each person depict what he/she likes most about this family and what he/she likes least. Developed plan for family fun night to increase cohesion.

Client Response/Feedback: Parents are eager to discuss problems but children can only listen for so long; all members actively engage in art activity, which brought out playfulness.

Plan: ☒ Continue with treatment plan; plan for next session: Parents only to begin working on increasing CM7 independence with homework.

☐ Modify plan: _____

Next session: Date: 5/19/09 Time: 4:00 am/**pm**
Crisis Issues: ☒ Denies suicide/homicide/abuse/crisis ☐ Crisis assessed/addressed:

_____

_____ , _____   _____
Therapist signature   License/Intern status   Date

◇◇◇

(continued)

PROGRESS NOTES *(continued)*

Case Consultation/Supervision Notes: Supervisor provided outline for operant conditioning related to homework.

Collateral Contacts: Date: 5/11/09 Time: 1:30 Name: Ms. Marshall

Notes: Teacher reports improved behavior in class and with schoolwork. Report continued talking during class but staying seated; less conflict with peers; turning in more classwork.

☒ Written release on file: ☒ Sent ☐ Received ☐ In court docs ☐ Other: _____

_____ , _____ _____
Therapist signature   License/Intern status   Date

_____ , _____ _____
Supervisor signature   License   Date

_____

Abbreviations: AM: Adult Male; AF: Adult Female; CM: Child Male; CF: Child Female; HW: Homework.

©2007. Diane R. Gehart

Solution-Based Therapies

"We intend to influence clients' perceptions in the direction of solution through the questions we choose to ask and our careful use of solution language. Reflection upon these questions helps clients to consider their situations from new perspectives."—O'Hanlon & Weiner-Davis, 1989, p. 80

Lay of the Land

The most well-known and arguably the first strength-based therapies, solution-based therapies are positive, active approaches that help clients move toward desired outcomes. The following three main strands of practice share many more similarities than differences:

- **Solution-Focused Brief Therapy (SFBT):** Developed by Steve de Shazer (1985, 1988, 1994) and Insoo Berg at the Milwaukee Brief Family Therapy Center, this therapy focuses on the future with minimal discussion of the presenting problem or the past; interventions target small steps in the direction of the solution.

- **Solution-Oriented Therapy:** This therapy (O'Hanlon & Weiner-Davis, 1989) and the related approach, *possibility therapy* (O'Hanlon & Beadle, 1999), were developed by Bill O'Hanlon and colleagues to incorporate a similar future orientation while drawing more directly from the language techniques used in Ericksonian trance. Solution-oriented therapy also uses more interventions that draw from the past and present to identify potential solutions than does solution-focused brief therapy.

- **Solution-Oriented Ericksonian Hypnosis:** Both solution-focused and solution-oriented therapies were inspired by the work of Milton Erickson, whose strength-oriented trance work is one of the most popular modern approaches to hypnosis.

Because of their numerous commonalities, this chapter presents solution-focused and solution-oriented therapies together under the general term *solution-based therapies;* it then discusses Ericksonian hypnosis.

Solution-Based Therapies
In a Nutshell: The Least You Need to Know

Solution-based therapies are brief therapy approaches that grew out of the work of the Mental Research Institute in Palo Alto (MRI) and Milton Erickson's brief therapy and trance work (de Shazer, 1985, 1988, 1994; O'Hanlon & Weiner-Davis, 1989). The first and leading "strength-based" therapies, solution-based therapies are increasingly popular with clients, insurance companies, and county mental health agencies because they are efficient and respectful of clients. As the name suggests, solution-based therapists spend a minimum of time talking about problems and instead focus on moving clients toward enacting *solutions*. Rather than being "solution-givers," solution-based therapists work with the client to envision potential solutions based on the client's experience and values. Once the client has selected a desirable outcome, the therapist assists the client in identifying small, incremental steps toward realizing this goal. The therapist *does not* solve problems or offer solutions but instead collaborates with clients to develop aspirations and plans that they then translate into real-world action.

Common Solution-Based Therapy Myths

More so than others, solution-based therapists are haunted by myths and misconceptions about what actually happens in session. So let's straighten these out before we go any further.

Myth: Solution-Based Therapists Propose Solutions (Give Advice)

Fact: Solution-based therapists do not suggest logical solutions to clients (O'Hanlon & Beadle, 1999). Instead, it is the client who identifies solutions with the help of the therapist, who identifies *exceptions* to the problem, descriptions of what is already working, and client resources to help the client envision potential solutions. Once a clear, behavioral goal is identified, the therapist works with the client to take small steps in this direction.

Myth: Solution-Based Therapists Never Talk About the Problem

Fact: Solution-based therapists are not psychic and therefore, like all therapists, must spend some time talking about the problem. However, they spend *less* time talking about the problem than most other therapists, especially SFBT therapists (De Jong & Berg, 2002). Solution-based therapists typically follow their clients' lead in determining how much and how often they need to talk about the problem versus the solution. To add further myth-busting evidence, hallmark techniques, such as *exception questions*, require talking about the problem as part of identifying the solution.

Myth: Solution-Based Therapists Never Talk About the Past

Fact: Again, solution-based therapists are not psychic, and they actually have numerous techniques that are grounded in talking about the past. However, when they talk about the past, they focus on strengths as well as the problem (Bertolino & O'Hanlon, 2002). Talking about the past is one of the most important means of identifying solutions: what has worked and what has not. The past is talked about in ways that facilitate the enactment of solutions.

Myth: Emotions Are Not Discussed

Fact: Emotions cannot be avoided in any therapy. However, solution-based therapists do not view the expression of emotion as curative in and of itself, as is assumed in humanistic therapies (Lipchik, 2002). Instead, emotions are used as clues to what works and what does not and where clients want to go.

The Juice: Significant Contributions to the Field

If you remember one thing from this chapter, it should be this:

Assessing Client Strengths

Assessing client strengths is one of the key practices in solution-based therapies (Bertolino & O'Hanlon, 2002; DeJong & Berg, 2002; O'Hanlon & Weiner-Davis, 1989). Strengths include resources in a person's life (personally, relationally, financially, socially, or spiritually) and may include family support, positive relationships, and religious faith. Most therapists *underestimate* the difficulty of identifying strengths. In fact, identifying client strengths is often harder than diagnosing pathology because clients come in with a long list of problems they want fixed and are thus prepared to discuss pathology. Surprisingly, many clients, especially those with depressive or anxious tendencies (the majority of outpatient cases), have great difficulty identifying areas without problems in their lives. Similarly, many couples who have been distressed and arguing for long periods of time, such as Suzie and Jorge in the case study at the end of this chapter, have difficulty identifying positive characteristics in their partners, happy times in the marriage, and, in the most desperate of cases, the reasons they got together in the first place. Therefore, therapists often have to ask more subtle questions and attend to vague clues in order to assess strengths well.

Solution-based therapists assess strengths in two ways: (a) by directly asking about strengths, hobbies, and areas of life that are going well, and (b) by listening carefully for *exceptions* to problems and for areas of unnoticed strength (Bertolino & O'Hanlon, 2002; De Jong & Berg, 2002). Furthermore, I have found that any strength in one context has the potential to be a liability in another context and that the inverse is also true: any weakness in one area is generally a *strength* in another area (see Client Strengths in Chapter 2). Therefore, if a client has difficulty identifying strengths and more readily discusses weaknesses and problems, a finely tuned solution-focused ear will be able to identify potential areas in which the "weakness" is a strength. For example, a person who is critical, anxious, or negative in a relational context typically excels at detailed or meticulous work and tasks. This insight can be useful in identifying ways for clients to move toward their goals. Solution-based therapists have been in the vanguard of a larger movement within mental health that emphasizes identifying and utilizing client strengths to promote better clinical outcomes (Bertolino & O'Hanlon, 2002). Increasingly, county mental health and insurance companies are requiring assessment of strengths as part of initial intake assessments. The key to successfully assessing strengths is having an unshakable belief that *all* clients have significant and meaningful strengths no matter how dire and severe their situations appear. It is helpful for therapists to remember that we see people typically in their worst moments; therefore, even if we are not seeing strengths in the present moment, they are undoubtedly there. Solution-based therapists maintain that all people have strengths and resources, and they make it their job to help identify and utilize those strengths toward achieving client goals.

Rumor Has It: The People and Their Stories

Behind-the-Scenes Inspiration: Milton Erickson

Milton Erickson served as an inspiration to Bill O'Hanlon's solution-oriented therapy and Steve de Shazer's solution-focused brief therapy. Trained in medicine as a psychiatrist, Erickson was a master therapist who was well known for his brief, rapid, and creative interventions (Erickson & Keeney, 2006; Haley, 1993; O'Hanlon & Martin, 1992). Rather than follow a specific theory, Erickson relied on keen observation while listening with an open mind to each patient's unique story. He frequently employed light trance work to evoke patient strengths and latent abilities (Haley, 1993; O'Hanlon & Martin, 1992). At a time when most therapies focused on the past, Erickson directed his clients to focus on the present and future, often envisioning times without the problem. Although others have meticulously studied his work, there has been no consensus or singular definition of Ericksonian therapy. The influence of his trance work is clearly evident in interventions such as the *miracle question* and the *crystal ball technique*, which rely on a pseudo-orientation to time and the implicit assumption that change *will* occur.

Solution-Focused Brief Therapy: Milwaukee Brief Family Therapy Center

Steve de Shazer

Steve de Shazer was a deeply thoughtful leader in the field. After his early work at the MRI with giants such as Jay Haley, Paul Watzlawick, John Weakland, and Virginia Satir, the late Steve de Shazer developed with his wife Insoo Kim Berg solution-focused brief therapy: "An iconoclast and creative genius known for his minimalist philosophy and view of the process of change as an inevitable and dynamic part of everyday life, he was known for reversing the traditional psychotherapy interview process by asking clients to describe a detailed resolution of the problem that brought them into therapy, shifting the focus of treatment from problems to solutions" (Trepper, Dolan, McCollum, & Nelson, 2006, p. 133). De Shazer was a prolific writer (de Shazer, 1985, 1988, 1994; de Shazer & Dolan, 2007), laying much of the philosophical and theoretical foundations for solution-focused work. His early work was influenced by the trance work of Milton Erickson (de Shazer, 1985, 1988) and his later work by Ludwig Wittgenstein, who viewed language as inextricably woven into the fabric of life (de Shazer & Dolan, 2007). With Insoo Kim Berg, de Shazer founded the Solution-Focused Brief Therapy Association and the Milwaukee Brief Family Therapy Center, where they trained therapists until their deaths in 2005 (Steve) and 2007 (Insoo).

Insoo Kim Berg

Warm and exuberant, Insoo Kim Berg was an energetic developer and leading practitioner of SFBT, co-founding the Milwaukee Brief Family Therapy Center and the Solution-Focused Brief Therapy Association with her husband, Steve de Shazer (Dolan, 2007). She was an outstanding clinician who furthered the development of SFBT, developing solution-focused approaches to working with drinking issues (Berg & Miller, 1992), substance abuse (Berg & Reuss, 1997), family-based services (Berg, 1994), child protective services families (Berg & Kelly, 2000), children (Berg & Steiner, 2003), and personal coaching (Berg & Szabo, 2005).

Scott Miller

Originally trained at the Milwaukee Brief Family Therapy Center with de Shazer and Berg, Scott Miller, along with his colleagues Barry Duncan and Mark Hubble, has been a strong proponent of the *common factors* movement (see Chapter 7; Miller, Duncan, & Hubble, 1997) and client-centered, outcome-informed therapy (see Chapter 5).

Yvonne Dolan

Yvonne Dolan studied and worked with de Shazer and Berg at the Milwaukee Brief Family Therapy Center, specializing in sexual abuse and trauma treatment (Dolan, 1991, 2000).

Linda Metcalf

Linda Metcalf applies solution-focused therapy in school counseling contexts, including solution-focused school counseling (Metcalf, 2008), solution-focused children's groups (Metcalf, 2007), solution-focused parenting (Metcalf, 1998), and solution-focused teaching (Metcalf, 2003).

Solution-Oriented Therapy

Bill O'Hanlon

A former student of Milton Erickson, Bill O'Hanlon is an energetic and popular leader in solution-oriented, strength-based therapies, including solution-oriented therapy and possibility therapy (O'Hanlon & Beadle, 1999; O'Hanlon & Weiner-Davis, 1989). A prolific and highly accessible writer and speaker, O'Hanlon emphasizes the significance of language, using subtle shifts in language to spark change. His work aims to transform client viewing as well as to solve the problem while attending to broader contextual issues that impact the client's situation (Bertolino & O'Hanlon, 2002). He has written extensively on numerous topics, including solution-oriented couples therapy (Hudson & O'Hanlon, 1991), solution-oriented approaches to treating sexual abuse (O'Hanlon & Bertolino, 2002), solution-oriented hypnosis (O'Hanlon & Martin, 1992), solution-oriented therapy with children and teens (Bertolino & O'Hanlon, 1998), and spirituality in therapy (O'Hanlon, 2006), as well as books for clients and popular audiences (O'Hanlon, 2000, 2005, 2006).

Michelle Weiner-Davis

Michelle Weiner-Davis developed a highly successful solution-oriented approach to working with divorce that she calls *divorce busting* (Weiner-Davis, 1992). She uses a brief, solution-oriented self-help approach for couples who want to prevent divorce.

Collaborative, Strength-Based Therapy

Matthew Selekman

Grounding his work in solution-oriented therapies and systems theory, Matthew Selekman has developed collaborative, strength-based therapies for working with children, adolescents, families, and self-harming adolescents (Selekman, 1997, 2005, 2006).

Solution-Focused Associations

SFBT has been influential in the United States, Europe, Latin America, and Asia:

- **European Brief Therapy Association:** Founded in 1994, the European Brief Therapy Association serves as a network of brief therapy practitioners in Europe who have worked closely with de Shazer and Berg over the years. They sponsor research projects in brief therapy and meet annually, bringing together therapists from across Europe and the world.

- **Solution-Focused Brief Therapy Association (SFBTA):** In 2001, Steve de Shazer and *Terry Trepper* began organizing SFBTA to bring together North American SFBT practitioners and researchers. Under the dynamic leadership of Thorana Nelson, Eric McCollum, Terry Trepper, Yvonne Dolan, and others, SFBTA is an active and engaged community of practitioners, educators, and researchers who work to further develop and refine SFBT practices.

The Big Picture: Overview of Treatment

Small Steps to Enacting Solutions

In broad strokes, solution-based therapists help clients identify their preferred solution (by talking about the problem, exceptions, and desired outcomes) and work with clients to take small, active steps in this general direction each week

(O'Hanlon & Weiner-Davis, 1989). In some cases, this is a very time-limited approach, often as few as 1 to 10 sessions; solution-focused therapists are advocates of the possibility of single-session therapy. In more complex cases, such as the treatment of sexual abuse or alcohol dependency, therapy may take years (O'Hanlon & Bertolino, 2002).

Making Connection: The Therapeutic Relationship

The Zen of Viewing: The Beginner's Mind

O'Hanlon and Weiner-Davis (1989) use the concept of a beginner's mind when forming a relationship, referring to the classic Zen saying "In the beginner's mind there are many possibilities; in the expert's mind there are few" (p. 8). Assuming a position of beginner's mind involves listening to each client's story as if you are listening for the first time, not filling in blanks with personal or professional knowledge. Most therapists underestimate how hard this is to do. When a client starts talking about "feeling depressed," most therapists believe they have useful diagnostic information, unthinkingly assuming that clients have read diagnostic manuals and use the term as a professional would. In contrast, solution-oriented therapists bring a beginner's mind to the conversation and are curious about *how this person experiences his/her unique depression.* If you get in the habit of asking, you will find that every depression is surprisingly "one of a kind." Thus, solution-oriented therapists make no assumptions when they are listening, asking to hear more about clients' unique experiences and understandings.

Echoing the Client's Key Words

Solution-based therapists carefully attend to *client word choice* and echo their key words whenever possible (De Jong & Berg, 2002). For example, rather than teaching clients to use psychiatric terms such as *depression* or *hallucinations* to describe their experience, the therapist prefers to use the clients' own language, such as "feeling blue" or "schizos." Using client language often makes the problem more solvable and engenders greater hope. For many, "ending the blahs" or "getting back to my old self" is a more attainable goal than treating a psychiatrically defined problem of "Major Depressive Disorder, Single Episode, Moderate."

Carl Rogers with a Twist: Channeling Language

O'Hanlon and Beadle (1999) describe how solution-oriented therapists use reflection, including reflection of feelings, with clients to build rapport. This approach is similar to humanistic approaches, such as Carl Rogers's client-centered therapy, but with a twist: solution-oriented reflections *delimit* the difficult feeling, behavior, or thought by reflecting on a time, context, or relational limit. Such reflections generally take three forms:

1. **Past Tense Rather than Chronic State or Characteristic:** Therapists reflect statements back to clients in the *past tense,* e.g., "You were feeling down yesterday."

2. **Partial Rather than Global:** Therapists reflect global statements back to clients as *partial* statements, e.g., "Your partner sometimes/often (instead of always) does things that annoy you."

3. **Perception Rather than Unchangeable Truth:** Therapists reflect a client's "truth" or "reality" claim as a *perception;* e.g., in response to "I'll never find anybody," they might say, "There does not seem to be anybody you are interested in right now."

For example, suppose a client is telling a story about how her boyfriend got angry at her for "no reason." A client-centered reflection would be something like "You aren't feeling understood" (present-focused statement about client's unexpressed emotion), whereas the solution-focus twist to delimit would be "You were not feeling understood *by your boyfriend last Saturday.*" The solution-oriented twist emphasizes the limited time and relational context in order to (a) define the problem in more solvable ways and (b) create hope. O'Hanlon and Beadle (1999) refer to this process as "channeling language." This technique helps both the client and therapist transition to desired outcomes.

Optimism and Hope

"Hope is like a road in the country; there was never a road, but when many people walk on it, the road comes into existence."—Lin Yutang

Optimism and hope are brilliantly palpable in solution-based therapies (Miller, Duncan, & Hubble, 1996, 1997). With all clients, solution-based therapists assume that change is inevitable and that improvement—in some form—is always possible (O'Hanlon & Weiner-Davis, 1989). Their optimism and hope do not stem from naïveté but rather from their ontology and epistemology: their theory of what it means to be human and how people learn. Because change is always happening—moods, relationships, emotions, and behaviors are in constant flux—change is inevitable (Walter & Peller, 1992). They have hope that the change will be positive because the client is in therapy to make an improvement and because over 90% of clients report positive outcomes in psychotherapy (Miller et al., 1997). Hope is cultivated early in therapy to develop motivation and momentum (Bertolino & O'Hanlon, 2002). For example, in the case study at the end of this chapter, the wife has little hope for the relationship; therefore, the therapist consciously tries to instill this hope early in treatment.

The Viewing: Case Conceptualization and Assessment

Strengths and Resources (see Juice)

Exceptions and "What Works"

Solution-based therapists listen for exceptions and examples of what works when clients are talking (de Shazer, 1985, 1988; O'Hanlon & Weiner-Davis, 1989). If you are listening closely, most clients spontaneously offer exceptions and examples of what works: "His ADHD is less of a problem in his math class" or "When his stepbrother helps him with homework, there does not seem to be much of a problem." These exceptions provide clues to what works and therefore what clients need to do more frequently.

Solution-based therapists identify exceptions and descriptions of what works in two ways: (a) indirectly, by listening for spontaneous descriptions, and (b) directly, by asking questions. They listen as carefully for exceptions as medical-model therapists listen for diagnostic symptoms. They then use these exceptions to help clients enact preferred solutions in their lives. They also ask exception questions to gather more information about what works.

EXAMPLES OF EXCEPTION QUESTIONS

- Are there any times when the problem is less likely to occur or be less severe?
- Can you think of a time when you expected the problem to occur but it didn't?
- Are there any people who seem to make things easier?
- Are there places or times when the problem is not as bad?

The vast majority of clients can identify exceptions with questions such as these. The underlying assumption is that the problem varies in *intensity*; the times when the problem is *less severe* are considered exceptions and generally provide clues to what works (de Shazer, 1985; O'Hanlon & Weiner-Davis, 1989). Especially with diagnoses such as depression, which are experienced most of the time on most days, therapists need to focus on variations of intensity rather than absence of the symptom to identify exceptions. With couples, such as in the case study for this chapter, the therapist listens for times when the couple are not fighting, "get along," or get things done, which may be in relation to children, work, extended family, and so forth.

Client Motivation: Visitors, Complainants, and Customers

Steve de Shazer (1988) assessed client motivation for change using three categories: visitors, complainants, and customers.

- **Visitors** do not have a complaint, but generally others have a complaint against them. They are typically brought to therapy by an outside other, such as courts, parents, or spouse.

- **Complainants** identify a problem but expect therapy or some other person to be the primary source of change. They are there to have their problems fixed by an expert.

- **Customers** identify a problem and want to take action toward the solution.

CLIENT MOTIVATIONS

	VISITOR	**COMPLAINANT**	**CUSTOMER**
Motivation	Low	Moderate to high	High
Source of Problem or Solution	Outside other (spouse, parent, court) thinks client has a problem.	Problem generally related to outside cause or person; expect therapist or another to be source of solution.	Self as part of problem and active agent in solution.
View of Who Needs to Change	Outside other needs to believe there is no problem.	Outside other needs to change and/or fix it.	Self needs to take action to fix things.
Building Therapeutic Alliance	Therapist identifies areas where client sees a problem and is willing to become a customer for change.	Therapist honors client's view of the situation while identifying specific instances where client can make a difference.	Therapist joins with client by complimenting readiness for change.
Focus of Interventions	Building alliance; understanding client perspective; framing outside request for change as "the problem."	Observation-oriented tasks (e.g., identifying exceptions over the week; Selekman, 1997).	Reframing; identifying what does not work; action-oriented tasks.
Readiness for Action	Not ready for making active changes in life until client believes there is some sort of problem and is motivated to change.	Not ready for action until open to the idea that client's actions can make a difference.	Ready to take action to make changes.

Assessing clients' motivation is helpful for knowing how to join with the client as well as knowing how to proceed. Many new therapists assume that all clients are customers for change: ready to take action to improve their situation simply because they showed up for a therapy session. However, this is often not the case. People come to therapy with mixed emotions and levels of motivation. Generally, most mandated clients are "visitors," and therapists need to find a way to connect with their agenda while still working with the referring party's agenda. This same dynamic is often the case with children, teens, and even one-half of a couple. With complainants, therapists need to either find ways that the client can contribute to making a difference or help shift the viewing of the problem to increase client willingness to take action. In the case study at the end of this chapter, Suzie is a complainant, seeing her husband as the problem, and Jorge is a visitor, not even aware there was a problem until now; thus the therapist will need to adjust the treatment plan to honor how each views the situation and motivate each accordingly.

Targeting Change: Goal Setting

Goal Language: Positive and Concrete

Solution-based therapists state their goals in positive, observable terms (De Jong & Berg, 2002). Positive goal descriptions emphasize what the client is *going to be doing* rather than focusing on symptom reduction, which is typical in the medical model and cognitive-behavioral therapies. Observable descriptions include clear, specific behavioral indicators of the desired change.

EXAMPLES OF OBSERVABLE AND NONOBSERVABLE GOALS

POSITIVE, OBSERVABLE GOALS	NEGATIVE (SYMPTOM-REDUCING), NONOBSERVABLE GOALS
Increase periods of enjoyable activity, social interaction, and hope for future	Reduce depression
Increase frequency of couple's emotionally intimate conversations	Reduce couple conflict
Increase cooperation and pro-social activities	Reduce defiance

You may have noticed that simply reading the left column generates more hope and provides greater direction for clinical change than the right column. Positive, observable goals provide a constant reminder to the therapist and client of the goal, and reinforce a solution-focused and solution-oriented perspective. Many solution-based techniques, such as scaling questions (discussed later in chapter), invite the client to measure goal progress weekly; thus carefully crafted goal language is particularly critical to success in solution-based therapies.

Solution-based goals should also have the following qualities (Bertolino & O'Hanlon, 2002; De Jong & Berg, 2002):

- **Meaningful to Client:** Goals must be personally important to the client.

- **Interactional:** Rather than reflect a general feeling (e.g., "feeling better"), the goals should describe how interactions with others will change.

- **Situational:** Goals are stated in situational terms (e.g., "improved mood at work") rather than global terms.

- **Small Steps:** Goals should be short-term and with identifiable small steps.

- **Clear Role for Client:** Goals should identify a clear role for the client rather than for others.

- **Realistic:** Goals need to be realistic for this client at this time.

- **Legal and Ethical:** Goals should be legal and adhere to client, therapist, and professional ethics.

Solution-Generating Questions

Solution-based therapists use several related questions to help generate solutions and identify goals early in therapy: miracle questions (de Shazer, 1988), crystal ball questions (de Shazer, 1985), magic wand questions (Selekman, 1997), and time machine questions (Bertolino & O'Hanlon, 2002). When successfully delivered, these questions help clients envision a future without the problem, generating hope and motivation. When poorly delivered, they can be quite awkward.

EXAMPLES OF SOLUTION-GENERATING QUESTIONS

- **Miracle Questions:** "Imagine that you go home tonight and during the middle of the night a miracle happens: all the problems you came here to resolve are miraculously resolved. However, when you wake up, you have no idea a miracle has occurred. What are some of the first things you would notice that would be different? What are some of the first clues that a miracle has occurred?"

- **Crystal Ball Questions:** "Imagine I had a crystal ball that allowed us to look into the future to a time when the problems you came here for are already resolved. I hold it up to you, and you look in. What do you see?"

- **Magic Wand Questions:** "Imagine I had a magic wand (or imagine that this magic wand I have actually works), and after you leave I wave it and all of the problems you came here for are resolved overnight. You of course have no idea that your problems have been solved. When you wake up in the morning, what would be the first clues that something is different? What would you be doing differently? What would others be doing differently?"

- **Time Machine Questions:** "Imagine I had a time machine that could propel you into the future to the point in time when the problems you came to see me for are totally resolved. Imagine you stepped in: Where do you end up? Who is with you? What is happening? How is your life different? How did your problems go away?"

I have found that the keys to making these questions work are (a) preparing clients for an unusual question, (b) creating a compelling vision, and (c) asking for specific behavioral changes in the follow-up questions.

- **Preparing Clients for a Solution-Generating Question:** You can prepare clients cognitively and emotionally for these questions by asking: "Is it okay if I ask you a kind of strange question?" or "Would you be willing to play along if I asked a somewhat odd question?"

- **Creating a Compelling Vision:** Because many solution-focused and solution-oriented therapists also have training in Ericksonian hypnosis, they are skilled in the important task of developing a compelling vision of the miracle, crystal ball, magic wand, or time machine. This can be done in many ways: having an actual object (all therapists should have a magic wand handy), imagining the object (pretend to have a crystal ball in your hand), describing actual details of their real life or imaginary details about the magic objects ("imagine I had a crystal ball sitting on the small table covered with red velvet"), and/or using humor ("imagine this magic wand actually worked").

- **Asking for Behavioral Changes:** Follow-up questions should focus on behavioral changes in the client and others; for example, "What might you find yourself doing differently?" "What will others be doing differently?" "What are some of the first clues that a miracle has happened?" When clients describe how others are behaving differently, therapists should follow up with circular questions to ask how they will respond to the others' new behavior.

In the case study at the end of the chapter, the therapist uses the miracle question to help Suzie, who is hopeless about her marriage, to develop a realistic vision of how things could improve and thus motivate her toward change.

Small Steps: Scaling Questions

Scaling questions invite clients to identify small steps toward goal attainment (de Shazer, 1994; O'Hanlon & Weiner-Davis, 1989; Selekman, 1997).

EXAMPLE OF A SCALING QUESTION

"On a scale from 1 to 10 with 10 being your desired goal, where are you this week? [Client responds and rates: e.g., 3]. If you are at a 3 this week, what things would need to be different for you to come in next week and rate it a 4 [or 3.5 if client tends toward pessimism or needs to keep goal smaller]?"

The response to the second question begins a discussion of small steps the client can take over the next week. The steps need to be *concrete* and *specific*. For example, if the client's initial response is "I would feel less depressed," the therapist needs to ask follow-up questions such as "How would you know you were less depressed?" "What would you be doing differently" "How would your days be different?" "What would other people notice?" These questions help the client identify specific small steps to be taken over the week, such as "call a friend," "get up and exercise," or "play guitar." The steps need to be small enough that the client thinks they are easily attainable, especially early in therapy. In the case study at the end of the chapter, the therapist plans to take very small steps toward change because Suzie's problems have been brewing for years and she is skeptical and hesitant.

One Thing Different: Client-Generated Change

In the beginning, the key is to do one small thing different—call one friend—rather than visit with someone every day (de Shazer, 1985, 1988; O'Hanlon, 2000; O'Hanlon & Weiner-Davis, 1989). Similarly, a goal such as "get up and exercise one day this week" is more likely to generate change and motivation for further change than a goal such as "get up and exercise every day this week." In most cases, making this one small change starts a cascade of change events that are inspired from the client's *own* motivation rather than the prescription of the therapist (or even the co-created solution with the therapist). Ideas generated in therapy are not viewed as the "best," "only," or "correct" solution but rather activities that will spark clients to identify what works for them.

The Doing: Interventions

Formula First Session Task

As the name implies, the formula first session task (de Shazer, 1985) is typically used in the first session with all clients, regardless of the issue, to increase client hope in the therapy process and motivation for change.

EXAMPLE OF A FORMULA FIRST SESSION TASK

Formula First Session Task: "Between now and the next time we meet, we [I] would like you to observe, so that you can describe to us [me] next time, what happens in your [pick one: family, life, marriage, relationship] that you want to continue to have happen" (de Shazer, 1985, p. 137).

(continued)

(continued)

> **Paraphrase with Introduction:** "As we are starting therapy, many things are going to change. However, I am sure that there are many things in your life and relationships that you do *not* want to have changed. Over the next week, I want (each of) you to generate a list of the things in your life and relationships that you *do not* want to have changed by therapy. Notice small things as well as big things that are working right now."

This directive stimulates clients to notice what is working, identifies their strengths and resources, and helps generate hope in their ability to change.

Scaling Questions for Weekly Task Assignments

Scaling questions are used for goal setting (see previous discussion) as well as for developing weekly tasks and homework (O'Hanlon & Weiner-Davis, 1989). Once a client has identified what behaviors would constitute moving up the scale, the therapist works with the client to identify specific activities and behaviors that will make the small changes needed to enact these behaviors. This intervention can be used weekly to develop homework assignments that will move clients step by step toward their goals. If clients do not follow through on the assigned tasks, therapists need to reassess by asking the following questions: (a) Am I expecting a complainant to be as motivated as a customer for change? (b) Was the task too big or can smaller steps be taken? (c) Are the right people involved? and (d) What actually motivates the client to take action and move toward change?

Asking Presuppositional Questions and Assuming a Future Solution

Presuppositional questions and talk that assumes future change help clients envision a future without the problem, generating hope and motivation (O'Hanlon & Beadle, 1999; O'Hanlon & Weiner-Davis, 1989). Solution-focused therapists assume change based on the observation that all things change: a client's situation cannot not change. Knowing that change is inevitable and that most clients benefit from therapy, therapists can be confident when they ask presuppositional questions such as the following:

- What will you be doing differently once we resolve these issues?
- Do you think there are other concerns you will want to address once we resolve these issues?
- When the problem is resolved, what is one of the first things you will do to celebrate?

Questions such as these can be very helpful in cases such as the one at the end of the chapter with Suzie and Jorge, when one or more parties are feeling hopeless.

Utilization

Drawing on the hypnotic work of Milton Erickson, de Shazer (1988) employed utilization techniques to help clients identify and enact solutions. *Utilization* refers to finding a way to use and leverage whatever the client presents as a strength, interest, proclivity, or habit to develop meaningful actions and plans that will lead in the direction of solutions. For example, if a client has difficulty making friends and close relations but has numerous pets, the therapist will utilize the client's interest in animals to develop more human connections, perhaps by having the client take a dog for a walk in public places, join a dog agility class, or volunteer at a pet shelter.

Coping Questions

Coping questions generate hope, agency, and motivation, especially when clients are feeling overwhelmed (De Jong & Berg, 2002; de Shazer & Dolan, 2007). They are used when the client is not reporting progress, describing an acute crisis, or otherwise feeling hopeless. Coping questions direct clients to identify how they have been coping with a current or past difficult situation.

EXAMPLES OF COPING QUESTIONS

- "This sounds hard—how have you managed to cope with this to the degree that you are?" (de Shazer & Dolan, 2007, p. 10)

- "How have you managed to prevent it from getting worse?" (p. 10)

Compliments and Encouragement

Solution-based therapists use compliments and encouragement to motivate clients and highlight strengths. The key with compliments is to compliment *only* when clients are making steps toward *goals that they have set* or to compliment *specific strengths that relate to the problem*. This is so important I am going to say it again and put it in a special box so you don't forget.

THERAPEUTIC COMPLIMENTS

Rule for Making Compliments

Compliment only when clients are making steps toward goals they have set, or compliment specific strengths that relate to the problem; compliment their progress, not their personhood.

Examples

Therapeutic compliment:

- *Wow! You made real progress toward your goal this week.*

Even better therapeutic compliment:

- *I am impressed; you not only followed through on the chart idea we developed last week but you came up with your own additional strategies—setting up a weekend outing with his friend—to improve your relationship with your son.* (compliments specific behavior toward goal)

Not-so-good therapeutic compliments:

- *I really admire what you have done with your life.* (too personal and does not clearly relate to the problem; sounds like you are buttering up client)

- *You really are a great mom.* (nonspecific; evaluating mother skills globally; discouraging client from evaluating her own behavior and performance as a mother)

When therapists compliment the client on anything other than the client's goals and strengths, they are setting up a situation in which they are rendering judgment, albeit a positive one, on the client or his/her life. Compliments should not be used to be "nice" to clients (De Jong &Berg, 2002). They should only be used to reinforce progress toward goals that clients have set for themselves and stated in such a way that they encourage clients to validate themselves rather than rely on an outside authority figure to do so. When clients can set goals and make progress toward them, they develop a greater sense of *self-efficacy* ("I can do this"), which is a greater predictor of happiness than self-esteem (Seligman, 2004).

Interventions for Specific Problems

Couples Therapy and Divorce Busting

Solution-oriented couples therapy is popular because the emphasis on strength and hope is well suited for working with negative, interpersonal conflict, especially with couples who are in crisis or considering divorce (Hudson & O'Hanlon, 1991; Weiner-Davis, 1992). These solution-oriented couples therapies have several unique interventions.

Videotalk

Videotalk is based on distinguishing between three levels of experience: facts, stories, and experience (Hudson & O'Hanlon, 1991). The *facts* are a behavioral description of what was done and said, what would be recorded on videotape during the couple's interaction. The *story* is the interpretation and meaning that a person associates with the behaviors and words. The *experience* is the internal thoughts and feelings each person had. When couples are having difficulty, therapists can help them sort through their differences by separating the facts from the story and the experience to increase each person's understanding of how he/she is interpreting the situation. Clients are encouraged to use videotalk (e.g., "She asked me three times" or "He went to his study after dinner without saying anything to me") instead of their default interpretations (e.g., "She was nagging" or "He is distant"). By using videotalk to separate the *behaviors* from the *interpretation of the behaviors*, couples become less defensive with one another and are able to engage in conversations in which they better understand each other and identify meaningful ways to reduce future conflict.

From Complaints to Requests

Solution-oriented therapists encourage clients to ask for what they want rather than what they don't want or, in other words, to move from making *complaints* to making *requests* (O'Hanlon & Hudson, 1991; Weiner-Davis, 1992). For example, instead of saying, "You don't do anything romantic anymore" (a global, overgeneralizing complaint), the partner would learn to rephrase the complaint as a request: "I would really enjoy adding romance back into our relationship." These requests need to be behavioral and specific. Thus the person in this example needs to add a specific behavioral request: "I'd like to go away for a weekend; go to dinner and a movie; go to the beach for a sunset walk" and/or "It would be nice if we went back to giving each other a kiss before we left the house, leaving little love notes, or giving each other massages."

Therapy for Sexual Abuse and Trauma

Yvonne Dolan (1991) and Bill O'Hanlon and Bob Bertolino (2002) use solution-based therapies with child and adult survivors of childhood sexual abuse. Solution-based approaches stand out from traditional approaches to sexual abuse treatment in their optimistic and hopeful stance that emphasizes the resiliencies of survivors. Given that these clients have *survived* such a difficult trauma, solution-oriented therapists harness those strengths in new ways to help them resolve current issues. Some of the distinctive qualities of these approaches include the following.

Honoring the Agency of Survivors

More so than traditional therapists, solution-based therapists honor the agency of survivors, allowing them to decide whether to tell their abuse stories and to determine the pacing of their treatment (Dolan, 1991; O'Hanlon & Bertolino, 2002). Although many therapists insist that survivors cannot heal without sharing the details of their abuse to their therapists, solution-based therapists would not readily agree. Instead, they work with clients to identify if, when, how, and to whom it is best to tell their stories. By fully honoring their agency, therapists create a relationship in which survivors regain full authority over the private aspects of their lives, reclaiming the autonomy that was lost through the abuse. Therapists who play a more directive role in working with a survivor may unintentionally replicate the abuse pattern by forcing clients to reveal parts of their sexual life in the name of treatment before they are ready, leaving them feeling violated and retraumatized.

The Recovery Scale: Focusing on Strengths and Abilities

Dolan (1991) uses the *Solution-Focused Recovery Scale* to identify what areas of the client's life were not affected by the abuse, thus reducing the sense that the client's whole life and self have been affected. The success strategies in these areas are used to address areas that are affected by the abuse.

3-D Model: Dissociate, Disown, and Devalue

O'Hanlon and Bertolino (2002) conceptualize the aftereffects of abuse and trauma using the 3-D model, which postulates that abuse leads people to dissociate, disown, and devalue aspects of the self, with the result that they develop symptoms that either inhibit experience (e.g., lack of sexual response, lack of memories, lack of anger) or that create intrusive experiences (e.g., flashbacks, sexual compulsions, or rage). The goal of therapy is to reconnect people with these disowned parts. O'Hanlon and Bertolino (2002) note that many of the symptoms related to sexual abuse are experienced as a sort of *negative trance*, a feeling that the experience is uncontrollable and involves only a part of the self. Solution-oriented therapists use *permissive, validating*, and *inclusive language* to encourage clients to revalue and include the devalued aspects of self that were disowned through the abuse.

Constructive Questions

Dolan (1991) uses constructive questions to identify the specifics of clients' unique solutions:

- What will be the first (smallest) sign that things are getting better, that this (the sexual abuse) is having less of an impact on your current life?
- What will you be doing differently when this (sexual abuse trauma) is less of a current problem in your life?
- What will you be doing differently with your time?
- What will you be thinking about (doing) *instead* of thinking about the past?
- Are there times when the above is already happening to some (even a small) extent? What is different about those times? What is helpful about those differences?
- What differences will the above healing changes make when they have been present in your life over an extended period of time (days, weeks, months, years)?
- What do you think your significant other would say would be the first sign that things are getting better? What do you think your significant other will notice first?
- What do you think your (friends, boss, significant other, etc.) will notice about you as you heal even more?
- What differences will these healing changes you've identified make in future generations of your family? (pp. 37–38)

Videotalk (Action Terms)

Because of the intense emotions that characterize abuse and trauma, survivors often have difficulty identifying the current effects of abuse in their present life. O'Hanlon and Bertolino (2002) use *videotalk* (previously discussed) with survivors to help identify specific actions and patterns of behavior that recreate the traumatic experience, including the sequence of events, antecedents, consequences, invariant actions, repetitive actions, and body responses. Once these recurrent patterns are identified, therapists help clients either change one part of the context to interrupt the cycle and create space for new responses or, if the client feels a certain degree of control over the symptoms, identify new, alternative solution-generating actions.

Solution-Oriented Ericksonian Hypnosis

Solution-oriented hypnosis, also known as Ericksonian hypnosis or naturalistic trance, is a unique form of hypnosis that aims to evoke client strengths and resources to resolve client problems (Erickson & Keeney, 2006; O'Hanlon & Martin, 1992). As the name suggests, solution-oriented Ericksonian hypnosis grew out of the work of Milton Erickson, *preceding* solution-focused and solution-oriented therapies. Many solution-focused premises and techniques directly evolved from Erickson's approach to hypnosis and therapy.

Difference from Traditional Hypnosis

Solution-oriented hypnosis is different from traditional hypnosis in two significant ways (O'Hanlon & Martin, 1992):

- **Permissive Rather than Hierarchical:** Traditional hypnosis is hierarchical; the therapist runs the show ("You 'vil become very sleepy"), whereas solution-oriented hypnosis is permissive: "You may find yourself wanting to close your eyes, or you may prefer to keep them open."

- **Evokes Client's Natural Resources:** In traditional hypnosis, the therapist effectively "reprograms" the client once he/she is in a trance; in solution-oriented therapy, the therapist tries to "evoke" or stimulate the client's natural resources for healing, serving more as a midwife who allows the natural process to occur.

The Big Picture: Overview of Treatment

Ericksonian therapy invites the client to go into a trance in order to evoke resources and strengths that the client already has: this may be done with or without a clear induction into a hypnotic trance state. Erickson was known for using stories, analogies, and directives to activate latent abilities that will enable clients to resolve their problems (O'Hanlon & Martin, 1992). His work was arguably the first *brief therapy*, developed during a time when psychiatry and psychotherapy were dominated by psychodynamic ideas about problem development and problem resolution (Erickson & Keeney, 2006; O'Hanlon & Martin, 1992). Many of his students have gone on to develop his work, including Richard Bandler, John Grinder, Jay Haley, Bill O'Hanlon, Ernest Rossi, and Jeffrey Zeig, and the Milton H. Erickson Foundation continues training in his approach.

The Doing: Interventions

Permission

When inviting clients to enter a trance state, Ericksonian therapists give their clients *permission* to think, experience, and feel whatever they are experiencing without any pressure to *do* something (O'Hanlon & Martin, 1992). Clients are given explicit permission to have doubts, allow their mind to chatter, lose focus, entertain distracting thoughts, and accept other thoughts or feelings.

Presuppositions

Ericksonian therapists who are inviting clients into a trance state *presuppose* that clients will enter a trance state by delivering certain questions and comments to the client (O'Hanlon & Martin, 1992); for example, "Have you ever been in a trance before today?" "You can choose to keep your eyes open or closed when you go into a trance." "Don't go into a trance too quickly" (p. 18).

Splitting

The therapist may split two things that the client may habitually consider as one thing, such as the conscious and unconscious mind or the left brain and right brain (O'Hanlon & Martin, 1992). Generally, problem-saturated thoughts and feelings are attributed to the conscious mind and positive thoughts to the unconscious to allow the person to trust the trance process. For example, the therapist may attribute doubt or apprehension to the conscious mind and trust to the unconscious mind: "Your conscious mind may doubt that trance is even possible, but your unconscious mind knows exactly what to do."

Class of Problems Versus Class of Solutions

To the untrained eye, Erickson often seemed to discuss issues and topics that were totally unrelated to the problem. For example, when working with a child with enuresis, he might spend the entire session chatting about seemingly unrelated topics, such as baseball and digestion, without ever discussing the presenting problem (O'Hanlon and Martin, 1992). Erickson would assess the class of problem (e.g., lack of muscle control) and then identify the class of solution that would most likely solve the problem (e.g., muscle control; O'Hanlon & Martin, 1992). Similarly, if a person's depressed mood was characterized by pessimism, he would find areas where the client had hope and optimism; if the client's depression was related to a recent failure, he would find ways to evoke a sense of success, whether actual or potential. Thus, for Erickson, the focus was on evoking the class of solution—*in any other area of the person's life*—rather than trying to solve the literal problem. He would focus on evoking the solution through both dialogue and trance.

The practice of identifying the class of solution is a particularly useful concept when assessing strengths because it highlights that all strengths are not created equal. Erickson draws our attention to the fact that it is most important *to identify client strengths that are in the same class of solutions that relate to the presenting problem.* Thus, if a child is having difficulty following parental requests at home, therapists should carefully listen for other situations in which the client is able to follow rules, whether playing on a soccer team, paying attention in class, or playing board games with a friend.

Snapshot: Research and the Evidence Base

Quick Summary: The evidence base for solution-focused therapy is strong and growing.

Solution-focused therapy has a quickly growing foundation of empirical support. In 2000, Gingerich and Eisengart published the first critical review of solution-focused outcome research, listing 15 controlled studies. Of the 5 well-controlled studies, 4 showed that solution-focused therapy was *better* than both treatment as usual and a no-treatment control group; 1 study found solution-focused therapy to be as effective as treatment as usual. The other 10 studies, which were moderately or poorly controlled, all supported the effectiveness of solution-focused therapy. As of November 2007, Gingerich and Patterson (2007) have identified 150 controlled outcome studies on the effectiveness of solution-focused therapy, a dramatic increase over seven years that attests to the increasing interest in establishing this therapy as an evidence-supported approach.

In his introduction to a special issue of the *Journal of Family Psychotherapy* in November 2007, McCollum (2007) identifies three key practical and philosophical challenges to establishing solution-focused therapy as an evidence-based approach. First, it is difficult to adequately manualize solution-focused therapy and capture not only the techniques, which are more easily quantified, but also the spirit and epistemological positioning that are the essence of the model. A rigid or shallow adherence to solution-focused techniques without grounding in the collaborative, strength-based mindset of the theory results in a pushy or Pollyanna approach that is not an accurate enactment of solution-focused therapy. Second, McCollum advocates for "streams" of studies that address particular populations or problems in greater depth. Finally, certain solution-focused philosophical principles, namely, honoring each client's uniqueness and recognizing change processes outside of therapy, are at odds with the broader research project, which aims to make global assessments of the effectiveness of this approach, thereby obscuring client uniqueness and extra-therapeutic factors that contribute to change.

Snapshot: Working with Diverse Populations

Quick Summary: Solution-focused therapy is widely used with diverse populations in the United States, Canada, and internationally and is easily adapted for a wide range of value systems and communication styles.

Because it does not use a theory of health to predefine client goals (O'Hanlon & Weiner-Davis, 1989), solution-focused therapy can be adapted to a wide range of populations and value systems. This therapy is widely used with diverse populations in North America, South America, Europe, the Middle East, Asia, and Australia (Gingerich & Patterson, 2007). It has also been studied with a range of clients, including immigrants, African-Americans, Hispanics, Saudi Arabians, Chinese, and Koreans; and in a wide range of contexts, such as schools, prisons, hospitals, businesses, and colleges (Gingerich & Patterson, 2007). When working with diverse clients, solution-focused therapists access their unique emotional, cognitive, and social resources, which often relate to issues of diversity. The case study that concludes this chapter applies solution-based therapy to a Caucasian-Chilean couple who are considering divorce.

ONLINE RESOURCES

Milton H. Erickson Foundation

www.erickson-foundation.org

Solution-Focused Brief Therapy Association

www.sfbta.org

Solution-Oriented, Possibility Therapy

www.billohanlon.com

Divorce Busting

www.divorcebusting.com

European Brief Therapy Association

www.ebta.nu

Review of Solution-Focused Therapy Research

gingerich.net/SFBT/2007_review.htm

REFERENCES

*Asterisk indicates recommended introductory books.

Berg, I. K. (1994). *Family based services: A solution-focused approach.* New York: Norton.

Berg, I. K., & Kelly, S. (2000). *Building solutions in child protective services.* New York: Norton.

Berg, I. K., & Miller, S. (1992). *Working with the problem drinker: A solution-focused approach.* New York: Norton.

Berg, I. K., & Reuss, N. H. (2007). *Solutions step by step: A substance abuse treatment manual.* New York: Norton.

Berg, I. K., & Steiner, T. (2003). *Children's solution work.* New York: Norton.

Berg, I. K., & Szabo, P. (2005). *Brief coaching for last solutions.* New York: Norton.

Bertolino, B., & O'Hanlon, B. (1998). *Therapy with troubled teenagers: Rewriting young lives in progress.* New York: Wiley.

*Bertolino, B., & O'Hanlon, B. (2002). *Collaborative, competency-based counseling and therapy.* New York: Allyn & Bacon.

*De Jong, P., & Berg, I. K. (2002). *Interviewing for solutions* (2nd ed.). New York: Brooks/Cole.

*de Shazer, S. (1985). *Keys to solution in brief therapy.* New York: Norton.

*de Shazer, S. (1988). *Clues: Investigating solutions in brief therapy.* New York: Norton.

de Shazer, S. (1994). *Words were originally magic.* New York: Norton.

*de Shazer, S., & Dolan, Y. (with Korman, H., Trepper, T., McCollum, & Berg, I. K.). (2007). *More than miracles: The state of the art of solution-focused brief therapy.* New York: Haworth.

*Dolan, Y. (1991). *Resolving sexual abuse: Solution-focused therapy and Ericksonian hypnosis for survivors.* New York: Norton.

Dolan, Y. (2000). *One small step: Moving beyond trauma and therapy into a life of joy.* New York: Excel Press.

Dolan, Y. (2007). Tribute to Insoo Kim Berg. *Journal of Marital and Family Therapy, 33,* 129–131.

Erickson, B. A., & Keeney, B. (Eds.). (2006). *Milton Erickson, M.D.: An American healer.* Sedona, AZ: Leete Island Books.

Gingerich, W. J., & Eisengart, S. (2000). Solution-focused brief therapy: A review of the outcome studies. *Family Process, 39,* 477–498.

Gingerich, W. J., & Patterson, L. (2007). *The 2007 SFBT effectiveness project.* Retrieved March 20, 2008, from www.gingerich.net/SFBT/2007_review.htm

Haley, J. (1993). *Uncommon therapy: The psychiatric techniques of Milton H. Erikson, M.D.* New York: Norton.

Hudson, P. O., & O'Hanlon, W. H. (1991). *Rewriting love stories: Brief marital therapy.* New York: Norton.

Lipchik, E. (2002). *Beyond technique in solution-focused therapy: Working with emotions and the therapeutic relationship.* New York: Guilford.

McCollum, E. (2007). Introduction to special issue. *Journal of Family Psychotherapy, 18*(3), 1–9.

Metcalf, L. (1998). *Parenting towards solutions.* Paramus, NJ: Prentice Hall.

Metcalf, L. (2003). *Teaching towards solutions* (2nd ed.). Wales, UK: Crown House Publishing.

Metcalf, L. (2007). *Solution-focused group therapy.* New York: Free Press.

Metcalf, L. (2008). *Counseling towards solutions: A practical solution-focused program for working with students, teachers, and parents* (2nd ed.). New York: Jossey-Bass.

Miller, S. D., Duncan, B. L., & Hubble, M. A. (1997). *Escape from Babel: Towards a unifying language for psychotherapy practice.* New York: Norton.

Miller, S. D., Duncan, B. L., & Hubble, M. (Eds.). (1996). *Handbook of solution-focused brief therapy.* San Francisco: Jossey-Bass.

O'Hanlon, B. (2000). *Do one thing different: Ten simple ways to change your life.* New York: Harper.

O'Hanlon, B. (2005). *Thriving through crisis: Turn tragedy and trauma into growth and change.* New York: Penguin/Perigee.

O'Hanlon, B. (2006). *Pathways to spirituality: Connection, wholeness, and possibility for therapist and client.* New York: Norton Professional.

*O'Hanlon, B., & Beadle, S. (1999). *A guide to possibilityland: Possibility therapy methods.* Omaha, NE: Possibility Press.

O'Hanlon, B., & Bertolino, B. (2002). *Even from a broken web: Brief and respectful solution-oriented therapy for resolving sexual abuse.* New York: Norton.

O'Hanlon, W. H., & Martin, M. (1992). *Solution-oriented hypnosis: An Ericksonian approach.* New York: Norton.

*O'Hanlon, W. H., & Weiner-Davis, M. (1989). *In search of solutions: A new direction in psychotherapy.* New York: Norton.

*Selekman, M. D. (1997). *Solution-focused therapy with children: Harnessing family strengths for systemic change.* New York: Guilford.

Selekman, M. (2005). *Pathways to change: Brief therapy with difficult adolescents.* New York: Guilford.

*Selekman, M. (2006). *Working with self-harming adolescents: A collaborative, strength-oriented therapy approach.* New York: Norton.

Seligman, M. (2004). *Authentic happiness.* New York: Free Press.

Trepper, T. S., Dolan, Y., McCollum, E. E., & Nelson, T. (2006). Steve de Shazer and the future of Solution-Focused Therapy. *Journal of Marital and Family Threapy, 32,* 133–140.

Walter, J. L., & Peller, J. E. (1992). *Becoming solution-focused in brief therapy.* New York: Brunner/Mazel.

Weiner-Davis, M. (1992). *Divorce busting.* New York: Summit Books.

SOLUTION-BASED THERAPY CASE STUDY

Suzie and Jorge Nunez are seeking therapy to keep their 10-year marriage together. Suzie reports that she has "had enough" of Jorge's selfishness and lack of support. He is a manager of a local rental car agency location, and she works as a secretary for an insurance agent and is the primary caretaker of their two children, Silvia, 6, and Albert, 3. Jorge is shocked to hear that Suzie is ready to leave as he feels he has been a good provider and treated her well. They have been arguing more and having sex less frequently over the past three years.

Based on interviews with this couple, Lilly, a solution-focused therapist, completed the following clinical documents.

Shaded Sections Emphasized in Solution-Focused Treatment Planning and Intervention

CASE CONCEPTUALIZATION FORM

Therapist: Lilly Ricard, MFT Trainee   **Client/Case #:** 1301   **Date:** 11/01/09

I. Introduction to Client and Significant Others *(Include age, ethnicity, occupation, grade, relevant identifiers, etc.). Put an * next to persons in session and/or IP for identified patient.*

AF†:   *(IP) 32, Caucasian, receptionist for insurance agency

AM: *(IP) 34, Chilean-American (parents immigrated), manager of rental car agency

CF: 61st grade, Dessert Sands Elementary

CM: 3 Daycare

II. Presenting Concern

Client's/Family's Descriptions of Problem(s):

AF or _____ : Believes AM is selfish and does not support her in parenting or household tasks; does not feel emotionally supported or appreciated by him.

AM or _____ : Believes AF has unrealistic expectations of him and perfectionist household standards.

CF or _____ :

CM or _____ :

Broader System Problem Descriptions (description of problem from referring party, teachers, relatives, legal system, etc.):

AF's family: View AM as a demanding husband.

AM's family: View AF as a demanding wife.

III. Background Information

Recent Background (recent life changes, precipitating events, first symptoms, stressors, etc.):

Although both were excited about having a second child, since his birth the couple have experienced increased tension, AF wanting more assistance from AM with the children; sex and intimacy have decreased in frequency. The couple currently do not live near either set of parents, having left their families when Jorge was promoted as manager shortly after the birth of the second child.

Related Historical Background (family history, related issues, past abuse, trauma, previous counseling, medical/mental health history, etc.):

The couple met in college and married without strong parental consent on either side; both families were concerned about the cultural difference between the two. However, they had a passionate connection that made them decide to "take a chance." Suzie's family has a history of independent working women,

† *Abbreviations:* AF: Adult Female; AM: Adult Male; CF#: Child Female with age, e.g., CF12; CM#: Child Male with age; Hx: History; Ex: Explanation or example; NA: Not applicable.

(continued)

III. Background Information *(continued)*

while in Jorge's family the women have typically stayed at home taking care of the children. No reports of past abuse, trauma, or prior treatment history.

IV. Systemic Assessment

Client/Relational Strengths

Personal/individual: AF is bright, articulate, and dedicated to raising her children. AM is strongly invested in the marriage and willing to do whatever it takes to improve things between them; he enjoys providing for his family.

Relational/social: Couple report strong passionate connection early in relationship; both have strong relationships with their family of origin, each having close sibling relationships; both are dedicated parents; they have one set of neighbors who have been helpful with watching the kids.

Spiritual: AM was raised Catholic and draws from this tradition for inspiration as a father and husband; AF is less religious but attends yoga practice regularly, which she finds calming.

Family Structure and Interaction Patterns

Couple Subsystem (to be assessed): ☒ Personal current ☐ Personal past ☐ Parents'

Couple Boundaries: ☐ Clear ☒ Enmeshed ☐ Disengaged ☐ Other: _____

Rules for closeness/distance: AF wants AM to feel the same parenting pressures she does and to have the same values and standards as she; AM experiences enmeshment in the sense that he has great difficulty accepting and understanding that AF has different needs and expectations.

Couple Problem Interaction Pattern (A ⇆ B):

Start of tension: AM does not contribute or help as AF has asked/anticipated.

Conflict/symptom escalation: AF becomes angry and tells AM how he has failed to help her; AM protests that he did not know.

Return to "normal"/homeostasis: Eventually AM says he is sorry and tries to make amends; AF is cool for several hours to a couple of days until things get back to normal.

Couple Complementary Patterns: ☒ Pursuer/distancer ☒ Over/under functioner
☐ Emotional/logical ☐ Good/bad parent ☐ Other: _____

Ex: AF pursues AM for greater participation as a parent; AM does not engage; AF overfunctions around house; AM underfunctions.

Satir Communication Stances:
AF: ☐ Congruent ☐ Placator ☒ Blamer ☐ Superreasonable ☐ Irrelevant
AM: ☐ Congruent ☒ Placator ☐ Blamer ☐ Superreasonable ☐ Irrelevant

Describe dynamic: AF tends to see faults in AM; AM more willing to placate.

Gottman's Divorce Indicators:

Criticism: ☒ AF ☐ AM. Ex: AF frequently and harshly criticizes AM.

Defensiveness: ☒ AF ☒ AM. Ex: Both defend their approach to the household.

Contempt: ☒ AF ☐ AM. Ex: AF often mocks AM; does not value his perspective.

Stonewalling: ☐ AF ☒ AM. Ex: AM sometimes ends arguments by refusing to look up or respond verbally.

Failed repair attempts: ☒ AF ☐ AM. Ex: AF unwilling to accept AM repair attempts.

Not accept influence: ☐ AF ☒ AM. Ex: Verbally AM accepts AF influence (agrees to make changes) to stop argument; however, never follows through.

Harsh startup: ☒ AF ☐ AM. Ex: AF starts criticism with "you always" or "you never".

Parental Subsystem: ☒ Family of procreation ☐ Family of origin

Membership in Family Subsystems: Parental: ☒ AF ☒ AM. ☐ Other: _____
Is parental subsystem distinct from couple subsystem? ☐ Yes ☒ No ☐ NA (divorce); Couple have not maintained strong couple alliance since birth of children.

Sibling subsystem: Two kids play together and are beginning to form more of a bond as CM3 gets older.

Special interest: _____

Family Life Cycle Stage:
☐ Single adult ☐ Marriage ☒ Family with young children
☐ Family with adolescent children ☐ Launching children ☐ Later life
Describe struggles with mastering developmental tasks in one of these stages:

Couple are having significant difficulty adjusting to having children, esp. related to the division of child-rearing tasks.

Hierarchy Between Child/Parents:
AF: ☐ Effective ☒ Insufficient (permissive) ☐ Excessive (authoritarian) ☐ Inconsistent
AM: ☐ Effective ☐ Insufficient (permissive) ☒ Excessive (authoritarian) ☐ Inconsistent

Ex: Have developed good/bad parent dichotomy.

Emotional Boundaries with Children:
AF: ☐ Clear/balanced ☒ Enmeshed (reactive) ☐ Disengaged (disinterested)
    ☐ Other: _____
AM: ☐ Clear/balanced ☒ Enmeshed (reactive) ☐ Disengaged (disinterested)
    ☐ Other: _____
Ex: Both easily angered when children misbehave; AM gets upset easily when children do not follow his requests.

(continued)

IV. Systemic Assessment *(continued)*

Problem Interaction Pattern (A ⇆ B):

Start of tension: <u>CF and CM start fighting.</u>

Conflict/symptom escalation: <u>AF tells them to stop; children each plead their case; AF tries negotiat-</u>
<u>ing and creating "fair" outcome; if this continues for several minutes, AM steps in and makes a "final</u>
<u>decision" based on what he sees in the moment.</u>

Return to "normal"/homeostasis: <u>Kids settle down after dad speaks; AF is then quietly angry at AM</u>
<u>for his harshness; the couple are "cool" toward each other for the rest of the day.</u>

Triangles/Coalitions:

☒ AF and CM/CF against AM: Ex: <u>AF often takes children's side against AM when he wants to set</u>
<u>harsh consequences.</u>

☐ AM and C _____ against AF: Ex: _____

☐ Other: Ex: _____

Communication Stances:

AF or _____ : ☐ Congruent ☐ Placator ☒ Blamer ☐ Superreasonable ☐ Irrelevant

AM or _____ : ☐ Congruent ☒ Placator ☐ Blamer ☐ Superreasonable ☐ Irrelevant

CF or _____ : ☐ Congruent ☐ Placator ☒ Blamer ☐ Superreasonable ☐ Irrelevant

CM or _____ : ☐ Congruent ☒ Placator ☐ Blamer ☐ Superreasonable ☐ Irrelevant

Ex: _____

Hypothesis (Describe possible role or function of symptom in maintaining family homeostasis):

<u>Couple have not adjusted to addition of children in their marriage, each having different expectations</u>
<u>for sharing these duties from their families and cultures of origin. The original passion between the</u>
<u>couple is now expressed in their "passionate" arguments.</u>

Intergenerational Patterns

Substance/alcohol abuse: ☒ NA ☐ Hx: _____

Sexual/physical/emotional abuse: ☒ NA ☐ Hx: _____

Parent/child relations: ☐ NA ☒ Hx: <u>Women close to children on AF side.</u>

Physical/mental disorders: ☒ NA ☐ Hx: _____

Historical incidents of presenting problem: ☐ NA ☒ Hx: <u>AF's parents had similar conflict.</u>

Family strengths: <u>AM's parents had low conflict, traditional relationship; despite conflict, AF's parents</u>
<u>stayed together and have been reasonably happy.</u>

Previous Solutions and Unique Outcomes

Solutions that DIDN'T work: AF making repeated requests of AM to help or do specific tasks; AM appeasing her in the moment but not following through; taking a "romantic" weekend ended in fighting.

Solutions that DID work: After big fights AM does more of what AF wants; AM more willing to help out with activity-based and "manlike" parenting tasks, such as teaching kids a sport, painting the baby's room, or setting up the car seats.

Narratives, Dominant Discourses, and Diversity

Dominant Discourses informing definition of problem:

Cultural, ethnic, SES, etc.: AF and AM have different cultural expectations regarding parenting and spousal roles; AM's family from a relatively wealthy South American family and AF from a middle-class family of northern European background.

Gender, sex orientation, etc.: AM adheres to more traditional gender roles; AF is wanting more egalitarian roles.

Other social influences: Couple live in a southwestern town in which highly contemporary and highly traditional family structures are equally common; thus both can point to other couples who do things the way each believes should be done.

Identity Narratives that have developed around problem for AF, AM, and/or CM/F:

AF feels more and more like a martyr to her husband and children because all of her energy is going toward raising the children. AF's constant criticism leaves AM feeling less and less like a man.

Local or Preferred Discourses: AF's preferred discourse is one of an egalitarian marriage; AM does not disagree in concept. AM wants to feel like a valued head of household and wants to feel loved by his wife.

Other Influential Discourses: Each family's discourse that the spouse is "not good enough" for their child adds extra pressure to the couple.

V. Genogram

Construct a family genogram and include all relevant information, including:

- ages, birth/death dates
- names
- relational patterns
- occupations
- medical history
- psychiatric disorders
- abuse history

Also include a couple of adjectives for persons frequently discussed in session (these should describe personal qualities and/or relational patterns, e.g., quiet, family caretaker, emotionally distant, perfectionist, helpless, etc.). Genogram should be attached to report.

(continued)

VI. Client Perspectives

Areas of Agreement: Based on what the client(s) has(ve) said, what parts of the above assessment do they agree with or are likely to agree with?

Clients in agreement with most of above, esp couple dynamic.

Areas of Disagreement: What parts do they disagree with or are likely to disagree with? Why?

AF not sure how much is cultural difference and how much is personality in regards to sharing of tasks.

How do you plan to respectfully work with areas of disagreement?

Explore culture and gender dynamics using open-ended questions, allowing clients to decide if this is useful for them in identifying potential solutions.

©2007. Diane R. Gehart

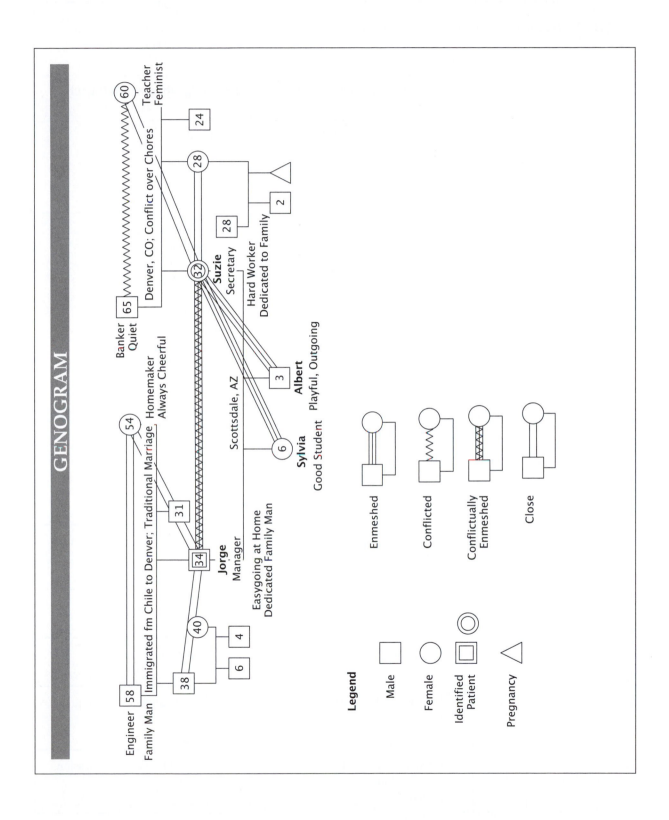

CLINICAL ASSESSMENT

Client ID # (do not use name): 1301.	Ethnicities: AF: Caucasian; AM: Children American	Primary Language: ☒ Eng ☒ Span ☐ Other: _____

List all participants/significant others: Put a [★] for Identified Patient (IP); [✔] for Sig. others who **WILL** attend; [×] for sig. others who will *NOT* attend.

Adult: Age: Profession/Employer	Child: Age: School/Grade
[★] AM† 34: Manager rental car agency	[×] CM 3: Daycare
[★] AF 32: Secretary at insurance agency	[×] CF 6: 1st grade
[ ] AF/M #2: _____	[ ] CF/M _____: _____

Presenting Problems

		Complete for children:
☐ Depression/hopelessness	☒ Couple concern	☐ School failure/decline
☐ Anxiety/worry	☒ Parent/child conflict	performance
☒ Anger issues	☐ Partner violence/abuse	☐ Truancy/runaway
☐ Loss/grief	☐ Divorce adjustment	☐ Fighting w/peers
☐ Suicidal thoughts/attempts	☐ Remarriage adjustment	☐ Hyperactivity
☐ Sexual abuse/rape	☒ Sexuality/intimacy concerns	☐ Wetting/soiling clothing
☐ Alcohol/drug use	☒ Major life changes	☐ Child abuse/neglect
☐ Eating problems/disorders	☐ Legal issues/probation	☐ Isolation/withdrawal
☐ Job problems/unemployed	☐ Other: _____	☐ Other: _____

Mental Status for IP (AF)

Interpersonal issues	☐ NA	☒ Conflict ☒ Enmeshment ☐ Isolation/avoidance ☐ Emotional disengagement ☐ Poor social skills ☒ Couple problems ☐ Prob w/friends ☐ Prob at work ☐ Overly shy ☐ Egocentricity ☐ Diff establish/maintain relationship ☐ Other: _____
Mood	☐ NA	☒ Depressed/sad ☒ Hopeless ☐ Fearful ☐ Anxious ☒ Angry ☒ Irritable ☐ Manic ☐ Other: _____
Affect	☐ NA	☐ Constricted ☐ Blunt ☐ Flat ☐ Labile ☒ Dramatic ☐ Other: _____
Sleep	☐ NA	☐ Hypersomnia ☒ Insomnia ☐ Disrupted ☐ Nightmares ☐ Other: _____
Eating	☐ NA	☒ Increase ☐ Decrease ☐ Anorectic restriction ☐ Bingeing ☐ Purging ☐ Body image ☐ Other: _____
Anxiety symptoms	☐ NA	☒ Chronic worry ☐ Panic attacks ☐ Dissociation ☐ Phobias ☐ Obsessions ☐ Compulsions ☐ Other: _____

---

† *Abbreviations:* AF: Adult Female; AM: Adult Male; CF#: Child Female with age, e.g. CF12; CM# Child Male with age; Hx: History; Cl: Client.

Trauma symptoms	☒ NA	☐ Acute ☐ Chronic ☐ Hypervigilance ☐ Dreams/nightmares ☐ Dissociation ☐ Emotional numbness ☐ Other:
Psychotic symptoms	☒ NA	☐ Hallucinations ☐ Delusions ☐ Paranoia ☐ Loose associations ☐ Other:
Motor activity/ speech	☐ NA	☐ Low energy ☐ Restless/hyperactive ☒ Agitated ☐ Inattentive ☐ Impulsive ☐ Pressured speech ☐ Slow speech ☐ Other:
Thought	☐ NA	☐ Poor concentration/attention ☐ Denial ☐ Self-blame ☒ Other-blame ☒ Ruminative ☐ Tangential ☐ Illogical ☐ Concrete ☐ Poor insight ☐ Impaired decision making ☐ Disoriented ☐ Slow processing ☐ Other:
Socio-Legal	☒ NA	☐ Disregards rules ☐ Defiant ☐ Stealing ☐ Lying ☐ Tantrums ☐ Arrest/incarceration ☐ Initiates fights ☐ Other:
Other symptoms	☒ NA	

Diagnosis for IP (AF)

Contextual Factors considered in making Dx: ☐ Age ☒ Gender ☒ Family dynamics ☒ Culture ☒ Language ☒ Religion ☐ Economic ☒ Immigration ☐ Sexual orientation ☐ Trauma ☐ Dual dx/comorbid ☐ Addiction ☐ Cognitive ability ☐ Other:

Describe impact of identified factors: Couple going through difficult time adjusting to having children; each has different gender role expectations for other as parent based on culturally informed gender roles.

Axis I

Primary: 309.28 Adjustment Disorder with Mixed Mood Anxiety and Depressed Mood, Chronic

Secondary: V61.10: Partner relational problem

Axis II: V71.09 None

Axis III: None reported

☒ Problems with primary support group Spouse; parenting
☒ Problems related to social environment/school: Move
☐ Educational problems
☐ Occupational problems
☐ Housing problems
☐ Economic problems
☐ Problems with accessing health care services
☐ Problems related to interactions with the legal system
☐ Other psychosocial problems

Axis V: GAF 60 GARF 55

List DSM symptoms for Axis I Dx (include frequency and duration for each). Client meets 5 of 5 criteria for Axis I Primary Dx.

1. Stressor: Birth of second child; couple still not adjusted to change

2. Periods of sadness/hopelessness; most days

3. Periods of irritability and poor impulse control; 1–2 times per week

4. Ongoing conflict with AM

5. Ongoing worry: most days

6. Does not qualify for mood/anxiety disorder; no bereavement

(continued)

Diagnosis for IP (AF) *(continued)*	
Have medical causes been ruled out? ☒ Yes ☐ No ☐ In process **Has patient been referred for psychiatric/ medical eval?** ☒ Yes ☐ No **Has patient agreed with referral?** ☐ Yes ☐ No ☒ NA; prior tx List psychometric instruments or consults used for assessment: ☐ None or _____ Outcome Rating Scale _____	**Medications (psychiatric & medical)** **Dose /Start Date** 1. <u>Celexa</u>/<u>40</u> mg; <u>9/1/09 (prior to start therapy)</u> 2. _____/ _____ mg; _____ 3. _____/ _____ mg; _____ Client response to diagnosis: ☒ Agree; ☐ Somewhat agree ☐ Disagree; ☐ Not informed for following reason: _____

Mental Status for IP (AM)

Interpersonal issues	☐ NA	☒ Conflict ☒ Enmeshment ☐ Isolation/avoidance ☐ Emotional disengagement ☐ Poor social skills ☒ Couple problems ☐ Prob w/friends ☐ Prob at work ☐ Overly shy ☐ Egocentricity ☐ Diff establish/maintain relationship ☐ Other: _____
Mood	☐ NA	☒ Depressed/sad ☐ Hopeless ☐ Fearful ☐ Anxious ☒ Angry ☒ Irritable ☐ Manic ☐ Other: _____
Affect	☐ NA	☒ Constricted ☐ Blunt ☐ Flat ☐ Labile ☐ Dramatic ☐ Other: _____
Sleep	☐ NA	☐ Hypersomnia ☐ Insomnia ☒ Disrupted ☐ Nightmares ☐ Other: _____
Eating	☒ NA	☐ Increase ☐ Decrease ☐ Anorectic restriction ☐ Bingeing ☐ Purging ☐ Body image ☐ Other: _____
Anxiety symptoms	☒ NA	☐ Chronic worry ☐ Panic attacks ☐ Dissociation ☐ Phobias ☐ Obsessions ☐ Compulsions ☐ Other: _____
Trauma symptoms	☒ NA	☐ Acute ☐ Chronic ☐ Hypervigilance ☐ Dreams/nightmares ☐ Dissociation ☐ Emotional numbness ☐ Other: _____
Psychotic symptoms	☒ NA	☐ Hallucinations ☐ Delusions ☐ Paranoia ☐ Loose associations ☐ Other: _____
Motor activity/ speech	☐ NA	☐ Low energy ☐ Restless/hyperactive ☐ Agitated ☐ Inattentive ☒ Impulsive ☒ Pressured speech ☐ Slow speech ☐ Other: _____
Thought	☐ NA	☐ Poor concentration/attention ☒ Denial ☐ Self-blame ☒ Other-blame ☐ Ruminative ☐ Tangential ☐ Illogical ☐ Concrete ☒ Poor insight ☐ Impaired decision making ☐ Disoriented ☐ Slow processing ☐ Other: _____
Socio-Legal	☒ NA	☐ Disregards rules ☐ Defiant ☐ Stealing ☐ Lying ☐ Tantrums ☐ Arrest/ incarceration ☐ Initiates fights ☐ Other: _____
Other symptoms	☒ NA	

Diagnosis for IP (AM)

Contextual Factors considered in making Dx: ☐ Age ☒ Gender ☒ Family dynamics ☒ Culture ☒ Language ☒ Religion ☐ Economic ☒ Immigration ☐ Sexual orientation ☐ Trauma ☐ Dual dx/comorbid ☐ Addiction ☐ Cognitive ability ☐ Other: _____

Describe impact of identified factors: Couple going through difficult time adjusting to having children; each has different gender role expectations for other as parent based on culturally informed gender roles.

Axis I

Primary: 309.4 Adjustment Disorder with Depressed Mood

Secondary: V61.10: Partner relational problem

Axis II: V71.09 None

Axis III: None reported

Axis IV:

☒ Problems with primary support group Spouse; parenting
☒ Problems related to social environment/school: Move
☐ Educational problems
☐ Occupational problems
☐ Housing problems
☐ Economic problems
☐ Problems with accessing health care services
☐ Problems related to interactions with the legal system
☐ Other psychosocial problems

Axis V: GAF 60 GARF 55

Have medical causes been ruled out?
☒ Yes ☐ No ☐ In process
Has patient been referred for psychiatric/ medical eval? ☐ Yes ☒ No
Has patient agreed with referral?
☐ Yes ☐ No ☒ NA
List psychometric instruments or consults used for assessment:
☐ None or _____ Outcome Rating Scale _____

List DSM symptoms for Axis I Dx (include frequency and duration for each). Client meets 5 **of** 5 **criteria for Axis I Primary Dx.**

1. Trigger: AF becoming increasingly unhappy with him following birth of second child; couple still not adjusted to change

2. Periods of sadness/hopeless following arguments (1–4 times/week)

3. Periods of irritability and poor impulse control; 1–4 days/week

4. On going conflict with AF

5. Does not qualify for mood disorder; no bereavement

Medications (psychiatric & medical) Dose /Start Date
☒ None prescribed

1. _____ / _____ mg; _____

2. _____ / _____ mg; _____

3. _____ / _____ mg; _____

Client response to diagnosis:
☒ Agree; ☐ Somewhat agree ☐ Disagree;
☐ Not informed for following reason:

_____

Medical Necessity *(Check all that apply):* ☐ Significant impairment ☒ Probability of significant impairment
☐ Probable developmental arrest
Areas of impairment: ☒ Daily activities ☒ Social relationships ☒ Health ☒ Work/school
☒ Living arrangement ☐ Other: _____

Risk Assessment

Suicidality
☒ No indication
☒ Denies
☐ Active ideation

Homicidality
☒ No indication
☒ Denies
☐ Active ideation

(continued)

Risk Assessment *(continued)*

Suicidality
☐ Passive ideation
☐ Intent without plan
☐ Intent with means
☐ Ideation past yr
☐ Attempt past yr
☐ Family/peer hx of completed suicide

Homicidality
☐ Passive ideation
☐ Intent without means
☐ Intent with means
☐ Ideation past yr
☐ Violence past yr
☐ Hx assault/temper
☐ Cruelty to animals

Hx Substance

Alc abuse:
☒ No indication
☒ Denies
☐ Past
☐ Current
Freq/Amt: _____

Drugs:
☒ No indication
☒ Denies
☐ Past
☐ Current
Drugs: _____
Freq/Amt: _____
☐ Family/sig other abuses

Sexual & Physical Abuse and Other Risk Factors
☐ Current child w abuse hx:
　☐ Sexual ☐ Physical ☐ Emotional ☐ Neglect
☐ Adult w childhood abuse:
　☐ Sexual ☐ Physical ☐ Emotional ☐ Neglect
☐ Adult w abuse/assault in adulthood:
　☐ Sexual ☐ Physical ☐ Current

☐ History of perpetrating abuse:
　☐ Sexual ☐ Physical
☐ Elder/dependent adult abuse/neglect
☐ Anorexia/bulimia/other eating disorder
☐ Cutting or other self-harm:
　☐ Current
　☐ Past; Method: _____
　☐ Criminal/legal hx: _____
　☒ None reported

Indicators of Safety: ☒ At least one outside person who provides strong support ☒ Able to cite specific reasons to live, not harm self/other ☐ Hopeful ☒ Has future goals ☐ Willing to dispose of dangerous items ☐ Willing to reduce contact with people who make situation worse ☐ Willing to implement safety plan, safety interventions ☐ Developing set of alternatives to self/other harm ☐ Sustained period of safety:_____ ☐ Other: _____

Safety Plan includes: ☒ NA ☐ Verbal no harm contract ☐ Written no harm contract ☐ Emergency contact card ☐ Emergency therapist/agency number ☐ Medication management ☐ Specific plan for contacting friends/support persons during crisis ☐ Specific plan of where to go during crisis ☐ Specific self-calming tasks to reduce risk before reach crisis level (e.g., journaling, exercising, etc.) ☐ Specific daily/weekly activities to reduce stressors ☐ Other:_____

Notes: Legal/Ethical Action Taken: ☒ NA: _____

Case Management

Date
1st visit: _11/1/09_____
Last visit: _11/14/09_____
Session Freq:
☒ Once week ☐ Every other week ☐ Other: _____
Expected Length of Treatment:
3 months

Modalities:
☐ Individual Adult
☐ Individual Child
☒ Couple
☐ Family
☐ Group:
_____

Is client involved in mental health or other medical treatment elsewhere?
☒ No
☐ Yes:
_____
If Child/Adolescent: Is Family Involved?
☐ Yes ☐ No

Patient Referrals and Professional Contacts

Has contact been made with social worker?

☐ Yes ☒ No: explain: _____ ☐ N/A

Has client been referred for medical assessment?

☒ Yes ☐ No evidence for need

Has client been referred for psychiatric assessment?

☐ Yes; cl agree ☐ Yes, cl disagree ☒ Not mec.

Has contact been made with treating physicians or other professionals?

☒ Yes ☐ No ☐ NA

Has client been referred for social services?

☐ Job/training ☐ Welfare/food/housing ☐ Victim services

☐ Legal aid ☐ Medical ☐ Other: _____ ☒ N/A

Anticipated forensic/legal processes related to treatment:

☐ No ☒ Yes: _____ Potential divorce _____

Has client been referred for group or other support services?

☐ Yes ☐ No ☒ None recommended

Client social support network includes:

☒ Supportive family; ☐ Supportive partner; ☒ Friends; ☐ Religious/spiritual organization; ☐ Supportive work/social group; ☐ Other: _____

Anticipated effects treatment will have on others in support system (parents, children, siblings, sig. others, etc.):

If couple issues not addressed, likely to affect children's behavior.

Is there anything else client will need to be successful?

_____

Client Sense of Hope: Little 1----- AF ---------- 5 ---- AM ----------10 High

Expected Outcome and Prognosis

☒ Return to normal functioning

☐ Expect improvement, anticipate less than normal functioning

☐ Maintain current status/prevent deterioration

Evaluation of Assessment/Client Perspective

How was assessment method adapted to client needs?

Used tone, language comfortable for couple; allow each person to share perspective.

Age, culture, ability level, and other diversity issues adjusted for by:

Provided opportunity for each to verbalize cultural/gender expectations.

Systemic/family dynamics considered in following ways:

Address over/underfunctioning dynamic by allowing each to speak for self; assign AM task of rescheduling appts.

Describe actual or potential areas of client-therapist agreement/disagreement related to the above assessment:

Couple seem to see situation as personality rather than cultural/gender conflict.

_____ , _____ _____

Therapist signature   License/Intern status   Date

_____ , _____ _____

Supervisor signature   License   Date

(continued)

TREATMENT PLAN

Therapist: Lilly Ricard, MFT Trainee   **Client ID #:** 1301

Theory: Solution-Based Therapy

Primary Configuration: ☐ Individual ☒ Couple ☐ Family Group: _____

Additional: ☒ Individual ☐ Couple ☒ Family ☐ Group: _____

Medication(s): ☐ NA ☒ AF: Celexa (began prior to therapy)

Contextual Factors considered in making plan: ☐ Age ☒ Gender ☒ Family dynamics

☒ Culture ☒ Language ☒ Religion ☐ Economic ☒ Immigration ☐ Sexual orientation

☐ Trauma ☐ Dual dx/comorbid ☐ Addiction ☐ Cognitive ability

☐ Other: _____

Describe how plan adapted to contextual factors: Plan includes exploring how gender, culture, immigration (language), and religious differences are informing each partner's expectations of the other as a parent; explore family dynamics (extended and with their children) that exacerbate couple relationship.

I. Initial Phase of Treatment (First 1–3 Sessions)

I.A. Initial Therapeutic Tasks

Therapeutic Relationship

> TT1: Develop therapeutic relationship with all members. Note: Attend to gender, culture, and tension
>
> I1: Intervention: Learn about each person's **strengths, hobbies, interests;** use **humor.**

Assessment

> TT2: Assess individual, system, and broader cultural dynamics. Note: Attend to culture, extended family.
>
> I1: Intervention: Assess **what works, exceptions** when couple get along; especially during former "passionate" phases of relationship.
>
> I2: Intervention: Assess client level of **motivation:** visitor, customer, complainant.

Note: **BOLD FACE** indicates Solution-Based Therapy assessment and techniques.

Abbreviations: TT: Therapeutic Task; I: Intervention; AM: Adult Male; AF: Adult Female; CM: Child Male; CF: Child Female; Dx: Diagnosis; NA: Not Applicable.

Set Goals

TT3: Define and obtain client agreement on treatment goals. Note: _____

I1: Intervention: Use **time machine question** to identify behavioral description of solution; **scaling questions** to break down into small steps. _____

Referrals and Crisis

TT4: Identify needed referrals, crisis issues, and other client needs. Note: _____

I1: Intervention: Identify social support and childcare assistance to enable couple to focus on relationship. _____

I.B. Initial Client Goals (1–2 Goals): Manage crisis issues and/or reduce most distressing symptoms.

Goal #1: ☒ Increase ☐ Decrease activities **that worked** for couple during dating and "good periods in relationship" (personal/relational dynamic) to reduce arguing/blaming (symptom).

Measure: Able to sustain positive affect activities for period of 4 ☐ wks ☒ mos with no more than 1 mild episodes of arguing per week.

I1: Intervention: Identify "**what worked**" while dating and use **scaling questions** to begin moving couple in this direction. _____

I2: Intervention: **Formula first session task** to identify what is working. _____

II. Working Phase of Treatment (Sessions 2+)

II.A. Working Therapeutic Tasks

Monitor Progress

TT1: Monitor progress toward goals. Note: Ensure both AF's and AM's complaints equally addressed. _____

I1: Intervention: Use **Outcome Rating Scale** to measure progress. _____

Monitor Relationship

TT2: Monitor quality of therapeutic alliance as therapy proceeds. Note: Focus on maintaining connection with both, esp. as discuss gender and cultural issues. _____

I1: Intervention: Use **Session Rating Scale** to measure alliance throughout. _____

II.B. Working Client Goals (2–3 Goals): Target individual and relational dynamics in case conceptualization using theoretical language (e.g., reduce enmeshment, increase differentiation, increase agency in relational narrative, etc.).

Goal #1: ☒ Increase ☐ Decrease cooperative co-parenting described in **miracle question** (personal/relational dynamic) to reduce couple arguing and triangulation of children (symptom).

(continued)

II. Working Phase of Treatment (Sessions 2+) *(continued)*

Measure: Able to sustain <u>agreed upon division of parenting tasks</u> for period of <u>3</u> ☐ wks ☒ mos with no more than <u>1</u> mild episodes of <u>arguing related to parenting per week.</u>

    I1: Intervention: **Miracle question** to identify expectations behaviorally, identifying cultural, gender, and family-of-origin issues related to expectations for partner's behaviors.

    I2: Intervention: **Scaling questions** to break goals down into small, easily achieved steps that enable AM to more directly increase role with children and reduce AF triangulation of children against AM.

Goal #2: ☒ Increase ☐ Decrease <u>emotional intimacy and sexual connection between couple</u> described in **miracle question** (personal/relational dynamic) to reduce <u>hopelessness and irritability</u> (symptom).

Measure: Able to sustain <u>emotional and sexual intimacy</u> for period of <u>3</u> ☐ wks ☒ mos with no more than <u>2</u> mild episodes of <u>not talking or avoiding sex for more than 2 weeks.</u>

    I1: Intervention: Use **videotalk** to reduce blame and increase positive affect communication and effective communication of requests.

    I2: Intervention: Create dedicated time for "**date night**" for couple to begin to reconnect.

Goal #3: ☒ Increase ☐ Decrease <u>couple agreement on each person's role in the marriage and family</u> (personal/relational dynamic) to reduce <u>arguing</u> (symptom).

Measure: Able to sustain <u>cooperative interactions</u> for period of <u>2</u> ☐ wks ☒ mos with no more than <u>1</u> mild episodes of <u>conflict.</u>

    I1: Intervention: Use **videotalk** to develop behavioral description of ideal partnership.

    I2: Intervention: Use **scaling questions** to help couple take small steps each week to realizing and maintaining desired relationship.

III. Closing Phase of Treatment (Last 2+ Weeks)

III.A. Closing Therapeutic Tasks
Termination Plan

    TT1: Develop aftercare plan and maintain gains. Note: _____

    I1: Intervention: Use **scaling** to develop "warning" behaviors and develop plan of action to prevent backslide.

III.B. Closing Client Goals: Determined by theory's definition of health.

Goal #1: ☒ Increase ☐ Decrease <u>couple's sense of solidarity as parents and as a couple</u> (personal/relational dynamic) to reduce <u>hopelessness, conflict, irritability</u> (symptom).

Measure: Able to sustain <u>positive interactions</u> for period of 2 ☐ wks ☒ mos with no more than 2 mild episodes of <u>conflict.</u>

    I1: Intervention: **Crystal ball question** to identify behavioral description of satisfying parenting and couple relationship.

    I2: Intervention: **Scaling questions** to identify small steps to move toward this goal.

IV. Client Perspective

Has treatment plan been reviewed with client? ☒ Yes ☐ No; If no, explain: _____

_____

Describe areas of client agreement and concern: <u>Although less optimistic than AM, AF is willing to try to make the marriage work; she wants to do so for the children and because they had a good relationship in the beginning.</u>

_____   , _____   _____
Therapist signature   Intern status   Date

_____   , _____   _____
Supervisor signature   License   Date

PROGRESS NOTES

Progress Notes for Client # 1301

Date: 12/4/09 **Time:** 4:00 am/pm   **Session Length:** ☒ 50 min or ☐ _____

Present: ☒ AM ☒ AF ☐ CM ☐ CF ☐ _____
Billing Code: ☐ 90801 (Assess) ☐ 90806 (Insight-50 min) ☒ 90847 (Family-50 min)

☐ Other _____

Symptoms(s)	Dur/Freq Since Last Visit	Progress: Setback----------Initial----------Goal
1. Conflict	2 moderate fights over past week	-5----------1---------X---5------------10
2. Irritability/anger (both)	Mild-moderate; worse on fight days	-5----------1-------X-----5------------10
3. Hopelessness (AF)	Mild, during fight days	-5----------1---------X---5------------10

Explanatory Notes: One fight related to children, one to extended family; followed typical fight pattern with slightly faster recovery. AF reports AM "slightly" more helpful with children around the house; couple had good night on "date night."

Interventions/HW: Used scaling question to identify how to move up from a 4 to a 5 over the next week: identified specific tasks for each and developed plan for implementing; used exception questions to identify small improvements in how couple handled arguments this week.

Client Response/Feedback: AM very responsive to compliments and exceptions; AF more hesitant to accept signs of progress, but is able to do so and reports seeing progress at home.

Plan: ☒ Continue with treatment plan: plan for next session: _____

☐ Modify plan: _____

Next session: Date: 12/11/09 Time: 4:00 am/pm
Crisis Issues: ☒ Denies suicide/homicide/abuse/crisis ☐ Crisis assessed/addressed:

_____

_____ , _____   _____
Therapist signature   License/Intern status   Date

◇◇

Case Consultation/Supervision Notes: Reported progress to supervisor who encouraged maintaining balance between AF pessimism and hope.

_____

Abbreviations: AM: Adult Male; AF: Adult Female; CM: Child Male; CF: Child Female; HW: Homework.

Collateral Contacts: Date: _____ Time: _____ Name: _____

Notes: _____

☐ Written release on file: ☐ Sent ☐ Received ☐ In court docs ☐ Other: _____

_____ , _____ _____
Therapist signature   License/Intern status   Date

_____ , _____ _____
Supervisor signature   License   Date

Collaborative and Narrative Therapies

"This kind of listening, hearing, and responding requires that a therapist enter the therapy domain with a genuine posture and manner characterized by an openness to the other person's ideological base—his or her reality, beliefs, and experiences. This listening posture and manner involve showing respect for, having humility toward, and believing that what a client has to say is worth hearing.... This is best accomplished by actively interacting with and responding to what a client says by asking questions, making comments, extending ideas, wondering, and sharing private thoughts aloud. Being interested in this way helps a therapist to clarify and prevent misunderstanding of the said *and learn more about the* unsaid."—Anderson, 1997, p. 153

Lay of the Land

The most recently developed family therapies are called "postmodern therapies," which can be broadly divided into two streams of practice:

- **Collaborative Therapy** developed by Harlene Anderson and Harry Goolishian in Texas (1988, 1992; Anderson, 1993, 1995, 1997; Goolishian & Anderson, 1987) and by Tom Andersen in Norway (1991, 1992)

- **Narrative Therapy** developed by Michael White and David Epston (1990) in Australia and New Zealand

These two approaches share many of the social constructionist premises described in Chapter 8, each being an approach to co-constructing new meanings with clients. Like solution-based therapists (Chapter 14), postmodern therapists optimistically focus on client strengths and abilities. Despite many similarities, however, collaborative and narrative therapies differ in significant ways, most notably in their philosophical foundations, the therapist's stance, the role of interventions, and the emphasis on political issues. Broadly speaking, narrative therapists have well-defined sets of questions and strategies for helping clients enact preferred narratives, whereas collaborative therapists avoid standardized techniques, instead using postmodern and social constructionist assumptions to facilitate a unique relational and dialogical process. The following table summarizes the difference between these two therapies.

COLLABORATIVE AND NARRATIVE THERAPIES

	COLLABORATIVE THERAPY	**NARRATIVE THERAPY**
Primary Philosophical Foundations	Postmodernism; social constructionism; hermeneutics (study of interpretation)	Foucault's philosophical writings; critical theory; social constructionism
Therapeutic Relationship	Therapist more facilitative; facilitates a dialogical process	Therapist more active: "co-editor," "co-author"
Therapeutic Process	No interventions; therapist focus is facilitating particular processes	Structured interventions
Politics and Social Justice	Political issues raised tentatively for client consideration	Social justice issues regularly included in therapy conversations

Collaborative Therapy and Reflecting Teams
In a Nutshell: The Least You Need to Know

Putting postmodern, social constructionist principles into action, collaborative therapy is a two-way dialogical process in which therapists and clients co-explore and co-create new and more useful understandings related to client problems and agency. Avoiding scripted techniques, therapists focus on the *process* of therapy, on *how* the client's concerns are explored and exchanged. They listen for how clients interpret the events of their lives and then ask questions and make comments to better understand how the client's story "hangs together." These questions and comments naturally emerge from conversation as the therapist strives to understand the values and internal logic of the client's perspective: to understand the client *from within the client's worldview.* As this process unfolds, the client is naturally invited to share in the therapist's curiosity, joining the therapist in a mutual or shared inquiry—a *mutual puzzling* about how things came to be and how things might best move forward. As therapist and client engage in this *shared inquiry*, asking questions and tentatively sharing their perspectives, alternative views and future options emerge on the client's situation. This process provides an opportunity for clients to see their situation differently, allowing them to make new interpretations and develop fresh ideas. Therapists do not try to control or direct the content of this meaning-making process; instead, they honor the client's ability to determine what to do with these new ideas (i.e., they honor the client's *agency*).

I am guessing this process still sounds vague, so perhaps it is best to offer an example. If a client says she is feeling "depressed," rather than hearing concrete, diagnostic information, collaborative therapists are profoundly aware of how little they know about *this* client's unique experience of depression, thus becoming sincerely curious about how the client came to this understanding of her experience. With no predetermined set of questions, the therapist asks questions that emerge from a genuine desire to better understand, such as: Does she cry often about something? About nothing? Has life gone to gray and nothing seems interesting anymore? Is her heart broken? Does she feel like a failure? There are as many unique depression stories as there are people who say they are depressed. As the therapist explores the client's view, the client is invited to join in the curiosity about her depression. Each new understanding informs alternative actions, thoughts, and feelings, thus shifting experience on multiple levels until the client has found a way to manage or resolve her initial concern.

The Juice: Significant Contributions to the Field

If you remember one thing from this chapter, it should be this:

Not Knowing and Knowing With

Perhaps one of the most frequently misunderstood concepts in collaborative therapy (Anderson, 2005), the idea of "not knowing" was first introduced by Goolishian and Anderson in 1988. At first blush, the not-knowing stance sounds contradictory: how can a paid professional like a therapist "not know"? Isn't that what they are paid for? What do you do with all that you have learned in graduate school? *Not knowing* refers to how therapists think about what they think they know and the intent with which they introduce this knowing (expertise, truths, etc.) to the client. Obviously, collaborative therapists are avoiding a particular type of knowing that Anderson calls "pre-knowing" (Anderson, 1997, 2007). In common English it's called *assuming:* believing that you can fill in the gaps or that you have enough information without sufficient evidence. Drawing from a postmodern social constructionist epistemology, collaborative therapists maintain that clients with apparently similar experiences, such as "psychosis," "mania," or "sexual abuse," have unique understandings of their situations (Anderson, 1997). Each client's understanding has evolved through conversations with significant others, acquaintances, professionals, and strangers, as well as through the larger societal discourse and stories in the media and literature. Therapists choose to *know with* and *alongside* clients as they engage in a process of better understanding clients' lives (Anderson, 1993, 2007). They view the client's knowledge as equally valid with their own.

This not-knowing, not-assuming stance requires the therapist to ask what on the surface appear as obvious or trivial questions: "You say you are sad about the loss of your mother. Can you tell me what aspects of her loss touch you most deeply?" or "Tell me how you experience that sadness in your daily life." When clients begin to explore the ideas, experiences, and influences that led to the perception of a problem, they often hear themselves saying things they have never told anyone before. Hearing these thoughts aloud for the first time inevitably shifts their perspective of the situation, sometimes subtly and sometimes dramatically. These new perspectives inform new action and identities related to the problem (e.g., from viewing her mother as an entirely separate person, the client may shift to seeing that she is part of how her mother lives on).

Rumor Has It: The People and Their Stories

Harlene Anderson and Harry Goolishian

Harlene Anderson and Harry Goolishian developed collaborative therapy with their colleagues at the University of Texas Medical Branch in Galveston and later established the *Houston Galveston Institute* (Anderson, 1997; Anderson, 2005, 2007). Their collaborative approach has roots in the early model developed by the Galveston group called "multiple impact therapy," a multidisciplinary approach to working with hospitalized adolescents, their families, and the broader social system. Their interest in hermeneutics, social construction, postmodern assumptions, and related social and natural science theories was initially fueled by their curiosity with the ideas of the Mental Research Institute (MRI), but in their work at Galveston they began to listen differently to what clients were saying rather than trying to learn clients' language to use it as a strategic tool. They noticed that it was not the family, but rather each *member* of the family, that seemed to have his/her own language, using words and phrases with unique meanings.

These interests naturally led to postmodern ideas, social construction theory, and then to the work of theorists such as Ludvig Wittgenstein, Mikhail Bakhtin, Ken Gergen, and John Shotter (see Chapter 8). As a result, Anderson and Goolishian began to conceptualize their work from a postmodern perspective, focusing on the construction of meaning in relationships. They also had a mutually influencing relationship with Tom Andersen, and over the years their therapy became known as collaborative language systems (Anderson, 1997) and, more recently, collaborative therapy (Anderson & Gehart, 2007).

After Harry's death in 1991, Harlene and her colleagues at the Houston Galveston Institute continued developing this internationally practiced approach. Ken Gergen (see Chapter 8), Harlene Anderson, Sheila McNamee, and others joined to form the *Taos Institute,* an organization of collaborative practitioners working in the fields of education, business, consultation, therapy, medicine, and other disciplines. Having found that the assumptions on which collaborative therapy is based have applications beyond therapy systems, Harlene currently refers to her work as "collaborative practices."

Tom Andersen

No relation other than a close friend to Harlene (note the "e" versus the "o" in Anders*e*n), Tom Andersen was a Norwegian psychiatrist who is best remembered for his gentle demeanor, respect for client privacy, and elegant therapeutic conceptions. Having originally studied with the Milan team using one-way mirrors, Tom transformed the systemic practice of the observation team using postmodern sensibilities that reduced the team-client hierarchy and made the process dialogical rather than strategic. His descriptions of *inner and outer dialogues* as well as *appropriately unusual comments* provide collaborative therapists with practical concepts that can be used to facilitate therapeutic conversations without the use of technique.

Lynn Hoffman

Known for her keen theoretical insights and broad vision, Lynn Hoffman has worked closely with many of family therapy's most influential thinkers, including Virginia Satir, Jay Haley, Paul Watzlawick, Salvador Minuchin, Dick Auserwald, Gianfranco Cecchin, Luigi Boscolo, Tom Andersen, Harlene Anderson, and Peggy Penn. Her first book, *Foundations of Family Therapy* (Hoffman, 1981), provides one of the most comprehensive overviews of systemic family therapy available. She began learning about family therapy at the MRI, where she served as an editor for Satir's books. She was so inspired by these ideas that she went on to pursue a career as a social worker, training in systemic family therapies. She befriended the Milan team, and along with Peggy Penn helped further their later development of the model (Boscolo, Cecchin, Hoffman, & Penn, 1987). In her later years, Hoffman became increasingly attracted to postmodern, collaborative approaches (Hoffman, 1990, 1993, 2001). She has detailed her remarkable journey in *Family Therapy: An Intimate History* (Hoffman, 2001), a favorite with my students who want to learn about the theories of family therapy yet prefer a little more "juice" and excitement than is offered in a textbook such as this. Hoffman is currently exploring the notion of rhizome theory in human systems.

Peggy Penn

A former training director of the Ackerman Institute and a published poet (Penn, 2002), Peggy Penn has developed unique approaches to using writing in collaborative therapy (Penn, 2001; Penn & Frankfurt, 1994; Penn & Sheinberg, 1991). Like Hoffman, Penn began her training in systemic therapies, most notably the Milan approach (Boscolo et al., 1987), but her work has since evolved into a more postmodern approach. She uses various forms of writing in therapy to help clients access multiple voices and perspectives.

Jaakko Seikkula

Psychologist Jaakko Seikkula and his colleagues (Haarakangas, Seikkula, Alakare, & Aaltonen, 2007) developed and researched the *open dialogue* approach to working with patients with psychotic symptoms in the Lapland region of Finland. As a result of 20 years of work, their hospital no longer has chronic cases of psychosis, and patients with psychotic symptoms need fewer medications and return to work more often. Jaakko's research provides some of the best empirical evidence for postmodern therapies (see Clinical Spotlight later in chapter).

Houston Galveston Institute

Originally founded by Harlene Anderson, Harry Goolishian, and their colleagues, the Houston Galveston Institute continues to be the premier training center for collaborative therapy, providing services to local child protection agencies, schools, and trauma survivors. Sue Levin currently serves as the executive director, and her research focuses on women who have been abused by their partners (Levin, 2007). Saliha Bava serves as the associate director of the institute, and her current work focuses on trauma (Bava, Levin, & Tinaz, 2002), qualitative research (Gehart, Tarragona, & Bava, 2007), and transformative performance.

Grupo Campos Elísios: Collaborative Therapy Training Center in Mexico City

Located in Mexico City and working closely with the Houston Galveston Institute, the bilingual faculty at Grupo Campos Elísios offer training in collaborative therapy and provide therapy and consultation services to local families, schools, and hospitals; the faculty and co-founders include Sylvia London, Margarita Tarragona, Irma Rodriguez-Jazcilevich, and Elena Fernandez.

Klaus Deissler: The Marburg Institute

Klaus Deissler and his colleagues at the Marburg Institute in Marburg, Germany, have developed a four-year postgraduate training program in collaborative therapy and collaborative business consultation, working closely with European businesses, school districts, and psychiatric hospitals.

The Big Picture: Overview of Treatment

Collaborative therapists do not have set stages of therapy or an outline for how to conduct a session. Instead, they use a single guiding principle: facilitate *collaborative relationships and generative, two-way dialogical conversations*, regardless of the topic and the participants. In short, they "keep the dialogue going." The key to facilitating dialogue is avoiding monologues.

Avoiding Monologues and the Therapeutic Impasse

Harry Goolishian often said that it is easier to identify what *not* to do as a therapist than what to do. Extending this logic, collaborative therapy is often easier to understand by identifying what is *not* a collaborative conversation, namely, a *monologue* (Anderson, 1997, 2007). A monologue can be a conversation with others or a silent conversation with oneself or an imagined other. In a spoken monological conversation between two people, each person is trying to sell his/her idea to the other person: a duel of realities. In such conversations, participants listen only to, or long enough, to plan their next defense—they are not trying to understand the other out of genuine curiosity or attempting to develop new understandings. In silent conversations, monologues occur when the same description, opinion, or thought consistently occupies one's thoughts, leaving no room for new ones or curiosity and being closed to other thoughts.

In therapy, monological conversations lead to a *therapeutic impasse*, at which point the therapeutic discussion no longer generates useful meanings or understandings. For most, it is easy to identify monological conversations because tension develops and the conversational task becomes trying to convince the other of a particular point. Therapists may also begin to have pejorative descriptions of clients, such as "resistant." When this happens—whether between therapist and client or between any two people in the room—the therapist's job is to gently shift the conversation back to a dialogical exchange of ideas. Therapists can achieve this by shifting back into a curious stance—asking to better understand the client's perspective or inquiring if there is a particular point that the client thinks the therapist is not fully understanding. However, to re-engage others in dialogue, the therapist must also be in an internal dialogical mode. In the simplest terms, a collaborative therapist's primary job is to ensure that the conversations in the room—whether between members of the client system or between the therapist and the client—do not become dueling monologues. As long as conversations are dialogical, change and transformation are inevitable.

Making Connection: The Therapeutic Relationship

Philosophic Stance

Collaborative therapists conceptualize the therapist's position as a philosophical stance, a particular *way of being in relation with others.* This stance informs how therapists speak, think about, act with, and respond in session, focusing their attention on the *person* of the client and shifting attention away from roles and functions. The philosophical stance essentially encompasses a sincere embodiment of the postmodern, social constructionist ideas that inform the collaborative approach, such as viewing the client as expert and valuing the transformative process of dialogue.

Conversational Partners: "Withness"

The therapeutic relationship in collaborative therapy is best described as a conversational partnership (Anderson, 1997), a process of being *with* the client. In this way of relating, sometimes referred to as "withness" (Hoffman, 2007), the conversational partners "touch" and move one another through their mutual understandings. Withness also involves a willingness to go along for the roller coaster ride (Anderson, 1993)—the ups and downs—of the client's transformational process, regardless of how uncomfortable, unpredictable, or scary it may be. It is a commitment to walk alongside the client, no matter where the journey leads.

Curiosity: The Art of Not Knowing

A hallmark of the collaborative therapeutic stance (Anderson, 1995, 1997), curiosity refers to the therapist's sincere interest in clients' unique life experiences and the meanings that are generated from these experiences. This curiosity is fueled by a *social constructionist epistemology* (assumptions about knowledge and how we know what we know; see Chapter 8), which posits that each person constructs a unique reality from the webs of relationships and conversations in which he/she is engaged. Thus no two people experience marriage, parenting, depression, psychosis, or anxiety the same. For example, in the case study at the end of this chapter, the therapist focuses on understanding 15-year-old Ashley's unique experience of being depressed and cutting, rather than filling in the blanks based on research or what she has learned from other teens with this problem.

Client and Therapist Expertise

In 1992, Anderson and Goolishian radically proposed, "The client is the expert." Although sometimes misunderstood to mean that the therapist has no opinion and no role in the therapeutic process, the concept of "client as expert" means that the therapist's attention is focused on sincerely valuing clients' thoughts, ideas, and opinions. Therapists ultimately have very limited information about the fullness and complexity of clients' lives; they can never acquire the complete history and "insider" perspective that clients themselves have (Anderson, 1997). Thus the concept of "client as expert" is more about respect for the client than a description of how the therapeutic process is conducted.

During the therapy session, however, therapists have a different expertise because they are responsible for ensuring that an effective and respectful dialogical conversation is conducted. They rely on the generative quality of the conversation to support client transformation rather than dictate the content, direction, or outcome of the conversation.

In broad strokes (which are always inaccurate), it may be helpful in the beginning to think of the client as holding more expertise in the area of *content* (what needs to be talked about) and the therapist as holding more expertise in the area of *process* (how things are talked about); however, in this collaborative process, both therapist and client have input on both content and process. If a collaborative therapist believes the client is not addressing an important area of content, the therapist will nonhierarchically raise the issue: "I know you prefer not to talk about the past, but I wonder if it might not be worthwhile to spend a little time exploring how your childhood abuse affects your marriage today." Such a comment is offered in such a way that the client feels truly free to say yes or no, and the therapist honors the client's wishes. For example, although the therapist in the case study at the end of the chapter suspects that Ashley's mother's decision to move in with her lesbian partner is affecting Ashley's reported feelings of depression, and although the therapist may invite Ashley to consider this link, he/she will not force the issue if the client does not think it is a useful line of conversation.

Conversely, the therapist is also open to client feedback about the therapeutic process, allowing clients' input on which processes work best for them, including who is in the room, the pacing, the types of homework or suggestions, the types of questions, and so forth. The therapist does not necessarily take the client's request as a dictate for how to do therapy, but thoughtfully considers the request and the need that underlies it and works to find the best possible ways to address it. This back-and-forth exchange is a sincere partnership in which the therapist works side by side with the client to find useful ways of talking. Anderson (1997) talks about this continual openness to client feedback as "research as part of everyday practice." The therapist uses the feedback to fine-tune the therapy process, lessening the opportunity for therapeutic impasse and ensuring that therapy is tailored to each client's unique needs.

Everyday, Ordinary Language: A Democratic Relationship

Collaborative therapists listen, hear, and speak in a natural, down-to-earth way that is more congruent with the client's language and more democratic than hierarchical (Andersen, 1991; Anderson, 2007). Although they are responsible for facilitating a dialogical process that clients find useful, they do not approach the task from a position of leadership or expertise. Instead, they assume a more humble position, using everyday language, a relaxed style, and a willingness to learn that invites clients to join them in exploring how best to proceed.

Inner and Outer Talk

Tom Andersen conceptualized conversations as involving both inner and outer talk (Andersen, 2007). In a conversation, we most quickly recognize the *outer talk*, the verbally spoken conversation between the therapy participants. Andersen also recognized that there were other dialogues going on, namely, *inner talk*, the thoughts and conversations each person has within while participating in a conversation. Thus, if a therapist is working with one client, at least three conversations are simultaneously occurring: (a) the client's inner dialogue, (b) the therapist's inner dialogue, and (c) the outer spoken dialogue. The therapist needs to allow space and time for each one of these conversations.

As Andersen (2007) pointed out, when clients are speaking, they are speaking not only to the therapist but, more importantly, *to themselves.* Often in therapy, clients are saying something aloud for the first time, and they may need time to reflect on the weight or unexpected content of what they hear themselves saying to the therapist. Andersen strongly admonished therapists to not pressure clients to share their inner dialogue, as is common in more content-based therapies. Thus, if a client does not want to speak about her sexual abuse or a difficult relationship, the therapist does not force the issue but instead leaves an open invitation for the client to speak about it when ready. Unlike most therapists, Andersen was a champion for client privacy and autonomy even in session, a reflection of his abiding faith that clients have the ability to navigate their lives in a way that works best for them.

In addition to tracking the outer dialogue with the client, Andersen encouraged therapists to track their own inner dialogues: their thoughts, feelings, and reactions to the client and the outer dialogue. The therapist's inner dialogue provides many forms of information that can facilitate the therapeutic relationship: the therapist's reaction to the client may provide information about how others are relating to the client, or it may indicate that the therapist is reacting to the client based on personal history or issues rather than professional knowledge. The therapist's inner dialogue might also include insights, ideas, or metaphors that could further the outer dialogue (Anderson, 1997). When the therapist's inner dialogue is distracting from the outer conversation—as in Anderson's notion of silent monologue—the therapist is encouraged to bring up the issue with the client if doing so furthers the dialogue in useful ways (Anderson, 1997). For example, if a client continually minimizes the role of alcohol in his stories of one-night stands and yet in each incident the therapist notices there is a clear link, the therapist can *gently* put forth this observation, while verbally and nonverbally giving permission for the client to maintain his/her opinion without feeling that the relationship is threatened (e.g., "I know from past conversations you don't think there is a link here, but I want to say that I keep seeing a link between your nights out partying and getting into these relationships you later regret. If you do not see alcohol as the main cause, is there a minor role it might be playing?"). The key is to offer the perspective in such a way that invites curiosity rather than defensiveness.

The Viewing: Case Conceptualization and Assessment

Case conceptualization in collaborative therapy involves asking two key questions:

- *Who* is talking about the problem?
- *How* does each understand the problem?

Therapists answer the first by assessing who is in the *problem-organizing system*, or who is in conversation with whom, about what. The second question is approached using the therapist's *philosophical stance* to understand the client's worldview.

Who's Talking? Problem-Organizing, Problem-Dissolving Systems

Anderson and Goolishian (1988, 1992) initially conceptualized therapeutic systems as *linguistic systems* that organize around the identification of a problem: therapists and clients come together because someone has identified a problem, issue, or concern; the word *problem* may not always be explicitly used by the client. They referred to these systems as problem-organizing, problem-dissolving systems. They are "problem-organizing" because they only come into being after someone has identified a problem. They are "problem-dissolving" in that they dissolve when the participants—therapists, clients, and interested third parties—no longer have a problem to discuss. Additionally, *dissolving* refers to the idea that the problem often is not "solved" in the traditional sense of finding a solution. Instead, the participants' understandings evolve through dialogue, allowing for new thoughts, feelings, and actions. In the end, the client may not feel that the problem was solved as much as it dissolved. For example, if a client initially reports feeling stressed because of a recent breakup, the problem is not solved, but rather the client comes to interpret the situation differently and therefore acts and feels differently.

Aware that all persons talking about the problem are part of the problem-organizing, problem-dissolving system, collaborative therapists ask the following questions:

QUESTIONS ABOUT THE PROBLEM

- Who is talking about the problem in session and outside of session?
- How does each define it?
- What does each think should be done about it?

As the understanding of the problem shifts and evolves through dialogue, the therapist continually assesses who is involved in talking about it outside of session and continually inquires about the multiple perspectives about the problem, encouraging all perspectives to be heard without trying to reconcile them or identify the "truth." Clients and therapists are most likely to generate new and more useful perspectives when they allow multiple, contradictory perspectives to constantly linger in the air. Thus, in the case study at the end of the chapter, the therapist seeks to understand not only the identified patient's perspective, the teen, but also the perspectives of her siblings, mother, mother's girlfriend, teachers, school counselor, and friends.

Philosophical Stance: Social Constructionist Viewing

As mentioned, collaborative therapists' primary tool in therapy is not a technique or intervention but a system of viewing, their philosophical stance (Anderson, 1997). Collaborative therapists work from a social constructionist, postmodern perspective, which maintains that our realities are constructed in language and through relationships. Rather than seeing identities and meanings as fixed, social constructionism describes how we engage in a constant process of revising and reinterpreting our personal identities and social realities by the way we tell ourselves what it means to be "a good person," "happy," "successful," "cared for," "living a meaningful life," "respected," and so forth. These stories are shaped by conversations with friends, news stories, fiction pieces, and any exchange of ideas, whether in person or through media. Rather than being bent on showing how clients are "incorrect" or "off," the therapist is curious about clients and focuses on *how clients construct meaning about the events in their lives.*

Assessing the Client's Worldview

This curiosity means that collaborative therapists focus on better understanding clients' worldview, their system for interpreting life events. They do not look for "errors" or even "the source of the problem" but rather approach clients with a gentle, nonjudging curiosity, much like a child exploring a tide pool for the first time, careful not to crush the intriguing creatures in this fascinating new world (Anderson, 1997; Hoffman, 2007). The therapist is looking for the internal logic that makes the client's world, hopes, problems, and symptoms make sense. For example, if a woman is feeling that her marriage is failing, how did she first get this idea? How did she respond? How did she make sense of her partner's changing behaviors and her own? What does she fear it says about her as a person? What does she think happened, and what does she see as the options from here? Why did her marriage work up until now, and what would it take to get it back to where it was or better? Such questions would not be in the therapist's toolbag but rather would be responses that remain congruent with the conversation at any point. Thus "assessment" in collaborative therapy is a continuous "co-assessment" that occurs through conversation. In the case study at the end of this chapter, the therapist asks with sincere not-knowing curiosity about how Ashley experiences and understands her feelings of sadness, how cutting "works" for her, what her mother's relationship means to her, and how she views her siblings.

Targeting Change: Goal Setting

Self-Agency

Like other postmodern approaches, collaborative therapists do not have a predefined model of health toward which they steer all clients in cookie-cutter fashion. Instead, the overall goal is to increase clients' sense of *agency* in their lives: the sense that they are competent and able to take meaningful action. Anderson (1997) believes that agency is inherent in everyone and can only be *self-accessed*, not given by someone else, as is implied in the concept of client "empowerment"; instead collaborative therapists see their role as participating in a process that maximizes the opportunities for agency to emerge in clients.

Transformation

Rather than conceptualizing the output of therapy as change, collaborative therapists conceptualize the process as transformation, emphasizing that some "original" aspects remain while other aspects are added or diminished. In therapy, clients' narrative of self-identity, who they tell themselves they are, is transformed through the dialogical process, opening new possibilities for meaning, relating to others, and future action. This transformational process is not controlled or directed by the therapist but emerges from within clients as they listen to themselves, the therapist, and others share their ideas, thoughts, and hopes.

The process of transformation through dialogue is inherently and inescapably *mutual*. When therapists participate in dialogical conversations, they risk being changed themselves because the same dialogical process that allows clients to change creates a context in which therapists are also transformed (Anderson, 1997). Although this transformation may not be as dramatic or immediately evident as the client's transformation, the worldview of therapists inevitably evolves and shifts as they learn from their clients about other ways to make sense of and engage life.

Setting Collaborative Goals

As the name implies, therapeutic goals are constructed collaboratively with clients using their everyday language rather than professional terms. In collaborative therapy, goals continually evolve as meanings and understandings change. The evolution of goals may be gradual—from arguing less to having more positive conversations—or dramatic—from focusing on school performance to focusing on emotionally connecting with one's parent. Therapists do not have a set of predefined goals they use with all clients. Instead, goals are negotiated with each client individually.

Examples of Middle-Phase Goals That Address Presenting Problems

- Reduce arguments between couple by increasing the number of conversations where they "get" each other
- Increase periods of "harmony" between the children
- Increase the times when the child can do his homework without being monitored
- Expand social network by reconnecting with old friends and family

Examples of Late-Phase Goals That Target Agency and Identity Narratives

- Increase sense of agency and assertiveness when relating to colleagues at work
- Increase the mother's sense of agency and ability to prioritize where her time and energy go
- Develop a family identity narrative that retains a strong sense of connection while allowing for individuality and differences of opinion
- Develop a sense of identity that honors the difficulties of the past without living in the shadow of the past

The Doing: Interventions and Ways of Promoting Change

Conversational Questions: Understanding from Within the Dialogue

Conversational questions are questions that come naturally from within the dialogue rather than from professional theory (Anderson, 1997). They are not canned or preplanned but instead follow logically from what the client is saying and are generated from the therapist's curiosity and desire to understand more. For example, if a client describes her frustration with her husband's lack of help around the house, the therapist asks questions that logically flow from the conversation in the moment, such as "What chores would you like help with? Has it always been this way?" rather than therapeutic or theoretically informed questions such as the miracle question in solution-based therapy (Chapter 14), externalizing questions in narrative therapy (see following text), or systemic interaction questions in a systems approach (Chapter 9).

Using the client's preferred words and expressions, therapists ask conversational questions, which help both the therapist and the client to better understand the client's situation. In research on the therapy process, clients reported that questions asked out of genuine curiosity are received quite differently than "conditional" or "loaded" questions, which are driven by a professional agenda to assess or intervene (Anderson, 1997). When the therapist in the case study at the end of this chapter asks the client to describe how and why she cuts, the therapist is genuinely curious about the meaning and reasoning Ashley attributes to her actions.

Making "Appropriately Unusual" Comments

One of the most elegant and practically useful therapeutic concepts, *appropriately unusual comments* enable therapists to offer clients reflections that make a difference. On the basis of his work with reflecting teams, Tom Andersen (1991, 1995) recommends that therapists avoid comments and questions that are "too usual" or "too unusual." Comments that are *too usual* essentially reflect the client's worldview, offering no possibility for generating new understanding or change: agreeing to or reflecting back the client's current perspective is not likely to promote change. Alternatively, comments that are *too unusual* are too different to be useful in developing new meanings. Some clients give immediate signals that a comment is too unusual by becoming "resistant," re-explaining themselves, or rejecting the comment or suggestion. Other clients give little indication in session that the comment is too unusual but afterward do not follow up on the comment and may even lose faith in the therapist and the therapy process.

Appropriately unusual comments are comments that clearly fit within the client's worldview while inviting curiosity and perhaps offering a new perspective that is easily digestible. For example, if a client comes in feeling overwhelmed with a new job that is more multifaceted than the previous job, an appropriately unusual response from the therapist might be: "It sounds like your new job may require skills in multitasking and prioritizing that weren't necessary in your old job," which speaks to the client's current experience while offering a slightly different viewpoint.

Such comments capture the client's attention because they are familiar enough to be safe and viable yet different enough to offer a fresh perspective (Anderson, 1997).

Listening for the Pause

When clients hear an appropriately unusual comment, suggestion, or question, they almost always have to pause and take time to integrate the new perspective with their current perspective: in these moments it is most important for the therapist to allow the client time for inner dialogue. Sometimes a client says, "I have to think about that" or "I never thought of it that way." A client's initial response may be "I don't know," but after taking a few moments to reflect on the new idea, the client usually begins to generate a response that reflects thoughts and ideas the client never had before.

How Far to Go?

How unusual is appropriately unusual? The trick here is that each client needs a different level of unusualness; alternatively stated, each client finds a different level of difference useful for generating new ideas. I often find that when I am first working with a teen, mandated client, or someone unsure of therapy, appropriately unusual comments cannot include significant differences from their current worldview until they have developed greater trust in me. Additionally, the more emotionally distraught clients are, the less useful they find highly unusual comments. Other clients require and prefer that the therapist deliver comments that are quite different from their own, often in a very direct manner that verges on being socially impolite. I have had clients, particularly men, say to me, "Just tell me where you think I got it wrong" or "Just tell it to me straight—don't sugarcoat it—I hate when therapists do that." Thus, "appropriately unusual" depends on the client's preferred style of communication and the quality of the therapeutic relationship. Collaborative therapists fine-tune their communication skills to deliver a range of appropriately unusual comments and carefully observe client responses to assess whether or not the comments are useful.

Mutual Puzzling Questions and Process: "Kicking Around" New Meanings

As already mentioned, the process by which collaborative therapists invite their clients to join them in becoming curious about clients' lives is referred to as "mutual puzzling" (Anderson, 1997). Anderson suggests that the therapist's curiosity becomes contagious, and clients are naturally invited into it. What begins, therefore, as the therapist's one-way inquiry shifts to a joint one. When clients join the therapist in the meaning-making process, their rate of talking may slow down, there may be more pauses in the conversation, and there is an inquisitive yet hopeful air to the conversation. Often the shift in clients is visible: their body posture softens, the head may tilt to the side, and they move more slowly or more quickly (Andersen, 2007). Mutual puzzling can occur only when therapists are successful in creating a two-way dialogical conversation in which both parties are able to sincerely take in and reflect on each other's contributions.

For example, if a client lives in daily fear of having another psychotic episode after not having one for over 10 years and says that it is her illness that keeps her from moving forward in life, the mutual puzzling process may be sparked by a question such as: "That's interesting. You say you haven't had an episode in 10 years, so hallucinations don't seem to be plaguing you these days. But it does sound like the *worry about* hallucinations is the problem at this point. Do you think of this as part of the original problem or is it a new problem that only developed after the first was resolved?" In this case, a new distinction is highlighted and the client is invited to "kick it around" and see what, if any, new ideas emerge and to follow where they lead. The therapist does not politely insist that worrying is the new problem but rather listens for how the client made sense of the comment and continues to follow the client's thinking, kicking around the next idea that evolves from the conversation. The therapist is always most curious about how the client is making sense of what is being discussed.

Being Public: Sharing One's Inner Dialogue

In "being public," therapists share their inner dialogue for two potential reasons: (a) to respect clients by honestly sharing their thoughts about significant issues affecting treatment, and (b) to prevent monological conversation by offering their private thoughts to the dialogue (Anderson, 1997, 2005). When therapists make their perspectives publicly known, they do so tentatively and, even when discussing professional knowledge, are careful not to overshadow the client's perspective (Anderson, 2007). When therapists are open with their silent thoughts, this helps prevent them from slipping into a monological view of the client and creates a situation where something different may be created for the therapist as well.

Being public generally occurs in two situations: (a) in communications about professional information with clients or outside agencies or professionals (e.g., courts, psychiatrists, etc.), and (b) when the therapist has significant differences from the client in values, goals, and purposes.

Being Public with Professional Communication

Whenever collaborative therapists handle professional matters, such as when making a diagnosis, speaking with a social worker, or filing a report with the court, they "make public" their thoughts, rationales, and intentions by discussing them *directly with clients*. Openly discussing what the therapist will reveal in an upcoming conversation with another professional and/or recapping what happened in the last conversation goes against traditional procedures, in which communications between professionals were kept confidential from the client, ostensibly because it could do "harm" to the client to know what professionals were actually thinking. The apparent "harm," however, was usually that clients would be angry.

In dramatic contrast, collaborative therapists have been pioneers in lifting the veil on dialogues between professionals, engaging in honest, direct conversation with clients about the contents of these conversations. Such conversations are not always easy, such as when a therapist has to tell a client that she cannot recommend unification through child protective services until x, y, and z happen (typically spelled out by the social worker or court). In the past, the parent learned this in court or from a social worker; in collaborative therapy, the therapist has an upfront conversation from the beginning, clearly laying out the types of behaviors that need to be seen for the desired recommendations, and then wholeheartedly and enthusiastically working with clients to reach this goal.

Most clients greatly respect the therapist's honesty and integrity and respond with increased motivation to make needed changes. They fully understand when they are not given the report they hoped for because the therapist and client have been discussing progress—or lack thereof—consistently along the way. When working with court-mandated clients, collaborative therapists St. George and Wulff (1998) have clients help write the first drafts of letters to the courts about their progress, including clinical recommendations, and then use the letters to discuss their progress and goals.

Similarly, when working with a teen such as the one in the case study at the end of this chapter, the therapist may "make public" her concern about the teen's safety and the potential for her to injure herself more than intended, especially if the client is not highly motivated to stop cutting. When the client is invited into a discussion to address the therapist's concern about the client's safety—without having rigid requirements for the client—the client and therapist can work together to develop a plan that is meaningful to the client while also addressing the therapist's safety concerns.

Being Public with Significant Differences in Values and Goals

The other situation in which collaborative therapists make public their voice is when there are significant differences in values or goals that make it hard for the therapist to move forward as an active participant in the conversation. For example, I recently had a teenager who discussed his plans to meet someone who had challenged him to a fight at a park and who had said, "Don't bring weapons or friends." The teen believed that if he didn't show up, more guys at school would gang up on him and that could lead to more events such as this. Although I saw his point, I also saw that he was at risk for seriously being hurt, a concern I decided to make "public." I invited him to explore my concerns: the guy might come with friends or weapons, there might be legal ramifications, and so forth. I offered my list of dangers from a place of serious concern without demanding a particular course of action on his part. Instead, I asked him how he would manage the dangers I saw; by the end of the conversation we arrived at a place where my concerns and his fears were addressed and we both felt good about his chosen course of action, namely, to avoid the park that day and to try to find out about this person's social network.

Accessing Multiple Voices in Writing

Peggy Penn and her associates (Penn, 2001; Penn & Frankfurt, 1994; Penn & Sheinberg, 1991) access multiple, alternative voices using various forms of writing (e.g., letters, poems, journals) to generate alternative perspectives and make room for silenced inner voices or the voices of significant persons not currently in the therapeutic dialogue. Penn and Frankfurt (1994) have found that "writing slows down our perceptions and reactions, making room for their thickening, their gradual layering" (p. 229). They have also found that the performative aspect, the reading aloud of letters to witnesses (the therapist, family, and others), makes things happen. Penn's writing has a different intent than writing in experiential therapies, which is meant to express repressed emotions, bring resolution to a past situation, or achieve a similar clinical aim. Instead, Penn's writing invites different voices into the conversation to generate alternative possibilities for understanding. Furthermore, writing promotes agency: "to write *gives us agency: we are not acted on by a situation, we are acting!*" (Penn, 2001, p. 49; emphasis in original). Clients may be asked to write the following:

- Letters to themselves from aspects of themselves and/or from newly emerging, future, or past selves
- Letters to themselves from significant others from the present, past, or future
- Letters to and from significant others (alive or dead) speaking from a voice or perspective that was formerly kept private
- Letters or journal entries to speak from parts of the self that are typically not expressed and/or are emerging in therapy
- Letters to the world or general audience
- Multivoiced biographies that describe one's life from various perspectives
- Poems that express inner voices and perspectives that are not readily articulated in other ways

Reflecting Teams and the Reflecting Process

Tom Andersen trained at the Milan Institute, where a small team of therapists would observe the therapist talking with families behind a one-way mirror, the preferred method for interviewing in early family therapy. Influenced by postmodern thinking as well as a gut feeling of discomfort because of the distance (Andersen, 1995), Andersen and his colleagues wanted to make the process more democratic and developed the idea of having the families listen to the team's conversation behind the mirror: thus, the reflecting team practice began. With the earliest reflecting teams, the family and team would literally switch rooms if sound could only be heard in one room, or they would turn off the lights in the family's room and turn on the lights in the team's room, reversing the one-way mirror. In later years, the team was invited to sit in the *same room but separate from* the family and therapist having a conversation. Over the years, the practice has developed into more of a general *process* of reflecting that is used for talking with clients, with or without a team.

The idea behind a collaborative reflecting team is to develop diverse strands of conversation so that the client can choose that which resonates and that which does not. This is in contrast to the private team conversations, which are synthesized by the team and in which the team chooses what is important for the client to hear. Collaborative reflecting teams avoid coming to agreement on any one description of what is going on with the client, allowing for *multiple, contradictory perspectives* to linger and promoting the development of new meanings and perspectives. Teams avoid comments that evaluate or judge the client in any way, positively or negatively. Instead, they focus on offering what is called *reflections*, observations, questions, or comments that are clearly owned by the person making them (e.g., "As I listened, I was wondering...").

General Guidelines for Reflecting Teams

Andersen (1991, 1995) provides the following guidelines for teams:

- **Only Use with the Client's Permission:** The therapist should obtain the client's permission to use a team *before* the session starts. When the therapist has a strong rapport with the client and confidently explains how the reflecting process works, most clients enthusiastically agree.

- **Give the Client Permission to Listen or Not to Listen:** Andersen gives the clients *explicit* permission to listen or not listen. I find it helpful to tell clients that they will probably hear some comments that resonate deeply and others that fit less well with their experience, and I recommend they focus on the comments that "strike a chord."

- **Comment on What Is Seen or Heard, Not What Is Observed:** Team members should comment on a specific event or statement in the conversation and then "wonder" or be "curious" about it. The wondering or curiosity statement should be *appropriately unusual* to help generate new perspectives.

- **Talk from a Questioning, Speculative, and Tentative Perspective:** Team members avoid offering opinions or interpretations and instead use "wondering" questions ("I am wondering if...") or offer a tentative perspective ("I am aware I don't know enough to know the whole story, but it seems like there might be..."). If a team member offers a strong opinion, another team member may ask, "What did you see or hear in the conversation that made you think that?" to open the conversation up and invite multiple perspectives.

- **Comment on All That You Hear but Not All That You See:** If the family members try to cover something up, allow them the *right to not talk about* all that they think and feel. Andersen warned: "Don't confuse therapy with confession." Unlike in psychodynamic and humanistic traditions, Andersen explicitly stated that if a client wants to hide an emotion or not say something, the client should be free to do so. He was a rare advocate for client privacy in therapy, believing that clients will share when they are ready. If a therapist notices a client getting agitated or holding back tears, he does not comment on it, allowing the client to speak about these emotions when he or she is ready to do so.

- **Separate the Team and the Family:** The team and family can be in the same room but should not talk to each other. Andersen believed that an important psychological space is created by the physical space between the team and client and by the two not talking directly; later research studies supported his view

(Sells, Smith, Coe, & Yoshioka, 1994). This space invites all participants to focus on their inner dialogue, stimulating new thoughts and ideas more readily.

- **Listen for What Is Appropriately Unusual:** *Avoid what is too usual or too unusual.* To identify useful reflections, Andersen asked himself: "Is what is going on now appropriately unusual or is it too unusual?" (Andersen, 1995, p. 21).

- **Ask: "How Would You Like to Use This Session Today?"** This question, although likely to be asked at the beginning of any session, is critical when a team is involved. If the client is nervous about using a reflecting team, the therapist can also add, "Are there particular topics you want to avoid with the team here?"

Related Reflecting Processes

Over time, the concept of the reflecting team has developed into a number of reflecting processes:

- **Multiple Reflectors:** A team of two to four therapists observe the therapist-client conversation, sitting either in a different room using a one-way mirror (or camera) or in a separate space in the same room.

- **Single Reflector:** If only one colleague is available, the therapist may turn and have a reflecting conversation with this one reflector while the client listens.

- **No Outside Reflector When Working with a Family:** When there is no outside colleague available, the therapist may choose to speak with a single family member while other family members listen.

- **No Outside Reflector When Working with an Individual:** When the therapist is working with an individual client, a reflective process can be created by talking about issues from the perspective of someone who is not present (e.g., a parent, friend, spouse, or famous person of personal significance).

- **With Young Children:** When working with children, reflections can include play media. A single therapist working with an individual child can create reflecting teams using puppets or other such media (Gehart, 2007a).

"As If" Reflecting

Developed by Anderson (1997), the "as-if" reflecting process involves having the team members or other witnesses to the conversation speak or reflect "as if" they are some of the people in the problem-organized system (i.e., the people talking about the problem), which includes the client, family members, friends, bosses, teachers, school personnel, medical professionals, probation officers, and so forth. This process can be used with clients or with supervisees staffing a case.

Clinical Spotlight: Open Dialogue, an Evidence-Based Approach to Psychosis

Using the collaborative approach described by Anderson, Goolishian, and Andersen, Jaakko Seikkula (2002) and his colleagues (Haarakangas et al., 2007) in Finland developed the open dialogue approach in their work with psychosis and other severe disorders. They report impressive outcomes in their 20 years of research, including 83% of first-episode psychosis patients returning to work and 77% with no remaining psychotic symptoms after two years of treatment. In comparison with standard treatment, the patients in the open dialogue treatment had more family meetings, fewer days of inpatient care, reduced use of medication, and a greater reduction in psychotic symptoms.

This approach uses collaborative dialogue and reflecting practices, as well as the following:

- **Immediate Intervention:** Within 24 hours of the initial call, the person who has had a psychotic break, the significant people in his/her life, and a treatment team of several professionals (e.g., for psychosis the team often includes a psychiatrist, psychotherapist, and nurse) meet to discuss the situation using collaborative dialogue.

- **Social Network and Support Systems:** Significant persons in the client's life and other support systems are invited to participate in all phases of the process.

- **Flexibility and Mobility:** Treatment is uniquely adapted to clients and their situations, with the treatment team sometimes meeting in their homes and sometimes in a treatment setting, depending on what is most useful.

- **Teamwork and Responsibility:** The treatment team is built on the basis of client needs; all team members are responsible for the quality of the process.

- **Psychological Continuity:** The team members remain consistent throughout treatment regardless of the stage of treatment.

- **Tolerance of Uncertainty:** Rather than employ set protocols, the team allows time to see how each situation will evolve and what treatment will be needed.

- **Dialogue:** The focus of each meeting is to establish an open dialogue that facilitates new meanings and possibilities. This process requires establishing a sense of safety for all participants to say what needs to be said.

Outside the Therapy Room

Because collaborative therapy is more a way of talking and being in the world, the collaborative conversational process has been applied to numerous other contexts, including education, research, and business consultation.

Education and Pedagogy

Collaborative practices have been used as a way to conceptualize educational pedagogy in K-12 and college settings (Anderson, 1997; Gehart, 2007b; London & Rodriguez-Jazcilevich, 2007; McNamee, 2007). Using social constructionist epistemology, educators use relational, collaborative practices to engage student curiosity and agency in the learning process, which is seen as a *community learning process* rather than an individual process. Students are invited to participate in designing the learning experiences, engage with multiple perspectives, and contribute to the learning of all class members.

Research

The same collaborative process used in therapy settings is used in research contexts to access client voices (Gehart, Tarragona, & Bava, 2007). Typically used in qualitative, interview studies, this form of research inquiry views data as co-constructed with participants, meaning that the participants play an active role not only in identifying what is important for the researchers to know about their experience but also in providing feedback on the final presentation of the results to ensure that they fairly represent the participants' intentions and meanings. Like the therapist, the researcher approaches clients from a not-knowing stance of curiosity, wanting to learn more about the participants' experiences rather than testing a preconceived hypothesis.

Business Consultation

Collaborative conversational and reflecting practices have also been used for consulting with businesses and other large systems (Anderson, 1997; Deissler, 2007).

The consultant approaches the system from a curious position, taking time to learn from those within it what they view as working and not working, what they value most, and what they would like to see happen. Much as in the therapy process, the consultant facilitates two-way dialogues in which members are able to hear and say things they were not able to before. Various reflecting processes are used to create forums for new dialogue and understanding.

Narrative Therapy
In a Nutshell: The Least You Need to Know

Developed by Michael White and David Epston in Australia and New Zealand, narrative therapy is based on the premise that we "story" and create the meaning of life events using available *dominant discourses*—broad societal stories, sociocultural practices, assumptions, and expectations about how we should live. People experience "problems" when their personal life does not fit with these dominant societal discourses and expectations. The process of narrative therapy involves *separating the person from the problem*, critically examining the assumptions that inform how the person evaluates himself/herself and his/her life. Through this process, clients identify alternative ways to view, act, and interact in daily life. Narrative therapists assume that all people are resourceful and have strengths, and they do not see "people" as having problems but rather see problems as being imposed upon people by unhelpful or harmful societal cultural practices.

The Juice: Significant Contributions to the Field

If you remember one thing from this chapter, it should be this:

Understanding Oppression: Dominant Versus Local Discourses

Narrative therapy is one of the few psychotherapeutic theories that integrates societal and cultural issues into its core conceptualization of how problems are formed and resolved. Narrative therapists maintain that problems do not exist separately from their sociocultural contexts, which are broadly constituted in what philosopher Michel Foucault called *dominant discourses* (Foucault, 1972, 1980; White, 1995; White & Epston, 1990). Dominant discourses are culturally generated stories about how life should go that are used to coordinate social behavior, such as how married people should act, what happiness looks like, and how to be successful. These dominant discourses organize social groups at all levels: large cultural groups down to individual couples and families. They are described as dominant because they are so foundational to how we behave and evaluate our lives that we are rarely conscious of their impact or origins.

Foucault contrasts dominant discourses with *local discourses*, which occur in our heads, our closer relationships, and marginalized (not mainstream) communities. Local discourses have different "goods" and "shoulds" than dominant discourses. A classic example is that women value relationships whereas men value outcome in typical work environments. Both discourses have a value they are working toward; however, men's discourse is generally privileged over women's and thus is considered a dominant discourse, with women's discourse being local. Narrative therapists closely attend to the fluid interactions of local and dominant discourses and how these different stories of what is "good" and valued collide in our web of social relationships, creating problems and difficulties. By attending to this level of social interaction, narrative therapists help clients become aware of how these different discourses are impacting their lives; this awareness increases clients' sense of agency in their struggles, allowing them to find ways to more successfully resolve their issues.

Rumor Has It: The People and Their Stories

Michael White

A pioneer in narrative therapy and the first to write about the process of *externalizing* problems, Michael White was based at the Dulwich Centre in Adelaide, Australia, which provides training and publishes books and newsletters on narrative therapy. Along with David Epston, he wrote the first book on narrative therapy, *Narrative Means to Therapeutic Ends* (White & Epston, 1990). His last publication, *Maps of Narrative Practice* (White, 2007), describes his later work before his death in 2008.

David Epston

From Auckland, New Zealand, David Epston worked closely with Michael White in developing the foundational framework for narrative therapy. His work emphasized creating unique sources of support for clients, such as writing letters to clients to solidify the emerging narratives and developing communities of concern or *leagues* (see discussion of leagues under Interventions) in which clients provide support to each other.

Jill Freedman and Gene Combs

Based in the United States, husband-and-wife team Jill Freedman and Gene Combs (1996) developed the narrative approach emphasizing social construction of realities and further developed the narrative metaphor for conceptualizing therapeutic intervention. They are the co-directors of the Evanston Family Therapy Center in Illinois.

Gerald Monk and John Winslade

After beginning their work in New Zealand, Gerald Monk and John Winslade now work in the United States and have developed narrative approaches for schools in counseling, multicultural counseling, mediation, and consultation (Monk, Winslade, Crocket, & Epston, 1997; Monk, Winslade, & Sinclair, 2008; Winslade & Monk, 2000, 2007, 2008).

The Big Picture: Overview of Treatment

Treatment Phases

The process of narrative therapy involves helping clients find new ways to view, interact with, and respond to problems in their lives by redefining the role of those problems (White, 2007). From a narrative perspective, persons are not the problem; problems are the problem. Although there is variety among practitioners, narrative therapy broadly involves the following phases (Freedman & Combs, 1996; White & Epston, 1990):

- **Meeting the Person:** Getting to know people as *separate* from their problems by learning about the hobbies, values, and everyday aspects of their lives

- **Listening:** Listening for the effects of dominant discourses and identifying times without the problems

- **Separating Persons from Problems:** Externalizing and separating people from their problems to create space for new identities and for life stories to emerge

- **Enacting Preferred Narratives:** Identifying new ways to relate to problems that reduce their negative effects on the lives of all involved

- **Solidifying:** Strengthening preferred stories and identities by having them witnessed by significant others in a person's life

Use of Thickening Descriptions

The narrative therapy process is a thickening and enriching of the person's identity and life accounts rather than a "story-ectomy." Instead of replacing a problem story with a problem-free one, narrative therapists *add* new strands of identity to the problem-saturated descriptions with which clients enter therapy. In any given day, an infinite number of events can be storied into our accounts of the day and who we are. When people begin to experience problems, they tend to notice only those events that fit with the problem narrative. For example, if they are feeling hopeless, they tend to notice when things do not go their way during the day and do not give much weight to the good things that happened. Similarly, when couples start a period of fighting, they start to notice only what the other person is doing that confirms their position in the fight and ignore and/or forget other events. In narrative therapy, the therapist helps clients create more balanced, rich, and appreciative descriptions of events that will enable them to build more successful and enjoyable lives.

Making Connection: The Therapeutic Relationship

Meeting the Person Apart from the Problem

Narrative therapists generally begin their first session with clients by meeting clients "apart from the problem," that is, as everyday people (Freedman & Combs, 1996). Therapists ask questions such as the following to familiarize themselves with clients' everyday lives:

> ### QUESTIONS FOR MEETING THE PERSON (NOT THE PROBLEM)
>
> - What do you do for fun? Do you have hobbies?
> - What do you like about living here? What don't you like?
> - Tell me about your friends and family.
> - What is important to you in life?
> - What is a typical weekday like? Weekend?

The answers to these questions enable narrative therapists to know and view their clients in much the same way that clients view themselves, as everyday people.

Separating People from Problems: The Problem Is the Problem

In narrative therapy, the motto is: "The problem is the problem. The person is not the problem" (Winslade & Monk, 1999, p. 2). Once therapists have come to know the client apart from the problem and have a clear sense of who the client is as a person, they begin to "meet" the problem in much the same way, keeping their identities separate. The problem—whether depression, anxiety, marital conflict, ADHD, defiance, loneliness, or a breakup—is viewed as a separate entity or situation that is *not* inherent to the person of the client. Therapists maintain a polite, social, "getting to know you" attitude.

> ### QUESTIONS FOR "MEETING" THE PROBLEM
>
> - When did the problem first enter your life?
> - What was going on with you then?
> - What were your first impressions of the problem? How have they changed?
> - How has your relationship with the problem evolved over time?
> - Who else has been affected by the problem?

Narrative therapists can take an adversarial stance toward the problem (wanting to outwit, outsmart, or evict it; White, 2007) or a more compassionate stance (wanting to understand its message and concerns; Gehart & McCollum, 2007).

Optimism and Hope

Because narrative therapists view problems as problems and people as people, they have a deep, abiding optimism and hope for their clients (Monk et al., 1997; Winslade & Monk, 1999). Their hope and optimism are not sugar-coated, naïve wishes but instead are derived from their understanding of how problems are formed—through language, relationship, and social discourse—having confidence that their approach can make a difference. Furthermore, by separating people from problems, they quickly connect with the "best" in the client, which reinforces a sense of hope and optimism.

Therapist as Co-Author and Co-Editor

The role of the therapist is often described as a *co-author* or *co-editor* to emphasize that the therapist and client engage in a joint process of constructing meaning (Freedman & Combs, 1996; Monk et al., 1997; White, 1995; White & Epston, 1990). Rather than attempting to offer a "better story," the therapist works alongside the client to generate a more useful narrative. Although the degree and quality of input vary greatly, narrative therapists tend to focus on the sociopolitical aspects of a client's life. Some narrative therapists maintain that therapists should take a stance on broader sociocultural issues of injustice with all clients (Zimmerman & Dickerson, 1996), but not all narrative therapists share this agenda (Monk & Gehart, 2003).

Therapist as Investigative Reporter

In his later works, White (2007) describes his relationship to problems as that of an *investigative reporter:*

> The form of inquiry that is employed during externalizing conversations can be likened to investigative reporting. The primary goal of investigative reporting is to develop an exposé on the corruption associated with abuse of power and privilege. Although investigative reporters are not politically neutral, the activities of their inquiry do not take them into the domains of problem-solving, of enacting reform, or of engaging indirect power struggles ... their actions usually reflect a relatively "cool" engagement. (pp. 27–28)

Thus, rather than rushing in to fix problems, the therapist uses a calm but inquisitive stance to explore the origins of problems and thus to inspire clients to develop a better understanding of their larger contexts.

The Viewing: Case Conceptualization and Assessment
Problem-Saturated Stories

As clients are talking, narrative therapists listen for the problem-saturated story (Freedman & Combs, 1996; White & Epston, 1990), the story in which the "problem" plays the leading role and the client plays a secondary role, generally that of victim. The therapist attends to how the problem affects the client at an *individual level* (health, emotions, thoughts, beliefs, identity, relationship with the divine) and at a *relational level* (with significant other, parents, friends, coworkers, teachers), as well as how it affects each of these significant others at a personal level. While listening to a client's problem-saturated story, the therapist listens closely for alternative endings and subplots in which the problem is less of a problem and the person is an effective agent; these are referred to as *unique outcomes.*

Unique Outcomes and Sparkling Events

Unique outcomes (White & Epston, 1990) or *sparkling events* (Freedman & Combs, 1996) are stories or subplots in which the problem-saturated story does not play out in its typical way: the child cheerfully complies with a parent's request; a couple are able to stop a potential argument from erupting with a soft touch; a teenager decides to call a friend rather than allow herself to cut. These stories often go unnoticed because they have no dramatic ending or particularly notable outcome that warrants attention, and therefore they are not "storied" in clients' or others' minds. These unique outcomes are used to help clients create the lives they prefer and to develop a more full and accurate account of their own and others' identities.

Dominant Cultural and Gender Discourses (see also Juice)

As already discussed, narrative therapists listen for dominant cultural and gender themes that have informed the development and perception of a problem (Monk et al., 1997; White & Epston, 1990). The purpose of all discourses is to identify the set of "goods" and "values" that organize social interaction in a particular culture. All cultures are essentially a set of dominant discourses: social rules and values that make it possible for a group of people to meaningfully interact (see Chapter 8).

Dominant discourses are the societal stories of how life "should" happen; for example, to be a happy and good person, you should get married, get a stable, high-paying job, have kids, get a nice car, buy a house, and volunteer at your child's school. Whether you comply with this vision of happiness, rebel against it, or are not even in the game because of social or physical limitations, problems can arise in relation to it. In working with clients, narrative therapists listen closely for the dominant discourses that are most directly informing the perception of a problem. In response, they inquire about *local* or *alternative discourses.*

Local and Alternative Discourses: Attending to Client Language and Meaning

Local and alternative discourses are those that do not conform to the dominant discourse (White & Epston, 1990): couples who choose not to have children, same-sex relationships, immigrant families wanting to preserve their roots, speaking English as a second language, teen subculture in any society, and so forth. The local discourses offer a different set of "goods," "shoulds," and ethical "values" than what is portrayed in the dominant discourse. For example, teens have created a subculture with different beauty standards, sexual norms, vocabulary, and friendship rules than are found in adult culture. The teen culture represents an alternative discourse that therapists can tap into to understand the teen's worldview and values, as well as to explore with the teen how this alternative discourse can successfully coexist with the dominant discourse. Thus the local discourse provides a resource for generating new ways of viewing the self and for talking and interacting with others around the problem.

Targeting Change: Goal Setting

Preferred Realities and Identities

As a postmodern approach, narrative therapy does not include a set of predefined goals that can be used with all clients. Instead, goal setting in narrative therapy is unique to each client. In the broadest sense, the goal of narrative therapy is to help clients *enact their preferred realities and identities* (Freedman & Combs, 1996). In most cases, enacting preferred narratives involves increasing clients' sense of *agency*, the sense that they influence the direction of their lives. When identifying preferred realities, therapists work with clients to develop thoughtfully reflected goals that consider local knowledges rather than simply adopting the values of the dominant culture.

Clients often redefine their preferred reality to incorporate these local knowledges and to lessen the influence of dominant discourses. For example, a couple may come in wanting things to go back to the way they were while dating, but as they move through the therapeutic process, they realize that they want and need something different than what they had before because they are entering a new chapter in their lives as individuals and as a couple.

Thus the key is defining the "preferred" reality and identity thoughtfully and with intention after considering the impact of dominant and local discourses as well as the meanings and impact of the proposed preferred reality. This process is often a gradual shift from "make this problem go away" to "I want to create something beautiful/meaningful/great with my/our life(ves)." The therapist allows the client to take the lead in defining the preferred realities and acts as a co-editor to help the client reflect on where the idea came from and the effects it will have on the client's life.

Middle-Phase Goals

Middle-phase goals target immediate symptoms and the presenting problem; the following are some examples:

- "Increase sense of agency in problem-resolution conversations with spouse"
- "Increase opportunities to interact with friends using 'confident, social' self"
- "Reduce number of times mother and father allow Anger to take over in response to child's defiance"
- "Increase instances of defiance in response to anorexia's directions to not eat"

Late-Phase Goals

Late-phase goals target personal identity, relational identity, and the expanded community:

- **Personal Identity:** "Solidify a sense of personal identity that derives self-worth from meaningful activities, relationship, and values rather than body size"

- **Relational Identity:** "Develop a family identity narrative that allows for greater expression of differences while maintaining family's sense of closeness and loyalty"

- **Expanded Community:** "Expand preferred 'outgoing' identity to social relationships and contexts"

The Doing: Interventions

Externalizing: Separating the Problem from the Person

The signature technique of narrative therapy, externalizing involves conceptually and linguistically separating the person from the problem (Freedman & Combs, 1996; White & Epston, 1990). To be successful, externalization requires a sincere belief that people are separate from their problems; thus the *attitude* of externalization is key to its effectiveness (Freedman & Combs, 1996). More than a single-session intervention, externalization is an organic and evolving process of shifting clients' perception of their relationship to the problem: from "having" it to seeing it as outside the self. Therapists can externalize by naming the problem as an external other or by changing a descriptive adjective into a noun (e.g., from a client being depressed to having a relationship with Depression, or changing from being a conflictual couple to having a relationship with Conflict). At other times, clients respond better by talking about "sides" of themselves or a relationship: "the little girl in me who is afraid" or "the competitive side of our relationship."

For externalization to work, it cannot be forced onto the client but rather needs to emerge from the dialogue or be introduced as a possibility for how to think about the situation. In most cases, techniques such as mapping the influence of persons and problem (see next section) invite a natural, comfortable process for externalizing the problem. Alternatively, therapists can ask clients if they want to refer to the problem as something separate from themselves when the conversation allows. If clients already have a name for the problem and conceptualize the problem as a sort of external entity or very discrete part of themselves, therapists need only build on the externalization process they have started.

Relative Influence Questioning: Mapping Influence of the Problem and Persons

Relative influence questioning was the first detailed method for externalization (White & Epston, 1990). Used early in therapy, it serves simultaneously as an assessment and an intervention and is composed of two parts: (a) mapping the influence of the problem and (b) mapping the influence of persons.

Mapping the Influence of the Problem

When mapping the influence of the problem, therapists inquire about how the problem has affected the lives of the client and significant others, often *expanding* the reach of the problem beyond how the client generally thinks of it; thus it is critical that this is followed up by *mapping the influence of person* questions to ensure that the client does not feel worse afterwards.

QUESTIONS FOR MAPPING THE INFLUENCE OF THE PROBLEM

How has the problem affected:

- Clients at a physical, emotional, and psychological level?
- Clients' identity stories and what they tell themselves about their worth and who they are?
- Clients' closest relationships: partner, children, parents?
- Other relationships in clients' lives: friendships, social groups, work or school colleagues, etc.?
- The health, identity, emotions, and other relationships of significant people in clients' lives (e.g., how parents may pull away from friends because they are embarrassed about a child's problem)?

Mapping the Influence of Persons

Mapping the influence of persons begins the externalization process more explicitly. This phase of questioning, which should immediately follow mapping the influence of problems, involves identifying how the person has affected the life of the problem, reversing the logic of the first series of questions.

QUESTIONS FOR MAPPING THE INFLUENCE OF PERSONS

When have the persons involved:

- Kept the Problem from affecting their mood or how they value themselves as people?
- Kept the Problem from allowing themselves to enjoy special and/or casual relationships in their lives?
- Kept the Problem from interrupting their work or school lives?
- Been able to keep the Problem from taking over when it was starting?

White and Epston (1990) report that externalization has the following beneficial effects:

- Decreases unproductive conflict and blame between family members
- Undermines sense of failure in relation to the problem by highlighting times the persons have had influence over it
- Invites people to unite in a struggle against the problem and reduce its influence
- Identifies new opportunities for reducing the influence of the problem
- Encourages a lighter, less stressed approach to interacting with the problem
- Increases interactive dialogue rather than repetitive monologue about the problem

Externalizing Conversations: The Statement of Position Map

White (2007) describes his more recently developed process for facilitating externalizing conversations as "the statement of position map." This map includes four categories of inquiry, which are used multiple times throughout a session and across sessions to shift the client's relationship with the problem and open new possibilities for action.

Inquiry Category 1: Negotiating an Experience-Near Definition

White begins by defining the problem using the client's language (experience-near language) rather than in professional or global terms (e.g., a "diagnosis"). Thus, "feeling blue" is preferred to "depressed."

Inquiry Category 2: Mapping the Effects

As in White's early work (White and Epston, 1990), mapping the effects of problems involves identifying how the problem has affected the various domains of the client's life: home, work, school, and social contexts; relationships with family, friends, and himself/herself; and the client's identity and future possibilities.

Inquiry Category 3: Evaluating the Effects

After identifying the effects of the problem, the therapist asks the client to evaluate these effects (White, 2007, p. 44):

- Are these activities okay with you?
- How do you feel about these developments?
- Where do you stand on these outcomes?
- Is the development positive or negative—or both, or neither, or something in between?

Inquiry Category 4: Justifying the Evaluation

In the final phase, the therapist asks about how and why clients have evaluated the situation the way they have (White, 2007, p. 48):

- Why is or isn't this okay for you?
- Why do you feel this way about this development?
- Why are you taking this stand or position on this development?

These "why" questions must be offered in a spirit of allowing clients to give voice to what is important to them rather than creating a sense of moral judgment. They should open up conversations about what motivates clients and how they want to shape their identities and futures.

Externalizing Metaphors

When externalizing using these four categories, White (2007, p. 32) employs various metaphors for relating to problems:

- Walking out on the problem
- Going on strike against the problem
- Defying the problem's requirements
- Disempowering the problem
- Educating the problem
- Escaping the problem
- Recovering or reclaiming territory from the problem
- Refusing invitations from the problem
- Disproving the problem's claims
- Resigning from the problem's service
- Stealing their lives from the problem
- Taming the problem
- Harnessing the problem
- Undermining the problem

Avoiding Totalizing and Dualistic Thinking

White (2007) avoids totalizing descriptions of the problem—the problem being all bad—because such descriptions promote dualistic, either/or thinking, which can be invalidating to the client and/or obscure the problem's broader context.

Externalizing Questions

Narrative therapists use externalizing questions to help clients build different relationships with their problems (Freedman & Combs, 1996). In most cases, these questions transform adjectives (e.g., *depressed, anxious, angry,* etc.) to nouns (e.g, *Depression, Anxiety, Anger,* etc.; capitalization is used to emphasize that the Problem is viewed as a separate entity). Externalizing questions *presume* that the person's are separate from the Problem and that they have a two-way relationship with the Problem: it affects them, and they affect it.

To experience the liberating effects of externalizing, Freedman and Combs (1996, pp. 49–50) have developed the following two sets of questions: one representing conventional therapeutic questions and the other externalizing questions. To do this exercise, choose a quality or trait that you or others find problematic, usually an adjective; substitute this for X in the questions below. Then find a noun form of that trait; substitute this for Y in the questions below. For example: X = depressed/Y = Depression; X = critical/Y = Criticism; X = angry/Y = Anger.

CONVENTIONAL VERSUS EXTERNALIZING QUESTIONS

Conventional Questions (insert problem description as *adjective* for X)	*Externalizing Questions* (insert problem description as *noun* for Y)
When did you first become X?	What made you vulnerable to the Y so that it was able to dominate your life?
What are you most X about?	In what contexts is the Y most likely to take over?
What kinds of things happen that typically lead to your being X?	What kinds of things happen that typically lead to the Y taking over?
When you are X, what do you do that you wouldn't do if you weren't X?	What has the Y gotten you to do that is against your better judgment?
Which of your current difficulties come from being X?	What effects does the Y have on your life and relationship?

What are the consequences for your life and relationships of being X?	How has the Y led you into the difficulties you are now experiencing?
How is your self-image different when you are X?	Does the Y blind you from noticing your resources, or can you see them through it?
If by some miracle you woke up some morning and were not X anymore, how, specifically, would your life be different?	Have there been times when you have been able to get the best of the Y? Times when the Y could have taken over but you kept it out of the picture?

Problem Deconstruction: Deconstructive Listening and Questions

Drawing from the philosophical work of Jacques Derrida, narrative therapists use deconstructive listening and questions to help clients trace the effects of dominant discourses and to empower clients to make more conscious choices about which discourses they allow to affect their life (Freedman & Combs, 1996). In deconstructive listening, the therapist listens for "gaps" in clients' understanding and asks them to fill in the details or has them explain the ambiguities in their stories. For example, if a client reports feeling rejected because friends did not call when they said they would, the therapist listens for the meanings that led to the sense of feeling "rejected."

Deconstructive questions help clients to further "unpack" their stories to see how they have been constructed, identifying the influence of dominant and local discourses. Typically used in externalizing conversations, these questions target problematic beliefs, practices, feelings, and attitudes by asking clients to identify the following:

- **History:** The *history of their relationship* with the problematic belief, practice, feeling, or attitude: "When and where did you first encounter the problem?"

- **Context:** The *contextual influences* on the problematic belief, practice, feeling, or attitude: "When is it most likely to be present?"

- **Effects:** The *effects or results* of the problematic belief, practice, feeling, or attitude: "What effects has this had on you and your relationship?"

- **Interrelationships:** The *interrelationship with other* beliefs, practices, feelings, or attitudes: "Are there other problems that feed this problem?"

- **Strategies:** *Tactics and strategies* used by the problem belief, practice, feeling, or attitude: "How does it go about influencing you?"

Mapping in Landscapes of Action and Identity or Consciousness

Based on the narrative theory of Jerome Bruner (1986), mapping the problem in the landscapes of action and identity (White, 2007) or consciousness (Freedman & Combs, 1996) is a specific technique for harnessing unique outcomes to promote desired change. Mapping in the landscapes of action and identity generally involves the following steps:

1. **Identify a Unique Outcome:** The therapist listens for and asks about times when the problem could have been a problem but was not.

2. **Ensure That the Unique Outcome Is Preferred:** Rather than assume, the therapist asks clients about whether the unique outcome is a preferred outcome: "Is this something you want to do or have happen more often?"

3. **Map in Landscape of Action:** First, the therapist begins by mapping the unique outcome in the landscape of action, identifying what actions were taken by

whom in which order. The therapist does this by asking about specific details: "What did you do first? How did the other person respond? What did you do next?" The therapist carefully plots the events until there is a step-by-step picture of the actions of the client and involved others, gathering details about the following:

- Critical events
- Circumstances surrounding events
- Sequence of events
- Timing of events
- Overall plot

4. **Map in the Landscape of Identity or Consciousness:** After obtaining a clear picture of what happened during the unique outcome, the therapist begins to map in the landscape of identity. This phase of mapping *thickens the plot* associated with the successful outcome, thus directly strengthening the connection of the preferred outcome with the client's personal identity. Mapping in the landscape of identity focuses on the psychological and relational implications of the unique outcomes. The following sample questions cover various areas of impact:

- "What do you believe this says about you as a person? About your relationship?"
- "What were your intentions behind these actions?"
- "What do you value most about your actions here?"
- "What, if anything, did you learn or realize from this?"
- "Does this change how you see life, God, your purpose, or your life goals?"
- "Does this affect how you see the problem?"

Intentional Versus Internal State Questions

White (2007) privileges intentional state questions (questions about a person's intentions in a given situation: "What were your intentions?") over internal state questions (questions about how a person was feeling or thinking: "What were you feeling?") because intentional state questions promote a sense of *personal agency*, whereas internal state questions can have the effect of diminishing one's sense of agency, increasing one's sense of isolation, and discouraging diversity.

Scaffolding Conversations

Drawing on Vygotsky's concept of *zones of proximal development*, White (2007) uses scaffolding conversations to move clients from that which is familiar to that which is novel. Vygotsky was a developmental psychologist who emphasized that because learning is relational, adults should structure children's learning in ways that help them interact with new information. The zone of proximal development is the distance between what the child can do independently and what the child can do in collaboration with others. *Scaffolding* is a term White developed with clients to describe five incremental movements across this zone of learning:

- **Low-Level Distancing Tasks:** These tasks *characterize a unique outcome*. Because they are at a low-level distance from the client (very close to what is familiar to him/her), they encourage the client to attribute meanings to events that have previously gone unnoticed: e.g., "Are there times when you don't seem to get into an argument even though there is tension?"

- **Medium-Level Distancing Tasks:** These tasks allow *unique outcomes to be taken into a chain of association*. They introduce greater "newness," encouraging more comparisons and contrasts with other unique outcomes: e.g., "How was last night's 'effective problem-solving conversation' similar or different from the one you described last week?"

- **Medium-High-Level Distancing Tasks:** These tasks *reflect on a chain of associations.* They encourage clients to reflect on, evaluate, and learn from the differences and similarities with other tasks: e.g., "Looking back over these examples of effective problem solving, is there anything that stands out as useful in preventing arguments?"

- **High-Level Distancing Tasks:** These tasks promote *abstract learning and realizations.* They require clients to assume a high level of distance from their immediate experience, promoting increased abstract conceptualization of life and identity: e.g., "What do these effective problem-solving conversations say about you as a person and about your relationship?"

- **Very-High-Level Distancing Tasks:** These are *plans for action.* They promote a high-level distancing from immediate experience to enable clients to identify ways of enacting their newly developed concepts about life and identity: e.g., "Do you have some ideas of how you want to translate these ideas into future action?"

Over the course of a conversation, therapists move back and forth between various levels of distancing tasks, progressively moving to higher levels of action planning.

Permission Questions

Narrative therapists use *permission questions* to emphasize the democratic nature of the therapeutic relationship and to encourage clients to maintain a clear, strong sense of agency when talking with the therapist. Quite simply, permission questions are questions therapists use to ask permission to ask a question. This goes against the prevailing assumption that therapists can ask any question they want to gather information they purportedly need to help the client. Socially, therapists are exempt from the prevailing social norms of polite conversation topics and are free to bring up taboo subjects such as sex, past abuse, relationship problems, death, fears, and weaknesses. Many clients feel compelled to answer these questions even if they are not comfortable doing so. Narrative therapists are sensitive to the power dynamic related to taboo and difficult subjects and therefore *ask for the client's permission* before asking questions that are generally taboo or that the therapist anticipates will make a particular client feel uncomfortable. For example, they might say, "Would it be okay if I ask you some questions about your sex life?"

In addition, permission questions are used throughout the interview regarding *what* is being discussed and *how* to ensure that the conversation is meaningful and comfortable for the client. For example, often when starting a session the therapist may briefly outline his/her ideas for how to use the time, asking for client input and permission to continue with a particular topic or line of questioning. Similarly, when therapists find themselves asking one person more questions than the others in a family session, they pause to ask permission to continue to ensure that everyone is okay with what is going on.

Situating Comments

Like permission questions, *situating comments* are used to maintain a more democratic therapeutic relationship and to reinforce client agency by ensuring that comments from the therapist are not taken as a "higher" or "more valid" truth than the client's (Zimmerman & Dickerson, 1996). Drawing on the distinction between dominant and local discourses, narrative therapists are keenly aware that any comment made by the therapist is often considered more valid than anything the client might say. Thus, therapists *situate* their comments by revealing the source of their perspective, emphasizing that it is only one perspective among others. When the source and context of a therapist comment are revealed, a client is less likely to overprivilege the comment.

EXAMPLES OF SITUATING COMMENTS

THERAPIST COMMENT WITHOUT SITUATING	SITUATING THERAPIST COMMENT
I am noticing that you tend to…	Having grown up on a farm, my attention is of course drawn to…
Research indicates that…	There is one therapist who has developed a theory (or done a study) that suggests.… Does this sound like something that would be true for you?
I suggest that you…	Since you are asking me for a suggestion, I can only tell you what I think as someone who believes action is more productive than talk…

Narrative Reflecting Team Practices

On the basis of Tom Andersen's collaborative practice of using reflecting teams (see earlier discussion), narrative therapists have developed a similar practice that supports their work. Using Andersen's format, Freedman and Combs (1996) assign the team *three primary tasks*:

1. Develop a thorough understanding by closely attending to details of the story
2. Listen for differences and events that do not fit the dominant problem-saturated narrative
3. Notice beliefs, ideas, or contexts that support the problem-saturated descriptions

In addition, they propose the following *guidelines* for the team:

1. During the reflecting process, the reflecting team members participate in a back-and-forth conversation rather than in a monologue.
2. Team members should not talk to each other while observing the interview.
3. Comments should be offered in a tentative manner (e.g., "perhaps," "could," "might").
4. Comments are based on what actually occurs in the room (e.g., "At one point mom got very quiet; I was wondering what was going on for her at that moment").
5. When appropriate, comments are situated in the speaker's personal experience (e.g., "Having been a teacher, I may have been the only one who focused on this…").
6. All family members should be responded to in some way.
7. Reflections should be kept short.

Re-Membering Conversations

White (2007) uses *re-membering conversations* to develop a multivoiced sense of personal identity that enables clients to make sense of their lives in a more coherent and orderly way. In these conversations, clients develop the sense of an identity that is grounded in *associations of life* rather than in a singular, core self. The associations of life include a "membership" of significant people and identities from the client's past, present, and projected future. In these conversations, clients are encouraged to identify who's a member, assess the influence of each member, and decide whether their membership should be upgraded, downgraded, or canceled (e.g., canceling the membership of a high school bully whose taunting still haunts the client). The process of re-membering includes the following components:

- Identifying the other person's contribution to the client's life
- Articulating how the other person may have viewed the client's identity

- Considering how the client may have affected the other person's life
- Specifying the implications for the client's identity (e.g., "I am a person who values justice")

Leagues

To solidify a new narrative and new identities, narrative therapists have created leagues (or clubs, associations, teams), membership in which signifies an accomplishment in a particular area. In most cases, leagues are virtual communities of concern (e.g., a Temper Tamer's Club to which a child is given a membership certificate), although some meet face to face or interact via the Internet (Anti-Anorexia/Anti-Bulima League; see www.narrativetherapy.com).

Definitional Ceremony

Generally used toward the end of therapy to solidify the emerging preferred narrative and identity, definitional ceremonies involve inviting significant others to *witness* the emerging story. This ceremony has three phases:

1. **The First Telling:** The client tells his/her life story, highlighting the emerging identity stories as the invited witnesses listen.

2. **Retelling:** The witnesses take turns retelling the story from their perspectives; they are prepared for the process by being asked to refrain from offering advice, making judgments, or theorizing and are asked to *situate* their comments.

3. **Retelling of the Retelling:** The client then retells the story incorporating aspects of the witnesses' stories.

Letters and Certificates

Narrative letters are used to develop and solidify preferred narratives and identities (White & Epston, 1990). Therapists can write letters detailing a client's emerging story after a session in lieu of doing case notes (unless they work in a practice environment that requires a specific format). Narrative letters use the same techniques used in session to reinforce the emerging narrative; they perform the following functions:

- **Emphasize Client Agency:** Letters highlight clients' agency in their lives, including small steps in becoming proactive.

- **Take Observer Position:** The therapist clearly takes the role of *observing* the changes the client is making, citing specific, concrete examples whenever possible.

- **Highlight Temporality:** The time dimension is used to plot the emerging story: where clients began, where they are now, and where they are likely to go.

- **Encourage Polysemy:** Rather than propose singular interpretations, multiple meanings are entertained and encouraged.

Letters can be used early in therapy to engage clients, during therapy to reinforce the emerging narrative and reinforce new preferred behaviors, or at the end of therapy to consolidate gains by narrating the change process.

Sample Letter

White and Epston (1990, pp. 109–110) offer numerous sample letters, such as the following:

Dear Rick and Harriet,

I'm sure that you are familiar with the fact that the best ideas have the habit of presenting themselves after the event. So it will come as no surprise to you that I often think of the most important questions after the end of an interview. ...

Anyway, I thought I would share a couple of important questions that came to me after you left our last meeting:

Rick, how did you decline Helen's [the daughter] invitation to you to do the reasoning for her? And how do you think this could have the effect of inviting her to reason with herself? Do you think this could help her to become more responsible?

Harriet, how did you decline Helen's invitations to you to be dependable for her? And how do you think this could have the effect of inviting her to depend upon herself more? Do you think that this could have the effect of helping her to take better care of her life?

What does this decreased vulnerability to Helen's invitations to have her life for her [e.g., take responsibility for her life by making decisions, solving problems, and handling consequences] reflect in you both as people?

By the way, what ideas occurred to you after our last meeting? M.W.

Certificates

Certificates are often used with children to recognize the changes they have made and to reinforce their new "reputation" as a "temper tamer," "cooperative child," and so forth.

Certified Temper Tamer

This is to certify that

_____

has proven himself as a skilled Tamer of Tempers,

having gone two months without temper problems at home or school

using the following taming techniques that he developed for himself:

1. Asking for help when confused

2. Taking three deep breaths when the scent of Temper appears

3. Using soft words to talk about anger and frustration

Date of award: _____

Witnessed by: _____ (therapist)

_____ (parents)

_____ (teacher)

Interventions for Specific Problems

Children

Numerous narrative therapists have developed interventions for working with children (Freeman, Epston, & Lobovits, 1997; Smith & Nylund, 2000; Vetere & Dowling, 2005; White & Morgan, 2006). The externalization process seems to come more naturally to children, perhaps because it is reflected so often in cartoons and children's literature (e.g., the devil and angel on a cartoon character's shoulders). Externalization adapts well to play and art therapies: externalized problems (e.g., Temper, Sadness, Anger) can be portrayed in art media (drawings, clay, paintings) or acted out with puppets and dolls. In addition to externalized problems, children enjoy drawing or acting out unique outcomes and preferred narratives; this process often accelerates their adaptation of new behaviors.

Domestic Violence

Narrative therapists have developed unique and promising alternatives to the standard treatment for those who batter (Augusta-Scott & Dankwort, 2002; Jenkins, 1990). Unlike the feminist-based Duluth model, which traces the cause of violence to men's attempts to gain power and control (Pence & Paymar, 1993; see Chapter 16), narrative approaches work from within clients' lived reality, which usually includes the experience of helplessness and powerlessness that they say leads them to try to regain control through violence (Augusta-Scott & Dankwort, 2002).

Jenkins (1990) warns therapists against accepting responsibility for the violence, which therapists inadvertently do when they challenge the man's explanations, give advice on how to stop abusive behavior, offer strong arguments against violence, or try to break down his denial, all of which are common therapist responses to violence. Instead Jenkins uses a nine-step model that requires the *client* to take full responsibility for the violence and for ending it. Throughout this process the therapist is supportive without condoning violence or attacking it; instead the focus is on facilitating the process in the nine-step model.

Jenkins's Nine-Step Model for Working with Men Who Batter

1. Invite the man to address his violence
2. Invite the man to argue for a nonviolent relationship
3. Invite the man to examine his misguided efforts to contribute to the relationship
4. Invite the man to identify time trends in the relationship
5. Invite the man to externalize restraints (note: he avoids externalizing anger and violence to prevent possible minimizing of responsibility)
6. Deliver irresistible invitations to challenge restraints
7. Invite the man to consider his readiness to take new action
8. Facilitate the planning of new action
9. Facilitate the discovery of new action (p. 63)

Throughout the process, the therapist identifies the dominant discourses, particularly patriarchal discourses, that have contributed to the violence; these are deconstructed and externalized to help the client develop more effective ways of relating. The narrative approach is careful not to replicate the abusive pattern of harshness and criticism in the therapeutic relationship and instead models the respect, tolerance, and boundaries that clients are aspiring to enact.

Snapshot: Research and the Evidence Base

Quick Summary: With the exception of the open dialogue approach for working with psychosis, most research on these approaches has focused on client experiences of therapy rather than outcome.

Consistent with their philosophical underpinnings, narrative and collaborative therapists have conducted more qualitative than quantitative investigations about their approaches to therapy (Anderson, 1997; Gehart et al., 2007). Qualitative research on postmodern therapies has focused on clients' lived experience of therapy and its effects on their lives, emphasizing the clients' experience over researcher-defined measures of successful therapy (Gehart & Lyle, 1999; Levitt & Rennie, 2004; London, Ruiz, Gargollo, & M.C., 1998). A notable exception, Finnish psychiatrist Jaakko Seikkula (2002) and his team (Haarakangas et al., 2007) have used qualitative and quantitative methods to study their open dialogue approach to working with psychosis and other severe diagnoses for the past 20 years, reporting significant evidence for their model's effectiveness (see Clinical Spotlight discussion).

Snapshot: Working with Diverse Populations

Quick Summary: Ideal for marginalized populations, these approaches focus on how the client's problems relate to the broader sociopolitical context.

Because postmodern therapies do not use pre-established theories of health to create predefined therapeutic goals, they are appropriate for working with a wide range of diverse populations. In fact, the broader questions of diversity and of how society, its norms, and the use of language affect individuals are the guiding questions in postmodern philosophical literature, making these therapies particularly suitable for clients from marginalized groups (for an in-depth discussion, see Monk et al., 2008: *New Horizons in Multicultural Counseling*). Unlike most mental health therapies, narrative therapy places societal issues of oppression at the heart of its therapeutic interventions, and many narrative therapists are active agents of social justice (Zimmerman & Dickerson, 1996). Collaborative therapy attends more to local discourses, working closely with the client and significant others to determine what the problem is (for the moment, knowing its definition will continually evolve) and how best to resolve it. This focus on local knowledges ensures that the client's cultural values and beliefs are a central part of the therapy process. Both narrative and collaborative therapy have international roots and are practiced in numerous countries around the world. The case study that concludes this chapter uses postmodern therapy to address a teen who began cutting after her mother moved in with her girlfriend and her son.

ONLINE RESOURCES

Harlene Anderson

www.harleneanderson.org

Anti-Anorexia/Anti-Bulima League

www.narrativeapproaches.com/antianorexia%20folder/anti_anorexia_index. htm

Dulwich Centre: Michael White's Narrative Therapy

www.dulwichcenter.com

Evanston Family Therapy Center: Freedman and Combs' Narrative Therapy

www.narrativetherapychicago.com

Grupo Campos Elíseos: Collaborative Therapy, Mexico City

www.grupocamposeliseos.com

Houston Galveston Institute: Collaborative Therapy

www.talkhgi.com

Marburg Institute: Collaborative Therapy, Germany

www.mics.de

Narrative Approaches

www.narrativeapproaches.com

Taos Institute: Collaborative Practices in Therapy, Consultation, Education, Business

www.taosinstitute.net

Yaletown Family Therapy: Narrative Therapy, Canada

www.yaletownfamilytherapy.com

REFERENCES

*Asterisk indicates recommended introductory readings.

*Andersen, T. (1991). *The reflecting team: Dialogues and dialogues about the dialogues.* New York: Norton.

Andersen, T. (1992). Relationship, language and pre-understanding in the reflecting process. *Australian and New Zealand Journal of Family Therapy, 13*(2), 87–91.

Andersen, T. (1995). Reflecting processes; acts of informing and forming: You can borrow my eyes, but you must not take them away from me! In S. Friedman (Ed.), *The reflecting team in action: Collaborative practice in family therapy* (pp. 11–37). New York: Guilford.

*Andersen, T. (2007). Human participating: Human "being" is the step for human "becoming" in the next step. In H. Anderson & D. Gehart (Eds.), *Collaborative therapy: Relationships and conversations that make a difference* (pp. 81–97). New York: Brunner/Routledge.

Anderson, H. (1993). On a roller coaster: A collaborative language systems approach to therapy. In S. Friedman (Ed.), *The new language of change* (pp. 323–344). New York: Guilford.

Anderson, H. (1995). Collaborative language systems: Toward a postmodern therapy. In R. Mikesell, D. D. Lusterman, & S. McDaniel (Eds.), *Family psychology and systems therapy* (pp. 27–44). Washington, DC: American Psychological Association.

*Anderson, H. (1997). *Conversations, language, and possibilities: A postmodern approach to therapy.* New York: Basic Books.

Anderson, H. (2005). Myths about "not knowing." *Family Process, 44,* 497–504.

Anderson, H. (2007). Historical influences. In H. Anderson & D. Gehart (Eds.), *Collaborative therapy: Relationships and conversations that make a difference* (pp. 21–31). New York: Brunner/Routledge.

*Anderson, H., & Gehart, D. (2007). *Collaborative therapy: Relationships and conversations that make a difference.* New York: Brunner/Routledge.

Anderson, H., & Goolishian, H. (1988). Human systems as linguistic systems: Preliminary and evolving ideas about the implications for clinical theory. *Family Process, 27,* 157–163.

*Anderson, H., & Goolishian, H. (1992). The client is the expert: A not-knowing approach to therapy. In S. McNamee & K. J. Gergen (Eds.), *Therapy as social construction* (pp. 25–39). Newbury Park, CA: Sage.

Augusta-Scott, T., & Dankwort, J. (2002). Partner abuse group intervention: Lessons from education and narrative therapy approaches. *Journal of Interpersonal Violence, 17,* 783–805.

Bava, S., Levin, S., & Tinaz, D. (2002). A polyvocal response to trauma in a postmodern learning community. *Journal of Systematic Therapies, 21*(2), 104–113.

Boscolo, L., Cecchin, G., Hoffman, L., & Penn, P. (1987). *Milan systemic family therapy.* New York: Basic Books.

Bruner, Jerome. (1986). *Actual minds, possible worlds.* Cambridge, MA: Harvard University Press.

Bruner, J. (1990). *Acts of meaning.* Cambridge, MA: Harvard University Press.

Deissler, K. (2007). Dialogues in a psychiatric service in Cuba. In H. Anderson & D. Gehart (Eds.), *Collaborative therapy: Relationships and conversations that make a difference* (pp. 291–309). New York: Brunner/Routledge.

Foucault, M. (1972). *The archeology of knowledge* (A. Sheridan-Smith, trans.). New York: Harper & Row.

Foucault, M. (1979). *Discipline and punish: The birth of the prison.* Middlesex: Peregrine Books.

Foucault, M. (1980). *Power/knowledge: Selected interviews and other writings.* New York: Pantheon Books.

*Freedman, J., & Combs, G. (1996). *Narrative therapy: The social construction of preferred realities.* New York: Norton.

*Freeman, J., Epston, D., & Lobovits, D. (1997). *Playful approaches to serious problems.* New York: Norton.

Gehart, D. (2007a). Creating space for children's voices: A collaborative and playful approach to working with children and families. In H. Anderson & D. Gehart (Eds.), *Collaborative therapy: Relationships and conversations that make a difference* (pp. 183–197). New York: Brunner/Routledge.

Gehart, D. (2007b). Process-as-content: Teaching postmodern therapy in a university context. *Journal of Systemic Therapies, 18,* 39–56.

Gehart, D. R., & Lyle, R. R. (1999). Client and therapist perspectives of change in collaborative language systems: An interpretive ethnography. *Journal of Systemic Therapy, 18*(4), 78–97.

Gehart, D., & McCollum, E. (2007). Engaging suffering: Towards a mindful re-visioning of marriage and family therapy practice. *Journal of Marital and Family Therapy, 33,* 214–226.

Gehart, D., Tarragona, M., & Bava, S. (2007). A collaborative approach to inquiry. In H. Anderson & D. Gehart (Eds.), *Collaborative therapy: Relationships and conversations that make a difference* (pp. 367–390). New York: Brunner/Routledge.

Goolishian, H., & Anderson, H. (1987) Language systems and therapy: An evolving idea. *Psychotherapy, 24*(3S), 529–538.

Haarakangas, K., Seikkula, J., Alakare, B., & Aaltonen, J. (2007). Open dialogue: An approach to psychotherapuetic treatment of psychosis in Northern Finland. In H. Anderson & D. Gehart (Eds.), *Collaborative therapy: Relationships and conversations that make a difference* (pp. 221–233). New York: Brunner/Routledge.

*Hoffman, L. (1981). *Foundations of family therapy: A conceptual framework for systems change.* New York: Basic Books.

Hoffman, L. (1990). Constructing realities: An art of lenses. *Family Process, 29,* 1–12.

Hoffman, L. (1993). *Exchanging voices: A collaborative approach to family therapy.* London: Karnac Books.

*Hoffman, L. (2001). *Family therapy: An intimate history.* New York: Norton.

Hoffman, L. (2007). The art of "withness": A bright new edge. In H. Anderson & D. Gehart (Eds.), *Collaborative therapy: Relationships and conversations that make a difference* (pp. 63–79). New York: Brunner/Routledge.

Jenkins, A. (1990). *Invitations to responsibility: The therapeutic engagement of men who are violent and abusive.* Adelaide, Australia: Dulwich Centre Publications.

Levin, S. (2007). Hearing the unheard: Advice to professionals from women who have been battered. In H. Anderson & D. Gehart (Eds.), *Collaborative therapy: Relationships and conversations that make a difference* (pp. 109–128). New York: Brunner/Routledge.

Levitt, H., & Rennie, D. L. (2004). Narrative activity: Clients' and therapists' intentions in the process of narration. In L. Angus & J. McLeod (Eds.), *The handbook of narrative and psychotherapy: Practice, theory, and research* (pp. 299–313). Thousand Oaks, CA: Sage.

London, S., & Rodriguez-Jazcilevich, I. (2007). The development of a collaborative learning and therapy community in an educational setting: From alienation to invitation. In H. Anderson & D. Gehart (Eds.), *Collaborative therapy: Relationships and conversations that make a difference* (pp. 235–250). New York: Brunner/Routledge.

London, S., Ruiz, G., Gargollo, M., & M.C. (1999). Clients' voices: A collection of clients' accounts. *Journal of Systemic Therapies, 17*(4), 61–71.

McNamee, S. (2007). Relational practices in education: Teaching as conversation. In H. Anderson & D. Gehart (Eds.), *Collaborative therapy: Relationships and conversations that make a difference* (pp. 313–336). New York: Brunner/Routledge.

Monk, G., & Gehart, D. R. (2003). Conversational partner or socio-political activist: Distinguishing the position of the therapist in collaborative and narrative therapies. *Family Process, 42,* 19–30.

Monk, G., Winslade, J., Crocket, K., & Epston, D. (1997). *Narrative therapy in practice: The archaeology of hope.* San Francisco: Jossey-Bass.

Monk, G., Winslade, J., & Sinclair, S. (2008). *New horizons in multicultural counseling.* Thousand Oaks, CA: Sage.

Pence, E., & Paymar, M. (1993). *Education groups for men who batter: The Duluth Model.* New York: Springer.

Penn, P. (2001). Chronic illness: Trauma, language, and writing: Breaking the silence. *Family Process, 40,* 33–52.

Penn, P. (2002). *So close.* Fort Lee, NJ: Cavankerry.

Penn, P., & Frankfurt, M. (1994). Creating a participant text: Writing, multiple voices, narrative multiplicity. *Family Process, 33,* 217–231.

Penn, P., & Sheinberg, M. (1991). Stories and conversations. *Journal of Systemic Therapies, 10*(3–4), 30–37.

Seikkula, J. (2002). Open dialogues with good and poor outcomes for psychotic crises: Examples from families with violence. *Journal of Marital and Family Therapy, 28*(3), 263–274.

Sells, S., Smith, T., Coe, M., & Yoshioka, M. (1994). An ethnography of couple and therapist experiences in reflecting team practice. *Journal of Marital and Family Therapy, 20,* 247–266.

Smith, C., & Nylund, D. (2000). *Narrative therapy with children and adolescents.* New York: Guilford.

St. George, S., & Wulff, D. (1998). Integrating the client's voice within case reports. *Journal of Systemic Therapies, 17*(4), 3–13.

Vetere, A., & Dowling, E. (2005). *Narrative therapies with children and their families: A practitioner's guide to concepts and approaches.* New York: Routledge.

Winslade, J., & Monk, G. (1999) *Narrative counseling in schools: Powerful and brief* (1st ed.). Thousand Oaks, CA: Corwin Press.

Winslade, J., & Monk, G. (2000). *Narrative mediation.* San Francisco: Jossey-Bass.

Winslade, J., & Monk, G. (2007) *Narrative counseling in schools: Powerful and brief* (2nd ed.). Thousand Oaks, CA: Corwin Press.

Winslade, J., & Monk, G. (2008). *Practicing narrative mediation: Loosening the grip of conflict.* San Francisco: Jossey-Bass.

White, M. (1995). *Re-authoring lives: Interviews and essays.* Adelaide, Australia: Dulwich Centre Publications.

*White, M. (2007). *Maps of narrative practice.* New York: Norton.

*White, M., & Epston, D. (1990). *Narrative means to therapeutic ends.* New York: Norton.

White, M., & Morgan, A. (2006). *Narrative therapy with children and their families.* Adelaide, Australia: Dulwich Centre Publications.

Zimmerman, J. L., & Dickerson, V. C. (1996). *If problems talked: Narrative therapy in action.* New York: Guilford.

POSTMODERN COLLABORATIVE CASE STUDY

Christie and Suzanne bring Christy's 15-year-old daughter, Ashley, in for therapy because Ashley has become increasingly depressed and has begun cutting to relieve pain. Ashley has always been a "sensitive" child and has a difficult time finding a place in high school. Suzanne and her 8-year-old son, Matt, moved in a little over a year ago, and they report that the transition has generally gone well. Ashley also has a half-brother from her father's second marriage, although they live five hours away and she visits only during the holidays. Ashley says she is "cool" with her mother's relationship with another woman and that she is "okay" with how often she sees her dad. Both Christie and her mother (Ashley's grandmother) have been treated for depression. Additionally, Christie was sexually abused by her brother while young, and her brother's son molested Ashley one time when she was 6 years old. Ashley's greatest passion is her art and writing music.

After meeting with the family, a postmodern, collaborative family therapist developed the following case conceptualization.

Shaded Sections Emphasized in Postmodern, Collaborative Treatment Planning and Intervention

CASE CONCEPTUALIZATION FORM

Therapist: Roxana Gilbert   **Client/Case #:** 1420   **Date:** 10/4/08

I. Introduction to Client and Significant Others *(Include age, ethnicity, occupation, grade, relevant identifiers, etc.). Put an * next to persons in session and/or IP for identified patient.*

*AF†: 47 High school music teacher, German-American, recently married AF40

*AF: 40 Bookkeeper, Irish-American, recently married AF47

*CF: 15 (IP) (AF47's daughter), 10th grade, artistic and musically talented

CM: 8 (AF40's son) 3rd grade; sports

AM: Ashley's father; High school math teacher; remarried with one child from second marriage.

II. Presenting Concern
Client's/Family's Descriptions of Problem(s):

AF: 47 Sees CF's depression as related to being shy and sensitive at a big high school; she relates this to her and her mother's depression and Ashley's sexual abuse at age 6.

AF: 40 Worries that CF's depression is related to her not accepting her and her mother's relationship; she feels guilt but is also frustrated with AF47 for not considering this as a factor.

CF: 15 Believes her depression stems from not having friends at school; feeling out of place at home and at school.

CM: 8 Is not quite sure why CF cries, but hopes it is not because of him.

Broader System Problem Descriptions (description of problem from referring party, teachers, relatives, legal system, etc.):

CF15's Father: Has not been made aware of her depression and cutting but believes it is "unhealthy" for her mother to be living with another woman with CF.

English teacher: CF's mentor: Believes CF is just a thoughtful young woman who is "too mature" for HS.

Best friend: Believes CF needs more friends at high school.

III. Background Information
Recent Background (recent life changes, precipitating events, first symptoms, stressors, etc.):

AF40 and CM moved in 15 months ago; CF began high school a year and half ago, leaving her best friend from middle school, who went to another high school. She takes art and works on the sets for plays.

---

† *Abbreviations:* AF: Adult Female; AM: Adult Male; CF#: Child Female with age, e.g., CF12; CM#: Child Male with age; Hx: History; Ex: Explanation or Example; NA: Not Applicable.

(continued)

III. Background Information *(continued)*

She has made a couple of friends at school, but she is closest to her old best friend, whom she sees on weekends. She had a crush on a guy at school in the fall, and he is now dating someone else. She often spends lunch and Friday night alone.

Related Historical Background (family history, related issues, past abuse, trauma, previous counseling, medical/mental health history, etc.):

CF was sexually abused by her cousin at age 6 (one incident); the father of that cousin sexually abused her mother when they were children. CF has lived with her mother since her parents' divorce when she was 3 years old. Her mother reports that she was an easy child to raise; CF's father moved away and she has visited him most holidays. AF47 started dating women 7 years ago and has been with AF40 for 3 years now.

IV. Systemic Assessment

Client/Relational Strengths

Personal/individual: CF is intelligent, artistic, and musically talented; she makes good choices socially and is a diligent student. AF47 is bright and a dedicated, caring mother. CF40 and CM are upbeat and bring liveliness to the home.

Relational/social: CF has a best friend from middle school who is supportive and an English teacher who is a great mentor. Her father is supportive when she invites him in. The family generally gets along well.

Spiritual: AF47 has a strong sense that "things happen for a reason" and has a strong nonreligious spirituality.

Family Structure and Interaction Patterns

Couple Subsystem (to be assessed): ☒ Personal current ☐ Personal past ☐ Parents'

Couple Boundaries: ☐ Clear ☒ Enmeshed ☐ Disengaged ☐ Other: _____

Rules for closeness/distance: AF47 and AF40 mildly enmeshed, each highly sensitive to the emotions and reactions of the other.

Couple Problem Interaction Pattern (A ⇆ B):

Start of tension: AF40 asks to spend a day alone with AF47.

Conflict/symptom escalation: AF47 says she needs to focus on CF15; AF40 feels rejected; AF47 defends her decision to put her child first; AF40 withdraws.

Return to "normal"/homeostasis: After a few hours, AF47 can't take it anymore and tries to make up to AF40 by offering to do something special; AF40 slowly comes around.

Couple Complementary Patterns: ☒ Pursuer/distancer ☐ Over/under functioner

☒ Emotional/logical ☐ Good/bad parent ☐ Other: _____ .

Ex: AF40 pursues AF47, who is generally "too stressed" or worried to fully engage. AF40 is the "logical and upbeat" one and AF47 is the "emotional and worried" one.

Satir Communication Stances:
AF47:   ☐ Congruent ☒ Placator ☐ Blamer ☐ Superreasonable ☐ Irrelevant
AF40:   ☐ Congruent ☐ Placator ☒ Blamer ☐ Superreasonable ☐ Irrelevant

Describe dynamic: AF47 is greatly distressed if others are not happy; AF40 is able to clearly state her needs and is less bothered by others not agreeing with her.

Gottman's Divorce Indicators:

Criticism: ☒ AF47 ☐ AM40. Ex: Tends to be the one to raise problem issues.

Defensiveness: ☒ AF47 ☒ AF40. Ex: Both are quick to defend themselves.

Contempt: ☐ AF47 ☐ AF40. Ex: _____

Stonewalling: ☐ AF47 ☒ AF40. Ex: When feels rejected.

Failed repair attempts: ☐ AF47 ☐ AF40. Ex: NA

Not accept influence: ☐ AF47 ☐ AF40. Ex: NA

Harsh startup: ☒ AF47 ☐ AF40. Ex: More likely to raise issue harshly.

Parental Subsystem: ☒ Family of procreation ☐ Family of origin

Membership in Family Subsystems: Parental: ☒ AF47 ☒ AF40 ☒ Other: AF40
Is parental subsystem distinct from couple subsystem? ☒ Yes ☐ No ☐ NA (divorce)

Sibling subsystem: CF has distant relationship from half-brother and CM8.

Special interest: AF47's family has generational pattern of close women.

Family Life Cycle Stage:
☐ Single adult ☐ Marriage ☐ Family with young children
☒ Family with adolescent children ☐ Launching children ☐ Later life
Describe struggles with mastering developmental tasks in one of these stages:

CF is cooperative at home but has not been able to develop successful social life or begin developing an individual identity.

Hierarchy Between Child/Parents:
AF47: ☒ Effective ☐ Insufficient (permissive) ☐ Excessive (authoritarian) ☐ Inconsistent
AM: ☒ Effective ☐ Insufficient (permissive) ☐ Excessive (authoritarian) ☐ Inconsistent

Ex: CF is very compliant with adults.

(continued)

IV. Systemic Assessment *(continued)*

Emotional Boundaries with Children:

AF47:   ☐ Clear/balanced ☒ Enmeshed (reactive) ☐ Disengaged (disinterested)

☐ Other: _____

AF40:   ☐ Clear/balanced ☐ Enmeshed (reactive) ☒ Disengaged (disinterested)

☐ Other: _____

Ex: CF and AF47 are "too close," more like sisters than mother-daughter. AM is emotionally detached from CF's life but is supportive when she opens up to him.

Problem Interaction Pattern (A ⇆ B):

Start of tension: AF47 suggests that CF15 visit with her friend over the weekend.

Conflict/symptom escalation: CF15 knows her mother is trying to help, but feels even more worthless inside; when she sees AF47 and AF40 together during dinner feels worse; feels like there is no place for her; cries and/or cuts late at night.

Return to "normal"/homeostasis: When AF47 discovers her crying or cutting, she puts everything else on hold to try to help CF15; she begins to feel better.

Triangles/Coalitions:

☒ AF47 and CF15 against AM: Ex: Although not hostile, AF47/CF have always been a team.

☐ AM and C _____ against AF: Ex: _____

☐ Other: Ex: _____

Communication Stances:

AF47 or ____: ☐ Congruent ☒ Placator ☐ Blamer ☐ Superreasonable ☐ Irrelevant

AM or AF40: ☐ Congruent ☐ Placator ☒ Blamer ☐ Superreasonable ☐ Irrelevant

CF15 or ____: ☐ Congruent ☒ Placator ☐ Blamer ☐ Superreasonable ☐ Irrelevant

CM8 or ____: ☐ Congruent ☒ Placator ☐ Blamer ☐ Superreasonable ☐ Irrelevant

Ex: _____

Hypothesis (Describe possible role or function of symptom in maintaining family homeostasis):

Prior to AF40 moving in, CF15 and AF47 were "best friends," and CF15 was the center of AF47's world. CF15 has not only had to adjust to AF47 being in a lesbian relationship, which is confusing, but also must adapt to going back to the child role. She has had difficulty making friends at her new school, creating additional loneliness in her life. Depression and cutting not only help deal with the pain but also help keep her connected to her mother.

Intergenerational Patterns

Substance/alcohol abuse: ☒ NA ☐ Hx: _____

Sexual/physical/emotional abuse: ☐ NA ☒ Hx: CF15 and cousin; AF47 and brother (cousin's father)

Parent/child relations: ☐ NA ☒ Hx: Close mother-daughter relationships on AF47 side.

Physical/mental disorders: ☐ NA ☒ Hx: AF47, her mother, and CF have had depression

Historical incidents of presenting problem: ☐ NA ☒ Hx: AF47 also had depression and was sexually abused

Family strengths: AF47 protected CF15 when learned of abuse; although not fully accepting, AF47's parents have also not cut her off once AF40 moved in.

Previous Solutions and Unique Outcomes

Solutions that DIDN'T work: AF47 trying to soothe CF15; trying to "cheer her up" by telling her things will all work out.

Solutions that DID work: CF15 less depressed when with best friend or when hanging out with friends from school. CF15 less depressed when mother spends time with her.

Narrative, Dominant Discourses, and Diversity
Dominant Discourses informing definition of problem:

Cultural, ethnic, SES, etc.: CF15 feels like she is "normal" on the outside but "abnormal" on the inside.

Gender, sex orientation, etc.: AF47's switch from heterosexual to same-sex relationships has felt "normal" to CF15 in that it was a gradual evolution as she grew up, but now that she is understanding more and having her own sexual feelings of attraction, it is confusing and embarrassing. CF15 and AF47 both feel safest in women to women relationships.

Other social influences: CF is trying to find a way to "fit in" in high school, a context in which her tendency for thoughtful reflection is not highly valued.

Identity Narratives that have developed around problem for AF, AM, and/or CM/F:

Since entering high school and having AF40 move in, CF is feeling increasing marginalized in all social worlds: "it's like there is no place for me anywhere." "No one wants me." AF47 feels like she is finally coming out and expressing her true self and that it is hurting her child.

Local or Preferred Discourses: AF47 describes CF as "mature for her age" and not fitting in because she is not "shallow" and "judgmental" like other kids. AF47 has always seen CF more as a peer than as a child.

(continued)

IV. Systemic Assessment *(continued)*

Other Influential Discourses: The family experiences ongoing discrimination due to the same-sex partnership. The effects of "being different" affect all members of the family.

V. Genogram

Construct a family genogram and include all relevant information, including:

- ages, birth/death dates
- names
- relational patterns
- occupations
- medical history
- psychiatric disorders
- abuse history

Also include a couple of adjectives for persons frequently discussed in session (these should describe personal qualities and/or relational patterns, e.g., quiet, family caretaker, emotionally distant, perfectionist, helpless, etc.). Genogram should be attached to report.

VI. Client Perspectives

Areas of Agreement: Based on what the client(s) has(ve) said, what parts of the above assessment do they agree with or are likely to agree with?

They readily describe AF40 moving in and CF15 changing schools as stressors related to CF's depression.

Areas of Disagreement: What parts do they disagree with or are likely to disagree with? Why?

AF47 feels that she has an appropriate level of closeness with CF and that treating her like a peer has been good because she is mature for her age.

How do you plan to respectfully work with areas of disagreement?

Avoid trying to find a cause or assign blame but instead have the family consider different ways of relating that might work better for CF.

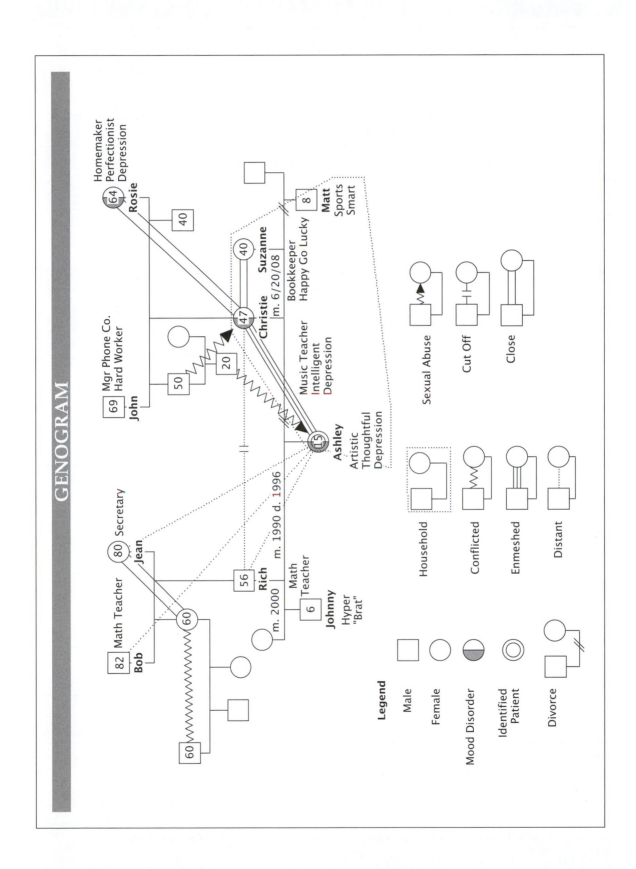

CLINICAL ASSESSMENT

Client ID # (do not use name): 1420	Ethnicities: Caucasian	Primary Language: ☒ Eng ☐ Span ☐ Other: _____

List all participants/significant others: Put a [★] for Identified Patient(IP); [✔] for sig. others who **WILL** attend; [✕] for sig. others who will **NOT** attend.

Adult: Age: Profession/Employer	Child: Age: School/Grade
[✔] AF† 47; High school music teacher; German-American; recently married AF40	[✔] CM 8 (AF40's son); 3rd grade; sports
[✔] AF 40; Bookkeeper; Irish-American; recently married AF47	[★] CF 15 (AF47's daughter); 10th grade; artistic; musically talented
[★] AF/M #2: AM; CF15's father; HS Math teacher	[ ] CF/M _____

Presenting Problems

		Complete for children
☒ Depression/hopelessness	☐ Couple concern	☒ School failure/decline performance
☐ Anxiety/worry	☐ Parent/child conflict	
☐ Anger issues	☐ Partner violence/abuse	☐ Truancy/runaway
☒ Loss/grief	☐ Divorce adjustment	☐ Fighting w/peers
☐ Suicidal thoughts/attempts	☒ Remarriage adjustment	☐ Hyperactivity
☐ Sexual abuse/rape	☐ Sexuality/intimacy concerns	☐ Wetting/soiling clothing
☐ Alcohol/drug use	☒ Major life changes	☒ Child abuse/neglect
☐ Eating problems/disorders	☐ Legal issues/probation	☒ Isolation/withdrawal
☐ Job problems/unemployed	☒ Other: Self Harm	☐ Other: _____

Mental Status for IP

Interpersonal issues	☐ NA	☐ Conflict ☒ Enmeshment ☒ Isolation/avoidance ☐ Emotional disengagement ☒ Poor social skills ☐ Couple problems ☒ Prob w/friends ☐ Prob at work ☒ Overly shy ☐ Egocentricity ☒ Diff establish/maintain relationship ☐ Other: _____
Mood	☐ NA	☒ Depressed/Sad ☒ Hopeless ☐ Fearful ☐ Anxious ☐ Angry ☐ Irritable ☐ Manic ☐ Other: _____
Affect	☐ NA	☒ Constricted ☐ Blunt ☐ Flat ☐ Labile ☐ Dramatic ☐ Other: _____
Sleep	☐ NA	☒ Hypersomnia ☐ Insomnia ☐ Disrupted ☐ Nightmares ☐ Other: _____
Eating	☐ NA	☒ Increase ☐ Decrease ☐ Anorectic restriction ☐ Bingeing ☐ Purging ☐ Body image ☐ Other: _____

† *Abbreviations:* AF: Adult Female; AM: Adult Male; CF#: Child Female with age, e.g., CF12; CM#: Child Male with age; Hx: History; CI: Client.

Anxiety symptoms	☐ NA	☒ Chronic worry ☐ Panic attacks ☐ Dissociation ☐ Phobias ☐ Obsessions ☐ Compulsions ☐ Other: _____
Trauma symptoms	☐ NA	☐ Acute ☒ Chronic ☐ Hypervigilance ☐ Dreams/nightmares ☐ Dissociation ☒ Emotional numbness ☐ Other:
Psychotic symptoms	☒ NA	☐ Hallucinations ☐ Delusions ☐ Paranoia ☐ Loose associations ☐ Other: _____
Motor activity/ speech	☐ NA	☒ Low energy ☐ Restless/hyperactive ☐ Agitated ☐ Inattentive ☐ Impulsive ☐ Pressured speech ☐ Slow speech ☐ Other: _____
Thought	☐ NA	☒ Poor concentration/attention ☐ Denial ☒ Self-blame ☐ Other-blame ☒ Ruminative ☐ Tangential ☐ Illogical ☐ Concrete ☐ Poor insight ☐ Impaired decision making ☐ Disoriented ☐ Slow processing ☐ Other: _____
Socio-Legal	☒ NA	☐ Disregards rules ☐ Defiant ☐ Stealing ☐ Lying ☐ Tantrums ☐ Arrest/incarceration ☐ Initiates fights ☐ Other: _____
Other symptoms	☒ NA	

Diagnosis for IP

Contextual Factors considered in making Dx: ☒ Age ☒ Gender ☒ Family dynamics ☐ Culture ☐ Language ☐ Religion ☐ Economic ☐ Immigration ☒ Sexual orientation ☒ Trauma ☐ Dual dx/comorbid ☐ Addiction ☐ Cognitive ability ☐ Other: _____

Describe impact of identified factors: Used age-appropriate language; considered gender and recent family changes, including mother's change in sexual orientation, when diagnosing mood and adjustment.

Axis I
Primary: 296.32 Major Depressive Disorder, Recurrent, Moderate

Secondary: 995.53 Sexual abuse of child

Axis II: V71.09 No diagnosis

Axis III: None reported

Axis IV:
☒ Problems with primary support group
☐ Problems related to social environment/school
☐ Educational problems
☐ Occupational problems
☐ Housing problems
☐ Economic problems
☐ Problems with accessing health care services
☐ Problems related to interactions with the legal system
☒ Other psychosocial problems Peer relations

Axis V: GAF 55 GARF 60

List DSM symptoms for Axis I Dx (include frequency and duration for each). Client meets 5 **of** 9 **criteria for Axis I Primary Dx.**

1. Depressed mood, most days, past 6 months
2. Loss of interest in pleasurable activities, most days
3. Hypersomnia, esp on weekends.
4. Feelings of worthlessness, most days
5. Lack of concentration, esp at school
6. No manic or mixed episodes; most recent episode 6 months

(continued)

Mental Status for IP *(continued)*

Have medical causes been ruled out?
☒ Yes ☐ No ☐ In process
**Has patient been referred for psychiatric/
medical eval?** ☒ Yes ☐ No
Has patient agreed with referral?
☒ Yes ☐ No ☐ NA
List psychometric instruments or consults used
for assessment:
☒ None or _____

**Medications (psychiatric & medical)
Dose /Start Date**
☐ None prescribed
1. _Zoloft/50 mg_ _____ ; _10/4/08_
2. _____ / _____ mg; _____
3. _____ / _____ mg; _____

Client response to diagnosis:
☒ Agree ☐ Somewhat agree ☐ Disagree
☐ Not informed for following reason:

_____

Medical Necessity *(Check all that apply):* ☒ Significant impairment ☒ Probability of significant impairment
☒ Probable developmental arrest
Areas of impairment: ☒ Daily activities ☒ Social relationships ☒ Health ☒ Work/school
☐ Living arrangement ☐ Other: _____

Risk Assessment

Suicidality:
☐ No indication
☐ Denies
☐ Active ideation
☒ Passive ideation
☐ Intent without plan
☐ Intent with means
☐ Ideation in past yr
☐ Attempt in past yr
☐ Family/peer hx of completed suicide

Hx Substance:

Alc abuse:

☒ No indication
☒ Denies

☐ Past
☐ Current

Freq/Amt: _____

Drugs:

☒ No indication

☒ Denies

☐ Past

☐ Current

Drugs: _____

Freq/Amt: _____

☐ Family/sig. other abuses

Homicidality:
☒ No indication
☒ Denies
☐ Active ideation
☐ Passive ideation
☐ Intent w/o means
☐ Intent with means
☐ Ideation in past yr
☐ Violence past yr
☐ Hx assault/temper
☐ Cruelty to animals

Sexual & Physical Abuse and Other Risk Factors:

☒ Current child w abuse hx:
 ☒ Sexual ☐ Physical ☐ Emotional ☐ Neglect
☐ Adult w childhood abuse:

 ☐ Sexual ☐ Physical ☐ Emotional ☐ Neglect
☐ Adult w abuse/assault in adulthood:
 ☐ Sexual ☐ Physical ☐ Current

☐ History of perpetrating abuse:
 ☐ Sexual ☐ Physical

☐ Elder/dependent adult abuse/neglect

☐ Anorexia/bulimia/other eating disorder

☒ Cutting or other selfharm: ☒ Current
 ☐ Past; Method: _Razor_ _____
 ☐ Criminal/legal hx: _____
 ☐ None reported

Indicators of Safety: ☒ At least one outside person who provides strong support ☒ Able to cite specific
reasons to live, not harm self/other ☐ Hopeful ☒ Has future goals ☒ Willing to dispose of dangerous items
☐ Willingness to reduce contact with people who make situation worse ☒ Willing to implement safety plan,
safety interventions

☐ Developing set of alternatives to self/other harm ☒ Sustained period of safety: 1 month.
☐ Other: _____

Safety Plan includes: ☒ Verbal no harm contract ☒ Written no harm contract ☒ Emergency contact card ☒ Emergency therapist/agency number ☒ Medication management ☒ Specific plan for contacting friends/support persons during crisis ☐ Specific plan of where to go during crisis ☐ Specific self-calming tasks to reduce risk before reach crisis level (e.g., journaling, exercising, etc.) ☒ Specific daily/weekly activities to reduce stressors ☐ Other: _____

Notes: Legal/Ethical Action Taken: ☐ NA Report past abuse to CPS; Riley West, 4:00 pm 10/4/08 _____

Case Management

Date
1st visit: 10/4/08
Last visit: 10/11/08
Session Freq:
☒ Once week ☐ Every other week ☐ Other: _____
Expected Length of Treatment:
_____

Modalities:
☐ Individual adult
☒ Individual child
☐ Couple
☒ Family
☐ Group: _____

Is client involved in mental health or other medical treatment elsewhere?
☒ No
☐ Yes:
_____
If Child/Adolescent: Is family involved?
☒ Yes ☐ No

Patient Referrals and Professional Contacts
Has contact been made with social worker?
☒ Yes ☐ No: explain: _____ ☐ NA

Has client been referred for medical assessment?
☒ Yes ☐ No evidence for need

Has client been referred for psychiatric assessment?
☒ Yes; cl agree ☐ Yes, cl disagree ☐ Not mec.

Has contact been made with treating physicians or other professionals?
☒ Yes ☐ No ☐ NA

Has client been referred for social/services?
☐ Job/training ☐ Welfare/food/housing ☒ Victim services
☐ Legal aid ☐ Medical ☐ Other: _____ ☐ NA

Anticipated forensic/legal processes related to treatment:
☒ No ☐ Yes: _____

Has client been referred for group or other support services?
☒ Yes ☐ No ☐ None recommended

Client social support network includes:
☒ Supportive family ☐ Supportive partner ☒ Friends ☐ Religious/spiritual organization ☐ Supportive work/social group ☐ Other: _____

Anticipated effects treatment will have on others in support system: (parents, children, siblings, sig. others, etc.):
Mother struggling with guilt for not protecting daughter better

Is there anything else client will need to be successful?
Mother may need individual therapy

Client Sense of Hope: Little 1-----X-----5----------10 High

Expected Outcome and Prognosis:
☒ Return to normal functioning
☐ Expect improvement, anticipate less than normal functioning
☐ Maintain current status/prevent deterioration

(continued)

Case Management *(continued)*

Evaluation of Assessment/Client Perspective

How was assessment method adapted to client needs?

Used age and gender appropriate language; created sense of safety, esp. reabuse assessment.

Age, culture, ability level, and other diversity issues adjusted for by:

Respectfully addressed sexual orientation of mother; used humor to connect with CF.

Systemic/family dynamics considered in following ways:

Invited AF40 to participate if interested; contacted AM to keep him involved also.

Describe actual or potential areas of client-therapist agreement/disagreement related to the above assessment:

AF47 wanted CF on medication because she found it helpful for herself and because CF is now cutting. No areas of identified disagreement.

_____ , _____   _____

Therapist signature   License/Intern status   Date

_____ , _____   _____

Supervisor signature   License   Date

TREATMENT PLAN

Therapist: Roxana Gilbert   **Client ID #:** 1420

Theory: Collaborative Therapy

Primary Configuration: ☐ Individual ☐ Couple ☒ Family ☐ Group: _____

Additional: ☒ Individual ☐ Couple ☐ Family ☐ Group: _____

Medication(s): ☐ NA ☒ Zoloft _____

Contextual Factors considered in making plan: ☒ Age ☒ Gender ☒ Family dynamics

☐ Culture ☐ Language ☐ Religion ☐ Economic ☐ Immigration ☒ Sexual orientation

☒ Trauma ☐ Dual dx/comorbid ☐ Addiction ☐ Cognitive ability

☐ Other: _____

Describe how plan is adapted to contextual factors: Use age and gender appropriate language and ways of talking; create space for family to explore dynamics and sexual orientation issues; extra attention on safety to address prior trauma.

I. Initial Phase of Treatment (First 1–3 Sessions)

I.A. Initial Therapeutic Tasks

Therapeutic Relationship

TT1: Develop therapeutic relationship with all members. Note: Emphasis on creating safety due to trauma and respectful and accepting space to discuss sexual orientation issues.

I1: Intervention: **Curious stance** and **everyday language** to create dialogical partnership with each member; allow all voices and perspectives to be heard; move slow enough for CF to feel safe.

Assessment

TT2: Assess individual, system, and broader cultural dynamics. Note: _____

I1: Intervention: Invite each participant to share **understanding of the problem** without privileging one over the other.

I2: Intervention: **Contact and inquire about** others talking about the problem, including psychiatrist, teacher, father, best friend.

Set Goals

TT3: Define and obtain client agreement on treatment goals. Note: _____

Note: **BOLDFACE** indicates Collaborative Therapy assessment and techniques.

(continued)

I. Initial Phase of Treatment *(continued)*

I1: Intervention: **Inquire about preferred way of meeting** (individually vs. family) and identify area(s) deemed most critical.

Referrals and Crisis

TT4: Identify needed referrals, crisis issues, and other client needs. Note: _____

I1: Intervention: Discuss potential of medication: discuss pros, cons, and family's perspectives and values.

I.B. Initial Client Goals (1–2 Goals): Manage crisis issues and/or reduce most distressing symptoms.

> **Goal #1:** ☒ Increase ☐ Decrease CF sense of having **agency** in relation to managing her feelings and emotions (personal/relational dynamic) to reduce cutting (symptom).
>
> *Measure:* Able to sustain safety for period of 4 ☒ wks ☐ mos with no more than 0 mild episodes of cutting.
>
> > I1: Intervention: Develop safety plan using scaling for safety; involve CF and AF47 in identifying level 7 and alternate plan.
> >
> > I2: Intervention: **Use conversational questions and mutual puzzling** to identify ways to increase social connection with best friend and new friends at school.

II. Working Phase of Treatment (Sessions 2+)

II.A. Working Therapeutic Tasks

Monitor Progress

TT1: Monitor progress toward goals. Note: _____

I1: Intervention: Check in each week on cutting, level of depression, and positive mood.

Monitor Relationship

TT2: Monitor quality of therapeutic alliance as therapy proceeds. Note: _____

I1: Intervention: Inquire frequently to ensure that the **pacing, form, and content** of therapy are working; create space for family to talk about what is not working.

II.B. Working Client Goals (2–3 Goals): Target individual and relational dynamics in case conceptualization using theoretical language (e.g., reduce enmeshment, increase differentiation, increase agency in relational narrative, etc.).

> **Goal #1:** ☒ Increase ☐ Decrease CF sense of belonging at home and school (personal/relational dynamic) to reduce social withdrawal and feelings of loneliness (symptom).

Measure: Able to sustain <u>sense of belonging</u> for period of 8 ☒ wks ☐ mos with no more than <u>2</u> mild episodes of <u>withdrawal.</u>

    I1: Intervention: **Invite all members** to share how they see family connections as well as CF's connection with each (esp AF47), allowing new **understandings of family connection to evolve.**

    I2: Intervention: **Appropriate unusual reflections** to invite CF to view her connections with friends in new ways and to identify potential action steps.

Goal #2: ☒ Increase ☐ Decrease <u>CF sense of **agency** in relationships and in life activities</u> (personal/relational dynamic) to reduce <u>depressed mood and hopelessnes</u> (symptom).

Measure: Able to sustain <u>agency</u> for period of <u>2</u> ☐ wks ☒ mos with no more than <u>1</u> mild episodes of <u>depressed mood.</u>

    I1: Intervention: **Access multiple voices through letter writing** to help CF identify current and preferred **identity narratives.**

    I2: Intervention: **Mutual puzzling** to identify small steps that CF is willing to take to move toward her **preferred self(selves)**.

III. Closing Phase of Treatment (Last 2+ Weeks)

III.A. Closing Therapeutic Tasks

Termination Plan

    TT1: Develop aftercare plan and maintain gains. Note: _____

    I1: Intervention: <u>Create long-term safety plan and identify early "warning signs" and how to manage.</u>

III.B. Closing Client Goals: Determined by theory's definition of health

---

Goal #1: ☒ Increase ☐ Decrease <u>family sense of **"normalcy" as they define and experience it**</u> (personal/relational dynamic) to reduce <u>social marginalization and adapt to new family structure</u> (symptom).

Measure: Able to sustain <u>sense of normalcy</u> for period of <u>8</u> ☒ wks ☐ mos with no more than <u>2</u> mild episodes of <u>disharmony.</u>

    I1: Intervention: <u>Create space for each member to **share inner talk** about the new family structure, including same-sex relationship.</u>

    I2: Intervention: **Conversational questions** <u>that encourage each person to share hopes and fears for the family structure; follow through on action plans based on this discussion.</u>

(continued)

TREATMENT PLAN *(continued)*

IV. Client Perspective

Has treatment plan been reviewed with client? ☒ Yes ☐ No; If no, explain: _____

_____

Describe areas of client agreement and concern: <u>Clients want to start with family for the first few</u> <u>weeks and later move to a mix of individual sessions with CF and family sessions.</u>

_____ , _____ _____

Therapist signature   Intern status   Date

_____ , _____ _____

Supervisor signature   License   Date

_____

Abbreviations: TT: Therapeutic Task; I: Intervention; AM: Adult Male; AF: Adult Female; CM: Child Male; CF: Child Female; Dx: Diagnosis; NA: Not Applicable.

PROGRESS NOTES

Progress Notes for Client # 1420

Date: 10/11/08 **Time:** 1:00 am/pm   **Session Length:** ☒ 50 min. or ☐ _____

Present: ☐ AM ☒ AF47 ☐ CM ☒ CF ☐ _____
Billing Code: ☐ 90801 (Assess) ☐ 90806 (Insight-50 min) ☒ 90847 (Family-50 min)

☐ Other _____

Symptoms(s)	Dur/Freq Since Last Visit	Progress: Setback----------Initial----------Goal
1. Cutting	Scratch arm (no blood) 1 x	-5------------------1-----X------5------10
2. Depressed mood	Mild, most days	-5------------------1------X------5-----10
3. Withdrawal	Moderate, most days	-5------------------1------X------5-----10

Explanatory Notes: CF reported greater hope after first session last week; did not "cut" because of safety plan but did scratch. Reports continued depressed mood but slightly more hopeful; continued hypersomnia and social withdrawal, although reports feeling more connected to AF47 after last session. Report saw psychiatrist and has begun taking Zoloft, 50 mg.

Interventions/HW: Developed detailed safety plan using scaling for safety; identified signals at 7 and strategies to manage mood at this point: call boy friend, talk with mom, play music, go for run. CF generated own plan easily and was open with AF47, who was supportive.

Client Response/Feedback: CF appeared motivated to change behavior and although hesitant when describing what she actually feels became more animated when identifying how to stop downward spiral.

Plan: ☒ Continue with treatment plan: plan for next session: Follow up on safety plan

☐ Modify plan: _____

Next session: Date: 10/18/08 Time: 2:00 am/pm
Crisis Issues: ☐ Denies suicide/homicide/abuse/crisis ☒ Crisis assessed/addressed:

Denies cutting (no evidence) but admits to scratching without drawing blood; developed safety plan and CF readily agreed to plan and was willing to include AF47.

_____ , _____   _____
Therapist signature   License/intern status   Date

(continued)

PROGRESS NOTES *(continued)*

◇◇◇

Case Consultation/Supervision Notes: Supervisor went over safety plan.

Collateral Contacts: Date: 10/12/08 Time: 5:00 Name: Dr. Lee

Notes: Consult with psychiatrist on medication, diagnosis (296.32), and safety plan.

☒ Written release on file: ☒ Sent ☐ Received ☐ In court docs ☐ Other: _____

_____ , _____ _____
Therapist signature   License/Intern status   Date

_____ , _____ _____
Supervisor signature   License   Date

_____

Abbreviations: AM: Adult Male; AF: Adult Female; CM: Child Male; CF: Child Female; HW: Homework.

Group Therapy with Couples and Families

Most parents with two or more children claim that adding a second child doesn't double the work—it quadruples it. The same can be said for clients: adding a second (e.g., a couple) or third (e.g., a family) person to the room exponentially increases the complexity of the situation. If you then add multiple couples and families into a single therapy session, things really get "rockin'." Remember the nursery tale about the old lady in the shoe: so many kids, she didn't know what to do. Well, this last chapter provides you with a basic overview of evidence-based group work with couples and families so that you will know what to do and will do what works best.

Lay of the Land

The first section of this chapter provides a brief overview of general group therapy, in case you skimmed most of your group therapy text or have not yet taken or will not be required to take a group therapy class. If you aced your group class, of course, you can go ahead and skip this section. The rest of the chapter focuses on evidence-based group therapy models for working with the following common client concerns:

- Severe mental illness
- Partner abuse and domestic violence
- Marital enrichment
- Parent training

Brief Overview of Types of Groups

Groups can be divided into three general categories based on their relative emphasis on *content* (information provided) versus *process* (emotional processing): psychoeducational groups, process groups, and combined groups.

Psychoeducational Groups or "Classes"

Psychoeducational groups, often referred to as "classes," are content-focused and educational, rooted in the cognitive-behavioral assumption that "if people just knew better, they'd do (i.e., behave or feel) better." In the arena of couple and family relations, research has particularly supported psychoeducational groups for the following problems:

- Families with members diagnosed with severe mental illness (McFarlane, Dixon, Lukens, & Lucksted, 2002)
- Domestic violence (Stith, Rosen, & McCollum, 2002)
- Marital enrichment (i.e., couples who do not present as distressed; Halford, Markman, Stanley, & Kline, 2002)
- Parent training (Northey, Wells, Silverman, & Bailey, 2002)

Process Groups

As the name suggests, process groups focus on *interpersonal process* rather than content. Although they are typically composed of individuals, increasingly they include couples and families. Process groups more closely address the goals targeted in experiential or psychodynamic forms of individual therapy, such as increasing insight into and confronting problematic interpersonal patterns. The group is often used as a forum for better understanding past or current couple and family relationships. Process groups are frequently used as an alternative to individual therapy or with clients coping with grief, divorce, loss, or abuse.

Yalom (1970/1985) identifies 11 elements that make process groups effective:

- **Instillation of Hope:** Gaining hopefulness for the future from meeting and interacting with others

- **Universality:** Realizing one is not alone in suffering or struggling with life

- **Imparting Information:** Benefiting from information shared by the therapist while facilitating the group

- **Altruism:** Learning how to give and receive from others without needing personal gain

- **The Corrective Recapitulation of the Primary Family Group:** Providing an opportunity to work through family-of-origin issues and respond in new ways

- **Development of Socializing Techniques:** Improving social skills by interacting intimately with others

- **Imitative Behavior:** Modeling self after chosen role models in the group

- **Interpersonal Learning:** Developing insight and working through transference issues in a group context

- **Group Cohesiveness:** Relating to the therapist and group as a whole to work through conflict and differences

- **Catharsis:** Experiencing and expressing emotions of deep significance, which, when combined with cognitive learning, predict positive outcomes

- **Existential Factors:** Recognizing existential truths, such as the inevitability of death and loss, the need for taking responsibility for one's own life, and the inescapability of suffering

Combined Groups

Combined psychoeducational-process groups generally include some psychoeducational instruction but reserve time for group members to share their thoughts, feelings, and internal processes related to the material, allowing members to address issues at a more personal and deeper level. Such groups are particularly common with victims of child abuse and domestic violence, and increasingly with perpetrators of abuse.

General Group Guidelines
Number of People

The number of people allowed into a group is the key to its success. Generally, for process groups, the limit is 4 children or 8 teens and adults. Combined psychoeducational-process groups can run with more, but the process element generally diminishes significantly once the group exceeds 12 people. Psychoeducational groups that do not include a process component can successfully run with 15 to 30 adults.

NUMBER OF PEOPLE IN GROUPS

	PSYCHOEDUCATIONAL GROUPS	COMBINED GROUPS	PROCESS GROUPS
Adults and Adolescents	2–30 adults	3–12 adults	3–8 adults
Elementary-Age Children	2–4 children	2–4 children	2–4 children
Middle-School–Age Children	2–6 children	2–6 children	2–6 children
Couples and Families	2–10 couples or families	2–7 couples or families	3–4 couples or families

Open Versus Closed Groups

Open groups are groups that can be joined at any time; closed groups are "closed" to new members once the group begins.

- **Open Groups:** The primary advantage of open groups is that clients do not have to wait to join; once referred, they can immediately start while their motivation is at its peak. Having an open group requires that all the psychoeducational components can be taken in any sequence, which is often difficult if you are trying to build on skills from the prior week.

- **Closed Groups:** Most process groups and court-mandated psychoeducational groups are closed groups. The closed format allows for the intimacy and trust necessary for process groups to function and also enables mandated groups to develop a coherent and in-depth curriculum that allows group facilitators to monitor individual members' progress.

Group Selection: Who's in Your Group?

As any group leader quickly realizes, who is in the group is a critical factor for success, not only for process-oriented groups but also for psychoeducational groups. For process and combined groups, most therapists screen potential group members to ensure that they are appropriate for the group. Group facilitators look at several different factors, depending on their group:

- **Presenting Problem:** When groups are organized around a presenting problem, such as sexual abuse or loss, the group facilitator screens to ensure that potential members are addressing the same general issue.

- **Level of Problem Resolution:** If a group is organized around a particular issue, the facilitator may want to assess the level of problem resolution so that participants are close enough in the recovery and healing process that they can meaningfully interact; this is particularly important when working with trauma victims (e.g., sexual abuse, national disaster recovery, loss, domestic violence) or substance abuse recovery (e.g., using versus sober and clean). Alternatively, some facilitators prefer to have a spectrum of problem resolution in the group so that members can learn from each other, in which case the group should be organized to accommodate these differences.

- **Ability to Meaningfully Contribute:** Most facilitators screen for a person's ability to meaningfully contribute, which is typically defined as being able to actively participate without dominating or developing hostile interactions with others. Therapists also consider the client's ability to speak and actively engage others in a group setting; clients who are unable to relate with others may not be good candidates for process groups.

Group Rules

Depending on the group situation, therapists may develop rules for how group participants interact in and out of the group session.

- **Confidentiality:** In most cases, as a condition for membership, group participants must agree to maintain the confidentiality of other members in a group, typically in writing. Although group participants cannot be held to the same legal standards as therapists for maintaining confidentiality, having a formal, written process increases members' awareness of the seriousness of the issue.

- **Respectfulness:** Most group leaders moderate discussion to ensure that members speak respectfully to one another and the group leaders, often directly intervening if a conflict gets out of control. However, in more traditional psychodynamic and experiential process groups, the facilitator does *not* interrupt certain conflicts, instead encouraging the members to grow by working through their issues together.

- **Punctuality and Attendance:** Often groups have rules for punctuality and attendance, especially if courts mandate treatment. In some cases, if members arrive after a designated time, they are not allowed to join that group session. Similarly, if the group has a set curriculum, a member may not be allowed to continue if he/she misses too many sessions.

Evidence-Based Couple and Family Groups
Psychoeducational Multifamily Groups for Severe Mental Illness

Numerous controlled, clinical studies have demonstrated that patients diagnosed with schizophrenia whose families receive psychoeducation have reduced incidents of psychotic relapse and rehospitalization (McFarlane et al., 2002). The relapse rate for these patients is about 15%, less than half the rate of those who receive individual therapy and medication or medication alone (relapse rate 30–40%). Several comparison studies indicate that multifamily groups are more effective than single-family sessions in which the family learns the same psychoeducational material, making groups not only the more cost-effective treatment but also the more effective overall. Multifamily groups lead to lower relapse rates and higher rates of employment than single-family sessions, probably because of the enhanced support that group settings offer. There is sufficient evidence at this time to consider family psychoeducation for families with a schizophrenic member as an *evidence-based practice* (McFarlane et al., 2002).

Multifamily psychoeducational groups currently focus on the following:

- Understanding schizophrenia as a brain disorder that is only partially remediable by medication
- Recognizing that the family has a significant role in the patient's recovery
- Educating families about which interactions impede and which facilitate recovery

Research indicates that psychodynamic and insight-oriented therapies are counterindicated (not recommended) with families who have a member diagnosed with schizophrenia.

The *psychoeducational curriculum* for multifamily groups typically includes the following:

- Education about the illness, prognosis, psychological treatment, and medication
- The biological, psychological, and social factors related to the illness
- Education on the role of high emotional expression in the home in increasing the likelihood of relapse (Hooley, Rosen, & Richters, 1995)
- Possible social isolation and stigmatization
- The financial and psychological burden on the family
- The importance of developing a strong social network to support the family
- Problem-solving skills

The *process* aspect of multifamily groups includes the following:

- Creating a forum for mutual aid and support
- Normalizing the family's experience
- Reducing the sense of stigma
- Creating a sense of hope by seeing how other families have coped
- Socializing with each other outside the group context

When families participate in these groups, the patient and the family have fewer social problems, fewer clinical management problems, reduced secondary stress (stress caused by the hospitalization of the patient), increased employment, and decreased relapse and rehospitalization.

Although most of the research on groups has been done with schizophrenic and schizoaffective disorders, several studies have used multifamily psychoeducation groups as a component of treatment for other severe mental health disorders (McFarlane et al., 2002), including the following:

- Bipolar disorder
- Dual diagnosis (e.g., substance abuse and an Axis I diagnosis)
- Obsessive compulsive disorder
- Depression
- Posttraumatic stress disorder in veterans
- Alzheimer's disease
- Suicidal ideation in adolescents
- Congenital abnormalities
- Intellectual impairment
- Child molesters and pedophilia
- Borderline personality disorder

Groups for Partner Abuse

A widespread and difficult-to-treat phenomenon with numerous physical and emotional effects on children, women, and families, physical abuse of one's partner is increasingly targeted for intervention by state and local authorizes. Today, most states mandate therapy in cases of partner abuse, a specific form of domestic violence. Treatment is most frequently delivered in the form of gender-based group therapy (i.e., groups for male batterers or female batterers and groups for male or female victims of abuse; Stith, Rosen, & McCollum, 2002). However, increasingly, couple-based approaches are being researched as alternative approaches, with initial studies indicating that carefully designed couple-based approaches to partner violence have comparable outcomes to the traditional gender-based groups, with no evidence of an increased potential for violence (Stith, McCollum, Rosen, & Locke, 2002; Stith, Rosen, & McCollum, 2002).

Traditional Gender-Based Groups for Partner Abuse

The traditional gender-based groups for partner abuse are based on the work of Lenore Walker (1979) and the closely related Duluth Model (Pence & Paymar, 1993). These models are psychoeducational cognitive-behavioral groups grounded in feminism that are widely used in the criminal justice system. Lenore Walker used the *cycle of violence* to describe the dynamics of the abuse relationship. The cycle has three phases: honeymoon, tension building, and acting out:

- **Honeymoon Phase:** This is the phase in which the batterer pursues the victim, asking forgiveness, promising to stop the violence, and attempting to woo the victim back.

- **Tension-Building Phase:** Victims often describe the tension-building phase as a state of "living on egg-shells." During this period, conflict and tension are rising and the victim tries to avoid behaviors that will "set off" the perpetrator.

- **Acting Out or Explosion:** The final phase is characterized by a physically violent episode; after this episode, the cycle repeats as the batterer tries to repair the relationship in the honeymoon phase.

In the early years of violent relationships, the cycle typically moves slowly, perhaps with only one or two mildly violent episodes per year (e.g., pushing, shoving, throwing objects, one slap). Over time, the frequency and severity of the violent episodes increase.

In addition to the cycle of violence, the Duluth Model uses the idea of the *wheel of power and control*, which describes the means by which batterers are believed to maintain control over their partners. The eight spokes of the wheel are as follows:

- Coercion and threats
- Intimidation
- Emotional abuse
- Isolation
- Minimizing, denying, and blaming
- Using children
- Economic abuse
- Male privilege

Critique of the Duluth Model

Although the Duluth Model is one of the most frequently used models for treating batterers, Dutton and Corvo (2006, 2007) note that the research literature has identified numerous and significant weaknesses with the model:

- **Poor Outcomes:** Studies on the effectiveness of batterer intervention groups indicate a high recidivism rate, with 40% of participants perpetrating again within six months of completing treatment.

- **De-emphasis on the Therapeutic Alliance:** One of the chief criticisms of the Duluth Model is that it fails to promote a supportive therapeutic alliance with clients and instead often involves an adversarial and blaming stance toward clients.

- **Unfounded Gender Bias:** The gender-based, feminist view is not supported by incidence statistics, which indicate that *personality* rather than gender predicts partner violence.

- **Unfounded Emphasis on Power:** The Duluth Model describes partner violence as an issue of power and male privilege; however, the research indicates that there is no clear correlation between violence and patriarchal privilege.

- **Unfounded De-emphasis on Anger:** In contrast to the Duluth position that partner violence is not related to anger but to power, research indicates that men who batter have significantly higher levels of anger and hostility than those who do not batter.

- **Ignoring Bidirectional Violence:** The Duluth Model is based on the assumption that violence is unilateral, whereas national surveys indicate that most domestic violence is *bidirectional*, with both partners acting violently; nonetheless, men are far more likely than women to severely injure their partners.

- **Unfounded Power and Control Assumptions:** The Duluth Model asserts that partner violence is due to the male's desire for power and control, whereas research indicates that both genders vie equally for power and control in relationships.

Thus, although the Duluth Model is the most common treatment model, the research literature does not support either the model's theoretical assumptions or its effectiveness.

Conjoint Treatment of Partner Abuse

Because of the limitations of the Duluth Model, therapists and researchers have explored other models of treatment, including conjoint couples therapy (Stith, McCollum, Rosen, & Locke, 2002), narrative therapy (Jenkins, 1990), and solution-focused therapy (Lipchik & Kubicki, 1996; Milner & Singleton, 2008; Stith, McCollum, Rosen, & Locke, 2002). Of these, conjoint couples therapy has been the best researched.

Until recently, couples therapy was considered "inappropriate" for the treatment of domestic violence, largely because of the assumption that there is a significant struggle for power, control, and dominance in all battering relationships. However, as already noted, there is little research to support this assumption (Dutton & Corvo, 2006, 2007). Instead, emerging research indicates that there is more than one type of batterer (Holtzworth-Munroe & Stuart, 1994): (a) those who are violent only within their families, (b) those who have more severe pathology, such as depression or borderline personality disorder, and (c) those who are generally violent and have antisocial characteristics. Conjoint couples therapy is designed for only one type of batterer: *family-only batterers without apparent psychopathology.* Arguments for using conjoint couples treatment for mild cases of family-only battering include the following (Stith, Rosen, & McCollum, 2002):

- It is estimated that as many as 67% of all couples presenting for couples therapy have a history of violence. Therapists may begin treating a couple for other issues before discovering violence; stopping therapy because of this revelation can result in the couple choosing to not pursue further treatment.
- Statistics show that 50–70% of wives who are battered return to the abusive partner after separating or going to a shelter; conjoint couples therapy provides one of the few safe forums for these couples to safely discuss their relationship.

- The majority of violent relationships are *bidirectional*, with both parties committing acts of violence. Because cessation of violence by one partner is highly dependent on the cessation of violence by the other, conjoint treatment, in which both parties are de-escalating violence, has a greater likelihood of reducing bidirectional violence.

Conjoint Couples Treatment

Several approaches for working conjointly with couples have been developed; most combine couple-only sessions with multicouple groups (Stith, Rosen, & McCollum, 2002). The common characteristics of conjoint couples treatment of partner violence include the following:

- Each partner is carefully screened to determine if the couple should participate in couple sessions or multicouple group sessions. Couples in which there has been serious injury to one or both partners are excluded. In addition, in private screening interviews, both partners must state that they prefer couples therapy and that they are not afraid of speaking freely in session with their partner.
- The primary goal is *decreasing violence and emotional abuse,* not saving the marriage or relationship.
- Partners are encouraged to take responsibility for their own violence.
- The skill-building component emphasizes identifying when one is angry, knowing how to de-escalate self and other, and taking time-outs.
- The effectiveness of the program is measured by reduction or elimination of violence.

Effectiveness of Conjoint Couples Treatment

Although the research is relatively sparse, conjoint couples treatment of partner violence appears to be *at least as effective* as more traditional gender-based models, with *no significant differences* in the effectiveness of individual couple sessions versus multicouple group sessions. In the carefully designed conjoint programs studied, there was no evidence that women in conjoint couples treatment for domestic violence were more likely to be abused than when the batterers were treated separately; thus, if thoughtfully approached, it does not appear that conjoint couples treatment increases the incidence of violence. Furthermore, using conjoint couples treatment when the batterer also had a substance abuse issue was *superior* to individual treatment in reducing violence.

Relationship Enhancement Programs

One of the most common forms of multicouple group sessions, relationship enhancement programs are preventive interventions for nondistressed couples who want to improve the quality of their relationship (Halford et al., 2002). These programs are typically offered as multicouple psychoeducational groups, which are generally grounded in cognitive-behavioral therapies. These groups may include lectures, demonstrations, audiovisual programs, practice, and discussion. Some of the more prominent programs have included the following:

- Relationship Enhancement (RE; Guerney, 1987)
- Prevention and Relationship Enhancement Program (PREP; Markman, Stanley, & Blumberg, 2001)
- Minnesota Couples Communication Program (MCCP; Miller, Nunnally, & Wackman, 1976)
- Practical Application of Intimate Relationship Skills (PAIRS; DeMaria & Hannah, 2002)

All these programs promote positive communication, conflict management, and positive expression of affection. Variations in the curriculum include the following:

- Preventing destructive conflict (emphasized in PREP)
- Developing empathy for one's partner (emphasized in RE)
- Strong emphasis on conflict management (emphasized in MCCP and RE)
- Commitment, respect, love, and friendship (emphasized in PREP)

Effectiveness of Multicouple Relationship Enhancement Programs

In the research literature on these programs, most couples report high satisfaction, rating skill training in communication as the most helpful intervention (Halford et al., 2002). In addition, skill-based relationship enhancement results in a significant increase in relationship skills upon completion of the program. Studies vary from no improvement to modest improvement in relationship satisfaction immediately following completion of a course. However, there is limited research on the long-term effectiveness of these programs. Such research has only been conducted on skill-based groups that met for four to eight sessions and that targeted dating, engaged, or recently married couples. These long-term studies indicate the following:

- Relational skills learned in the group are maintained for a period of several years but begin to trail off in 5 to 10 years.
- PREP participants reported enhanced relationship satisfaction and functioning 2 to 5 years after the course.
- PREP participants reported fewer incidents of violence at the 5-year follow-up than those who did not participate.
- Certain effects, such as increased satisfaction and decreased divorce rate, seemed to become evident at the 4- to 5-year mark, meaning that the difference between couples who participated in PREP and those who began marriage without an enrichment program became *detectable only several years later.*
- In one study involving older, more distressed couples, PREP was not effective, indicating that enrichment programs that work early in a relationship might not be equally effective for more established or more distressed couples.

Guidelines

Based on their review of the research literature, Halford et al. (2002) propose the following as best practices in relationship enhancement:

- **Assess Risk and Protective Factors:** Before admitting couples to a relationship enhancement group, therapists should screen them for risk factors associated with higher stress and divorce, such as parental divorce, age, previous marriages, length of time the partners have known each other, cohabitation history, and the presence of stepchildren. Additionally, therapists should consider protective factors and strengths, such as clear communication and realistic relationship expectations.

- **Encourage High-Risk Couples to Attend:** Relationship enhancement is more likely to benefit high-risk couples early in their relationships because they are more likely to need better skills to manage their stressors.

- **Assess and Educate About Relationship Aggression:** Because physical and verbal aggression occur at high rates early in couple relationships, education about aggression and how to handle it can better prepare couples to reduce hostile and dangerous behavior.

- **Offer Relationship Education at Change Points:** In addition to the beginning of a relationship, couples can benefit from relationship enhancement at numerous other life and developmental transition points, such as the birth of a child, relocation, major illness, and unemployment.

- **Promote Early Presentation of Relationship Problems:** Because long-standing distress predicts poor response to couples therapy, couples should be encouraged to address mild distress as it emerges rather than allow the relationship to further deteriorate.

- **Match Content to Couples with Special Needs:** Program enhancement needs to be adapted to fit a couple's special needs, such as a major mental health diagnosis, alcohol or substance abuse, and stepfamily issues.

- **Enhance Accessibility of Evidence-Based Relationship Education Programs:** Programs can be made more accessible by increasing the formats in which they are offered: weekly, on weekends, or online.

Parent Training

Described in Chapter 13, parent training is a cognitive-behavioral intervention that has shown effectiveness in treating a wide range of childhood problems. It is the treatment of choice for oppositional defiant disorder (ODD) and the *only treatment that produces normalization of child functioning with attention-deficit, hyperactivity disorder* (ADHD; Northey et al., 2002). Parent training has been shown to be effective with both individual families and multifamily groups (DeRosier & Gilliom, 2007; van den Hoofdakker, van der Veen-Mulders, & Sytema, 2007).

Parent training group curricula include similar elements to parent training with individual families (see Chapter 13):

- Encouraging positive reinforcement to shape desired behaviors
- Using natural and logical consequences whenever possible
- Improving parents' ability to listen and communicate understanding to their child
- Increasing parents' use of "I" statements
- Providing multiple-choice options for children in negotiations when appropriate
- Training parents in emotional coaching to help their children identify, express, and appropriately manage their emotions
- Contingency contracting and point systems to motivate children
- Training in how to use time-outs and other punishments to reduce negative behaviors

Summary

Group therapy with couples and families is gaining recognition as an evidence-based approach for working with a number of common clinical issues, including schizophrenia, bipolar disorder, domestic violence, ADHD, and ODD. Most evidence-based forms of couple and family group psychotherapy are psychoeducational groups that integrate a cognitive-behavioral, family systems approach. New therapists are strongly encouraged to seek advanced training in groups they plan to lead and, whenever possible, co-facilitate groups to "learn the ropes."

Compared with other forms of therapy, psychoeducational groups require a unique set of skills:

- The ability to build rapport with an entire group rather than an individual or a family
- Public speaking skills

- An understanding of curriculum design
- Technical skills to produce overheads and handouts
- Creativity to select and design engaging group activities
- The ability to manage conflict between unrelated persons

Although initially challenging, learning to facilitate couple and family groups adds refreshing diversity to one's clinical workload and provides numerous opportunities for further professional growth.

ONLINE RESOURCES

Minnesota Couples Communication Program (MCCP)

www.couplecommunication.com

Relationship Enhancement Program (PE)

National Institute for Relationship Enhancement

www.nire.org

Practical Application of Intimate Relationship Skills (PAIRS)

www.pairs.com

Prevention and Relationship Enhancement Program (PREP)

www.prepinc.com

SAMHSA Description of PREP

Review of Evidence-Based Program

www.nrepp.samhsa.gov/programfulldetails.asp?PROGRAM_ID=86

SAMHSA Family Psychoeducation Toolkit

www.mentalhealth.samhsa.gov/cmhs/communitysupport/toolkits/family

REFERENCES

DeMaria, R., & Hannah, M. (2002). *Building intimate relationships: Bridging treatment, education and enrichment through the PAIRS Program.* New York: Brunner/Routledge.

DeRosier, M. E., & Gilliom, M. (2007). Effectiveness of a parent training program for improving children's social behavior. *Journal of Child and Family Studies, 16,* 660–670.

Dutton, D. G., & Corvo, C. (2006). Transforming a flawed policy: A call to revive psychology and science in domestic violence research and practice. *Aggression and Violent Behavior, 11,* 457–483.

Dutton, D. G., & Corvo, C. (2007). The Duluth Model: A data-impervious paradigm and a failed strategy. *Aggression and Violent Behavior, 12,* 658–667.

Guerney, B. G. (1987). *Relationship enhancement manual.* Bethesda, MD: Ideal.

Halford, W. K., Markman, H. J., Stanley, S., & Kline, G. H. (2002). Relationship enhancement. In D. Sprenkle (Ed.), *Effectiveness research in marriage and family therapy* (pp. 191–222). Alexandria, VA: American Association for Marriage and Family Therapy.

Holtzworth-Munroe, A., & Stuart, G. L. (1994). Typologies of male batterers: Three subtypes and the differences among them. *Psychological Bulletin, 116,* 476–497.

Hooley, J. M., Rosen, L. R., & Richters, J. E. (1995). Expressed emotion: Toward clarification of a critical construct. In G. A. Miller (Ed.), *The behavioral high-risk paradigm in psychopathology* (pp. 88–120). New York: Springer Verlag.

Jenkins, A. (1990). *Invitations to responsibility: The therapeutic engagement of men who are violent and abusive.* Adelaide, Australia: Dulwich Centre Publications.

Lipchik, E., & Kubicki, A. (1996). Solution-focused domestic violence views: Bridges toward a new reality in couples therapy. In S. D. Miller, M. A. Hubble, & B. L. Duncan (Eds.), *Handbook of solution-focused brief therapy* (pp. 65–97). San Francisco: Jossey-Bass.

Markman, H., Stanley, S., & Blumberg, S. (2001). *Fighting for your marriage.* San Francisco: John Wiley.

McFarlane, W. R., Dixon, L., Lukens, E., & Lucksted, A. (2002). Severe mental illness. In D. Sprenkle (Ed.), *Effectiveness research in marriage and family therapy* (pp. 255–288). Alexandria, VA: American Association for Marriage and Family Therapy.

Miller, S. L., Nunnally, E. W., & Wackman, D. B. (1976). A communication training program for couples. *Social Casework, 57,* 9–18.

Milner, J., & Singleton, T. (2008). Domestic violence: Solution-focused practice with men and women who are violent. *Journal of Family Therapy, 30*(1), 29–53.

Northey, W. F., Wells, K. C., Silverman, W. K., & Bailey, C. E. (2002). Childhood behavioral and emotional disorders. In D. Sprenkle (Ed.), *Effectiveness research in marriage and family therapy* (pp. 89–122). Alexandria, VA: American Association for Marriage and Family Therapy.

Pence, E., & Paymar, M. (1993). *Education groups for men who batter: The Duluth Model.* New York: Springer.

Stith, S. M., McCollum, E. E., Rosen, K. H., & Locke, L. D. (2002). Multicouple group treatment for domestic violence. In F. Kaslow (Ed.), *Comprehensive textbook of psychotherapy* (Vol. 4). New York: Wiley.

Stith, S. M., Rosen, K. H., & McCollum, E. E. (2002). Domestic violence. In D. Sprenkle (Ed.), *Effectiveness research in marriage and family therapy* (pp. 223–254). Alexandria, VA: American Association for Marriage and Family Therapy.

van den Hoofdakker, B. J., van der Veen-Mulders, L., & Sytema, S. (2007). Effectiveness of behavioral parent training for children with ADHD in routine clinical practice: A randomized controlled study. *Journal of the American Academy of Child and Adolescent Psychiatry, 46,* 1263–1271.

Walker, Lenore E. (1979). *The battered woman.* New York: Harper & Row.

Yalom, I. D. (1970/1985). *The theory and practice of group psychotherapy* (3rd ed.). New York: Basic Books.

Closing Thoughts: Where to Go from Here?

You have just finished a grand tour of the pragmatic and theoretical aspects of family therapy practice in the 21st century. You have been introduced to the clinical skills you will be expected to perform in field placements: case conceptualization, clinical assessment, treatment planning, and progress assessment. You have also been introduced to the most established therapeutic models in the field of family therapy, including the new evidence-based models. So, where do you go from here? The next step in mastering the competencies is to enter the real world of clinical practice, where you will learn to walk the talk.

Getting Started: Working with a Supervisor

If you have started field placement, you already know that your supervisor is the key to meaningfully mastering competencies. More so than your professors, your supervisor is the one who helps you translate book knowledge into action. Thus, it is important to learn how to "use" supervision well.

Realistic Expectations

Perhaps it is easiest to start with what *not* to do, which is *not* to expect your supervisor to be omniscient and omnipotent—in other words, don't confuse a supervisor with God, a common misunderstanding. New trainees often expect their supervisors to have mastered all aspects of the profession: all theories, all techniques, all laws, all ethic codes, all diagnoses, all referral possibilities, all research methods—in short, everything. It's just not possible—at least I have not met anyone who has. Instead, it is useful to approach each supervisor with the attitude that you have *something* to learn from him/her—it might be diagnosis, a specific theory, case notes, law and ethics, or group work. Every supervisor has something valuable to teach. Many of my trainees find that approaching their supervisors with more realistic expectations not only reduces their frustration with their supervisor but also gives them more realistic expectations of what they themselves should be mastering in the first few years of training.

Asking for What You Need

If for some reason you believe your supervisor is not helping you in a particular area—perhaps with treatment plans, diagnosis, or a specific theory—it often helps to *directly ask* for what you want. Most supervisors are more than happy to work such requests into the supervision process. If not, know that you will have many more supervisors who will provide further opportunities for learning.

Seeking Advanced Training

Another frequent misunderstanding new trainees have is thinking that they are done with academic training once they receive a master's degree or license. A master's degree is the *minimal* training you need to prepare you for licensure, and a license simply certifies that the state does not think you will hurt anybody without direct supervision. Those are pretty low standards. To become a competent therapist, you will need a minimum of 5 to 10 years of postdegree training in a specialty. Most importantly, it takes this level of training to provide the knowledge and skill foundations you will need to *prevent burnout*. Becoming a skilled therapist is a *long-term project*; a master's degree and license are just the first steps in the process.

The greatest barrier to advanced training is time and money. Once you graduate and have to start paying back student loans, it is hard to afford conferences and workshops because they are expensive, at least in the short term; however, they are an *investment*. Investing in advanced training is investing in your future and opens new opportunities to expand your practice. There are state and national conferences, special in-depth trainings offered by institutes specializing in particular approaches or populations, and an increasing number of quality online programs. You do not have to go broke, but you do need to put some time and money aside to ensure that you develop fully as an independent, creative professional. I have never met anyone who regretted investing in training. I recommend you get to as many trainings as possible while you are in school and still qualify for the "student" discount: those will look like bargain-basement prices once you graduate.

Belonging: Professional Organizations

Almost all professionals belong to professional organizations. But for therapists in the 21st century, membership is a matter of survival: namely, the ability to get hired and paid. Why? National professional organizations, such as the American Association for Marriage and Family Therapy (for LMFTs), the American Counseling Association (for LPCs), the National Association of Social Workers (for social workers), and the American Psychological Association (for psychologists), are the people who lobby in Congress, in state legislatures, and with third-party payers to ensure that their licensees have jobs and get reimbursed. Without these organizations working on behalf of their members, therapists would not be able to survive in today's marketplace. So, depending on which license you intend to pursue, it is important to join—and membership is always cheapest as a student.

Besides the not-so-minor issue of ensuring a paycheck, these organizations offer some of the best training and networking opportunities available. Attending national conventions and trainings keeps you on the cutting edge of the profession. Most also have state-level and regional meetings that keep you up to date. The local meetings are often the source of great networking connections, whether you are just starting out and looking for a job or have been in the field for years and want to market or hire. All have opportunities to join boards of directors and subcommittees, where you have the opportunity to shape the future direction of the profession. Professional organizations also provide free legal consultation—and if you have ever had to pay a lawyer, you know that one phone call pays for three years of membership. In the end, professional organizations are where it is all happening—so don't miss the party!

Self-Supervision

In addition to using your supervisor and knowledge from advanced training, it is still helpful to learn how to help yourself. Whether a veteran therapist or the new kid on the block, one of the most exciting parts of learning how to complete a case conceptualization (Chapter 2) is that you can provide yourself with outstanding supervision at a moment's notice, without paying a fee or waiting until next week's supervision session. You can use the case conceptualization form to walk yourself through the case and identify the core issues and dynamics you can use to focus your treatment. This is most useful when you are feeling stuck but also helpful with new cases or cases that you have been seeing for long periods of time with minor to moderate change. As simple as it may sound, this exercise has often helped me and my supervisees identify more useful ways to proceed—and all we did was answer questions we asked ourselves.

Last Words

I hope this introduction to family therapy has inspired you to work creatively and hopefully with individuals, couples, and families using family therapy theories, all of which view individuals and their problems as part of larger relational and social contexts. I trust you will find that they provide a remarkably rich foundation for helping people with all forms of suffering and life struggles. Most importantly, I hope the depth and humanity of these ideas translate off the pages of this book and into your work with clients, so that with each interaction you touch that ineffable part of their being that brings forth the best of who they are—and in doing so brings forth the best in you.

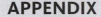

CACREP
Competency-Based Standards

Below you will find the new CACREP competency-based standards for master students in marriage and family counseling. Students should be able to demonstrate these competencies prior to graduating. Faculty in CACREP programs can download scoring rubrics with the CACREP standards from the textbook web page hosted by the publisher.

Marriage, Couple, and Family Counseling

Students who are preparing to work as marriage, couple, and family counselors are expected to possess the knowledge, skills, and practices necessary to address a wide variety of issues in the context of relationships and families. In addition to the common core curricular experiences outlined in Section II.F [of the CACREP 2009 Standards], programs must provide evidence that student learning has occurred in the following domains:

Foundations

A. Knowledge

1. Knows the history, philosophy, and trends in marriage, couple, and family counseling.
2. Understands the ethical and legal considerations specifically related to the practice of marriage, couple, and family counseling.
3. Knows the roles and functions of marriage, couple, and family counselors in a variety of practice settings and in relation to other helping professionals.
4. Knows the professional organizations, preparation standards, and credentials relevant to the practice of marriage, couple, and family counseling.
5. Understands a variety of models and theories of marriage, couple, and family counseling.
6. Understands family development and the life cycle, sociology of the family, family phenomenology, contemporary families, family wellness, families and culture, aging and family issues, family violence, and related family concerns.
7. Understands the impact of crises, disasters, and other trauma-causing events on marriages, couples, families, and households.

B. Skills and Practices

1. Demonstrates the ability to apply and adhere to ethical and legal standards in marriage, couple, and family counseling.
2. Demonstrates the ability to select models or techniques appropriate to couples' or families' presenting problems.

Counseling, Prevention, and Intervention

C. Knowledge

1. Understands issues of marriage, couple, and family life-cycle dynamics; healthy family functioning; family structures; and family of origin and intergenerational influences in a multicultural society.
2. Recognizes specific problems (e.g., addictive behaviors, domestic violence, suicide risk, immigration) and interventions that can enhance family functioning.
3. Understands human sexuality (e.g., gender, sexual functioning, sexual orientation) and its impact on family and couple functioning.
4. Understands professional issues relevant to the practice of marriage, couple, and family counseling, including recognition, reimbursement, and right to practice.

D. Skills and Practices

1. Uses preventive, developmental, and wellness approaches in working with individuals, couples, families, and other systems such as premarital counseling, parenting skills training, and relationship enhancement.
2. Uses systems theory to conceptualize issues in marriage, couple, and family counseling.
3. Uses systems theories to implement treatment, planning, and intervention strategies.
4. Demonstrates the ability to use procedures for assessing and managing suicide risk.
5. Adheres to confidentiality responsibilities, the legal responsibilities and liabilities of clinical practice and research, family law, record keeping, reimbursement, and the business aspects of practice.
6. Demonstrates the ability to recognize his or her own limitations as a marriage, couple, and family counselor and to seek supervision or refer clients when appropriate.

Diversity and Advocacy

E. Knowledge

1. Understands how living in a multicultural society affects couples and families.
2. Recognizes societal trends and treatment issues related to working with multicultural and diverse family systems (e.g., families in transition, dual-career couples, blended families, same-sex couples).
3. Understands current literature that outlines theories, approaches, strategies, and techniques shown to be effective in working with diverse family systems.
4. Understands the effects of racism, discrimination, sexism, power, privilege, and oppression on one's own life and that of the client(s).
5. Understands the effect of local, state, and national policies, programs, and services on diverse family systems.

F. Skills and Practices

1. Demonstrates the ability to provide effective services to clients in a multicultural society.
2. Maintains information regarding community resources to make appropriate referrals.
3. Advocates for policies, programs, and services that are equitable and responsive to the unique needs of couples and families.
4. Demonstrates the ability to modify counseling systems, theories, techniques, and interventions to make them culturally appropriate for diverse couples and families.

Assessment

G. Knowledge

1. Knows principles and models of assessment and case conceptualization from a systems perspective, including diagnostic interviews, mental diagnostic status examinations, symptom inventories, and psychoeducational and personality assessments.
2. Understands marriage, couple, and family assessment tools and techniques appropriate to clients' needs in a multicultural society.
3. Understands the impact of addiction, trauma, psychopharmacology, physical and mental health, wellness, and illness on marriage, couple, and family functioning.

H. Skills and Practices

1. Applies skills in interviewing, assessment, and case management for working with individuals, couples, and families from a system's perspective.
2. Uses systems assessment models and procedures to evaluate family functioning.
3. Determines which members of a family system should be involved in treatment.

Research and Evaluation

I. Knowledge

1. Understands how to critically evaluate research relevant to the practice of marriage, couple, and family counseling.
2. Knows models of program evaluation relevant for the practice of marriage, couple, and family counseling.
3. Knows evidence-based treatments and basic strategies for evaluating counseling outcomes in marriage, couple, and family counseling.

J. Skills and Practices

1. Applies relevant research findings to inform the practice of marriage, couple, and family counseling.
2. Develops measurable outcomes for marriage, couple, and family counseling programs, interventions, and treatments.
3. Analyzes and uses data to increase the effectiveness of marriage, couple, and family counseling interventions and programs.

Index

U

V

W